MRI Bioeffects, Safety, and Patient Management

MRI Bioeffects, Safety, and Patient Management

Frank G. Shellock, Ph.D. - Editor

Adjunct Clinical Professor of Radiology and Medicine
Keck School of Medicine
University of Southern California

Director of MRI Studies of Biomimetic MicroElectronic
Systems (BMES) Implants, National Science Foundation
BMES Engineering Research Center
University of Southern California

Adjunct Professor of Clinical Physical Therapy, Division of Biokinesiology and Physical
Therapy, School of Dentistry
University of Southern California

Founder, Institute for Magnetic Resonance Safety, Education, and Research

President, Shellock R & D Services, Inc.
Los Angeles, California

John V. Crues, III, M.D. - Editor

Medical Director and MRI Fellowship Director
Radnet, Inc.
Los Angeles, CA

Professor of Radiology
University of California, San Diego

Alexandra M. Karacozoff - Associate Editor

Los Angeles, California

Biomedical Research Publishing Group
Los Angeles, CA

Made in the United States of America

Library of Congress Cataloging-in-Publication Data
Frank G. Shellock and John V. Crues, III

MRI Bioeffects, Safety, and Patient Management

p. cm.

Includes bibliographical references and index.

ISBN-10   0989163202

ISBN-13   978-0-9891632-0-0

1.   Magnetic resonance imaging. 2. Magnetic resonance imaging—safety measures. 3. Magnetic resonance imaging—Health aspects. 4. Magnetic resonance imaging—Complications.   I. Shellock, Frank G.   II. Crues, John V.   III. Title.

Great care has been taken to assure the accuracy of the information contained in this textbook that is intended for educational and informational purposes, only. Neither the publisher nor the authors assume responsibility for errors or for any consequences arising from the use of the information contained herein.

Important Note: The development of this textbook was supported, in part, by an Unrestricted Educational Grant provided by Bracco Diagnostics, Inc.

Disclaimer

This textbook was designed to provide a reference for radiologists, MRI technologists, facility managers, MRI physicists, MRI researchers, engineers, and others. The information is current through the publication date of this textbook. The content of this book is designed for general informational purposes only and is not intended to be nor should it be construed to be technical or medical advice or opinion on any specific facts or circumstances.

The authors and publisher of this work disclaim any liability for the acts of any physician, individual, group, or entity acting independently or on behalf of any organization that utilizes information for a medical procedure, activity, service, or other situation through the use of this textbook. The content of this textbook makes no representations or warranties of any kind, expressed or implied, as to the information content, materials or products, included in this textbook. The authors and publisher assume no responsibilities for errors or omissions that may include technical or other inaccuracies, or typographical errors. The authors and publisher of this work specifically disclaim all representations and warranties of any kind, expressed or implied, as to the information, content, materials, or products included or referenced in this textbook.

The authors and publisher disclaim responsibility for any injury and/or damage to persons or property from any of the methods, products, instructions, or ideas contained in this publication. The authors and publisher disclaim liability for any damages of any kind arising from the use of the book, including but not limited to direct, indirect, incidental, punitive and/or consequential damages.

The information and comments provided in this book are not intended to be technical or medical recommendations or advice for individuals or patients. The information and comments provided herein are of a general nature and should not be considered specific to an individual or patient, whether or not a specific patient is referenced by a physician, technologist, individual, group, or other entity seeking information.

The authors and publisher assume no responsibility for the accuracy or validity of the information contained in this book nor the claims or statements of any manufacturer or website that is referenced. Manufacturers' product specifications are subject to change without notice. Always read the product labeling, instructions and warning statements thoroughly before using any medical product or similar device.

Preface

Since its introduction into clinical practice in the early 1980s, magnetic resonance imaging (MRI) has exhibited exceptional growth and created a paradigm shift in medicine. Not only has this imaging modality markedly expanded the roles of imaging in medical diagnoses, opening up vistas in neurological, musculoskeletal, oncological, cardiovascular and a variety of other diseases not accessible to prior imaging techniques, but it has also had a profound impact on our basic understanding of the pathophysiologic mechanisms of abnormal conditions and disease processes.

The continuous growth of MRI has led to an explosion in the number of patients, healthcare professionals, and other individuals exposed to the powerful static magnetic fields, rapidly changing magnetic fields, and intense radiofrequency fields used during the procedures. Numerous investigations have been performed during the past three decades in an effort to characterize the bioeffects and safety aspects of MRI. However, the interactions of the MRI-related electromagnetic fields with biologic tissues are still incompletely understood and safety issues persist despite best efforts to implement preventive practices. Unfortunately, this has led to many adverse consequences, including injuries to patients and healthcare workers as well as several patient deaths.

The transformative impact of MRI on medicine continues to progress and advances in technology continue unabated. Whereas the highest magnetic field used in routine clinical imaging was 1.5-Tesla during most of the 1990s, 3-Tesla is currently the standard. Research is routinely performed at 7-Tesla and an 11.7-Tesla MR system was recently developed to scan human subjects. In addition to the high static magnetic fields, both the speed of magnetic field gradient switching and the levels of radiofrequency field exposures are pushing limits well beyond what was possible just a few years before. Therefore, we strongly believe that, for progress to continue in this field, appropriate safeguards must be in place to protect all human subjects exposed to MRI. This is best accomplished by conducting careful research directed towards studying the effects of the electromagnetic fields used in clinical and research MRI settings and implementing cautionary measures based on the knowledge acquired during the last 30 years.

Ultimately, MRI safety must begin with understanding. At the present time, there are thousands of articles in the scientific literature detailing MRI safety issues from every conceivable approach. Importantly, this textbook brings together an internationally respected group of experts who are directly involved in the areas of MRI bioeffects, safety, and patient management. The unique collective expertise of these physicians (radiologists, cardiologists, anesthesiologists, etc.), scientists, engineers, and other professionals resulted in vital contributions to this well-organized resource of essential scientific knowledge that covers all critical topics of interest to physicians, physicists, scientists, healthcare professionals, imaging center managers, bioengineers, regulatory affairs professionals, and laypersons. The ambitious purpose of this textbook is to provide actionable information that will be used to ensure that the MRI environment is as a safe as possible under all circumstances. We hope that we've accomplished this important goal and that the MRI community will benefit from the indispensable content of this textbook.

Frank G. Shellock

John V. Crues, III

The Editors

Frank G. Shellock, Ph.D. is a physiologist with more than 25 years of experience conducting laboratory and clinical investigations in the field of magnetic resonance imaging (MRI). He is an Adjunct Clinical Professor of Radiology and Medicine at the Keck School of Medicine, University of Southern California, Adjunct Professor of Clinical Physical Therapy, Division of Biokinesiology and Physical Therapy, School of Dentistry, University of Southern California, the Director of MRI Studies at the Biomimetic Microelectronic Systems, National Science Foundation (NSF), Engineering Research Center, University of Southern California,

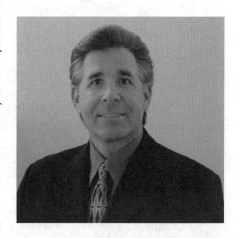

and the Founder of the Institute for Magnetic Resonance Safety, Education, and Research (www.IMRSER.org). As a commitment to the field of MRI safety, bioeffects, and patient management, he created and maintains the internationally popular web site, www.MRIsafety.com.

Dr. Shellock has authored or co-authored more than 230 publications in the peer-reviewed literature. He co-authored the MRI safety section of the Cardiovascular MR Self-Assessment Program (CMR-SAP) for the American College of Cardiology and three of his medical textbooks are considered best sellers - *Reference Manual for Magnetic Resonance Safety, Implants and Devices*; *Magnetic Resonance Procedures: Health Effects and Safety*; and *Kinematic MRI of the Joints: Functional Anatomy, Kinesiology, and Clinical Applications*.

Dr. Shellock serves in advisory roles to government, industry, and other policy-making organizations. Recently, the American College of Radiology (ACR) appointed him to the ACR Subcommittee on MR Safety and the Joint Commission appointed him to the Diagnostic Ionizing Radiation and Magnetic Resonance Expert Panel.

Dr. Shellock is an Associate Editor for the Journal of Magnetic Resonance Imaging and a Reviewing Editor for several medical journals including Radiology, Investigative Radiology, Magnetic Resonance in Medicine, Magnetic Resonance Imaging, the Journal of Cardiovascular Magnetic Resonance, Circulation, the American Journal of Neuroradiology, Neurosurgery, the Journal of the American College of Cardiology, and the Journal of Magnetic Resonance Imaging.

Memberships in professional societies include the American College of Radiology, the International Society for Magnetic Resonance in Medicine (ISMRM), the Radiological Society of North America, the California Radiological Society, the Hawaii Radiological Society, and the Society for Cardiovascular Magnetic Resonance. He is also a member and Fellow of the American College of Cardiology and the American College of Sportsmedicine.

In 1994, the Crues-Kressel Award was given to Dr. Shellock for his outstanding contributions to the education of MRI Technologists. In 2003, the Section for Magnetic Resonance Technologists (SMRT) further recognized him by presenting the Honorary Member Award to him for his extraordinary achievement and exceptional level of service and support of the SMRT.

In 2004, the International Society for Magnetic Resonance in Medicine recognized the significant contributions Dr. Shellock has made to the scientific and educational mission of the ISMRM by designating him a Fellow of the Society. The American College of Radiology awarded him a Distinguished Committee Service Award for years of dedicated service to the Practice Guidelines and Technical Standards Committee, Body MRI.

Dr. Shellock has lectured both nationally and internationally and has provided plenary lectures to numerous organizations including the Radiological Society of North America, the International Society for Magnetic Resonance in Medicine, the American College of Radiology, the American Roentgen Ray Society, the American Society of Neuroradiology, the Environmental Protection Agency, the Oklahoma Heart Institute, the Head and Neck Radiology Society, the Center for Devices and Radiological Health (CDRH) of the FDA, the Magnetic Resonance Managers Society, the American Heart Association, the American College of Cardiology, the American Society of Neuroimaging, the Society for Cardiovascular Magnetic Resonance, the Heart Rhythm Society, the Finnish Radiological Society, the International Congress of Radiology, the Japanese Society of Neuroradiology, the British Chapter of the International Society for Magnetic Resonance in Medicine, the Royal Australian and New Zealand College of Radiologists, and the Institute of Physics and Engineering in Medicine.

His company, Magnetic Resonance Safety Testing Services, specializes in the assessment of MRI safety for implants and devices as well as the evaluation of electromagnetic field-related bioeffects and the development of new clinical MR imaging applications for low-field (0.2-Tesla), high-field, and very-high-field strength MR systems.

John V. Crues, III, M.D., M.S. is a radiologist with more than 27 years experience in magnetic resonance imaging (MRI). He is the Medical and MRI Fellowship Director for Radnet, Inc., the largest owner and operator of outpatient imaging centers in the United States; President of Pronet Imaging; and a Clinical Professor of Radiology at the University of California, San Diego (UCSD), School of Medicine. His undergraduate degree was in physics at Harvard University and he obtained a masters degree in solid-state physics (MR spectroscopy) with Professor Charles Slichter at the University of Illinois before attending Harvard Medical School.

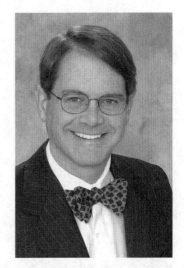

Dr. Crues has authored more than 100 papers in the medical literature, 13 textbooks and CDs, 27 books chapters, and over 100 abstracts. He is a member of numerous professional societies, including being a past President of the International Society for Magnetic Resonance in Medicine (ISMRM) and a previous Chairperson of the Subcommittee on Magnetic Resonance Biological Effects of the Commission on Neuroradiology and Magnetic Resonance of the American College of Radiology (ACR). Contributions towards the development of clinical magnetic resonance led to his selection as a Fellow of both the ISMRM and the ACR. Dr. Crues has also served on the ACR's MRI Accreditation Committee, the Board of the Intersocietal Commission for the Accreditation of Magnetic Resonance Imaging Laboratories, and the Diagnostic Ionizing Radiation and Magnetic Resonance Expert Panel for the Joint Commission. For six years he represented the ACR on the American Registry of Radiological Technologists, MRI Examination Committee.

Dr. Crues has presented over 2,000 invited lectures on five continents, including plenary lectures for the Society of Nuclear Medicine, Society of Magnetic Resonance in Medicine, Radiologic Society of North America, Colorado Radiologic Society, National Academy of Sciences Second Annual Symposium on Frontiers of Science, American Roentgen Ray Society, Society of Magnetic Resonance Imaging, MR '93 Internationales Kernspintomographic Symposium, German Orthopaedic Society, Austral-Asian Radiological Society, Scandinavian Congress of Radiology, International Skeletal Society, American Society of Emergency Radiology, Brasilian Radiologic Society, Swedish Society of Medical Radiology, International Society for Extremity MRI in Rheumatology, Society of Radiology Physician Extenders, and the Professional Hockey Athletic Trainers Association. As a Visiting Professor, he has been hosted by more than twenty academic institutions world-wide.

Contributors

Gregory Brown, A. Dip. Rad. Tech., FSMRT
Centre for Advanced Imaging
The University of Queensland
St. Lucia, Queensland and
Department of Radiology
Royal Adelaide Hospital
Adelaide, South Australia
Australia

Ji Chen, Ph.D.
Professor of Engineering
Department of Electrical and Computer Engineering
University of Houston
Houston, TX

Patrick M. Colletti, M.D.
Professor of Radiology
Professor of Medicine
Professor of Biokinesiology
Professor of Pharmacology and Pharmaceutical Sciences
Chief of MRI
Director Nuclear Medicine Fellowship
University of Southern California
LAC+USC Medical Center
Los Angeles, CA

John V. Crues, III, M.D.
Medical Director and MRI Fellowship Director
Radnet, Inc.
Los Angeles, CA and
Professor of Radiology
University of California, San Diego
San Diego, CA

Laura Foster, J.D., M.P.H.
Vice President, Regulatory Affairs
Radnet, Inc.
Los Angeles, CA

Yan Liu, Ph.D.
Postdoctoral Fellow
Department of Electrical and Computer Engineering
University of Houston
Houston, TX

Janice Fairhurst, B.S., R.T. (R)(MR)
Lead Technologist
Radiology Department
Brigham and Women's Hospital
Harvard Medical School
Boston, MA

Christine Harris, R.T. (R)(MR)
MRI Safety Officer
Radiology Manager
Department of Radiology/MRI
Children's Hospital of Philadelphia
Philadelphia, PA

Henry Halperin, M.D., M.A., FAHA
Professor of Medicine, Biomedical Engineering and Radiology
Johns Hopkins Hospital
Baltimore, MD

Nobuhiko Hata, Ph.D.
Director, Surgical Navigation and Robotics Lab
Radiology Department
Brigham and Women's Hospital
Harvard Medical School
Boston, MA

Randy L. Gollub, M.D., Ph.D.
Associate Professor of Psychiatry
Associate Director of Psychiatric Neuroimaging
Massachusetts General Hospital
Charlestown, MA

Ferenc A. Jolesz, MD.
B. Leonard Holman Professor of Radiology
Director, Division of MRI and National Center for Image Guided Therapy. Department of Radiology
Brigham and Women's Hospital
Harvard Medical School
Boston, MA

Robert Junk, AIA, AHRA
President
JUNK Architects, PC and Radiology Planning
Kansas City, MO

Daniel F. Kacher, M.S.
Clinical Engineers
Biomedical Engineering Department
Brigham and Women's Hospital
Harvard Medical School
Boston, MA

Wolfgang Kainz, Ph.D.
Research Biomedical Engineer
Division of Physics
Office of Science and Engineering Laboratories
Center for Devices and Radiological Health
Food and Drug Administration
Silver Spring, MD

Angela Kanan, R.N., BSN, CRN, CNOR
Nurse-In-Charge, Amigo Suite
Radiology Department
Brigham and Women's Hospital
Harvard Medical School
Boston, MA

Alayar Kangarlu, Ph.D.
Director of MRI Physics
Columbia University
New York, NY

Mark N. Keene, Ph.D.
Chief Technology Officer
Metrasens, Ltd.
Worcestershire
United Kingdom

Stephen F. Keevil, Ph.D.
Consultant Physicist
Head of Magnetic Resonance Physics
Department of Medical Physics
Guy's and St. Thomas' NHS Foundation Trust
London, England and

Professor of Medical Physics
Department of Biomedical Engineering
King's College of London
London, England, United Kingdom

Steven G. Manker, BSME
Program Director, MRI Conditionally Safe Systems
Medtronic Neuromodulation
Minneapolis, MN

Michael Manzano, M.D.
Musculoskeletal MRI Fellow
Radnet, Inc.
Los Angeles, CA

Ramon F. Martin, M.D., Ph.D.
Director, Out of OR Anesthesia
Brigham and Women's Hospital
Harvard Medical School
Boston, MA

Mark McJury, Ph.D.
Consultant Clinical Scientist
Department of Clinical Physics and Bio-Engineering
Beatson Cancer Centre
Glasgow, Scotland
United Kingdom

Donald W. McRobbie, Ph.D.
Senior Lecturer in Imaging
Imperial College London
United Kingdom and
Chief Physicist
South Australia Medical Imaging
Adelaide, Australia

Saman Nazarian, M.D., Ph.D., FHRS, FACC
Director, Ventricular Arrhythmia Ablation Service
Cardiac Electrophysiology
Johns Hopkins Hospital
Baltimore, MD

Moriel NessAiver, Ph.D.
Simply Physics
Baltimore, MD

John Nyenhuis, Ph.D.
Professor of Electrical and Computer Engineering
Purdue University
School of Electrical and Computer Engineering
West Lafayette, IN

Lawrence P. Panych, Ph.D.
Director, MRI Physics Research Group
Radiology Department
Brigham and Women's Hospital
Harvard Medical School
Boston, MA

John Posh, R.T. (R)(MR)
Director, MRI Internship and
RT Continuing Education
Faculty, RT Education
Penn Medicine
Hospitals of the University of Pennsylvania
Philadelphia, PA

Debra Reinking, M.D.
Anesthesiologist
Aptos, CA

Ashok K. Saraswat, M.S., B.Ed., R.T. (R)(MR)
MRI Educational Program Director
Ohio State University
Wexner Medical Center
Clinical Instructor
Health & Rehabilitation Sciences
Columbus, OH

Anne Marie Sawyer, B.S., R.T. (R)(MR), FSMRT
Manager, MR Whole Body Research Systems
Radiological Sciences Laboratory
Richard M. Lucas Center for Imaging
Stanford University School of Medicine
Stanford, CA

Daniel J. Schaefer, Ph.D.
Retired, Formerly Principal Engineer
MR Systems Engineering
General Electric Healthcare
Waukesha, WI

John F. Schenck, M.D., Ph.D.
Principal Scientist
General Electric Corporate Research and Development Center
Schenectady, NY

Ehud J. Schmidt, Ph.D.
Radiology Department
Brigham and Women's Hospital
Harvard Medical School
Boston, MA

Frank G. Shellock, Ph.D.
Adjunct Clinical Professor of Radiology and Medicine
Keck School of Medicine, University of Southern California
Adjunct Professor of Clinical Physical Therapy
Division of Biokinesiology and Physical Therapy
School of Dentistry, University of Southern California
Director for MRI Studies of Biomimetic MicroElectronic Systems
National Science Foundation, Engineering Research Center
University of Southern California
Institute for Magnetic Resonance Safety, Education, and Research
President, Shellock R & D Services, Inc.
Los Angeles, CA

Jerold S. Shinbane, M.D., FACC, FHRS, FSCCT
Associate Professor of Clinical Medicine
Director, USC Arrhythmia Center
Director, Cardiovascular Computed Tomography
Division of Cardiovascular Medicine
Cardiovascular and Thoracic Institute
Keck School of Medicine
University of Southern California
Los Angeles, CA

Karen Smith, M.S., RTMR, ACR, RTR
Life Member
Canadian Association of Medical Radiation Technologists
Regional Practice Lead, MRI
Integrated Medical Imaging
Vancouver Coastal Health Authority
Instructor, MRI Program
British Columbia Institute of Technology
Burnaby, British Columbia, Canada

Mark A. Smith M.S., ABMP, R.T. (R)(MR)
MRI Physicist
Nationwide Children's Hospital
Clinical Instructor, Adjunct Faculty
Ohio State University
Wexner Medical Center
Columbus, OH

Rosa Babbitt Spaeth, B.S.
Research Assistant
Laboratory of Pain, Placebo and Acupuncture Imaging
Department of Psychiatry
Massachusetts General Hospital
Charlestown, MA

Alberto Spinazzi, M.D.
Senior Vice President
Head, Global Medical and Regulatory Affairs
Bracco Group
Monroe, NJ

John Summers, M.D., FACC
Electrophysiology Fellow
Division of Cardiovascular Medicine
Cardiovascular and Thoracic Institute
Keck School of Medicine
University of Southern California
Los Angeles, CA

Nanda Deepa Thimmappa, M.D.
Fellow, Body MRI
Department of Radiology
Weill Cornell Medical College
New York, NY

Dedications

This book is dedicated to the many patients suffering from Lupus, including my dear wife, Jaana. Notably, the color orange is the awareness color for Lupus and, as such, orange was selected for the cover of this textbook in an effort to raise awareness of this chronic autoimmune disease.

A portion of the proceeds from the sale of this textbook will be donated to *Lupus LA* to support the *Lupus Research Institute*. To make a donation or to obtain information about Lupus LA and the research supported by this organization, please visit: www.lupusla.org

Frank G. Shellock, Ph.D.

First and foremost I dedicate this book to my wife, Maribeth, without whose support my involvement would have been impossible. Secondly, I dedicate this project to Radnet, a company and environment that has provided extensive tolerance and support for my involvement in MRI practice, teaching, and research.

John V. Crues, M.D., III

Acknowledgments

We are especially indebted to Alexandra M. Karacozoff, the Associate Editor of this textbook, for her exceptional editing and proofreading capabilities, as well as her other vital contributions. To the extent that there are any errors remaining in this book, they are our responsibility alone. Special thanks to Mark Bass for his extensive experience and great efforts that helped to make this textbook possible by taking care of the overall production of this project and providing careful attention to an amazing list of details.

Table of Contents

Chapter 1   Basic MRI Physics: Implications for MRI Safety

MORIEL NESSAIVER, PH.D.

Simply Physics
Baltimore, MD

INTRODUCTION

Most medical professionals today are well aware that magnetic resonance imaging (MRI) technology uses systems with powerful magnets that may make considerable noise and that you generally cannot bring ferromagnetic object or patients with certain implants into the scanner room. They may or may not be aware that the MR systems use relatively safe radiofrequency (RF) radiation instead of ionizing radiation (e.g., X-rays, gamma rays, etc.) to create images. Nor do they understand just how powerful the magnets are, why they may always be "on" and why they make so much noise. This chapter provides simple explanations for these matters by presenting information pertaining to basic MRI physics.

MRI has at its root the chemical technique known as nuclear magnetic resonance or NMR (1, 2). As every chemist knows, the use of the word "nuclear" has nothing to do with radioactivity, but since the general population is not composed of mostly chemists, the medical community has dropped that emotionally laden word to become, simply, MRI. For most MRI examinations, the word "nuclear" has to do with the nucleus of the hydrogen atom, which consists of a single proton. The content of this chapter will begin by examining the magnetic properties of protons and then continue with an explanation of the MRI signal, some basic tissue properties, spin echo formation, and conclude with a brief discussion of MRI hardware issues. Much of the information in this chapter is adapted from *All You Really Need to Know About MRI Physics* (3). Several other textbooks also cover this introductory material (4-7).

Note: Throughout this chapter, "Key Definitions" are designated in bold print.

MAGNETIC PROPERTIES OF PROTONS

Spinning Protons Act Like Little Magnets

A moving electric charge, be it positive or negative, produces a magnetic field. The faster a charge moves or the larger the charge, the larger the magnetic field it produces. Think back to when you were a child and would make a crude electromagnet by wrapping wire around a nail and connecting it to a battery. The larger the voltage of the battery, the larger the current and the stronger the magnet.

Some of the basic properties of a simple proton include mass, a positive electric charge and spin. Granted, a proton does not have a very large electric charge, but it does spin very fast and, therefore, does produce a small, but noticeable, magnetic field. Water is the largest source of protons in the body, followed by fat. Normally, the direction that these tiny magnets point in is randomly distributed (**Figure 1A**).

Key Definition: Spinning protons are little magnets which are frequently referred to as "spins".

Just as a compass aligns with the Earth's magnetic field, a spinning proton placed near (or within) a large external magnetic field (called $B_{\emptyset}$) will align with the external field. Unfortunately, it is not quite so simple. At the atomic level, some of the protons align with the field and some actually align against the field, cancelling each other out. A slight excess will align with the field so that the net result is an alignment with the external field. **Figure 1B** depicts nine protons, four of which have aligned *against* $B_{\emptyset}$ and five have aligned *with* $B_{\emptyset}$ resulting in an excess of one proton. (To be honest, this diagram showing the protons

Figure 1. (A, left) Protons that are randomly oriented in the absence of an external magnetic field. **(B, right)** Protons are now aligned either with (slight majority) or against (slight minority) an external magnetic field.

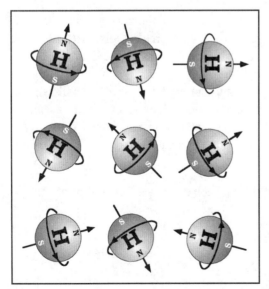
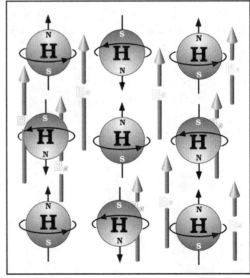

aligning perfectly with or against $B_\emptyset$ is not completely accurate. This will be addressed further when dealing with **Figure 3**.)

Some Quantum Physics

A complete explanation of why the protons align both with and against the external magnetic field would require a study of quantum mechanics. Suffice it to say that both alignments are possible but the one with the field is at a lower energy state. The protons are continually oscillating back and forth between the two states but at any given instant, and with a large enough sample, there will be a very slight majority aligned with the field. The larger the external static magnetic field, the greater the difference in energy levels and the larger the excess number aligned with the field. **Figure 2** demonstrates this for a sample of two million protons. At 1-Tesla there are just six extra protons. At 1.5-Tesla, the most common field strength used in the clinical setting, there are only nine extra protons for every two million. At 3-Tesla, the highest field strength used in the clinical setting, there are 18 excess

Figure 2. At 1.5-Tesla, for every two million protons there are nine more protons aligned with the field than there are aligned against the field.

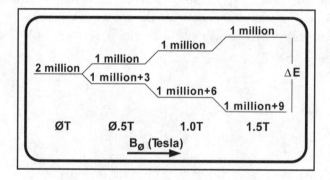

Figure 3. Dreidles (toy tops) rapidly spin about their axis while at the same time they wobble or "*precess*" at a rate that depends on the strength of the gravity field.

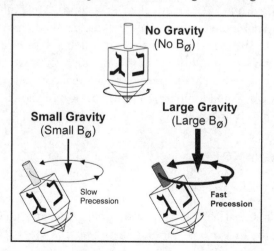

protons for every two million. Therefore, the number of excess protons is proportional to the strength of the static magnetic field.

As will be discussed more fully later in this chapter, the NMR or MRI signal comes from just these excess protons. With only nine out of two million protons in excess, one might ask how can we even detect such a small signal? We shall answer that question by first asking a different question: How many excess protons are there in a single imaging voxel? (A voxel is a three-dimensional or volume pixel.) Without going into the math in great detail, assume a voxel dimension of 2-mm x 2-mm x 5-mm = 0.02-cm^3 or 0.02-ml. Using Avogadro's Number, we can calculate that there are a total of 1.34×10^{21} water protons in a 0.02-ml voxel. If nine out of every two million protons are in excess, then there are a total of 6.02×10^{15} protons in every voxel that will contribute to the MRI signal. The important lesson here is that even though a spinning proton is a very poor magnet, the number of excess protons that align with the field is so large that we can pretty much ignore quantum mechanics and focus on the classical mechanics description.

Key Definition: The total magnetic field of the excess protons is defined as $M_{\emptyset}$.

While it was stated above that due to the large number of excess protons we can pretty much ignore quantum physics, there is still one issue that is best discussed using quantum physics terminology. The relationship between the energy (**E**) of a photon or a unit of electromagnetic radiation and its frequency (*v*) (the Greek symbol 'nu') is described by the Planck's equation:

$$E = h\,v \tag{1}$$

Where *h* is known as Planck's constant. (This is the only place where we will use either *h* or *v*.) In simple words, the energy of electromagnetic radiation goes up directly with the frequency of the radiation. **Table 1** lists the approximate frequency ranges for different types of electromagnetic radiation. As will be discussed in detail shortly, MRI uses radio waves with frequencies around 10^7-Hz (cycles per second). Most other radiology imaging techniques (e.g., X-ray, computed tomography, and nuclear medicine) use ionizing radiation with frequencies in the 10^{18}- to 10^{19}- Hz range or roughly 10^{12} larger than those used in MRI. Accordingly, X-rays are roughly a trillion times more energetic (and potentially damaging) than radio waves. MRI is able to provide such great pictures not because of the high energy involved (like computed tomography) but because of the large number of protons found in the body, primarily in water and fat.

MAGNETIC RESONANCE

Spinning Protons Act Like Dreidles

Three spinning Dreidles (i.e., a toy top traditionally used during Chanukah) are shown in **Figure 3**. Imagine the first one is spinning on the international space station. In the ab-

Table 1. Frequencies associated with different types of electromagnetic radiation.

Types of Radiation	Approximate Frequency in Hz
Radio Waves	10^7
Visible Light	10^{14}
Ultraviolet	10^{16}
X-Rays	10^{18}
Gamma Rays	$>10^{19}$

sence of gravity, it behaves just like a gyroscope and spins without wobbling. Imagine the second one is spinning on the moon. In the low gravity of the moon the Dreidle will wobble rather slowly. The third Dreidle is spinning on the Earth and wobbles faster than the Dreidle on the moon. Imagine a fourth Dreidle somewhere on Jupiter (if you could find a solid surface.) That Dreidle would be spinning the fastest yet.

Previously, a spinning proton was described as being a very tiny magnet. Just as a spinning Dreidle wobbles about its axis, so do spinning protons wobble, or precess, about the axis of the external $B_\emptyset$ field. The frequency of the precession is directly proportional to the strength of the magnetic field and is defined by the Larmor Equation:

Memorize this! ➡️
$$\omega_\emptyset = \gamma B_\emptyset$$
(2)

Where, $\omega_\emptyset$ is known as either the precessional, Larmor or resonance frequency and γ (gamma) is the gyromagnetic ratio and is a constant unique to every atom. For a simple proton $\gamma = 42.56$-MHz/Tesla. As before, $B_\emptyset$ represents the external applied magnetic field. At the magnetic field strengths used in clinical MR systems, 0.2- to 3-Tesla, the resonance frequency of hydrogen ranges from 8.5-MHz to 128-MHz (8.5 x 10^6-Hz to 1.28 x 10^8-Hz). In **Table 1**, it is shown that this range is in the radiofrequency (RF) range of the electromagnetic spectrum.

As such, it is now apparent how **Figure 1B** was slightly inaccurate. The spins do align roughly with (or against) the magnetic field but, if you could take a freeze frame snapshot of all of the protons in a voxel, you would see that each individual proton is slightly tilted. However, remember that the protons are each precessing at faster than ten million times per second, so if you take the average position of the vectors over even a very short amount of time, they will each be aligned either perfectly with, or perfectly against, the main magnetic field.

APPLY AN RF EXCITATION PULSE

If an electromagnetic radiofrequency (RF) pulse is applied at the resonance (Larmor, precession, wobble) frequency, then the protons can absorb that energy. At the quantum level, a single proton "jumps" to a higher energy state. At the macro or classical level, to an

Figure 4. Radiofrequency (RF) energy is absorbed. **(A, left)** An observer in the surrounding laboratory will see $M_\emptyset$ spiral down to the XY-plane (or even down to the negative Z-axis.) **(B, right)** An observer riding on the $M_\emptyset$ vector sees the external world rotating about him. The $M_\emptyset$ vector tips $\alpha°$ (alpha degrees) towards the Y'-axis.

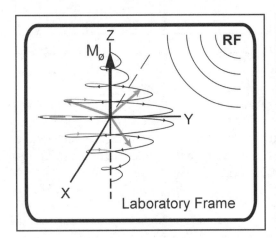 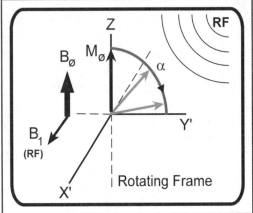

observer in the external laboratory frame of reference, the magnetization vector, $M_\emptyset$, (roughly six million, billion protons) spirals down towards the XY plane (**Figure 4A**). If you could somehow jump aboard $M_\emptyset$, just like a merry-go-round, the laboratory would be rotating around you. In this rotating frame of reference, $M_\emptyset$ would seem to smoothly tip down (**Figure 4B**). The tip angle, α, is a function of the strength and duration of the RF pulse. The absorption of the energy from the applied RF excitation pulse can be roughly compared to shining a light onto phosphorescent paint. The stronger the light or the longer it is applied, the more energy is absorbed (up to a point, that is).

Key Definition: Laboratory Frame. The viewpoint of an observer in the laboratory. The laboratory is stationary, the protons are spinning.

Key Definition: Rotating Frame. The viewpoint of an observer riding along on the protons. The protons appear stationary, the laboratory is rotating.

Key Definition: M_Z. The component of the net magnetization vector that points in the Z or $B_\emptyset$ direction.

Key Definition: M_{XY}. The component of the net magnetization vector that resides in or projects onto the XY-plane.

TURN OFF THE TRANSMITTER – WHAT HAPPENS?

Once the RF transmitter is turned off, three things begin to happen simultaneously: (1) The absorbed RF energy is re-transmitted (at the resonance frequency). (2) The excited spins begin to return to the original M_Z orientation (i.e., T_1 recovery to thermal equilibrium)(3). Initially in-phase, the excited protons begin to dephase (i.e., T_2 and T_2^* relaxation).

Figure 5. With the RF transmitter turned off, the M_{XY} vector continues to rotate about the Z-axis ($B_{\varnothing}$) emitting RF energy at the resonance frequency $\omega_{\varnothing}$.

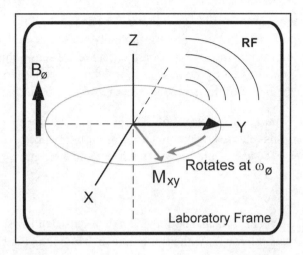

Figure 6. When a proton flips from aligning *against* $B_{\varnothing}$ (high energy state) to aligning *with* $B_{\varnothing}$ (low energy state) it emits a photon at the resonance frequency, $\omega_{\varnothing}$.

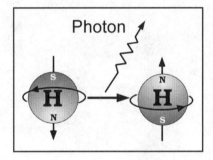

RF Energy Is Re-Transmitted

Continuing the analogy of phosphorescent paint, when the light is turned off the paint will re-emit the absorbed energy and "glow". Once $M_{\varnothing}$ has been tipped away from the Z-axis and the RF transmitter is turned off, the vector will continue to precess around the external $B_{\varnothing}$ field at the resonance frequency, $\omega_{\varnothing}$ (**Figure 5**). Any rotating magnetic field produces electromagnetic radiation. Since $\omega_{\varnothing}$ is in the radiofrequency portion of the electromagnetic spectrum, the rotating vector is said to give off RF waves. These re-emitted RF waves are the MRI signal.

M_Z Recovers Via T_1 Relaxation

The rotating M_{XY} vector shown in **Figure 5** will continue to give off RF waves as long as it continues to rotate. However, to give off energy it has to come from somewhere. The process of giving off RF energy occurs as the spins drop from a high energy state to a low energy state, realigning with $B_{\varnothing}$ and releasing a photon (**Figure 6**). The RF emission is the net result of the **Z** component (**M**$_Z$) of the magnetization recovering back to **M**$_\varnothing$ while the **M**$_{XY}$ component gets smaller and smaller (**Figure 7**).

Not all of the energy given off is detectable as an RF signal. Some of the energy is re-absorbed by nearby protons. Most of the energy actually goes to heating up the surrounding tissue, referred to as the lattice. In a global, or rather, universal sense, this system can be divided into the spins, and the rest of the universe, or a very large lattice. This type of spin-lattice interaction is the result of the excited system returning to thermal equilibrium.

Key Definition: Spin-Lattice Relaxation. The process whereby energy absorbed by the excited protons or spins is released back into the surrounding lattice re-establishing thermal equilibrium. In general, T_1 values are longer at higher field strengths.

Figure 7. As the **M**$_{XY}$ vector rotates about the Z-axis it gets steadily smaller, spiraling inwards, as RF energy is released. At the same time an **M**$_Z$ component starts to recover. This is the exact reverse of the process depicted in **Figure 4A**.

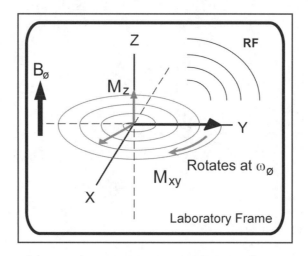

Figure 8. Recovery of Z-magnetization of tissues with two different T_1 time constants. Roughly 63% of Z-magnetization recovers during one T_1 time period.

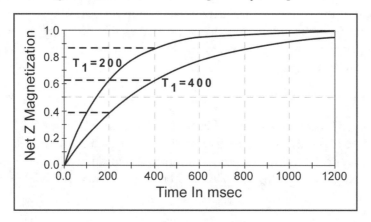

Table 2. MZ recovery fractions at different multiples of T_1 times.

t/T_1	M_Z
-1	0.6321
-2	0.8646
-3	0.9502
-4	0.9816
-5	0.9932

The time course whereby the system returns to thermal equilibrium, or M_Z grows to $M_{\emptyset}$, is mathematically described by an exponential curve (Equation 3) (**Figure 8**).

$$M_Z = M_{\emptyset} \cdot (1 - e^{-t/T_1}) \tag{3}$$

This recovery rate is characterized by the time constant T_1, which is unique to every tissue. This uniqueness in M_Z recovery rates is one of the mechanisms that enables MRI to differentiate between different types of tissue. At a time $t = T_1$ after the excitation pulse, 63.2% of the magnetization has recovered alignment with $B_{\emptyset}$. Full recovery of M_Z to $M_{\emptyset}$ is considered to occur at a time $\geq 5\ T_1$ (**Table 2**).

Key Definition: T_1 Relaxation: Spin-Lattice relaxation. The exponential recovery of longitudinal (aligned with $B_{\emptyset}$) magnetization. M_Z returns to $M_{\emptyset}$.

M_Z Recovers Via T_1 Relaxation

When the spins are first tilted down to the XY-plane, they are all in-phase. Think of a playground with a million swings. If all of the children are going up and down together, at exactly the same rate, then they are swinging in-phase. Assuming that all the children are pumping their legs with the same force and frequency, then they will stay in-phase. But if one child stops pumping for a few seconds and another child pumps a little harder or a little faster, then they will start to get out of sync with everyone else. The same type of thing happens to the spins. For reasons that will be described later, some protons spin a little faster while others spin a little slower (**Figure 9**). Very quickly, they get out of phase relative to some reference (usually the spins at the center of the magnet).

As another analogy, think of a room filled with a million (or six million, billion) people, all of them whispering "Mary had a little lamb". As long as they are all speaking in-phase with each other, you hear a very loud "MARY HAD A LITTLE LAMB". But what usually happens in a room full of people where those at one end of the room can't hear those at the other, some people start speaking a little faster and others a little slower. Soon the words start to become harder to make out until eventually all you hear is some low, background noise (**Figure 10**). The same happens to the spins and the resulting MRI signal.

Figure 9. Immediately after the $M_{\varnothing}$ vector is tipped to the XY-plane all of the six million, billion or so spins that make up the vector start to spread out.

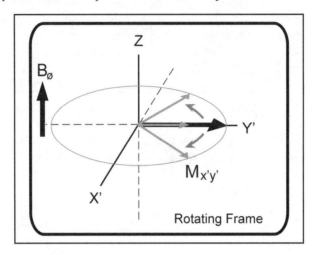

Figure 10. With a room full of people whispering "MARY HAD A LITTLE LAMB" they may all start at the same time and an outside observer can clearly hear the phrase. But what usually happens is that, those at one end of the room can't hear those at the other, so some people start speaking a little faster and others a little slower. Soon the words start to become harder to make out until eventually all you hear is some low, background noise. The same happens to the spins and the resulting MRI signal.

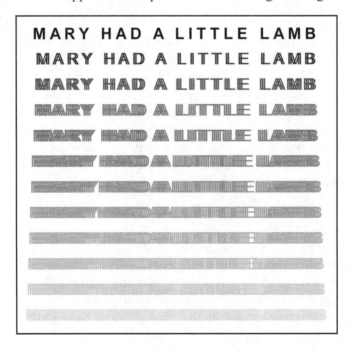

Figure 11. As two spins (or protons) approach each other, the magnetic fields produced by each will either add to or subtract from the main external field ($B_Ø$) causing the other to precess either faster or slower. **(A, left)** The case where one proton is aligned against the main field while the other is aligned with the main field. **(B, right)** The case where both spins are aligned against the main field.

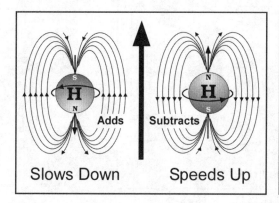 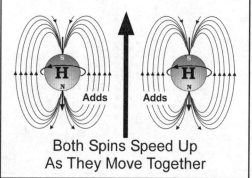

How fast a proton wobbles or precesses depends on the magnetic field that it experiences. An isolated proton, far from any other proton (or electron), is only affected by the main magnetic field, $B_Ø$. As protons (or spins) move together (e.g., due to random motion), their magnetic fields begin to interact. If the field from one proton increases the field that the second proton feels, while the field from the second proton reduces the field that the first proton feels, then the second proton will precess at a slightly faster rate, while the first proton will precess slightly slower (**Figure 11A**). If the fields from both protons add to the main field, then both protons will precess more rapidly (**Figure 11B**). As soon as the spins move farther apart, their fields no longer interact and they both return to the original frequency but at different phases. This type of interaction is called spin-spin interaction. These temporary, random interactions cause a cumulative loss of phase across the excited spins resulting in an overall loss of signal.

Key Definition: Spin-Spin Relaxation. The temporary and random interaction between two spins that causes a cumulative loss in-phase resulting in an overall loss of signal, also known as transverse or T_2 relaxation.

Similar to T_1 relaxation, the signal decay resulting from transverse or spin-spin relaxation is described mathematically by an exponential curve, identical in concept to radioactive decay with a half-life measured in tens of milliseconds (Equation 4) (**Figure 12**).

$$M_{xy} = M_Ø \bullet e^{-t/T_2} \tag{4}$$

The value T_2 is the time after excitation when the signal amplitude has been reduced to 36.8% of its original value or has lost 63.2%. This is the opposite of T_1 where 63.2% of M_z is *recovered* in one T_1 period. By three times T_2 there is less than 5% of the original signal

Figure 12. Graphs depicting the exponential loss of signal from two different tissues with T_2 time constants. Similar to the T_1 recovery curve (**Figure 8**) where 63% of magnetization is recovered in one T_1 time period, here 63% of magnetization is dephased or lost during one T_2 time period.

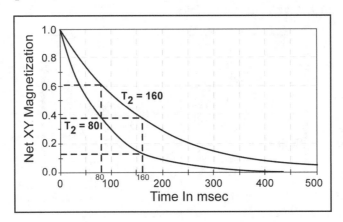

remaining (**Table 3**). The value of T_2 is unique for every kind of tissue and is determined primarily by its chemical environment with little relation to field strength. This uniqueness in T_2 decay rates is one of the other mechanisms that enables MRI to differentiate between different types of tissue.

Key Definition: T2 Decay. The exponential loss of signal resulting from purely random spin-spin interactions in the transverse or XY-plane. In general, T2 values are unrelated to field strengths (unlike T1 values).

FREE INDUCTION DECAY (FID) AND SPIN ECHO FORMATION

To summarize what has been covered so far, after the RF transmitter is turned off, the protons immediately begin to re-radiate the absorbed energy. If nothing is affecting the homogeneity of the magnetic field, all of the protons will spin at the same resonance frequency. The initial amplitude of the signal is determined by the portion of the magnetization vector ($M_\emptyset$) that has been tipped onto the XY-plane. This, in turn, is determined by the sine of the flip angle, α. The maximum signal is obtained when the flip angle is 90°. (Note: sine (0°) = 0, sine (90°) = 1.0) The signal unaffected by any gradient is known as a Free Induction Decay (FID) (**Figure 13**). The time constant that determines the rate of decay is called T_2.

Table 3. M_{XY} residual fractions at different multiples of T_2 times.

t/T_2	M_{xy}
-0.5	0.6065
-1	0.3679
-2	0.1354
-3	0.0498
-4	0.0184

Figure 13. A graph depicting how, while the NMR signal oscillates rapidly at the resonance frequency, $\omega_{\varnothing}$, the amplitude or signal envelope decays at a rate dependent on the T_2 time constant. This type of signal is known as Free Induction Decay or FID.

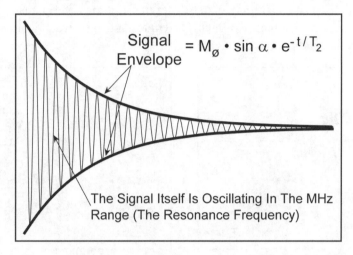

$$\text{Signal Envelope} = M_{\varnothing} \cdot \sin \alpha \cdot e^{-t/T_2}$$

The Signal Itself Is Oscillating In The MHz Range (The Resonance Frequency)

Figure 14. The graph of Figure 13 represents the ideal case. In the real world the FID decays much more rapidly with a time constant of T_2^* (T_2-star).

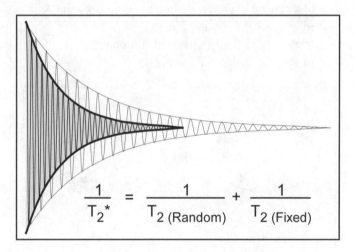

$$\frac{1}{T_2^*} = \frac{1}{T_{2\,(Random)}} + \frac{1}{T_{2\,(Fixed)}}$$

Key Definition: Free Induction Decay (FID). An NMR signal in the absence of any magnetic gradients. The decay curve is the signal envelope. The actual signal is oscillating at the resonance frequency which is in the MHz range.

In the real world, the NMR signal decays faster than T_2 would predict. Pure T_2 decay is a function of completely random interactions between spins. The assumption is that the main external $\mathbf{B_{\varnothing}}$ field is absolutely homogeneous. In reality, there are many factors creating imperfections in the homogeneity of a magnetic field. The main magnet itself will have flaws related to the manufacturing process. Every tissue has a different magnetic susceptibility which distorts the field at tissue borders, particularly at air/tissue interfaces. Additionally, patients may have some type of metallic implants (e.g., clips, staples, heart valves,

Figure 15. Excited spins can be compared to contestants in a race. The car in the middle represents the pace car or spins at exactly the resonance frequency. Some spins are at a lower frequency (the bicyclist and the turtle) while others are at a higher frequency (the plane and the rocket.) **(A, left)** Immediately after the start the contestants spread out. **(B, right)** After some sort of signal (Go Back) the contestants turn around and head back to the Start/Finish line ending in a tie.

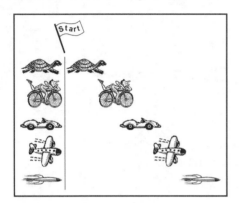 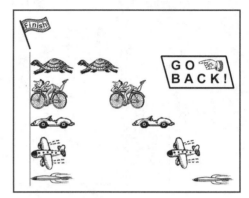

Figure 16. Spin echo formation. **(A)** $M_{\emptyset}$ is flipped down onto the X'Y' plane. **(B)** Spins dephase (T_2^*) followed by a 180° RF pulse flipping them to the other side of the X' axis. **(C)** The spins continue moving at their individual frequencies resulting in them moving back together. **(D)** Forming the re-phased spin echo.

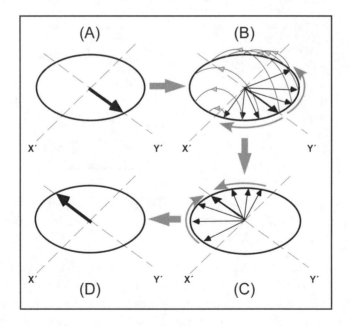

Figure 17. Application of multiple 180° RF pulses will create multiple spin echoes, the amplitude of which is limited by the T_2 decay envelope.

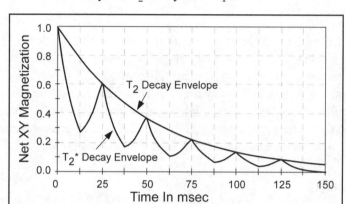

etc.) which cause disruptions of the magnetic field. The sum total of all of these random and fixed effects is called T_2* (pronounced "T-two star") (**Figure 14**).

Thus, T_2 relaxation comes from random causes while T_2* comes from a combination of both random and fixed causes. There is nothing that can be done to prevent or compensate for random losses in-phase, but what about the fixed effects? Can anything be done about these losses? The answer is yes.

Consider the following race (**Figure 15A**). The contestants are a turtle, a bicyclist, a pace car, an airplane, and a rocket. At the start of the race, everyone is together (in-phase.) Once the race starts (at t = 0), the contestants all move out, each at their fastest pace. Soon, there is a noticeable distance between them.

After some time, let's call it TE/2, a signal is given for everyone to turn around and go back. Assuming that everyone is still going at the same rate as before, then after an additional time, TE/2, they all arrive at the starting/finish line together (**Figure 15B**).

In terms of MRI, at the time TE (TE/2 + TE/2) all the spins are back in-phase, producing a large signal. This large signal is called a spin echo and the time TE is called the echo time (8).

Key Definition: Echo. The reflection (mirror image) of a signal caused by some sort of reversal of direction. (e.g., the sound bouncing off of a cliff). In MRI, there are spin echoes and gradient echoes.

The principle of spin echo formation in the rotating frame is presented in **Figure 16:** (**A**) At time t = 0, immediately after a 90° RF pulse, $\mathbf{M_0}$ points along the Y'-axis. (**B**) A time of TE/2 is allowed to elapse while the spins dephase (T_2* mechanisms). At t = TE/2, a 180° RF pulse is given which flips the dephased vectors about the X' axis. (**C**) Another TE/2 time is allowed to pass while the vectors rephase. (**D**) At t = TE, the vectors have rephased and an echo of opposite sign forms. (The astute observer will note that the arrows drawn to represent the 180° rotation about the X'-axis go above the X'Y'-plane, not below it. This is true only if a negative 180° pulse is what is actually used. Whether a positive or negative 180° is used, or one that rotates about the Y'-axis instead of the X'-axis, the end result is the same.)

As described above, a 180° pulse can be used to reverse the T_2* dephasing process and, thereby, produce a spin echo. As soon as the spins all come back into phase at the echo time, they immediately start to go out of phase again. A second 180° pulse will generate a second echo. This process can be repeated many times, producing many echoes, as long as the pure T_2 decay mechanisms have left some signal to work with (**Figure 17**). This repeating echo train can be used to produce multiple images or can be used to greatly speed up the acquisition time using a method known as fast or turbo spin echo imaging.

MRI HARDWARE

In order to perform MRI, the patient must be placed inside of some sort of magnet. There are many factors that go into the design of a magnet used in an MR system. As stated above, the higher the strength of the static magnetic field, the larger the number of excess protons there are to produce the NMR signal (which usually means better quality images). Also, in order to reduce T_2* signal dephasing the magnetic field in the imaging volume should be as homogeneous as possible over as large a volume as possible.

A third issue that has not been discussed, nor will it be possible to discuss in any great detail, is the need to be able to change the magnetic field at will. Equation 2 states that the resonance frequency is directly proportional to the strength of the magnetic field. By changing the strength of the magnetic field in some sort of known or predictable fashion, different resonance frequencies can be assigned to different locations in the magnet. This is accomplished using what are known as the X-, Y- and Z-gradients.

Figure 18. The magnet field for most MR systems is produced using large electromagnets. The main working field is concentrated in the center and the fringe field can extend far outside the imaging region.

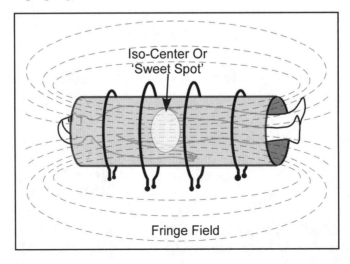

The Magnet and the Fringe Field

Horizontal field magnets produce magnetic field lines that go out one end of the magnet, loop around and go back the other end. Areas with the highest density of field lines have the highest strength. However, it is the areas that have the most rapidly changing density of field lines (i.e., the largest spatial gradients) that produce the greatest forces that can act on ferromagnetic materials. In other words, it is these areas that represent the greatest danger for items to become projectiles. Examples of projectiles that occurred in the MRI environment may be seen at www.simplyphysics.com (9).

The vast majority of high field strength MR scanners use superconducting electromagnets to produce the main magnetic field. [Note that some low field MR systems use permanent magnets, which are limited to fields less than 0.3-Tesla (10)]. A simple four loop design of such a magnet used in an MR system is depicted in **Figure 18**. The two central loops produce the majority of the field and the two outer loops help to shape it, to make it more homogeneous. Note that the center of the magnet is where the field lines are most closely packed meaning this is where the highest field strength is. The area marked as "iso-center" is also referred to as the "sweet spot", the region with the greatest magnetic field uniformity.

A current running through a loop of wire wrapped around a nail and attached to a battery produces a small magnetic field. (Actually the nail isn't needed, it just acts to intensify the field.) The larger the current flowing, the greater the magnetic field produced. This type of magnet is called a resistive electromagnet because the wire resists the flow of electrons. This resistance to the current flow also produces heat. So while larger currents can generate higher magnetic fields, they will also produce considerable heat.

Similar to resistive magnets, the field from a superconducting magnet is produced by current flowing in multiple loops of wires. The wires are made out of niobium-titanium which, when cooled to 9.5°-K (9.5° above absolute zero), lose all resistance to current flow. The coils are surrounded by liquid helium which boils at 4.2° K (**Figure 19**). When the scanner is first installed, a power supply is utilized to slowly build up the current and, thus, the magnetic field. This can take several hours to accomplish. Once it is up to full field, the power supply is disconnected and the current will continue virtually for centuries (as long as it's kept cold, of course). This is why you will typically see signs outside MR system rooms that state, "Danger! This Magnet is Always On!"

The magnetic field lines depicted in **Figure 18** that extend outside of the magnet are known as the fringe field. It is this fringe field that can cause problems with ferromagnetic objects. In general, the five gauss line is the demarcation between what is considered safe or a danger for certain objects. Modern-day MR systems use what is know as "active shielding". An actively-shielded magnet has an inner or primary set of field coils that produces more than the desired field with an outer or secondary set of field coils with a lower current going in the opposite direction (**Figure 20**). The smaller opposite field partially cancels the field at the center of the magnet but cancels a much larger portion on the outside. For example, the primary set coils might produce a positive 2-Tesla field while the secondary coils produce a negative 0.5-Tesla, resulting in a net 1.5-Tesla field at the center of the magnet

Figure 19. A cross section through a typical superconducting, high field strength MR scanner.

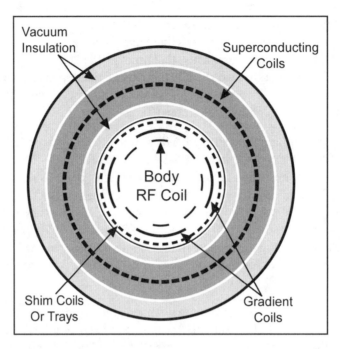

Figure 20. A cross section through a superconducting, high field strength MR system with active shielding. The current in the secondary field coils flow in the opposite direction from the current in the primary field coils.

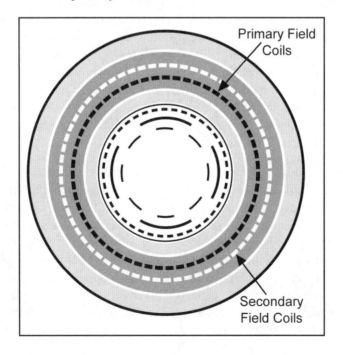

Figure 21. A hospital bed stuck to the front of a 3-Tesla MR system. (Photograph provided courtesy of Simply Physics.)

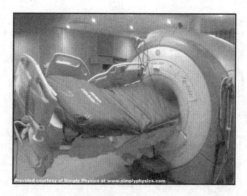

Figure 22. (A, left) The magnetic field produced by a current in a simple loop of wire is at a maximum at the center of loop and drops off rapidly (and non-linearly) as you move away. **(B, right)** Using two loops of wire separated by roughly the diameter of the coil and with currents flowing in opposite direction results in a region in-between where the strength or amplitude of the magnet field varies in a linear fashion.

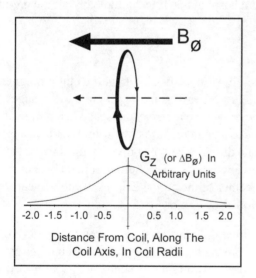 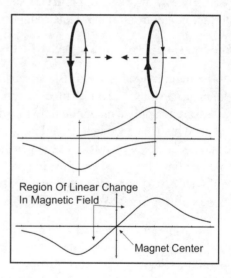

but, because the secondary coils are closer to the outside, they create a greater amount of cancellation.

The advantage of modern actively-shielded magnets is that the five gauss line can be restricted relatively close to the magnet. However, this also means that as a ferromagnetic object gets closer to the bore of the magnet, the field strength rises rapidly over a relatively short distance (i.e., a high spatial gradient magnetic field is present). Understandably, a relatively high spatial gradient magnetic field can produce substantial issues for ferromagnetic

Figure 23. X-, Y- and Z-gradient coils mounted on the gradient tube of an MR system.

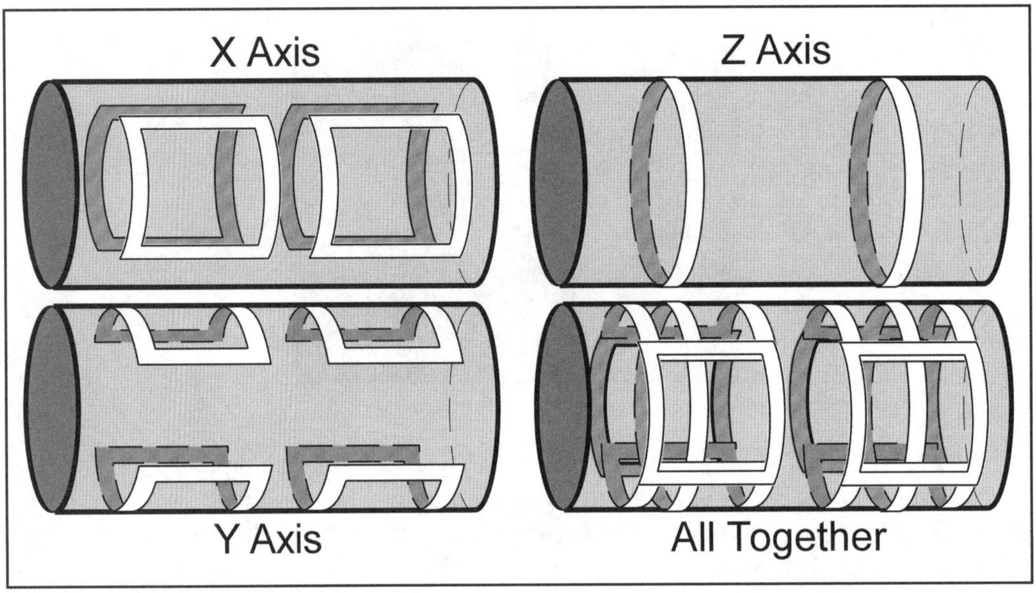

objects. By way of example, **Figure 21** shows a hospital bed lifted completely off the ground and stuck to the front of a 3-Tesla scanner.

Time-Varying Gradient Magnetic Fields

The main magnetic field, $B_{\emptyset}$, discussed above is also known as the static magnetic field, meaning that it never changes over time. In order to actually produce MR images, it is necessary to apply a magnetic field that does change over time and space in a predictable fashion. What is needed is to be able to produce a change that is linear moving away from the magnet center, with positive changes in one direction and negative changes in the other. (Note, the field at the center of the magnet never changes.) The field produced by a current in a single loop of wire reaches a peak at the center of the coil and drops off non-linearly as it move out (**Figure 22A**). Obviously, this won't suffice for MRI.

However, if a second coil with a current flowing in the opposite direction is placed one coil diameter away from the first, the fields from each coil totally cancel each other at the point midway between them (**Figure 22B**). The fields interact in such a way that they produce an almost perfectly linear change in the area midway between them. The field change then drops off as you move outside of the coils. This linear change (also known as a gradient) is not only along the centerline between the two coils but remains linear for about half of the center volume. If properly designed, this region of reasonable linearity corresponds with the "sweet spot" or most homogeneous portion of the magnet. Note that the locations with the greatest offset from the field at the center of the magnet are located near the center of each loop. This is also the location of the greatest change in magnetic field per unit time, dB/dt, during an imaging sequence.

Every MR system has three orthogonal (perpendicular) sets of gradient coils (i.e., X-, Y-, and Z-gradient coils) that are mounted on what is referred to as the "gradient tube" (11)

Figure 24. A pulse profile is a diagram that depicts gradient (or RF) activity during an MRI pulse sequence.

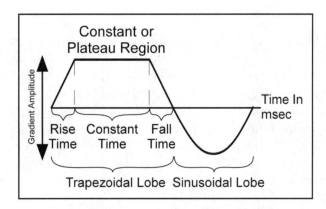

(**Figure 23**). Current passing through these coils is rapidly turned on and off during the imaging process and are referred to as time-varying gradient magnetic fields. A diagram depicting the gradient activity during an MRI sequence showing how the gradient is turned on and off, is known as the "pulse profile" (**Figure 24**). A typical imaging sequence diagram will use pulse profiles to show the temporal relationship between each "gradient channel", X-, Y-, Z- and the RF transmitter/receiver (**Figures 25 to 28**).

Every gradient system is characterized by two parameters: (1) the peak gradient amplitude, which primarily determines how small the field of view (FOV) may be and (2) the peak slew rate, which is how fast the gradients can be turned on and off, which affects things like minimum echo and/or repetition times. Between the two, a fast slew rate is better from an MRI consideration than a high peak amplitude, however, faster slew rates cause more safety-related issues, as will be discussed below.

From the standpoint of MRI safety, these time-varying gradients raise two primary areas of concern. The first is acoustic noise that is associated with the gradient magnetic fields (12-14). An MR system can be compared to a giant speaker system. In a typical stereo speaker, there is a small permanent magnet with loops of wire wrapped around it and a magnet attached at the center of a diaphragm. When an oscillating current is applied through the wire, it creates a time-varying gradient magnetic field that pushes and pulls on the permanent magnet causing the supporting speaker diaphragm to vibrate.

The static $B_{\emptyset}$ magnet of the MR system is like the speaker's permanent magnet. The imaging gradients are like the loop of wire wrapped around the permanent magnet. The gradient tube is like the diaphragm. During the imaging process, the imaging gradient can be turned on and off in as little as 1-msec (corresponding to 1000-Hz) or as much as 20-msec (corresponding to 50-Hz). This causes the imaging gradients to push and pull against the main magnetic field, and the physical supporting structures, resulting in vibrations that occur in the typical audio range. The higher the magnetic field, $B_{\emptyset}$, and the faster the imaging sequence (higher slew rates), the louder the noise is that will be produced. The resulting acoustic noise can be at levels that may cause hearing damage if hearing protection is not used in the MR system room. As shown in the pulse profile of **Figure 24**, imaging gradients can be turned on and off rather abruptly (i.e., the trapezoidal lobe) or more gradually (i.e., the sinusoidal lobe). There are always trade-offs when designing an imaging sequence (see below), but using the lowest amplitude and lowest slew rates possible helps to minimize acoustic noise.

One of the important properties of electromagnetism is, just as an electric current creates a magnetic field, a time-varying gradient magnetic field can produce an electric current in any nearby conductor. This brings us to the other issue that is associated with time-varying gradient magnetic fields. The human body is an electrical conductor. If a patient undergoing MRI has crossed-arms or crossed-legs, these may create a closed loop for current to flow under certain imaging conditions. The rapidly changing imaging gradients can induce current to flow across the body and peripheral nerve stimulation may occur (15). The area near the center of the coils in **Figure 22B** is the location of the largest dB/dt so it is at this location where the greatest danger of induced currents exists with respect to peripheral nerve stimulation.

To summarize, the potential problems caused by time-varying gradient magnetic fields are, as follows: (1) acoustic noise and (2) peripheral nerve stimulation. The more rapidly the gradients change and the higher the amplitude, the greater the risks. Importantly, for patients with electronically-activated devices, the location of the greatest risk is not at the center of the MR system but at the outer edges of the gradient coils where the absolute changes in the magnetic fields per unit time (i.e., dB/dt) is the highest.

RF Coils and RF Power Deposition

As discussed above, MRI requires the use of a radio transmitter to provide the RF excitation pulses. Every scanner has a built in body RF coil (**Figure 19**) which is used for many of the imaging sequences. Alternatively, the RF excitation pulses can be applied by a smaller transmit RF coil, most commonly designed for imaging either the patient's head or knee. While some of the applied RF energy that is absorbed ends up producing the MRI signal, most of it actually results in tissue heating (16). The amount of RF power absorbed by the body increases approximately with the square of the field strength. Accordingly, at higher static magnetic fields, there can be an inherent danger of over-heating the patient (16). The mass normalized rate at which RF energy is coupled to biological tissue is characterized by the specific absorption rate (SAR) and is reported in W/kg relative to the use of a particular pulse sequence and the body weight of the patient.

The built in transmit body RF coil deposits RF energy over a relatively large area of the patient. Even if only a small amount of tissue is actually being imaged, a large amount of tissue will absorb much of the transmitted energy. By comparison, smaller transmit/receive RF coils have a limited volume of coverage and result in greatly reduced RF power deposition. Additionally, a class of RF coils known as quadrature (quadrature is an engineering term that has nothing to do with the number four) coils result in less power deposition than comparably-sized linear coils. Notably, this information has implications for scanning patients with certain types of biomedical implants insofar as it may be necessary to prevent substantial implant heating by limiting the MRI examination to the use of a transmit/receive head RF coil only, versus performing the MRI procedure using a transmit body

Figure 25. This diagram shows the temporal relationship between activity on the X-, Y-, and Z-gradients as well as the RF transmitter and receiver during a simple gradient echo pulse sequence. E.A.O.S. stands for Equal Area Opposite Sign.

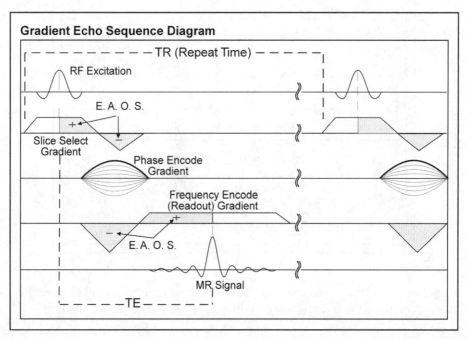

Figure 26. The same diagram as shown in **Figure 25** except for a simple spin echo pulse sequence.

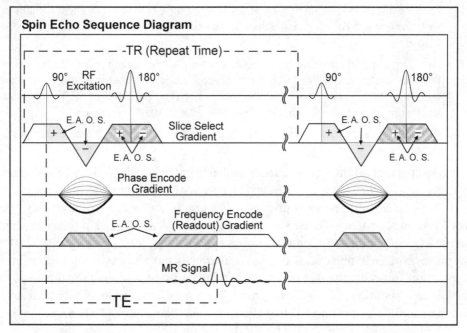

Figure 27. The same diagram as shown in **Figure 26** except for a fast spin echo pulse sequence.

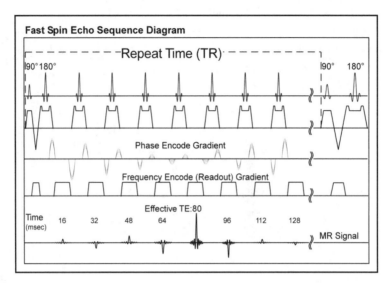

RF coil and a receive-only head coil (e.g., certain neurostimulation systems used for spinal cord stimulation have these particular conditions specified in the MRI labeling).

Imaging Sequences

While there are many different types of imaging sequences used for MRI, they all have three basic steps in common which are:

(1) Exciting a section location or slice of tissue by using a slice select gradient combined with one or more RF excitation pulses. In an axial image, the Z-gradient is the slice select gradient.

(2) Applying a spatial encoding gradient known as a phase encoding pulse. The details of how this works are beyond the scope of this chapter. In an axial plane image, the phase encoding direction can be in either the X-direction (i.e., left/right) or the Y-direction (i.e., anterior/posterior). For the moment, let's assume it is in the Y-direction.

(3) Reading out the MRI signal while applying a third spatial encoding gradient known as the frequency encoding gradient.

Two simplest of all imaging sequences, a basic gradient echo (GRE)(17), also known as a field echo (FE) and a basic spin echo (SE) are shown in **Figure 25** and **Figure 26**, respectively (8). As was previously discussed (**Figure 16**), a SE sequence requires two RF pulses while, as shown in **Figure 25**, a GRE sequence uses a single RF pulse. The SE pulse sequence is most commonly used for T1-weighted imaging incorporating a 90°/180° pair of RF pulses. The GRE pulse sequence can use virtually any flip angle, which then impacts the type of image-weighting that results, in part, by the combination of the flip angle, echo time (TE) and repetition time (TR). Typically, flip angles from 20° to 40° are used for T2*-weighting and flip angles from 70° to 90° are used for T1-weighting. The key point here is that, with only one RF pulse, the RF power deposition, or SAR, is substantially lower with

Figure 28. The same as shown in **Figure 26** except for a spin echo sequence with an echo planar imaging (EPI) readout.

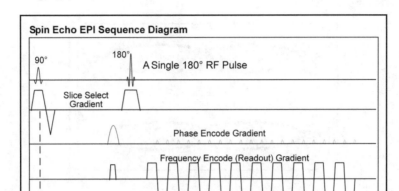

GRE sequences than with SE sequences. This is particularly important on MRI examinations using MR systems operating at 3-Tesla or higher.

Figure 17 illustrates how it is possible to obtain multiple spin echoes using a train of 180° RF pulses. **Figure 27** shows how a train of eight 180° RF pulses, combined with appropriate slice select, phase encode and frequency encode gradients, comprise what is known as a fast spin echo (FSE) pulse sequence (18) (also known as turbo spin echo, or TSE). This type of sequence can have an echo train length (ETL) as short as two to four for T1-weighted or proton density-weighting, or moderate echo train lengths of eight to 32 for T2-weighted imaging or as long as 128 to 256 for MRI procedures such as single shot myelograms or cholangiograms (20, 21). The advantage of using a FSE pulse sequence is the decreased acquisition time that is due to acquiring multiple echoes or lines of data during one repetition time (TR) interval.

With all of the associated gradient activity, a FSE pulse sequence may suffer from the consequences of time-varying gradient magnetic fields discussed earlier. More importantly, particularly at 1.5-T and higher fields, all of the 180° RF pulses significantly increase the SAR level. Accordingly, the MR system reported SAR may exceed the recommended FDA limits for specific absorption rate. When this happens, there are four possible options: (1) Increase the repetition time (TR) so that the average power per unit time goes down. (2) Decrease the total number of slices acquired per repetition time (TR)(3, 16). Half the number of slices means half the RF power. (3) Use the technique known as Half-Fourier imaging (22). This takes advantage of the symmetry in MRI raw data to reduce the number of lines of data required (and the associated acquisition time and RF power) by roughly one half. The disadvantage to this is that it reduces the signal-to-noise ratio (SNR) by the square root of two. (4) Use refocusing RF pulses less than 180°. The amount of RF energy per RF pulse is directly proportional to the flip angle. Reduce flip angle of a large number of RF pulses and the total SAR will be decreased.

Figure 29. A diagram showing a four-channel phased array coil. This is typical configuration for a torso phased-array coil.

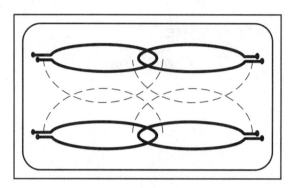

Reducing the flip angle of the refocusing pulse does reduce the SAR, but with all things in MRI, there are tradeoffs. In terms of refocusing spins that are going out of phase due to T2* affects (**Figure 16**), a 180° pulse is optimal. Reducing the refocusing flip angle from 180° to 140° for a single echo will reduce the effectiveness by about 12%. The effect of involving multiple refocusing pulses becomes very complicated but suffice to say that the SNR is maximum with 180° pulses and goes down from there. While RF power deposition is mainly a problem at higher static magnetic field strengths, higher fields have higher SNR starting points so they can better afford some loss in SNR in order to minimize the SAR.

Figure 28 depicts the last imaging sequence to be discussed in this chapter, a spin echo -echo planar imaging (SE-EPI) pulse sequence (19). This type of sequence is most commonly used for diffusion-weighted imaging (DTI) or functional MRI (fMRI). The RF excitation utilizes a single 90°/180° pair so the SAR levels associated with these pulse sequences are usually not a problem. However, these sequences use the absolute fastest changing gradients so they have the greatest potential for creating the possible problems related to the time-varying gradient magnetic fields discussed above.

Parallel Imaging Reconstruction

The goal of most clinical MRI examinations is to achieve the best quality that is possible in the shortest acquisition time. Over the years, gradient slew rates have increased dramatically, improving the imaging speed of many techniques (such as FSE and EPI discussed above). However, there is still a physical limit as to how fast gradients can be turned on and off as well as the practical limit that exists to prevent problems such as peripheral nerve stimulation. The main purpose of the imaging gradients is to impart spatial information to the MRI signal. One might ask is there any other way of obtaining at least some of the spatial information?

As discussed earlier, with the exception of transmit/received RF coils such as those used for the knee or head, most MRI procedures use the body RF coil for excitation and passive receive-only coils to detect the MRI signal. Modern-day MR systems use multichannel phased-array (PA) RF coils that are designed for specific, limited anatomical coverage. These PA coils consist of multiple small coils (anywhere from two to 32) where each coil is sensitive to signal from only a portion of the FOV. A four channel configuration typical of a torso phase-array coil is shown in **Figure 29**. In this case, four images are produced, one from the signal obtained from each coil, which are then combined to make a single composite image.

Without going into the mathematical details which are beyond the scope of this chapter, techniques such a SENSE (23), SMASH (24), GRAPPA (25), all members of a class of parallel imaging reconstruction methods utilize the known or measured sensitivity profile of each individual coil to impart some spatial information. This makes it possible to reduce the number of phase encoding (PE) steps that are required for virtually any imaging technique. As the number of PE steps goes down, so does the total SAR. If the acquisition time is reduced by a factor of two, then the SAR is cut in half. If the acquisition time is reduced by a factor of four, then the SAR is cut to one-fourth. Theoretically, while it is possible to "speed up" a scan by a factor equal to the number of different coil elements, in practice the speed up factors are usually two or four. The main reason for this limitation is that while the acquisition time may be faster, the SNR of the final image is proportional to the square root of the number of actual phase encoding views used. If the scan is speeded up by a factor of four, the SNR is cut in half. Therefore, while high field strength MR systems have an initially high SNR, there is a limit as to how much SNR can be "thrown away".

One final cautionary note about parallel imaging techniques: some MRI centers may decide to use "speed up" factors of two or three but then are not happy with the SNR of the final images. Therefore, these MRI facilities use two or three signal averages for the pulse sequence. Of course, that just takes the acquisition time back to what it would have been without the use of parallel imaging. In fact, parallel imaging reconstruction can actually add artifacts to the image, particularly if the patient moves. Thus, parallel imaging should only be used with one signal average. If better SNR is desired, it is best to not use parallel imaging.

CONCLUSIONS

This chapter presented information on the basic MRI physics that are involved in creating exquisite images of human anatomy. The same physics helps us to understand the potential risks and problems associated with MRI technology and guides us in how to deal with those issues. MRI is a safe and effective imaging modality as long as careful attention is given to established safety policies and procedures (26). Other chapters in this textbook provide comprehensive details related to the bioeffects, safety, and patient management aspects of MRI.

REFERENCES

1.   Block F, Hanson WW, Packard ME. Nuclear induction. Phys Rev 1946;69:127-138.

2.   Purcell EM, Torrey HC, Round RV. Resonance absorption by nuclear magnetic moments in solid. Phys Rev 1946;69:37.

3.   NessAiver MS. All You Really Need to Know About MRI Physics. Chapters 2 and 3. Baltimore: Simply Physics; 1997.

4.   Abragam A. The Principles of Nuclear Magnetism. Oxford: Oxford University Press, 1978.

5. Mansfield P, Morris PG. NMR Imaging in Biomedicine. New York: Academic Press; 1982.

6. Stark D. Bradley WG. Magnetic Resonance Imaging. St. Louis: Mosby Year Book; 1992.

7. McRobbie DW, Moore EA, Graves MJ, Prince MR. MRI From Picture to Proton. Second Edition, Cambridge: Cambridge University Press; 2007.

8. Hahn EL. Spin echoes. Phys Rev 1950;20:580.

9. NessAiver MS. "Flying Objects" slide show. Available at: http://www.simplyphysics.com/flying_objects.html

10. Zijlstra H. Permanent magnetic systems for NMR tomography. Philips Journal of Research 1985;40:259-288.

11. Turner R. Gradient coil design, a review of methods. Magn Reson Imaging 1993;11:903-920.

12. Cho ZH, Park SH, Kim JH, et al. Analysis of acoustic noise in MRI. Magn Reson Imaging 1997;15:815-22.

13. Price DL, De Wilde JP, et al. Investigation of acoustic noise on 15 MRI scanners from 0.2T to 3T. J Magn Reson Imaging 2001;13:288-93.

14. Cho ZH, Chung SC, et al. Effects of the acoustic noise of the gradient systems on fMRI: a study on auditory, motor, and visual cortices. Magn Reson Med 1998;39:331-5.

15. Ham CL, Engels JM, et al. Peripheral nerve stimulation during MRI: effects of high gradient amplitudes and switching rates. J Magn Reson Imaging 1997;7:933-7.

16. Bottomley PA. Turning up the heat on MRI. J AM Coll Radiol 2008;5:853-855.

17. Meulen PD, Groen JP, Cuppen JM. Very fast MR Imaging by field echoes and small angle excitation. Magn Reson Imaging 1985;3:297-299.

18. Hennig J, Nanert A, Friedburg H. RARE imaging, a fast imaging method for clinical MR. Magn Reson in Med 1986;3:823-833.

19. Mansfield P. Real time echo planar imaging by NMR. Br Med Bull 1984;40:187-90.

20. Aggarwal A, Azad R, et al. Additional merits of two-dimensional single thick-slice magnetic resonance myelography in spinal imaging. J Clin Imaging Sci 2012;2:84.

21. Van Epps K, Regan F. MR cholangiopancreatography using HASTE sequences. Clin Radiol 1999;54:588-94.

22. Runge VM, Wood ML. Half-Fourier MR imaging of CNS disease. Am J Neuroradiol 1990;175:77-82.

23. Pruessmann KP, Weiger M, Scheidegger MB, et al. SENSE: sensitivity encoding for fast MRI. Magn Reson Med 1999;42:952-962.

24. Sodickson DK, Manning WJ. Simultaneous acquisition of spatial harmonics (SMASH): fast imaging with radiofrequency coil arrays. Mag Reson Med 1997;38:591-603.

25. Griswold MA, Jakob PM, Heidemann RM, et al. Generalized autocalibrating partially parallel acquisitions (GRAPPA). Magn Reson Med 2002;47:1202-1210.

26. Shellock, FG. Reference Manual for Magnetic Resonance Safety, Implants and Devices, 2013 Edition. Los Angeles: Biomedical Research Publishing Group; 2013.

Chapter 2   Bioeffects of Static Magnetic Fields

ALAYAR KANGARLU, PH.D.

Director of MRI Physics
Columbia University
New York, NY

JOHN F. SCHENCK, M.D., PH.D.

Principal Scientist
General Electric Corporate Research and Development Center
Schenectady, NY

INTRODUCTION

For the three different types of electromagnetic fields associated with magnetic resonance imaging (MRI), the static magnetic field has been a primary focus of safety considerations. The need for intermittent exposure to the powerful static magnetic field of the MR system is at the base of safety concerns, from the pioneers working on developing nuclear magnetic resonance (NMR), to the diagnostic imaging technique that is currently in use today, as magnetic resonance imaging (MRI). Since the early 1970s, when Raymond Damadian's pioneering work on animal tumor imaging and Paul Lauterbur's application of gradient magnetic fields in combination with a strong magnetic field to generate images marked the birth of MRI (1, 2), the safety implications for human subjects has been a constant preoccupation of practitioners (1, 2). This has been the case in spite of the lack of any unpreventable safety incidents for patients and others in the MRI environment (3). The safety record of scanning hundreds of millions of human subjects imaged in MR systems around the world indicates a relative lack of an inherent risk being associated with MRI.

Although the static magnetic field (B_0) is not the only source of safety concern, the other two, that is, the radiofrequency (RF) electric field (B_1-field) and gradient switching (dB/dt), warrant their own safety evaluations. Considering that all three of these electromagnetic fields act simultaneously on the human body and understanding their interactions constitutes the first order of business in quantifying safety implications. In so doing, in the present chapter, we exclusively focus on the harder task of understanding the interaction of the static magnetic field with the human body. The other two, RF and dB/dt, are easier to quantify since a large part of their interactions is manifestation of Faraday's Law of Induction. These effects are functions of easily controlled characteristics of transmit RF coils and the gradient fields, such as amplitude and frequency. It is far easier to build an RF coil operating at high frequencies greater than 300-MHz and gradients operating at greater than 50-mT/m with slew rates of greater than 200-T/m/s than to build a whole-body magnet operating at greater than 7-Tesla (T). Furthermore, computations of specific absorption rate (SAR) and dB/dt induced voltage and subsequent nerve stimulations are readily carried out. On the other hand, the limiting physiological effects of static magnetic fields on biological tissues have not been quantified because the observable effects on tissues are very small and it is difficult to estimate the field strengths at which these will become significant hazards (**Table 1**)(3).

However, since developing the technological capability of manufacturing powerful magnets, scientists have begun to understand the mechanisms of interactions with biological tissues at different levels. To date, the strongest of these effects, the attractive force on ferromagnetic materials has demonstrated the most ominous of all safety risks to the life and well being of patients and other individuals (4, 5). However, this effect, also known as the projectile or missile effect, is a secondary effect meaning that it is easily avoidable and is not inherent to the interaction of the static magnetic with the human body. As far as the hazards associated with inherent interactions, the scientific community has yet to establish an upper limit for the static magnetic field designed for exposure of human subjects. Considering the difficulty of building whole-body magnets operating at field strengths much higher than currently recommended by the United States, Food and Drug Administration (FDA) presently standing at 8-Tesla (5), it is conceivable that there would be many opportunities and available hardware to test viable hypotheses for such effects. Proliferation of 7-T whole-body magnets (subsequent to the success of the 8-T scanner, designed by the team at Ohio State University in 1998) has offered a fertile ground to study the interactions of static magnetic fields with biological tissues using all available techniques, in addition to the imaging capabilities that such scanners afford the scientists. The safe operation of the fifty or so 7-T scanners around the world has encouraged scientists to dream of higher fields. NeuroSpin in Orsay, France, and the National Institutes of Health (NIH) are in the process of installing 11.7-T whole-body MR systems. This is the result of successful exposures of thousands of

Table 1. Comparison of the physical effects of the various fields applied to patients during MRI.

Type of Field	Physical Limitation on Human Exposure
Switched Gradient Fields	Peripheral Nerve Stimulation[1,2]
Radiofrequency B_1 Fields	Tissue Heating[1]
Static B_0 Fields	Unknown

[1] The origin of both effects can be attributed to the electric field that accompanies all time-dependent magnetic fields and not the magnetic field itself.
[2] Both the rate of change of the field and the duration of the change must be above threshold values for stimulation to occur.

human subjects to 7-, 8-, and 9.4-T fields since 1998. There have been many safety investigations carried out on ultra-high-field (UHF) magnets, to date (5-10). But, as the number of high-field (HF) magnets (less than 4-T) increase in medical settings and the number of UHF magnets (higher than 4-T) increase in research facilities, the opportunity is created for more complex safety studies that could investigate the interactions of strong magnets with matter at molecular, cellular, tissue, and systems levels.

HISTORIC PERPECTIVE

Over more than a century of recorded research on the effect of static magnetic fields on human subjects, there have been a vast number of publications (11-98). The end result of these works has been that no verifiable harmful effect can be attributed to exposure to strong static magnetic fields. This is attributed to the diamagnetic nature of human tissues and the small amount of paramagnetic elements present in the human body. Nevertheless, the fact that, following the introduction of MRI as a dominant medical imaging device, an ever larger segment of human population is being exposed to powerful magnetic fields each year and this warrants additional research in this area. It is conceivable that, as MRI becomes available to more developing countries, a time will be reached that most human beings will be exposed to strong magnetic fields at some time in their lives.

There have been few reports of deaths associated with MRI procedures and the MRI environment (99-101). A close look at these fatalities reveals that they were all caused by controllable factors and involved implanted or other extraneous devices that interacted strongly with the magnetic field. In fact, knowing that life on our planet is formed in the magnetic field of about 0.5-gauss indicates that the probable interaction of molecules building life with the magnetic field at this field strength is incorporated in the structure and function of biological tissues. Although the earth's magnetic field is relatively weak, it is sufficient to put a proton of hydrogen to a precession of about 2-kHz. Thus, the Larmor precession that takes into account the torque imparted on nuclear spins and formulates their rotational motion will allow the use of the gyromagnetic ratio (γ) of a hydrogen proton to yield its frequency of rotation. This is the magnetic effect that is at the basis of the mechanism of signal generation in MRI. Attraction by natural magnets had been discovered and cited in many ancient treatises (11). Chinese (102), Greek (103), and Persian (103) scientists discovered the unique properties of magnets and offered various treatments for diseases more than a thousand years ago. However, since natural ores can produce magnets with field strength less than 0.5-T, these materials do not produce very high magnetic polarization. Furthermore, the field distributions of natural magnets are inhomogeneous, producing a strong field in small regions unsuitable for observation of any effects that would otherwise require establishing strong fields in larger areas. This is why magnets were not used in many tools before the 19th century. Electromagnets provided the opportunity of manufacturing magnets stronger than 1-T, but the resistive heat in these magnets places an upper limit on their applications.

At the present time, the most powerful electromagnet in the world generates a continuous field of 35-T, which is a Bitter magnet located at the U.S. National High Magnetic Field Laboratory in Tallahassee, Florida. Such magnets allow scientists to study exotic effects exhibited by matter only under extreme conditions. The possibility that metallic hydrogen may be a superconductor at room temperature was put forward in 1968 and its potential technological applications initiated interest in even stronger magnets. Because compact high field magnets made of high temperature superconductors may offer highly efficient transportation systems and quantum leaps in computational power of computers, research on the health implications of strong magnets go well beyond their application to MR scanners. Today, the magnets for MR systems use special Niobium-Titanium alloys, which are capable of producing magnetic fields up to approximately 10-Tesla at liquid helium temperatures (104). These so-called type II superconductors are only one class of alloys that reveal superconductivity at cryogenic temperatures. Other materials, such as bismuth alloys, have been used to construct test coils that can achieve 32-Tesla. While strong magnets have been built for research in charged particle accelerators and in electromagnetic ore extraction, their use has not produced a widespread exposure of human subjects to such magnetic fields. The introduction of MRI as the standard of medical diagnosis started the era of pervasive human exposure to strong magnetic fields in the early 1980s.

From the time of magnetotherapy, when magnets were used for therapeutic purposes, some scientists believed in the capability of magnetic effects on the body. Centuries ago, magnets were used for their presumed effectiveness in remedying headache, pain, and other conditions (105). However, in light of the diamagnetic property of human tissues, the interaction with magnetic fields is negligible for most tissues. Because of its iron content and different susceptibility state between oxyhemoglobin and deoxyhemoglobin, there is a slight magnetic interaction with hemoglobin. However, this effect has not been large enough for bulk measurement other than its effect on functional MR images, or fMRI. The need for a high static magnetic field and high homogeneity in MR systems requires that these magnets be much larger than they need to be to simply produce a given field strength. MR system magnets are designed to produce a field homogeneity on the order of 10 parts per million (ppm) over the diameter of spherical volumes (DSV) of 50-cm. Producing a highly homogeneous DSV50 with a solenoid magnet is the primary requirement of MRI scanners.

Cylindrical superconducting geometries are the most abundant form of "closed" scanners, while permanent and hybrid magnets are often used for "open" MR systems. An account of the dates when MR systems with various magnetic fields were debuted is listed in **Table 2** (106-115). In this table, the timing of major increases in field strength has been presented but it is not meant to be a catalogue of improvement in all aspects of magnet technology.

In assimilation of new MRI technology, three factors have dominated the introduction of new scanners: engineering innovation, safety, and an advantage in clinical diagnostics. The complexity of scientific, financial, and technical factors involved in justifying, funding, and manufacturing whole-body scanners with ever higher field strengths is indicated by the eleven years that were required from the installation of the first 4-T human scanners to the introduction of the first 8-T whole-body MR system (98).

Currently, a 9.4-T at the University of Illinois in Chicago is the highest field strength whole-body MR system. Furthermore, a 10.5-T head-only scanner at the University of Minnesota and 11.7-T whole-body scanners are being installed at the National Institutes of Health and at NeuroSpin in Orsay, France, thus, increasing the range of proton frequency

Table 2. Historical development of MRI-related static magnetic field strengths (data adapted from references 63, 65, 76, 77, 93-101).

Field Strength (Tesla)	Date of Introduction	Institution	Type	Comments
0.05 to 0.10	1977	State University of New York, Brooklyn	superconducting	This MR system produced an early image of the human thorax.
0.7	1977	University of Nottingham	iron core electromagnet	This machine, with a 13-cm gap, produced an early wrist image.
0.04	1980	Aberdeen	air core electromagnet	This machine was used for the first clinical MRI studies.
0.35	1981	Hammersmith, Diasonics	whole-body, superconducting	These MR systems were the first whole-body superconducting scanners.
1.5	1982	General Electric	whole-body, superconducting	Whole-body MR systems at 1.5-T have been in widespread clinical use since the mid-1980s.
4.0	1987	Siemens, General Electric, Philips	whole-body, superconducting	During the late 1990s 3-T and 4-T scanners became widely available at research institutions.
8	1998	Ohio State University	whole-body, superconducting	This MR system was used for many UHF safety studies.
9.4	2004	University of Illinois (Chicago)	whole-body, superconducting	This is the highest field strength, whole-body MR system currently operating.

for MR scanners use in human subjects toward 500-MHz. The economics of magnet technology and the scientific capabilities and image resolution of MR systems are on the opposite sides of the trend toward higher field strengths. In one analysis published in 2002 that was based on sales activity at that time, it was predicted that 3-T would displace 1.5-T MR systems and become the dominant field strength by 2012 (115). This prediction has only been realized to some degree as approximately one-quarter of new installations in 2012 were at 3-T. By the same token, UHF units are being installed in more research facilities and, as their technological challenges are met, they will provide the incentive for pushing field strength beyond 3-T for clinical applications during the next decade.

At this point, it is worth remembering the prediction of early MRI pioneers that declared MRI a safe modality for scanning humans. That no major, unavoidable incidents have occurred in association with MRI is a testimony to the sound basis of analyzing the interactions of static magnetic fields with human subjects (35-37). Similar studies have been conducted at UHF ranges, indicating that the magnetic interactions with biological tissues are safe up to and including 8-T (98). However, it should be noted that, the consequence of taking ferromagnetic materials into the fringe fields of a UHF MR system will create more serious problems than has been predicted by many authors (57, 62, 63, 66, 83). Similar facts are at work regarding medical implants in patients within fringing fields of the MR scanners.

INTERACTIONS WITH HUMAN TISSUE

The mechanisms of interactions between static magnetic fields and biological tissues can be used as the basis for assessing the potential damage in human subjects. Understanding these mechanisms will allow use of the benefits of MRI, while avoiding the possible hazards of exposure to strong magnetic fields. The major effects that have been researched to date are described below.

Magnetic Forces

High magnetic fields will exert an attractive force on tissues with permanent magnetic dipoles. Tissues with higher magnetic susceptibilities than water will repel diamagnetic materials (116-117). High field regions are centers of attraction and this is a way for separating tissues with higher paramagnetic susceptibilities. But, this effect is too weak for practical use in living tissues even in high magnetic fields. The absence of permanently magnetized tissues in the human body makes this force of lesser concern in assessing the safety of these fields, except where materials with permanent magnetic properties are present (e.g., ferromagnetic foreign bodies), as they experience displacement forces in regions of magnetic field, spatial gradients.

Magnetic forces can produce torques on permanently magnetized materials that will tend to rotate them to align their magnetic moment with the magnetic field. Magnetic torques will rotate magnetic materials to make the long axis of the object parallel to the applied field. Foreign objects that are ferromagnetic can experience a sizable torque posing even a greater potential hazard than the translational forces on such materials. For materials with different paramagnetic susceptibilities in different directions with respect to the magnetizing field, the anisotropic susceptibility will lead to a torque on the axis of the most positive susceptibility tending to align it with the field. Diamagnetic susceptibility anisotropy (DSA) observed in some materials has the effect of rotating them to align the axis of least negative susceptibility with the field. Observation of DSA can only be made *in vitro* because the effect is too weak *in vivo* for quantitative measurement.

Flow and Its Consequences

In the human body, electric fields are normally produced by processes such as the depolarization of the heart tissue that produces current flow, which is the basis of the electrocardiogram (ECG). In addition to the normal static field currents producing the ECG, any motion by the tissue will produce an additional term in the expression for the current density, $\mathbf{J} = \sigma\,(\mathbf{E} + \mathbf{v} \times \mathbf{B})$ where $\mathbf{v}$ is the velocity of the moving tissue relative to the static magnetic field. The term, $\mathbf{v} \times \mathbf{B}$, is the consequence of motion and can be viewed as a motion-induced electric field.

Motion of conductive tissues within a magnetic field will produce a force perpendicular to the direction of motion. There are many different types of motions by internal organs in the human body, including those associated with the beating heart and blood flow. The currents produced by blood flow in the presence of powerful magnetic fields are large enough that its effect on body surface potentials has long ago been proposed to be used for a flow meter (118-119).

The electromotive force (emf) induced as a result of blood flow in the heart produces a large signal during the T-wave phase of the cardiac cycle. In the 1960s, it was shown that the electrocardiograms of monkey hearts in strong magnetic fields displayed a field-induced amplified T-wave (44). Subsequent studies have shown this T-wave amplification to result from blood flow and not from a direct magnetic field effect on cardiac muscle (120-121). This effect is easily demonstrated in patients in clinical MR systems and contributes to the difficulty in obtaining acceptable electrocardiograms during MRI procedures.

Dependence of the induced emf on the velocity of blood flow and the strength of the static magnetic strength has been visualized in humans at field strengths as high as 8-Tesla (98). There is no evidence of flow-induced nerve or muscle stimulation for fields as high as 9.4-T, as the induced emf is below the threshold levels required for such stimulations (122). As the magnetic field strengths of MR scanners increase, the flow-induced currents near blood vessels could eventually reach levels capable of inducing nerve stimulation and this may determine the upper limit of human tolerance for exposure to extremely high static magnetic fields (87-88). However, all currently planned MR systems operate well below these levels.

Interactions with Metabolic Reactions

Chemical reactions are at the core of metabolic function of tissues. The massive number of chemical reactions required for normal function indicates that any external factor, such as an applied static magnetic field, which is capable of altering the rate of these reactions, could affect their equilibrium positions (123-130). This condition prevails, for example, in those chemical reactions in which the products are more paramagnetic than the reactants. Such reactions will respond to the presence of a magnetic field by shifting the reaction equilibrium towards an increase in the concentration of the products, displacing the equilibrium position of the reaction.

The presence of molecules of different magnetic properties on opposite sides of a reaction is among the class of reactions that will be affected by magnetic fields. For example, the dissociation of oxygen from hemoglobin as oxyhemoblobin is diamagnetic, and both oxygen and hemoglobin are paramagnetic. However, although the applied field will lower the energy barrier for the dissociation of diamagnetic molecules to paramagnetic molecules, calculations show that the free energy barrier to dissociation of oxyhemoglobin (about 64,000-J/mol) will only be changed by about 1-J/mol at a field strength of 4-T. Such disturbances of oxygen dissociation are comparable to a temperature change of only 0.01°C making it unable to significantly modify the reaction equilibrium (87).

Another possible magnetic field effect on a chemical reaction involves the dissociation of a binary molecule, AB (124-130). If the bond between A and B is non-magnetic (electron-pair bond) but the dissociated radicals A and B have unpaired electrons, then the magnetic field will favor dissociation of the bound state as the two electrons in the bond will have opposite spins and a total spin of zero while the free spins of individual radicals will be nonzero. Precession of the A and B spins subsequent to dissociation will limit to some extent the tendency toward re-bonding. However, no significant effects on reactions of biochemical significance have been reported from this effect.

Ferromagnetic Tissue Components

The magnitude of interaction of materials with magnetic fields is directly proportional to their magnetic susceptibility. The human body is diamagnetic which makes its interaction with external magnetic fields inherently weak. However, there are small amounts of tissue components that are paramagnetic, which allows them to couple more strongly with magnetic fields (131-136). There is about 3.7-grams of iron in the body of a 70-kg adult human. Fortunately, the iron in the human body is in weak paramagnetic form incorporated in various chemical compounds such as hemoglobin, ferritin and hemosiderin, which are spread throughout the body preventing strong interactions with applied fields. The small concentration of these paramagnetic substances is insufficient to make the overall susceptibility of the tissues, including blood, paramagnetic (90). Obviously, exogenous paramagnetic materials can enter the human body causing interaction with a magnetic field. Studies on coal miners exposed to rock dust have detected small amounts of particulate magnetite in their lungs. Other forms of deliberate addition of iron oxides compounds to the body, such as in tattooing involving iron oxide-based pigments, will similarly increase the possibility of magnetic interactions.

The presence of particles of iron oxides less than 500-angstroms in diameter has been reported in the human brain and other tissues using electron microscopy in autopsy studies (136). The source and function of such particles are unclear and determination of their origin requires further investigations. The small size of these particles makes their artifacts on MR images too small to be detected at the range of field strengths used for human imaging. Perhaps at higher field strengths, susceptibility enhanced pulse sequences would permit visualization of these particles. Such artifacts will most likely induce sub-voxel signal dropout and require rigorous quantification methods to measure their interactions with magnetic fields.

MRI examinations of patients with tattoos or permanent eye makeup using iron oxide-based pigments have shown artifacts around those regions as well as local edema in some cases. This effect does not appear to be caused by the static magnetic field but, rather, results from interactions with the RF field used during MRI (65, 68, 70-72). However, it may be possible that irregularly shaped iron oxide particles in the implanted pigments experience a torque in the magnetic field that rotates them making their long axis parallel to applied field. The image artifact is caused by the magnetic fields of these particles resulting in signal losses, while the torque that forces their alignment with that static magnetic field may be the cause of local tissue irritation, resulting in localized edema. Such tissue irritation could be exacerbated by motion of the patients inside the magnetic field of the MR system.

Magnetoresistance

The magnitude of the electrical resistance of a material will change when it is placed in an external magnetic field. This phenomenon, called magnetoresistance, is caused by the forces exerted on ions in solutions moving through strong magnetic fields. Depolarizing currents associated with the propagation of nerve and muscle action potentials could be modified by such a field-dependent effect. However, since electrical resistance is a function of dynamics of current-carrying particles, the mean free path (MFP) of these carriers and the time between their collisions plays an important role in determining the size of the magnetoresistance effect.

For sufficiently long MFP, an electric field perpendicular to the direction of current will be established increasing the effective resistivity of the conductors when they are placed in a magnetic field. This phenomenon is called the Hall Effect and, in nerve and muscle tissues, could modify the transmission of currents. However, ions whose flow determines the action potentials of nerve and muscle tissue have extremely short mean MFP ($\sim$ 1-angstrom) and collision times (10^{-12}-seconds), drastically reducing the effect of magnetoresistance on the associated action potentials (60). Neurocognitive studies inside magnetic fields of up to 8-T have not detected a decrease in the performance of motor, sensory, and cognitive tasks (10).

Magnetohydrodynamics (MHD)

Currents flowing in tissues experience a body force. The resulting pressures and forces are transmitted to the tissues. These forces can be substantial in flowing liquid metals such as mercury. However, flowing physiological fluids such as blood have much lower electrical conductivities than mercury and MHD forces on flowing blood are relatively small compared to the naturally occurring hemodynamic forces in the vascular system. Therefore, contrary to early speculations, there is no requirement for increased heart activity to maintain the cardiac output in the presence of a strong static magnetic field (59,71). On the other hand, it may be that very small MHD forces operating on the endolymphatic tissues of the inner ear are the source of the sensations of nausea and vertigo sometimes reported by human subjects in the presence of higher static magnetic fields (86,87). Recently, the feasibility of using MHD effects at 7-T for synchronization of MRI with the cardiac cycle has been reported (136).

Magnetostriction

A substantial force acting on an object can change its size and shape. Among the three types of magnetic properties, ferromagnetism produces by far the largest magnetostrictive forces. Therefore, in consideration of the range of susceptibility of biological tissues, their size and shape change only slightly when exposed to strong magnetic fields (137). Since human tissues do not normally contain ferromagnetic materials, magnetostriction is negligible. Furthermore, compared to the naturally occurring forces (i.e., thermal expansion and mechanical stresses), any effect in human tissue would be insignificant.

CALCULATION OF STATIC MAGNETIC FIELD EFFECTS

Magnetic susceptibility is the term used to define the quantification of the effect of static magnetic fields on matter. Analysis of the magnetic response of tissues through the concept of magnetic susceptibility is a simple method that will be discussed in this section. In this analysis, it will be shown that the large differences between the magnetic properties of biological tissues and those of ferromagnetic materials governs their different responses to magnetic fields. This difference is so profound that, in many cases, this makes their response to applied magnetic fields qualitatively different. This is why extrapolation of our daily experiences with ferromagnetic materials has been the source of the many concerns with the safety of powerful static magnetic fields in predicting the response of tissues to such fields. In this section, the concept of magnetic susceptibility is discussed and the calculations of magnetic forces and torques are presented. The quantitative response of tissues to applied magnetic fields will then be formulated in these terms.

Magnetic Susceptibility

Magnetic susceptibility is a quantity that describes the response of materials, which are not permanently magnetized to applied magnetic fields (90). The discussion in this chapter will not consider permanent magnets, such as bar magnets, because their strong interaction with magnetic fields makes them extremely hazardous in the MRI environment. Thus, except in rare situations, permanent magnets are not allowed in the MR system room. Biological tissues have very small magnetic susceptibilities and that is the reason why they do not interact strongly with applied magnetic fields. This fact is supported by noting the high quality of MR images due to the highly uniform magnetic field inside the human body within the MR scanner (i.e., due to the small variation in susceptibility in biological tissues).

Polarization of materials in an applied magnetic field is measured by a quantity called the magnetization, defined as the magnetic dipole moment per unit volume. To provide a quantitative account of the response to magnetic fields in terms of magnetization, System International (SI) units will be used along with the standard mathematical convention of using bold face symbols to designate vector quantities. If matter of susceptibility, χ, is placed in magnetic field $\mathbf{H}$, it will develop a magnetization $\mathbf{M}$ given by the equation $\mathbf{M} = \chi \mathbf{H}$. The susceptibility, χ, is a dimensionless quantity as both $\mathbf{M}$ and $\mathbf{H}$ represent the strength of magnetic fields, $\mathbf{H}$ for external field and $\mathbf{M}$ for induced field. $\mathbf{B}$, the magnetic flux density is given by $\mathbf{B} = \mu_0 (\mathbf{H} + \mathbf{M})$. As the induced field is a property of the magnetized object, while the applied field only modulates that property, interaction between them is best managed if we designate the total field with $\mathbf{B}$ and the applied field with the symbol $\mathbf{B}_o = \mu_r \mu_o \mathbf{H}$, where, μ_r, is called the relative permeability.

In an isotropic material, χ is a scalar quantity, meaning that it has the same value in all directions. This is the case in most materials. In isotropic materials, the induced magnetization $\mathbf{M}$ is parallel to $\mathbf{H}$, which makes $\mathbf{M}$, $\mathbf{B}$, and $\mathbf{H}$ all parallel to each other. If matter has a preferred direction in which it magnetizes more easily than in other directions, the resultant magnetization is not necessarily parallel to the magnetic field. Such materials are represented by an anisotropic χ in the form of a symmetric tensor.

In this chapter, aside from the discussion about the weak torques formed in certain biological crystals, the analysis is limited to isotropic materials. For materials with large susceptibilities, the magnetization is found by taking into account the effects of the induced as well as the applied field in a self-consistent way. This is due to the fact that in the definition of χ, **H** is the sum of the applied and induced fields. The example of ellipsoidal objects using demagnetizing coefficients is worked out in this section to demonstrate such calculations. For biological tissues with very small susceptibility, however, the fields induced by the magnetization are much smaller than the applied field, which makes them negligible. For such material, the magnetization is determined entirely by the applied field and the more complex self-consistent method is not necessary for their calculations.

In isotropic material, **M**, **H**, and **B** are parallel and, as shown in the following discussion, no torques will be formed to align the object with the local fields. In reality, the negligible magnitude of the torques due to the applied field compared to other biological forces acting on the tissue component allows us to ignore them in our calculations.

The magnitude and sign of χ determines the extent of the interaction with the applied field. In this regard, materials are classified into three large groups: diamagnetic, paramagnetic and ferromagnetic. Conservation of energy requires that only χ with values $\chi > -1$ are possible (140). Diamagnetic materials have negative susceptibilities (i.e., $-1.0 < \chi < 0$). This property causes them to be magnetized in the direction opposite to the applied magnetic field, causing them to be repelled from regions of strong magnetic fields. All materials have diamagnetic properties if they do not possess components, such as the magnetic ions in transition elements, which make a larger positive contribution to χ. Paramagnetic materials have positive χ that makes them attracted to regions of strong magnetic fields. Materials with $|\chi| < 0.01$ or so do not respond to weak sources of magnetic fields such as hand-held magnets and, as such, are classified as non-magnetic. Most common materials, including all living beings, with the exception of magnetotactic bacteria, are in this group.

Ferromagnetic materials with $|\chi| \geq 0.01$ constitute the third group of materials to which we will refer as ferromagnetic or magnetic. These materials exhibit a strong response to an applied magnetic field and the large attractive force induced on them poses the biggest danger if taken into the vicinity of an MR system. Some ferromagnetic materials do not appear magnetic until they are exposed to an external field, and they are called "soft magnets" to distinguish them from permanent magnets or "hard" magnetic materials.

The enormous range of susceptibility values of all matter in nature is shown in **Figure 1** (90). As is seen in this figure, the vast majority of materials have susceptibility values much less than 0.001, making the magnetic forces on such materials very weak and not easily observable. Relevant to this discussion are the vast majority of biological tissues with susceptibilities very close to the susceptibility of water, $\chi_{H2O} = -9.05 \times 10^{-6}$ in SI units. In fact, χ of most biological tissues differs from that of water by about $\pm 20\%$. This narrow range of variation of χ is the primary reason why exquisite MR images are acquired from biological tissues. In regions of the human body where large variation in susceptibility is present (e.g., the air/tissue interfaces between the sinuses and the orbitofrontal regions of the brain), high field MRI causes large position-dependent variations in the Larmor frequency that results in severe signal losses.

Figure 1. Spectrum of magnetic susceptibilities. The upper diagram uses a logarithmic scale to indicate the full range of observed magnetic susceptibility values: it extends from $\chi = -1.0$ for superconductors to $\chi > 100,000$ for soft ferromagnetic materials. The bottom diagram uses a linear scale (in ppm) to indicate the properties of some materials with $|\chi| < 20$ ppm. The susceptibilities of most human tissues are in the range from -7.0 to -11.0 ppm (90).

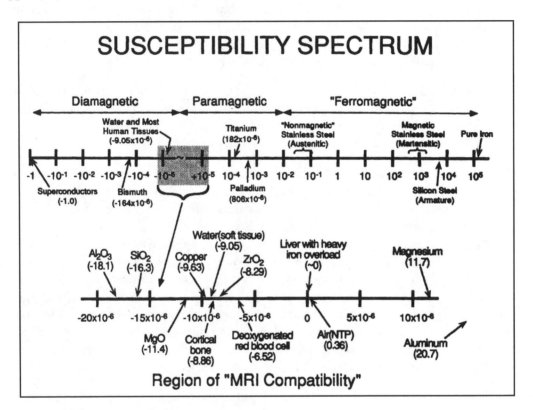

Because of diamagnetism, small forces act on the patients as they are inserted into MR systems. This force is so small that it cannot be perceived. Normal magnetic materials, on the other hand, have susceptibility values much larger than those of diamagnetic materials, usually a factor of 1000 or more, that lead to much stronger responses in the presence of magnetic fields. The large variation in the magnitude of susceptibility causes qualitatively differing responses by ferromagnetic and diamagnetic materials to applied fields, as discussed later in this section.

A demonstration of the existence of repulsive diamagnetic forces exerted on living beings by strong magnets has been made by suspending small frogs and other diamagnetic objects in midair in the vertical bore of a magnet operating at 16-T (116, 117). In achieving such suspension, the diamagnetic force counters the weight of the frog. It is worth noticing that even in the presence of very high magnetic fields, there was no harm done to the frog.

Magnetic Energy

The force of the magnetic field on matter could cause two types of motion, translational and rotational. An object, like an aneurysm clip with a long blade, if placed in a strong magnetic field, experiences a magnetic force that could cause translational and rotational motions that can be measured. In the human body, depending on its shape, the object could experience translational attraction and torque that could cause it to move and rotate with respect to the direction of the field. The size of the translational forces and/or torques depends on the applied field strength, the susceptibility, and the shape of the material. This could vary from no observable effect, to forces large enough to produce injury or even lethal consequences. Typically, to understand whether these forces and torques will be at a level to significantly alter the structure or function of tissues, we need to develop rigorous mathematical expressions based on the physical properties of the material.

The work required to move magnetic dipoles within a magnetic field is independent of path. Therefore, a magnetic potential energy function, U, can be defined that depends on the field strength (position), magnetic dipole moment of the object, the relative angle between the field and the dipole orientation, and the magnetic properties of the medium (139-142). For magnetization, $\mathbf{M}$, the total dipole moment of a volume, V, for a uniformly magnetized object is $\mathbf{m} = \mathbf{M}\,V$. The energy required to bring an object with permanent dipole moment $\mathbf{m}$ to a point within a magnetic field $\mathbf{B_0}$ is $U = \mathbf{m} \bullet \mathbf{B_0}$. But to assess the energy of a non-permanently magnetized object, as is the case for the human body in an MR system, we have to take into account the fact that biological tissues within a magnetic field acquire a magnetic moment that is proportional to the applied field. If biological tissues are brought within a magnetic field, $\mathbf{B_0}$, they acquire an induced moment, $\mathbf{m}$, and an energy

$U = \dfrac{1}{2}\mathbf{m} \bullet \mathbf{B}_o$. The reason for the presence of the factor 1/2 for the second case (although

the magnetic field was assumed to be the same $\mathbf{B_0}$ and does not change after the introduction of the material in both cases at the point where energy was calculated) is the following. When biological tissues with no permanent magnetic dipole (the second case) are brought into the magnetic field, their magnetic moment increases from zero (where the magnetic field is zero) to $\mathbf{m}$ (where the magnetic field is $\mathbf{B_0}$). This is in contrast with the case of permanently magnetized objects, in which magnetization is $\mathbf{m}$ all along the path. The magnetic field energy increases through the work of forces and torques on objects introduced in them. Magnetic forces attract paramagnetic materials and repel diamagnetic ones. Also, if $\mathbf{m}$ is not aligned with $\mathbf{B_0}$, the magnetic field will produce a torque on it to make it parallel to $\mathbf{B_0}$.

So using the expression for the force, $\mathbf{F} = \nabla U$ and the torque $\tau = \dfrac{\partial U}{\partial \theta}\mathbf{u} = \mathbf{M} \times \mathbf{B}_o$

where $\mathbf{u}$ is the unit vector perpendicular to the plane of $\mathbf{M}$ and $\mathbf{B}$ and θ is the angle between $\mathbf{M}$ and $\mathbf{B_0}$, the expression for energy for an object of volume V and susceptibility χ, is then

found to be $\mathbf{m} = \mathbf{M}V = \chi V \mathbf{H}_o = \dfrac{\chi}{\mu_o}V\mathbf{B}_o$ and $U = \dfrac{1}{2}\mathbf{M} \bullet \mathbf{B}_o = \dfrac{1}{2}\dfrac{\chi V}{\mu_o}B_o^2$. This ex-

pression applies to situations where the magnitude of the susceptibility is much less than one and that $\mathbf{B_0}$ is uniform over the volume of the object. The square dependence of energy on B_0 has implications on both energy deposition and the magnitude of the attractive or re-pulsive force that magnetic fields exert on diamagnetic objects within them.

Demagnetizing Factor

In this chapter, we are concerned with the effect of magnetic fields on biological tissues, which do not have fixed dipole moments. For these materials, the evaluation of the translational attractions and torque must take into account the fact that magnetization is induced by the applied field. This makes it necessary to determine the field-induced dipole moment that must be inserted back into the above formulas to find forces and torques. In general, this is a complex mathematical process. However, for certain simple shapes, such as ellipsoids, the mathematics is simple. Once results for ellipsoids, such as spheres, cylinders, and plates are calculated, they offer a good measure of the size of this effect for more complex objects. Below a simple analysis for ellipsoids is presented.

If an ellipsoid object with isotropic susceptibility is placed in a field along its principal axis, an internal field parallel to the applied field will be induced in the object. This field, called demagnetization field, H_{dm}, is given by $H_{dm} = -D M$ where the demagnetizing factor, D, is a number that depends on the shape of the object and it varies between zero and one (90-138). In general, the sum of the three demagnetizing factors along all axes of an object is equal to one. Spherical objects for which the three principal axes of a sphere are equivalent making the demagnetizing factor for any direction equal to 1/3 constitute the simplest case. In contrast, ellipsoids have three distinct principal axes. For a cylinder placed in a magnetic field so that its long axis is parallel to this field, $D = 0$. However, if the long axis is perpendicular to the applied field, $D = 1/2$. To find the total internal field H the demagnetizing field, H_{dm} must be added to the applied field, $H_o = B_0/\mu_o$. Replacing the expression for magnetization, $M = \chi H$, in the formula for magnetic flux, $B = \mu_o (H + M)$, the total internal fields can be found in terms of the applied field B_0, as follows:

$B = \mu_o H (1 + \chi)$,

$H = H_o + H_{dm} = H_o - D M = H_o - D \chi H$,

$H_o = H + D \chi H = H (1 + D\chi)$,

$H = H_o/(1 + D\chi)$,

$B = \mu_o H (1 + \chi) = B_0 (1 + \chi) / (1 + D\chi)$,

$\mu_o H = B_0 / (1 + D\chi)$,

$\mu_o M = B_0 \chi / (1 + D\chi)$.

To derive these results, D is assumed to be the demagnetizing factor for the principal axes parallel to B_0. This result can be extended to cases where B_0 is not along a principal axis by resolving it into components along these axes to find the resulting fields, which is the sum of the fields along each axis. These expressions for the magnetic response of the object to an applied field work well as they take into account the interaction of B_0 with both the shape of an object, as is represented by D, and the magnetic properties, as is represented by χ.

   Ellipsoids of revolution, with two equivalent axes and two identical demagnetization factors, are a simpler form of the more general ellipsoids that have three independent principal axes and three different demagnetizing factors. For most cases, however, it is adequate to consider only ellipsoids of revolution. Deduction of important trends for the behavior of non-isotropic objects in a magnetic field is evidence to the utility of the above results. For example, it can be stated that for strongly magnetic materials with $\chi > 1$, to the first order, the internal field **B** and the magnetization are independent of the susceptibility and only depend on the shape of the object, D. For materials with $|\chi| \ll 1$, however, magnetization **M**=χ**B**$_0$/μ_o which makes it parallel to the applied field and independent of the shape of the ellipsoid. Thus, forces and torques on ferromagnetic objects in a magnetic field critically depend on the object's shape. For biological tissues with tiny susceptibilities, these same equations predict that the forces and torques induced by the magnetic fields will be independent of the shape of the tissues.

Quantification of Forces

   If a magnetic force induces magnetization in a direction, say along z-axis, on an isotropic object its magnitude will be given by $F_z = \dfrac{\partial U}{\partial z} = \dfrac{\chi V}{\mu_o} B \dfrac{\partial B}{\partial z}$. For paramagnetic materials with positive χ, the force will be in the direction of increasing **B**$_0$ and for diamagnetic material with negative χ, force will be in the direction of decreasing **B**$_0$. This means that in MR scanners, paramagnetic materials are pushed towards the center of the magnet while diamagnetic materials are pushed out of the magnet. This effect could have implications on the signal-to-noise ratio for a functional MRI (fMRI) examination in which the signal is largely determined by the replacement of paramagnetic deoxyhemoglobin with diamagnetic oxyhemoglobin. This force will have a retarding effect on the direction of flow for both oxyhemoglobin into the brain and deoxyhemoglobin out of the brain, thereby reducing the fMRI signal. For medical implants, such as ferromagnetic aneurysm clips that have high magnetic susceptibility, $F_z = \dfrac{V}{2\alpha\mu_o} B_z \dfrac{\partial B_z}{\partial z}$ and for weakly magnetic objects

$F_z = \dfrac{V}{2\mu_o} \chi B_z \dfrac{\partial B_z}{\partial z}$. The torque, τ, is given by τ = **M** x **B**$_0$ or, if the y-axis is perpendicular to **B**$_0$ and **M** , $\tau_y = \dfrac{\partial U}{\partial \theta} = MB_o \sin\theta$, where, θ, is the angle between **M** and **B**$_0$.

Risks Posed By Translational Forces And Torques

   Since ellipsoids of revolution illustrate most of the important features of magnetic interaction with matter, a summary of the expressions for the quantities derived in this chapter including magnetic energy, force and torque are listed in **Table 3**. Also, the asymptotic limits of these expressions for extreme values of the susceptibility predict behaviors that are qualitatively different from one other. Designating the demagnetizing factor along the axis of symmetry of the object as D_a and the radial demagnetizing factor in the transverse direction

Table 3. Magnetic properties of ellipsoids of revolution.

Qty	Full Expression	Soft Magnetic Materials	"Non-Magnetic" Materials
U	$\dfrac{\chi V B_o^2}{2\mu_o}\left[\dfrac{\cos^2\theta}{1+\chi D_a}+\dfrac{\sin^2\theta}{1+\chi D_r}\right]$	$\dfrac{V B_o^2}{2\mu_o}\dfrac{\cos^2\theta}{D_a}+\dfrac{\sin^2\theta}{D_r}$	$\dfrac{\chi V B_o^2}{2\mu_o}$
F_z	$\dfrac{\chi V}{\mu_o}B_o\dfrac{\partial B_o}{\partial z}\left[\dfrac{\cos^2\theta}{1+\chi D_a}+\dfrac{\sin^2\theta}{1+\chi D_r}\right]$	$\dfrac{V}{\mu_o}B_o\dfrac{\partial B_o}{\partial z}\left[\dfrac{\cos^2\theta}{D_a}+\dfrac{\sin^2\theta}{D_r}\right]$	$\dfrac{\chi V}{\mu_o}B_o\dfrac{\partial B_o}{\partial z}$
M_x	$\dfrac{\chi B_o}{\mu_o}\left[\dfrac{D_r-D_a}{(1+\chi D_a)(1+\chi D_r)}\right]\cos\theta\sin\theta$	$\dfrac{B_o}{\mu_o}\dfrac{D_r-D_a}{D_a D_r}\cos\theta\sin\theta$	$\dfrac{\chi^2 B_o}{\mu_o}(D_r-D_a)\cos\theta\sin\theta$
M_z	$\dfrac{\chi B_o}{\mu_o}\left[\dfrac{\cos^2\theta}{1+\chi D_a}+\dfrac{\sin^2\theta}{1+\chi D_r}\right]$	$\dfrac{B_o}{\mu_o}\left[\dfrac{\cos^2\theta}{D_a}+\dfrac{\sin^2\theta}{D_r}\right]$	$\dfrac{\chi B_o}{\mu_o}$
τ_y	$\dfrac{\chi^2 V B_0^2}{\mu_o}\dfrac{D_a-D_r}{(1+\chi D_a)(1+\chi D_r)}\cos\theta\sin\theta$	$\dfrac{V B_o^2}{\mu_o}\dfrac{D_a-D_r}{D_a D_r}\cos\theta\sin\theta$	$\dfrac{\chi^2 V B_o^2}{\mu_o}($

The first column gives the complete expression for the magnetic potential energy (U), force (F_z), magnetization (M_x and M_z) and torque (T_y) for an ellipsoid of revolution in a magnetic field along the z-axis. The symmetry axis is in the x-direction and θ is the angle between this axis and the magnetic field. The second column gives approximations appropriate for soft magnetic materials and the third column gives approximations appropriate to materials, such as biological tissues, with very small susceptibilities. For objects inside a medium of uniform susceptibility, such as water or tissue with $\chi = \chi_{H2O}$, χ should be replaced by $\Delta\chi = \chi - \chi_{H2O}$. It is assumed that B_z is the only non-zero component of $\mathbf{B}_0$ at the location of the object and that the spatial derivatives of the transverse components, $\dfrac{\partial B_x}{\partial x}, \dfrac{\partial B_y}{\partial x}$, are all zero. This is the case along the central axis of the magnets commonly used in MRI. At other points in the field there may be non-zero force components in addition to F_z, but the qualitative physical principles are unchanged.

as D_r from the earlier discussion we have $D_a + 2 D_r = 1$. The relative values of D_a and D_r offer simple results with powerful implications. For needle-like ellipsoids with one very long axis of symmetry and isotropic radial directions, $D_a \to 0$ and $D_r \to \frac{1}{2}$. For a sphere, $D_a = D_r = 1/3$. For flat ellipsoids, $D_a \to 1$ and $D_r \to 0$. These case examples are useful to provide an insight in the behavior of biological tissues in magnetic fields. Expressions for demagnetization factors for a broad range of ellipsoids of revolution are available in the published literature (90).

Certain metallic implants have magnetic properties that could put the patient at risk from translational and rotational forces in association with exposure to the powerful magnetic field of an MR system. If the combination of the geometrical and magnetic properties produces substantial translational forces, then the object could move in the presence of a powerful static magnetic field. If the same combination results in a torque, then the object could be rotated into alignment with the static magnetic field. The factors determining the relative strength of these two effects are magnetic susceptibility and the shape of the object as well as its position in the magnetic field that determines the magnitude and the field's spatial gradient. Notice that the force does not just depend on the field strength but the product of field spatial gradient by field strength, $B\partial B/\partial dz$. So, in the regions of a homogeneous magnetic field where $\partial B/\partial dz \sim 0$, the translational forces are negligible. This does not mean that such metallic devices are safe, as the patient has to pass through the entry regions of the MR system where $B\partial B/\partial dz$ is large and the object could experience a large force during this time. As expressions for torque reveal, even for metallic devices with low translational force, the torque could pose a greater hazard than the translational force in some cases. A discussion of such cases is warranted here.

A cylindrical magnet, such as that often used in a high field MR system, offers an opportunity to look in more detail at the analysis of magnetic forces as regions near its central axis have a uniform magnetic field and small field spatial gradients. For spherically symmetrical objects, there are no torques acting on the object. So, the translational forces are caused by the induced magnetization, which is parallel to the applied magnetic field. In the cases of non-isotropic objects like long, thin needles or thin and flat plates, then large torques may be formed on these objects. The forces will rotate elongated objects, to make the long axis of the object parallel to the direction of the magnetic field. On a flat object, however, the magnetic field will exert a torque turning it parallel to the field lines of the magnet. The following quantitative analysis is meant to support these predictions.

The large disparity between demagnetizing factors along axial (a) and radial (r) axes of a needle-like object ($D_r >> D_a$) when placed in the magnet, with the long axis of the object parallel to the z-axis of the magnet, produces the maximum translational force when the needle is aligned with the field ($\theta = 0$) and at a location where the product $B_z \dfrac{\partial B_z}{\partial z}$ is maximum. Regions at the isocenter of MR system's magnet (i.e, where MR imaging occurs) have a very homogenous magnetic field ($\dfrac{\partial B_z}{\partial z}=0$), although the magnitude of the magnetic field in these regions is highest. These facts mean that no translational forces will form on the objects in the central, homogenous regions of the magnet where $B_z \dfrac{\partial B_z}{\partial z}$ is zero. These conditions are created in two distinct regions, one outside and far from the magnet where $B = 0$ and, another, in the central regions where $\dfrac{\partial B_z}{\partial z}= 0$. The product of magnetic field with field spatial gradient falls to zero at the center of the magnet and regions far outside the magnet and goes through a maximum near the opening of the bore, say z_{max}. These conditions cause the attractive translational force to reach a maximum value at z_{max}.

A plot of $B_z \dfrac{\partial B_z}{\partial z}$ for an 8-Tesla MR system with a 90-cm bore diameter and 3.4-meter length is shown in **Figure 2**. If magnetic objects get pulled into the magnet of the MR sys-

Figure 2. Force by magnetic field spatial gradient. The product of the spatial gradient of the magnetic and the magnetic field (BdB/dz) produces a large force that rises to a maximum value around the entry point on either end of the magnet of the MR system. A plot of BdB/dz for the 8-T whole-body magnetic field is shown here. The origin corresponds to the center of the magnet.

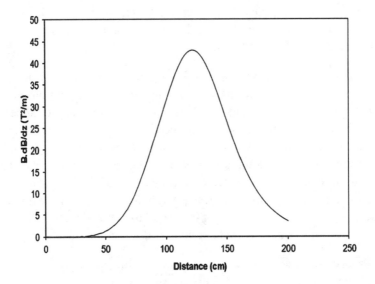

tem, they will be lodged at the center of the magnet, where the force drops to zero. To dislodge such objects, the maximum force needs to be overcome, which could be enormous depending on the magnitude of the variables determining the force. The maximum value

of the quantity $\left[B_z \dfrac{\partial B_z}{\partial z}\right]_{max}$ determines the maximum value of the translational force

for a needle-like object when it resides on the axis of the magnet and is given by

$$F_{trans}^{max} = \frac{V}{\mu_o D_a}\left[B_z \frac{\partial B_z}{\partial z}\right]_{max}$$. To determine the torque on the same object, the strength

of the force couple applied to both ends of the symmetry axis, say F_{torque}, can be defined as the force necessary to prevent the ellipsoid from being twisted and aligned with $\mathbf{B_0}$. The maximum torque along the main axis of the magnet (z-axis) will occur at the isocenter,

when the angle between the long axis of the ellipsoid and the magnet is $\theta = \dfrac{\pi}{4}$. If the total

length of the ellipsoid is 2 L, then the absolute value of the forces creating the torque is

$$F_{trans}^{max} = \frac{V}{\mu_o D_a}\left[B_z \frac{\partial B_z}{\partial z}\right]_{max}$$. Therefore, the rotational force and translation force will

be $\dfrac{F^{max}_{torque}}{F^{max}_{trans}} = \dfrac{1}{2L} B_z^2\big|_{max} \Big/ \left[B_z \dfrac{\partial B_z}{\partial z}\right]_{max}$. For the 8-T whole-body MR system (5) these

values are $B_z^{max} = 8\,\text{T}$ and $\left[B_z \dfrac{\partial B_z}{\partial z}\right]_{max} = 42.6\,\text{T}^2/\text{m}$. The ratio (R) of

$B_z^2\big|_{max} \Big/ \left[B_z \dfrac{\partial B_z}{\partial z}\right]_{max}$ for this magnet was 1.5/m while, for most superconducting cylin-

drical magnets, regardless of their field strengths, this ratio will be comparable to that of

the 8-T scanner. For an ellipsoid of length $L = 1$-cm in this magnet the $\dfrac{F^{max}_{torque}}{F^{max}_{trans}} = 75$. Since

the 8-T magnet was unshielded, for shielded magnets, the ratio, R, would be smaller because

the value $\left[B_z \dfrac{\partial B_z}{\partial z}\right]_{max}$ is larger for such magnets. The large ratio of rotational and trans-

lational force indicates that elongated ferromagnetic implants must be tightly anchored to or retained in the patient's tissues because a much larger force is required to prevent rotation as opposed to translational attraction. This is particularly true for implants such as a ferro-magnetic aneurysm clip with one dimension longer than the other (i.e., an aneurysm clip with a long blade). These calculations indicate that the possibility of patient injury from aneurysm clips in magnetic fields is much higher due to rotational force than by translational motion. This is notable, as estimations of the effect of magnetic fields have traditionally been focused on translational forces.

Hairpins or paper clips are occasionally lodged inside the MR system. As the clip is being pulled out of the magnet, the small attractive translational force is at a maximum near the opening of the magnet where the patient is inserted into the scanner. The torque, however has different positional dependence and has it maximum value near the center of the magnet when the axis of the paper clip is at a direction of 45-degrees with respect to the z-axis of the magnetic field.

A close examination of the behavior of biological tissues, with $|\chi| \ll 1$ by using the expressions listed in **Table 3**, demonstrates that the magnitude of the torques acting on these tissues are proportional to χ^2. Due to the opposite signs of the susceptibilities of diamagnetic and paramagnetic materials, they are expected to point in opposite directions when lined up in a uniform magnetic field. However, the χ^2-dependence of the torque causing the alignment means that the direction of alignment would be the same for both types of materials. A more important consequence of the χ^2-dependence of the torque is that, for very small values of χ, the alignment torque that is caused by the shape-dependence is negligible. As shown by the above analysis, materials with high susceptibility and those of very low susceptibilities show qualitatively different responses to magnetic fields. Thus, strong magnetic fields apply strong forces on flat magnetic objects, such as magnetic washers, that could align their face parallel to the field. Since red blood cells basically have the same geometry as washers, they were expected to experience a torque large enough to align them with their flat side parallel to the magnetic field. But, due to the small magnitude of their susceptibility, $\chi^2 \approx 10^{-10}$, the torque acting on red blood cells is exceedingly low and unable to cause any shape-dependent effect.

Diamagnetic Susceptibility Anisotropy

The shape-dependence of torque due to field inhomogeneity and demagnetizing factors were shown to be negligible on biological materials due to χ^2-dependence of the torque expression. However, another mechanism through which magnetic fields can interact with biological tissues is diamagnetic susceptibility anisotropy (DSA). This effect has been observed in assembly of large numbers of macromolecules when they are bound together in a crystalline structure. This effect is present when all the molecules in a crystal are twisted in the same orientation by the applied magnetic field. Such conditions allow the torques on individual elements in all the molecules or cells in a volume V to add up to a measurable level. If susceptibility is anisotropic in a tissue, then we can designate its magnitude in one direction of this tissue as χ_1 and the angle between this direction and the applied field as θ. For tissues in which susceptibility in both orthogonal directions is the same and equal to χ_2, we can assume that for diamagnetic tissues $|\chi_1|, |\chi_2| \ll 1$. For such tissues, the magnetic

energy is given by $U = \dfrac{1}{2} V \mathbf{M} \bullet \mathbf{B_o} = \dfrac{V B_o^2}{2\mu_o} \left[\chi_1 \cos^2 \theta + \chi_2 \sin^2 \theta \right]$, and the expression of

torque will be $T = \dfrac{\partial U}{\partial \theta} = \dfrac{V B_o^2}{\mu_o} (\chi_2 - \chi_1) \sin \theta \cos \theta$.

Biological materials usually have negative χ_1 and χ_2 of the order of -10^{-5} that in magnetic fields will experience a torque that tends to rotate the object in a direction that aligns the axis with the least negative value of χ with the field. The difference of susceptibility between the two axes is $\Delta\chi = \chi_1 - \chi_2$ that is about 1% to 10% of the average susceptibility, $(\chi_1 + 2\chi_2)/3$. For biological tissues, $\Delta\chi$ is of the range of 10^{-7} to 10^{-6}, which is much larger than the shape-dependent torque that has an order of magnitude of 10^{-10}. Prediction of the analysis presented here (i.e. the four order of magnitude larger value of anisotropy-dependent torques than shape-dependent torques) is confirmed by observation in biological materials (143). Another important factor governing the size of the torque in the expressions derived in this chapter is the volume, V, of the tissue, which indicates that aggregation of anisotropic molecules to form larger assemblies will increase the torque that can, in turn, enhance the size of the effect of the magnetic field on these tissues.

Among biological tissues, red blood cells of sickle cell anemia have received much attention as they have been shown that they align in a field of 0.5-T *in vitro* (45-46). The lack of observation of alignment of the hemoglobin molecules in normal red blood cells is due to the fact that they are free in solution that makes them randomly oriented. But, the hemoglobin S molecules in sickle cell red blood cells have a tendency to stick together. This binding tendency makes them aggregate, polymerize, form fibers, and gel-like structures that are made up of similarly oriented hemoglobin molecules bound together. The anisotropic molecules in these structures and their binding in an aligned formation increase the anisotropy of the overall structure that have revealed anisotropy-dependent orientation in these studies (45-46). However, this effect has only been reported based on laboratory studies. Unlike the conditions *in vitro*, where there is no force competing with magnetic force, the forces experienced by red blood cells in flowing blood are much larger than the magnetic forces of orientation (61, 74, 77, 85). Experiments that would allow observation of magnetic orientation in the presence of flow, however slow, would shed light on the necessary conditions for red blood cell orientation *in vivo*.

Other structures, such as retinal rod cells, nucleic acid solutions, and fibrin gels have revealed similar orientation effects *in vitro* (144-149). As in red blood cells, we are unaware of a report of magnetic orientation effects by these structures *in vivo* for the same reason that flow forces overwhelm the magnetic orientation forces preventing any alignments. The size of the magnetic torque, however, as is shown by our equations depends on $B_o{}^2$. This fact points to a rapidly growing orientation torque as the magnetic field strength increases. Since the trend in MRI is relentlessly pushing for higher static magnetic fields, studies of orientation effects at these fields are warranted to enable us to reveal them *in vivo* and to incorporate them in plans for safe exposure of human subjects to such high static magnetic fields. In fact, experiments have already been performed in which 16-T magnets were used to demonstrate that cleavage planes of the developing frog embryo orient in such high fields (150). Anisotropy-dependent alignment of tubulin molecules has been presented as the cause of this observation (151). Independent confirmation of these effects would validate the effect and the explanation as many magnetic field effects on biological tissues have proven to be difficult to reproduce.

Alignment of Water Molecules

We need to be aware of the magnetic field strength required to align water molecules, *in vivo*. Although not reported, the far reaching consequence of such effect on life justifies the vigilance. The possibility of aligning of water molecules in magnetic fields and its ability in altering the biological and physiological processes in tissues are already proposed as a rationale for magnetotherapy, a commercial venture with some success in convincing its followers of its efficacy. This is in consideration of the fact that physics allows us to estimate the extent of alignment of water molecules inside magnetic fields. The random orientation of water molecules is the cause of its small magnetic susceptibility of $\chi = -9.05 \times 10^{-6}$. A variation of about one-percent in χ along the principal axes of the molecule is caused by the asymmetry of the water molecule (152). As we have discussed before, susceptibility anisotropy is the basis of the development of magnetic torques. So we need to calculate the magnetic alignment energy of a water molecule. Here we will present such calculation for an applied field of 10-Tesla as is presently close to the upper range of field strengths of research scanners to which human subjects may be exposed. Inserting the susceptibility of water and field strength of B=10-T in the expression for magnetization yields

$$M = \chi H = \frac{\chi}{\mu_o} B = -72 \text{ A/m}$$. This is the magnetization, which is the sum of magnetic

dipole moments of 3.34×10^{28} water molecules per cubic meter. So, the average dipole moment per water molecule in a field of 10-Tesla is calculated to be $m = -2.16 \times 10^{-27}$ J/T.

The implication of 1% anisotropy of the molecular magnetization is that a maximum magnetic energy change due to change in molecular orientation is calculated to be $\Delta E = 2.16$ x 10^{-29} J. To compare this magnetic energy with thermal energy of the human body at 38°C

yields $kT = 4.28$ x 10^{-21} J that leads to a ratio of $\dfrac{\Delta E}{kT} = 5.0 \times 10^{-9}$ for a 10-T magnet.

This indicates that the magnetic energy is 200 million times smaller than thermal energy at 10-Tesla. Such little energy is unlikely to cause significant biological or physiological changes in water molecules *in vivo*.

These results indicate that for a 0.01% deviation from random orientation of water molecules, a static magnetic field strength of 450-Tesla is needed. This is in spite of the B^2-dependence of the magnetic energy. By comparison, the expected alignment within the fields of even ultra-high-field-strength MR systems is negligible. To our knowledge, no observation of magnetic field-induced alignment of water molecules has been reported at the static magnetic field strengths used for MR scanners, to date. This is in agreement with the model presented above for magnetic alignment of diamagnetic molecules in strong magnetic fields.

Translational Forces

Injury can be caused by application of forces on tissues. For tissue components with large differences in magnetic properties, such forces could develop in non-uniform magnetic fields. As it was shown earlier, diamagnetic tissue components tend to move toward lower fields and paramagnetic tissue components will be forced to higher field regions. The formation of such opposing forces on components of the same tissue could interfere with the physiological function of the tissue and lead to injury. It is conceivable that under normal circumstances, biological structures have greater internal forces, such as electric forces involved in chemical reactions, than magnetic forces due to susceptibility variations (34, 87). Furthermore, gravitational forces and forces produced by acceleration and other motions during routine activities produce considerable forces on tissue components. The evolution of life under gravitational action of the Earth and routine life activities must have resulted in development of the "means" to incorporate these forces in the inner working of living beings. These "means" will be unable to identify the source of the force and end up preventing tissue function from being substantially affected by magnetic forces.

As it was shown in the examples above for UHF magnets, say 10-T, for the magnetic torque on water molecules, the differential magnetic forces can be shown to be much smaller than differential gravitational forces. This is important since even the larger differential gravitational forces are too small to disturb physiological processes. Here, too, red blood cells can be used to as a quantitative analysis of the role of magnetic translational forces. Behavior of red blood cells in the blood is affected by its higher density than plasma density that makes them sink in the blood in the absence of larger hemodynamic forces. This effect called erythrocyte sedimentation rate (ESR) is used in the laboratory to test for abnormalities of blood proteins. While gravitational forces are useful for separation of blood ingredients in test tubes, they are too small to make red blood cells sink *in vivo*.

The molecule, hemoglobin, has four iron atoms in each molecule that reduces the diamagnetic properties of red blood cells making it slightly less than that of surrounding plasma. This pushes red blood cells toward regions of strong magnetic fields relative to the plasma. Using the expression for magnetic force from **Table 3**, the magnitude of this differential force is given by $\dfrac{(\chi_{rbc} - \chi_{plasma})V_{rbc}}{\mu_o} B_o \dfrac{\partial B_o}{\partial z}$.

Working this example for the 8-T whole body scanner the maximum value of $B_o \dfrac{\partial B_o}{\partial z}$ is 42.6-T^2/m. To find the susceptibility of deoxygenated hemoglobin, participation of four iron atoms per molecule is taken into account to get χ_{rbc} = -6.53 x 10^{-6}. Taking the susceptibility of plasma to be the same as water -9.05 x 10^{-6}. In addition, the mass densities of red blood cells and plasma are given by ρ_{rbc} = 1.093 g/cc and ρ_{plasma} = 1.027-g/cc. Inserting these quantities in the ratio equation will give the ratio of the magnetic and gravitational forces at 8-T to be,

$$\frac{F_m}{F_g} = \frac{1}{\mu_o g} B \frac{\partial B}{\partial z} \frac{\chi_{rbc} - \chi_{plasma}}{\rho_{rbc} - \rho_{plasma}} = 0.13$$

where gravitational acceleration is taken to be g = 9.8-m/s^2. As is seen from these calculations, even at the highest static magnetic field strength available for MRI research, the maximum magnetic force capable of separating the red blood cells from the plasma is about 13 percent of the gravitational forces. Considering that gravitational forces have negligible effects *in vivo*, the effect of magnetic forces is even smaller by almost an order of magnitude for static magnetic fields of up to 8-T.

Discussions and calculations in this section show that, while finite magnetic effects act on tissues in magnetic fields, their magnitude for fields available for MRI procedures in human subjects are very small when compared to other known forces, such as gravitational and routine physical activities, and these forces are clearly incapable of causing injury to biological tissues. Forces maintaining the integrity of molecular and cellular structures of biological tissues appear to be orders of magnitude larger than the forces that magnetic fields can exert on living beings.

SENSORY EFFECTS OF STATIC MAGNETIC FIELDS

Static magnetic effects on stationary tissues were presented in previous sections. Here we will analyze the interaction of sensory tissues with magnetic fields. Research in this area has revealed that motion in strong magnetic fields could induce mild sensory effects that are transient and not harmful (44, 48, 80, 86). These reports rely on a subjective description of sensory stimulations and their effects have to be interpreted with great caution, as the number of studies of these effects is limited. On the issue of subjectivity of this effect, reports have documented static magnetic field-induced sensory effects by staff members working around superconducting magnets, even during the time when the magnets were "off" (89). Nevertheless, comparisons of incidents at different field strengths show that human subjects exposed to higher fields (9.4-Tesla) reported higher rates of sensory stimulation than those subjected to a 0.5-Tesla field (5, 86, 153). Field-dependence of sensory effects has been both expected and reported by workers on high field magnets. Particularly, sensations of nausea, vertigo and metallic taste sensations related to exposures to static magnetic fields at 4-, 8-, and 9.4-Tesla have been reported (5, 86, 153). However, effects such as headache, tinnitus, vomiting, hiccups, and numbness that have sometimes been attributed to magnetic field exposures have not been observed for the same field strengths.

Magnetophosphenes, sensations of light flashing when the eyes are moved rapidly while inside the magnetic field in a dark room, have been reported in field strengths of up to 9.4-Tesla. Computational results have confirmed the factors involved in observation of magnetophosphenes and have provided quantitative models for this phenomenon (154).

Sensory experiences in static magnetic fields form 0.5- to 9.4-Tesla have been reported and shown that avoiding rapid body movements inside these magnetic fields may reduce these sensations. In addition, lower field strengths are associated with lower peripheral nerve stimulation. However, there is substantial evidence that magnetic field-induced sensory effects are caused by activation of highly excitable sensory systems by weak electrical currents which can be induced by moving the body part inside the magnetic fields (154-156). Sensations, such as nausea, have been reported which are probably caused by magnetic forces exciting motion sensors in the semicircular canals of the inner ear (98). This specific effect may be created due to a conflict in the position information supplied by the visual systems and vestibular position-sensing system. A possible source of vertigo could be magnetic forces caused by diamagnetic anisotropy of the inner ear receptors. Small torques acting on these receptors could induce a small level of sensory effects. Notably, slow movements of the patient inside or around a very strong magnetic field drastically reduces sensory stimulations and provides comfort in association with the performance of an MRI examination using a UHF MR system.

HEATING EFFECTS

Studies using laboratory animals have reported the effect of static magnetic fields on body and skin temperatures (157-162). However, these investigations do not offer an unequivocal conclusion about this issue. One report indicated that exposure to static magnetic fields can change body temperature depending on the orientation of the animal with respect to the magnetic field (157). Another report presented measurements performed on small animals and made specific comments about their mechanism of action (161). Still other studies of mammals, including those involving human subjects, report the absence of an effect of static magnetic fields on skin and body temperatures (158-160).

Most reports of temperature changes related to static magnetic fields have not proposed a plausible mechanism for these observations. The choice of animals as well as the temperature measuring devices could affect the results of such studies because, in some of the reports of static magnetic field-induced temperature changes, the investigations used temperature-labile mammals or problematic instrumentation. Also, the possibility of the effect of strong static magnetic fields causing erroneous readings on the temperature recording devices was not addressed.

Various investigations performed using laboratory animals and human subjects exposed to high static magnetic fields have reported that there are no changes in skin or body temperatures (6, 158-160). Utilizing a fluoroptic thermometry system known to be impervious to strong magnetic fields to record temperatures in laboratory animals and human studies ensures that accurate temperature readings are achieved inside the bore of the MR system. In consideration of the above, exposure to static magnetic fields is not believed to alter human body temperatures.

SAFETY REGULATIONS

The safety of human exposure in MR systems is the responsibility of the Food and Drug Administration (FDA) in the United States (U.S.) and other similar agencies outside of the U.S. The FDA provides guidelines for the limits of safe exposures to static magnetic fields as well as the other electromagnetic fields use for MRI (i.e., gradient magnetic fields and radio frequency power deposition). The FDA's assessment of the health risks associated with exposure to static magnetic fields was last updated in 2003 when the upper limit was set at 8-Tesla. The World Health Organization (WHO) has also established health criteria for static magnetic fields within the Environmental Health Criteria Program (WHO 2006)(163). The International Commission on Non-Ionizing Radiation Protection (ICNIRP) report, along with other similar documents, offer insight and regulatory guidelines pertaining to the biological effects of exposure to static fields (163-176). The regulatory body in the United Kingdom for medical device safety is the National Radiological Protection Board (NRPB) and in the European Union this task is carried out by the International Electrotechnical Commission (IEC). All these regulatory bodies evaluate the available scientific database and develop rationale for the guidelines that are updated as new data and technology becomes available (169-179).

The Medical Devices Act passed by the U.S. Congress in 1977 required MRI for the first time to demonstrate its viability as an imaging modality and safety. Subsequent to the discovery of MRI as a viable medical imaging device, major manufacturers introduced their products and applied for FDA approval. Rapid success in demonstrating its safe operation led in 1987 to the FDA designation of a static magnetic field strength of 2-T as the limit below which MR systems will pose a non-significant risk to human subjects. Proliferation of MR scanners and research systems helped to support an increase in the non-significant field strength risk to 4-T in 1996 and 8-T in 2003. As such, since 2003, exposure of research subjects to static magnetic fields above 8-T in the U.S. requires approval of the research protocol by an Institutional Review Board (IRB) with informed consent of the subjects.

Occupational Exposure

Exposure to strong magnetic fields is often greater for workers involved with manufacturing and testing magnet-based instruments and devices than it is for patients. In addition to workers involved in the manufacturer of MR systems, MRI researchers, MRI technologists in hospitals and imaging centers, and experimental high-energy physicists are among the populations with chronic exposures to strong static magnetic fields. To regulate chronic exposure, guidelines have been developed in some countries. Proposed in Europe, a time-weighted-average field exposure of 0.20-T/8-hour would limit the workers to 0.2-T field for an eight-hour day or 8-T for 12-minutes. A higher limit of 2-T/8-hour limit was proposed for the extremities by these guidelines. The lack of confirmed evidence for harmful cumulative effects of exposures to static magnetic fields has made these limits less consequential than the limit on the highest field strength used for human subjects. This is especially true as the fields outside magnets are highly inhomogeneous. This strong spatial variation of the magnetic fields is not usually specified for MR systems. Because of this sharp variation of the magnetic field outside the magnet (i.e., the fringe field), workers are not within a constant magnetic field, making it difficult to average the values over a workday period. For these workers, still the most ominous potential hazard remains any inadvertent introduction of ferromagnetic tools or other objects into the areas with strong fringe fields.

Experiments are continuing to investigate the chronic effects of any mechanisms of tissue injury at the field strengths currently available for human magnets. Expanding the number of controlled studies that involve long-term exposures of animals and human subjects to strong magnetic fields may offer valuable insight into the safety of chronic magnetic field exposures. Furthermore, the collection of safety data from MR system manufacturers, researchers, and medical staff will be helpful for the analysis of the effects of static magnetic fields on human subjects.

CONCLUSIONS

According to OECD Health Data 2009, published by the Organization for Economic Co-operation and Development (OECD), the average number of MRI examinations performed per 1,000-population per year for the thirty countries of the OCED was forty-one. Considering the population of the OCED to be 1.2 billion means that approximately 54 million MRI exams were performed in the thirty OCED countries (179) each year. In the United States, 91.2 MRI procedures per 1,000-population equates to about 28 million examinations each year. Nevertheless, no unpreventable harm to the patients from exposure to the static magnetic field has been reported. As previously indicated, all serious accidents associated with MR systems, to date, have been caused by involuntary introduction of ferromagnetic materials or medical devices into the magnetic field. In addition to clinical scanners, research scanners operating at fields of up to 11.7-Tesla for humans and up to 16.4-Tesla for animals have shown no major safety incidents, which has laid the foundation for clinical scanners to be designed for operation at these higher field strengths. There is still much fertile ground for research in studying the interaction of biological tissues with stronger fields regardless of how safe the record of operation at high static magnetic fields is at the present time.

Keeping in mind that the spatial gradient magnetic field will be larger for higher field strength magnets, more stringent measures to exclude the presence of ferromagnetic objects from MRI suits will be needed. In spite of the existence of approximately fifty 7-T human MR systems around the world, a number of technological issues such as RF inhomogeneity, susceptibility artifacts, and RF power deposition (i.e., SAR) issues will have to be worked out before their introduction to clinical settings. But, the relentless drive for higher fields is achieving new milestones, such as the 21.1-T, 105-mm magnet located at the National High Magnetic Field Laboratory in Tallahassee, Florida (which is the strongest MR system in the world used for animal imaging). Nuclear magnetic resonance (NMR) magnets operating at 23.5-T with a hydrogen proton Larmor frequency of 1-GHz and a bore size of 54-mm are now commercially available. This trend will continue and the safety studies involving small animals will add valuable information on our understanding of the mechanisms of interactions of these fields with living beings (178-179).

Research on the effect of strong magnetic fields on tissues, cells, and molecules has not produced evidence for its harm to human life. The forces analyzed in many publications as the possible mechanisms of interactions have proven to be insignificant compared to the natural forces that maintain the structural integrity of the tissues and in consideration of the routine forces to which the human body is exposed to through everyday activities.

Regulatory bodies have rightly taken the attitude of requiring verification of any claim of adverse effects of static magnetic fields before they can be incorporated into the safety guidelines. This is a reasonable approach that has proven to demonstrate attention to scientific findings, while preventing unnecessary impediments to research and exploration of benefits of magnetic fields for the good of society.

Fortunately, the physics of such interactions are straightforward and simple calculations provide insight into the order of magnitude of magnetic field effects. So far, such calculations have indicated that forces exerted on diamagnetic materials, of which biological tissue are overwhelmingly made, are insignificant compared to other forces involved in maintaining their structure and function. It seems that all the major revisions in the FDA guidelines for assessing non-significant risk involved in the exposure of human subjects to static magnetic fields have followed this course of action. The present FDA guidelines recommend 8-T as the strongest magnetic field with non-significant risk. As the field strengths are increasing for whole body scanners, it is conceivable that sensory effects such as vertigo, metallic taste and magnetophosphenes may become more prevalent. However, no permanent harm from these effects has been presented. Transient effects caused by movement inside the magnetic field can be minimized through training. The long-term, cumulative effect of exposures to static magnetic fields is a topic requiring more research to confirm any adverse effects.

As the field strength of MR systems increases, it is conceivable that eventually one of the forces of interaction will become large enough to require limiting its effect on human life. Diamagnetic susceptibility is not likely to be the limiting factor. However, the effect of field inhomogeneity and the magnetic effect on the blood flow could limit the persistent drive towards higher fields. For now, even research magnets seem to be far from that limit and we are fortunate to be able to safely explore the benefits of higher static magnetic fields to visualize the structure and function of the human body. If more complex safety studies confirm no significant adverse effects, then much higher magnetic fields could become available for human MR imaging to continuously enhance our ability to "see" naturally opaque biological structures and functions. Such observations may lead to better healthcare for future generations and offer understanding of the mysteries of life.

[Portions of this chapter were excerpted with permission from Schenck, JF. Safety of strong static magnetic fields. Journal of Magnetic Resonance Imaging 2000;12:2-19.]

REFERENCES

1. Damadian R. Tumor detection by nuclear magnetic resonance. Science 1971; 171:1151-1153.

2. Lauterbur PC. Image formation by induced local interactions: Examples employing nuclear magnetic resonance. Nature 1973;242:190 -191.

3. McRobbie DW. Occupational exposure in MRI. Br J Radiol 2012;85:293-312.

4. U.S. Department of Health and Human Services, Food and Drug Administration, Center for Devices and Radiological Health, Radiological Devices Branch, Division of Reproductive, Abdominal, and Radiological Devices, Office of Device Evaluation, Guidance for MRI Industry and FDA Staff, Criteria for Significant Risk Investigations of Magnetic Resonance Diagnostic Device. Document issued on: July 14, 2003.

5. Kangarlu A, Robitaille PML. Biological effects and health implications in magnetic resonance imaging. Concepts in Magnetic Resonance 2000;12:321–359.

6. Kangarlu A, Shellock FG, Chakeres DW. 8.0-Tesla human MR system: temperature changes associated with radiofrequency-induced heating of a head phantom. J Magn Reson Imaging 2003;17:220-6.

7. Kangarlu A, Shellock FG. Aneurysm clips: evaluation of magnetic field interactions with an 8.0 T MR system. J Magn Reson Imaging 2000;12:107-11.

8. Heinrich A, Szostek A, Meyer P, et al. Cognition and sensation in very high static magnetic fields: a randomized case-crossover study with different field strengths. Radiology 2013;266:236-45.

9. Chakeres DW, Kangarlu A, Boudoulas H, Young DC. Effect of static magnetic field exposure of up to 8 Tesla on sequential human vital sign measurements. J Magn Reson Imaging. 2003;18:346-52.

10. Chakeres DW, Bornstein R, Kangarlu A. Randomized comparison of cognitive function in humans at 0 and 8 Tesla. J Magn Reson Imaging 2003;18:342-5.

11. Mottelay PF. Bibliographical History of Electricity and Magnetism Chronologically Arranged. Charles Griffin & Co, London, 1922.

12. Davis LD, Pappajohn K, Plavnieks IM, Spiegler PE, Jacobius AJ. Bibliography of the biological effects of magnetic fields. Fed Proc Suppl 1962;2:1-38.

13. Gross L. Bibliography of the Biological Effects of Static Magnetic Fields. In: Barnothy MF, Editor. Biological Effects of Magnetic Fields. Plenum Press, New York, 1964, pp. 297-311.

14. Gartrell RG. Electricity, Magnetism, and Animal Magnetism: A Checklist of Printed Sources, 1600-1850. Scholarly Resources, Inc., Wilmington, DE, 1975.

15. Mourino MR. From Thales to Lauterbur, or from the lodestone to MR imaging: magnetism and medicine. Radiology 1991;180;593-612.

16. Binet A, Féré C. Animal Magnetism. Kegan Paul, Editor. London, 1887. Reprinted, Gryphon Editions, New York, 1993.

17. Barnothy MF. Editor, Biological Effects of Magnetic Fields. Plenum Press, New York, 1964.

18. Kholodov YA. The effect of electromagnetic and magnetic fields on the central nervous system. NASA Technical Translation F-465, Clearing House for Federal Scientific and Technical Information, Springfield, VA, 1967.

19. Barnothy MF. Editor, Biological Effects of Magnetic Fields. Volume 2, Plenum Press, New York, 1969.

20. Pressman AS. Electromagnetic Fields and Life. Sinclair FL, Brown FA Jr, Translators, Plenum Press, New York, 1970.

21. Kholodov YA. Editor, Influence of Magnetic Fields on Biological Objects. JPRS 63038, National Technical Information Service, Springfield, VA, 1974.

22. Llaurado JG, Sances A, Battocletti AJH, Editors. Biologic and Clinical Effects of Low-Frequency Magnetic and Electric fields. Thomas, Springfield, IL, 1974.

23. Buranelli V. The Wizard from Vienna: Franz Anton Mesmer. Coward, McCann and Geohagen, New York, 1975.

24. Tenforde TS. Editor. Magnetic Field Effect on Biological Systems. Plenum Press, New York, 1979.

25. Herlach F. Editors, Strong and Ultrastrong Magnetic Fields and Their Applications. Springer-Verlag, Berlin, 1985.

26. Maret G, Boccara N, Kiepenheuer J, Editors. Biophysical Effects of Steady Magnetic Fields, Springer-Verlag, Berlin, 1986.

27. Polk C, Postow E. Handbook of Biological Effects of Electromagnetic Fields. CRC Press, Boca Raton, FL, 1986.

28. Crabtree A. From Mesmer to Freud: Magnetic Sleep and the Roots of Psychological Healing. Yale University Press, New Haven,1993.

29. Shellock FG, Kanal E, Magnetic Resonance: Bioeffects, Patient Safety, and Patient Management. 2nd Edition, Lippincott-Raven, Philadelphia, PA, 1996.

30. Whitaker J, Adderly B. The Pain Relief Breakthrough: The Power of Magnets to Relieve Backaches, Arthritis, Menstrual Cramps, Carpal Tunnel Syndrome, Sports Injuries and More, Little Brown, Boston, 1998.

31. Quinan JR. The use of the magnet in medicine: a historical study. Maryland Med. J 1886;14,:460-465.

32. Schaefer DJ. Safety Aspects of Magnetic Resonance Imaging. In: Wehrli FW, Shaw D, Kneeland JB, Editors. Biomedical Magnetic Resonance Imaging: Principles, Methodology and Applications. VCH Verlagsgesellschaft, Weinheim, 1988, pp. 553-578.

33. Shellock FG, Kanal E, Moscatel M. Bioeffects and Safety Considerations. In: Atlas SW, Editor. Magnetic Resonance Imaging of the Brain and Spine. 2nd Edition. Lippincott-Raven, Philadelphia, PA, 1996, pp. 109-148.

34. Schenck JF. MR Safety at High Magnetic Field Strengths. In: Kanal E. Editor. Magnetic Resonance Imaging Clinics of North America: MR Safety. Volume 6, Saunders, Philadelphia, PA, 1998, pp. 715-730.

35. Hermann L. Hat das magnetische Feld directe physiologische Wirkungen? Pflügers Arch. Gesammte Physiol Menschen Thiere 1888;43:217-234.

36. Peterson F, Kennelly AE. Some physiological experiments with magnets at the Edison Laboratory. NY Med J 1892;56:729-734.

37. Drinker CK, Thomson RM. Does the magnetic field constitute an industrial hazard? J Ind Hyg 1921;3:117-129.

38. American Medical Association. Theronoid and vitrona: the magic horse collar campaign continues. JAMA 931;96:1718-1719.

39. Barnothy MF, Barnothy JM, Boszormenyi-Nagy I. Influence of magnetic field upon the leucocytes of the mouse. Nature 1956;177: 577-578.

40. Barnothy MF, Barnothy JM. Biological effect of a magnetic field and the radiation syndrome. Nature 1958;181:1785-1786.

41. Freeman MW, Arrott A, Watson JHL. Magnetism in medicine. J Appl Phys 1960;31: 404S-405S.

42. Eiselein TE, Boutell HM, Biggs MW. Biological effects of magnetic fields – negative results. Aerospace Medicine 1961;32:383-386.

43. Beischer DE. Human tolerance to magnetic fields. Astronautics 1962;7:24-25, 46,48.

44. Beischer DE, Knepton Jr JC. Influence of strong magnetic fields on the electrocardiogram of squirrel monkeys (Saimiri sciureus). Aerospace Medicine 1964;35: 939-944.

45. Murayama M. Orientation of sickled erythrocytes in a magnetic field. Nature 1965; 206:420-422.

46. Murayama M, Molecular mechanism of red cell "sickling." Science 1966;153:145-149.

47. Malinin GI, Gregory WD, Morelli L, Sharma VK, Houck JC. Evidence of morphological and physiological transformation of mammalian cells by strong magnetic fields. Science 1976;194:844-846.

48. St. Lorant SJ. Biomagnetism: A Review. In: SLAC Publication, 1984. Stanford Linear Accelerator, Stanford, CA, 1977, pp. 1-9.

49. Ketchen EE, Porter WE, Bolton NE. The biological effects of magnetic fields on man. Am Ind Hyg Assoc J 1978;39:1-11.

50. Budinger TF. Threshold for physiological effects due to RF and magnetic fields used in NMR imaging,IEEE Trans. Nucl Sci 1979;NS-26:2821-2825.

51. Saunders RD. Biological Hazards of NMR. In: Witcofski RL, Karstaedt N, Partain CL, Editors. Proceedings of an International Symposium on Nuclear Magnetic Resonance Imaging. Bowman Gray School of Medicine, Winston-Salem, NC, 1981, pp. 65-71.

52. Battocletti JH, Salles-Cunha S, Halbach RE, et al. Exposure of rhesus monkeys to 20000 G steady magnetic field: effect on blood parameters. Med Phys 1981;8:115-118.

53. Budinger TF. Nuclear magnetic resonance (NMR) *in vitro* studies: known thresholds for health effects. J Comput Assisted Tomog 1981;5:800-811.

54. Hong C-Z, Lin JC, Bender LF, et al. Magnetic necklace: its therapeutic effectiveness on neck and shoulder pain. Arch Phys Med Rehabil 1982;63:462-466.

55. Budinger TF. Hazards from DC and AC magnetic fields. In: Book of Abstracts, Society of Magnetic Resonance in Medicine, Berkeley, CA, 1982, pp. 29-30.

56. Milham S. Mortality from leukemia in workers exposed to electrical and magnetic fields (Letter). N Engl J Med 1982;307:249.

57. New PF, Rosen BR, Brady TJ, et al. Potential hazards and artifacts of ferromagnetic and nonferromagnetic surgical and dental materials and devices in nuclear magnetic resonance imaging. Radiology 1983;147:139-148.

58. Saunders RD Smith H. Safety aspects of NMR clinical imaging. Br Med Bull 1984;40:148-154.

59. Budinger TF, Bristol KS, Yen CK, Wong P. Biological effects of static magnetic fields. In: Book of Abstracts, Society of Magnetic Resonance in Medicine, Berkeley, CA, 1984, pp. 113-114.

60. Budinger TF, Cullander C. Health Effects of *In Vivo* Nuclear Magnetic Resonance. In: Biomedical Magnetic Resonance. James CE, Margulis A. Editors. Radiology Research and Education Foundation, San Francisco, 1984, pp. 421-441.

61. Brody AS, Sorette MP, Gooding CA, et al. Induced alignment of flowing sickle erythrocytes in a magnetic field: a preliminary report. Invest Radiol 1985;20:560-566.

62. Kelly WM, Paglen PG, Pearson JA, San Diego AG, Soloman MA. Ferromagnetism of intraocular foreign body causes unilateral blindness after MR study. Am J Roentgenol 1987;149:1080. 1986;7:243-245.

63. Gleick J. Man hurt as medical magnet attracts forklift. New York Times, June 5, 1986, A21.

64. von Klitzing L. Do static magnetic fields of NMR influence biological signals? Clin Phys Physiol Meas 1986;7:157-160.

65. Lund G, Nelson JD, Wirtschafter JD, et al. Tattooing of eyelids: magnetic resonance imaging artifacts. Ophthalmic Surg 1986;17:550-553.

66. Fowler JR, Ter Penning B, Syverud SA, Levy RC. Magnetic field hazard (Letter). N Engl J Med 1986;314:1517.

67. Miller G. Exposure guidelines for magnetic fields. Am Ind Hyg Assoc J 1987;48: 957-968.

68. Jackson JG, Acker JD. Permanent eyeliner and MR imaging (Letter). Am J Roentgenol 1987;149:1080.

69. Budinger TF. Magnetohydrodynamic retarding effect on blood flow velocity at 4.7 Tesla found to be insignificant. In: Book of Abstracts, Society of Magnetic Resonance in Medicine, Berkeley, CA, 1987, pp.183.

70. Jackson JG, Acker JD. Permanent eyeliner and MR imaging (Letter). Am J Roentgenol 1987;149:1080.

71. Sacco DC, Steiger DA, Bellon EM, et al. Artifacts caused by cosmetics in MR imaging of the head. Am J Roentgenol 1987;148:1001-1004.

72. Wolfley DE, Flynn KJ, Cartwright J. Eyelid pigment implantation: early and late histopathology. Plast Reconstr Surg 1988;82:770-774.

73. Schenck JF, Dumoulin CL, Mueller OM, et al. Proton imaging of humans at 4.0 Tesla. In: Book of Abstracts, Society of Magnetic Resonance in Medicine, Berkeley, CA, 1988; pp. 153.

74. Brody AS, Embury SH, Mentzer WC, Winkler M, Gooding CA. Preservation of sickle cell bloodflow patterns during MR imaging: an *in vivo* study. Am J Roentgenol 1988;151:139-141.

75. Redington RW, Dumoulin CL, Schenck JF, et al. MR imaging and bio-effects in a whole-body 4.0 Tesla imaging system. In Book of Abstracts, Society of Magnetic Resonance in Medicine, Berkeley, CA, 1988, pp. 20.

76. Wahlund L-O, Agartz, I, Almqvist, O, et al. The brain in healthy aged individuals. Radiology 1990;174:674-679.

77. Mankad VN, Williams JP, Harpen MD, et al. Magnetic resonance imaging of bone marrow in sickle cell disease: clinical, hematological, and pathologic correlations. Blood 1990;75:274-283.

78. Hong C-Z, Shellock F. Short term exposure to a 1.5 Tesla static magnetic field does not affect somato-sensory-evoked potentials in man. Magn Reson Imaging 1990;8:65-69.

79. Muller S, Hotz M. Human brainstem auditory evoked potentials (BAEP) before and after MR examinations. Magn Reson Med 1990;16:476-480.

80. Schenck JF, Dumoulin CL, Souza SP. Health and physiological effects of human exposure to whole-body 4 Tesla magnetic fields during magnetic resonance scanning. In: Book of Abstracts, Society of Magnetic Resonance in Medicine, Berkeley, CA 1990, pp. 277.

81. Keltner JR, Roos MS, Brakeman PR, Budinger TF. Magnetohydrodynamics of blood flow. Magn Reson Med 1990;16:139-149.

82. Phillips ME. Industrial hygiene investigation of static magnetic fields in nuclear magnetic resonance facilities. Appl Occup Environ Hyg 1990;5:353-358.

83. Kelsey CA, King JN, Keck GM, et al. Ocular hazard of metallic fragments during MR imaging at 0.06 T. Radiology 1991;180:282-283.

84. Buettner UW. Human interactions with ultra high fields. In: Magin RL, Liburdy RP, Persson B, Editors. Biological and Safety Aspects of Nuclear Magnetic Resonance Imaging and Spectroscopy. Annals of the New York Academy of Sciences, Volume 649. New York Academy of Sciences, New York, 1992, pp. 59-66.

85. Schenck JF. Quantitative assessment of the magnetic forces and torques in red blood cells: implications for patients with sickle cell anemia. In: Book of Abstracts, Society of Magnetic Resonance in Medicine, Berkeley, CA, 1992, pp. 3405.

86. Schenck JF, Dumoulin CL, Redington RW, et al. Human exposure to 4.0-Tesla magnetic fields in a whole-body scanner. Med Phys 1992;19:1089-1098.

87. Schenck JF. Health and physiological effects of human exposure to whole-body four-Tesla magnetic fields during MRI. In: Magin RL, Liburdy RP, Persson B. Editors. Biological and Safety Aspects of Nuclear Magnetic Resonance Imaging and Spectroscopy. Annals of the New York Academy of Sciences, Volume 649. New York Academy of Sciences, New York, 1992, pp 285-301.

88. Macklis RM. Magnetic healing, quackery, and the debate about the health effects of electromagnetic fields. Ann Int Med 1993;118:376-383.

89. Erhard P, Chen W, Lee J-H, Ugurbil K. A study of effects reported by subjects at high magnetic fields. In: Book of Abstracts, Society of Magnetic Resonance in Medicine, Berkeley, CA, 1995, pp. 1219.

90. Schenck JF. The role of magnetic susceptibility in magnetic resonance imaging: magnetic field compatibility of the first and second kinds. Med Phys 1996;23:815-850.

91. Shermer M, Salas C, Salas D. Testing the Claims of Mesmerism: Commissioned by King Louis XVI: Designed, Conducted and Written by Benjamin Franklin, Antoine Lavoisier and Others. Translation of the 1784 Report of the Commissioners Charged by the King to Examine Animal Magnetism. Skeptic 1996;4:66-83.

92. Minczykowski A, Wlodzimierz P, Smielecki J, et al. Effects of magnetic resonance imaging on polymorphonuclear neutrophil functions. Acad Radiol 1996;3:97-102.

93. Vallbona C, Hazlewood CF, Jurida G. Response of pain to static magnetic fields in postpolio patients: a double-blind pilot study. Arch Phys Med Rehabil 1997;78:1200-1203.

94. Horstman J. Explorations: magnets. Arthritis Today 1988;12:48-51.

95. Ramey DW. Magnetic and electromagnetic therapy. Sci Rev Alt Med 1998;2:13-19.

96. Kinouchi Y, Yamaguchi H, Tenforde TS. Theoretical analysis of magnetic field interactions with aortic blood flow. Bioelectromagnetics 1996;17:21-32.

97. Feingold L. Magnet therapy. Sci Rev Alt Med 1999;3:26-33.

98. Kangarlu A, Burgess RE, Zhu H, et al. Cognitive, cardiac, and physiological safety studies in ultra high field magnetic resonance imaging. Magn Reson Imaging 1990;17:1407-1416.

99. Klucznik RP, Carrier DA, Pyka R, et al. Placement of a ferromagnetic intracerebral aneurysm clip with a fatal outcome. Radiology 1993;187:587-599.

100. Kanal E, Shellock FG. MR imaging of patients with intracranial aneurysm clips. Radiology 1993;187:612-614.

101. Gimbel JR, Johnson D, Levine PA, et al. Safe performance of magnetic resonance imaging on five patients with permanent cardiac pacemakers, PACE (Pacing and Clinical Electrophysiology) 1996;19: 913-919.

102. Becker RO. Cross Currents. The Promise of Electromedicine, the Perils of Electropollution. Torcher, Los Angeles, 1990.

103. Davis AR, Rawls WC. Magnetism and Its Effects on the Living System. Exposition Press, Smithtown, NY, 1975

104. Wilson MN. Superconducting Magnets. Clarendon Press, Oxford, 1983.

105. Vallbona C, Richards T. Evolution of magnetic therapy from alternative to traditional medicine. Phys Med Rehabil Clin N Am 1999;10(3):729-54.

106. Hinshaw WS, Bottomley PA, Holland GN. Radiographic thin-section image of the human wrist by nuclear magnetic resonance. Nature 1977;270:722-723.

107. Hinshaw WS, Andrew ER, Bottomley PA, et al. Display of cross sectional anatomy by nuclear magnetic resonance imaging. Br J Radiol 1978;51:273-280.

108. Damadian R, Minkoff L, Goldsmith M. Field-focusing nuclear magnetic resonance (FONAR). Naturwissenschaften 1978;65:250-252.

109. Edelstein WA, Hutchison JMS, Johnson G, et al. Spin warp NMR imaging and applications to human whole-body imaging. Phys Med Biol 1980;25:751-756.

110. Vetter J, Siebold H, Söldner L. A 4 -T superconducting whole-body magnet for MR-imaging and spectroscopy. In: Book of Abstracts, Society of Magnetic Resonance in Medicine, Berkeley, CA, 1987, pp. 181.

111. Vetter J, Ries G, Reichert T. A 4-Tesla superconducting whole-body magnet for MR imaging and spectroscopy. IEEE Trans Magn 1988;24:1285-1287.

112. Barfuss H, Fischer H, Hentschel D et al. Whole-body MR imaging and spectroscopy with a 4-T system. Radiology 1988;169: 811-816.

113. Barfuss H, Fischer H, Hentschel D, et al. *In vivo* magnetic resonance imaging and spectroscopy of humans with a 4T whole-body magnet. NMR in Biomed 1990;3:31-45.

114. Chu SC. The development of a 4T whole body system for clinical research. Jap J Magn Reson Med 1990:10:63-64.

115. Bell RA. Economics of MRI technology. J Magn Reson Imaging 1996;6:10-25.

116. Berry MV, Geim AK. Of flying frogs and levitrons. Eur J Phys 1997;18:307-313.

117. Geim AK, Simon MD, Boamfa MI, Heflinger LO. Magnet levitation at your fingertips. Nature 1999;400:323-324.

118. Kolin A. Improved apparatus and technique for electromagnetic determination of blood flow. Rev Sci Instr 1952;23:235-242.

119. Kanai H, Yamano E, Nakayama K, Kawamura N, Furuhata H. Transcutaneous blood flow measurement by electromagnetic induction. IEEE Trans Biomed Engin 1974;BME-21:144-151.

120. Togawa T, Okai O, Ohima M. Observation of blood flow e.m.f. in externally applied strong magnetic fields by surface electrodes. Med Biol Engineer 1967;5:169-170.

121. Tenforde TS, Gaffey CT, Moyer BR., Budinger TF. Cardiovascular alterations in Macaca monkeys exposed to stationary magnetic fields: experimental observations and theoretical analysis. Bioelectromagnetics 1983;4:1-9.

122. Winfrey AT. The electrical thresholds of ventricular myocardium J Cardiovascular Physiol 1990;1:393-410.

123. Haberditzl W. Enzyme activity in high magnetic fields. Nature 1967;213:72-73.

124. Atkins PW. Magnetic field effects. Chem Brit 1976;12:214-218.

125. Atkins PW, Lambert TP. The effect of a magnetic field on chemical reactions. Ann Rep Prog Chem 1976;A72:67-88.

126. Brocklehurst B. Spin correlation in the geminate recombination of radical ions in hydrocarbons. Part I - theory of the magnetic field effect. J Chem Soc Faraday Trans 1976;72:1869-1864.

127. McLauchlan KA. The effects of magnetic fields on chemical reactions. Sci Prog (Oxford) 1981;67:509-529.

128. Turro NJ. Influence of nuclear spin on chemical reactions: magnetic isotope and magnetic field effects (a review). Proc Natl Acad Sci 1983;80:609-621.

129. Gould IR, Turro NJ, Zimmt MB. Magnetic Field and Magnetic Isotope Effects on the Products of Organic Reactions. In: Gold V, Bethel D, Editors. Advances in Physical Organic Chemistry, Volume 20. Academic Press, New York, 1984.

130. Steiner UE, Ulrich T. Magnetic field effects in chemical kinetics and related phenomena. Chem Rev 1989;89:51-147.

131. Cohen C. Ferromagnetic contamination in the lungs and other organs of the body. Science 1973;180:745-748.

132. Freedman AP, Robinson SE, Johnston RJ. Non-invasive magnetopneumographic estimation of lung dust loads and distribution in bituminous coal workers. J Occupational Med 1980;22:613-618.

133. Cohen D, Nemoto I. Ferrimagnetic particles in the lung part 1: the magnetizing process. IEEE Trans Biomed Engineer 1984;31:261-273.

134. Cohen D, Nemoto I, Kaufman L, et al. Ferrimagnetic particles in the lung part 2: the relaxation process. IEEE Trans Biomed Engineer 1984;31:274-284.

135. Moatamed F, Johnson FB. Identification and significance of magnetite in human tissues. Arch Pathol Lab Med 1986;110:618-621.

136. Kirschvink JL, Kobayishi-Kirschvink A, Woodford BJ. Magnetite biomineralization in the human brain. Proc Natl Acad Sci 1992;89:7683-7687.

137. Frauenrath T, Fuchs K, Dieringer MA, et al. Detailing the use of magnetohydrodynamic effects for synchronization of MRI with the cardiac cycle: a feasibility study. J Magn Reson Imaging 2012;36:364-72.

138. Bozorth RM. Ferromagnetism. Van Nostrand, New York, 1951. Reprinted, IEEE, Piscataway, NJ, 1993, pp. 627-699.

139. Scott WT. The Physics of Electricity and Magnetism. 2nd Edition. Wiley, New York, 1966, pp. 323-368.

140. Landau LD, Lifshitz EM, Pitaevskii LP. Electrodynamics of Continuous Media, 2nd Edition, Pergamon Press, Oxford 1984, pp. 105-128 and 217-222.

141. Bleaney BI , Bleaney B. Electricity and Magnetism. 3rd Edition, Oxford University Press, Oxford, 1976, pp. 101-107.

142. Jackson JD. Classical Electrodynamics. 3rd Edition, Wiley, New York, 1999, pp. 214.

143. Hong FT, Magnetic anisotropy of the visual pigment rhodopsin Biophysical Journal, Volume 29, Issue 2, 343-346,1980.

144. Torbet J, Freyssinet J-M, Hudry-Clergeon G. Oriented fibrin gals formed by polymerization in strong magnetic fields. Nature 1981;289;91-93.

145. Maret G, von Schickfus M, Mayer A, Dransfeld K. Orientation of nucleic acids in high magnetic fields. Phys Re Lett 1975;35:397-400.

146. Worcester DL. Structural origins of diamagnetic anisotropy in proteins. Proc Natl Acad Sci 1978;75: 5475-547.

147. Hong FT. Photoelectric and magneto-orientation effects in pigmented biological membranes. J Colloid Interface Sci 1977;58:471-497.

148. Geacintov NE, Van Nostrand F, Becker JF, Tinkel JB. Magnetic field orientation of photosynthetic systems. Biochem Biophys Acta 1972;267:65-79.

149. Hong FT, Mauzerall D, Mauro A. Magnetic anisotropy and the orientation of retinal rods in a homogeneous magnetic field. Proc Natl Acad Sci 1971;68:1283-1285.

150. Denegre JM, Valles JM, Lin K, Jordan WB, Mowry KL. Cleavage planes in frog eggs altered by strong magnetic fields. Proc Natl Acad Sci 1998;95:14729-14732.

151. Bras W, Diakun GP, Diaz JF, et al. The susceptibility of pure tubulin to high magnetic fields: a magnetic birefringence and x-ray fiber diffraction study. Biophys J 1998;74:1509-1521.

152. Kern CW, Karplus M. The Water Molecule. In: Franks F, Editor. Water: A Comprehensive Treatise. Volume 1. The Physics and Physical Chemistry of Water. Plenum Press, New York, 1972, pp. 21-91.

153. Patel M, Williamsom RA, Dorevitch S, Buchanan S. Pilot study investigating the effect of the static magnetic field from a 9.4-T MRI on the vestibular system. J Occup Environ Med 2008;50:576-83.

154. Laakso I, Hirata A. Computational analysis of thresholds for magnetophosphenes. Phys Med Biol 2012;7;57:6147-65.

155. Jokela K, Saunders RD. Physiologic and dosimetric considerations for limiting electric fields induced in the body by movement in a static magnetic field. Health Phys 2011;100:641-53.

156. Hirata A, Takano Y, Fujiwara O, Dovan T, Kavet R. An electric field induced in the retina and brain at threshold magnetic flux density causing magnetophosphenes. Phys Med Biol 2011;7;56:4091-101.

157. Gemmel H, Wendhausen H, Wunsch F. Biologische effekte statischer magnetfelder bei NMR-tomographie am menschen, Radiologische Klinik Wiss Mitt Univ. Kiel, 1983.

158. Shellock F, Schaefer D, Crues J. Exposure to a 1.5 T static magnetic fields does not alter body and skin temperatures in man. Magnetic Resonance in Medicine 1989;11: 371.

159. Shellock F, Schaefer D, Gordon C. Effect of a 1.5-T static magnetic field on body temperature of man. Magnetic Resonance in Medicine 1986;3:644.

160. Tenforde T, Levy L. Thermoregulation in rodents exposed to homogeneous (7.55 Tesla and gradient (60 Tesla/per second) DC magnetic fields. Proceedings of the Bioelectromagnetics Society, 7th Annual Meeting Abstracts, 1985, pp. 7.

161. László JF, Hernádi L. Whole body static magnetic field exposure increases thermal nociceptive threshold in the snail, Helix pomatia. Acta Biol Hung 2012;63:441-52.

162. Yan Y, Shen G, Xie K, Tang C, Wu X, Xu Q, Liu J, Song J, Jiang X, Luo E. Wavelet analysis of acute effects of static magnetic field on resting skin blood flow at the nail wall in young men. Microvasc Res 2011;82:277-83.

163. Environmental Health Criteria, Static fields, Geneva: World Health Organization, Monograph, Vol. 232, 2006.

164. Noble D, McKinlay A, Repacholi M. Effects of static magnetic fields relevant to human health. Prog Biophys Mol Biol 2005;87:171–372.

165. McKinlay AF, Allen SG, Cox R, et al. Review of the scientific evidence for limiting exposure to electromagnetic fields (0–300 GHz). Chilton: National Radiological Protection Board (NRPB), Docs NRPB, 15(3); 2004.

166. Goyan JE. Medical devices; procedures for investigational device exemptions. Fed Regist 1980;45:3732-3759.

167. National Radiological Protection Board (NRPB), Exposure to nuclear magnetic resonance clinical imaging, Radiography, 1980;47:258-260.

168. Gundaker WE, Guidelines for Evaluating Electromagnetic Risk for Trials of Clinical NMR Systems. U.S. Food and Drug Administration, Rockville, MD, 1982.

169. National Radiological Protection Board (NRPB). Revised guidance on acceptable limits of exposure during nuclear magnetic resonance clinical imaging. Br J Radiology 1982;56:974-977.

170. Villforth JC. Guidelines for Evaluating Electromagnetic Exposure Risk for Trials of Clinical NMR Systems. U.S. Food and Drug Administration, Rockville, MD, 1982.

171. Medicine and Healthcare Products Medical Agency (MHRA) Safety Guidelines for Magnetic Resonance Imaging Equipment in Clinical Use, DB2007 (03), December, 2007.

172. U.S. Food and Drug Administration, Magnetic resonance diagnostic device; panel recommendation and report on petitions for MR reclassification. Fed Regist 1988;53:7575-7579.

173. Young FE. Magnetic resonance diagnostic device; panel recommendation and report on petitions for MR reclassification. Fed Regist 1988;53:7575-7579.

174. Department of Health and Human Services, Guidance for Content and Review of a Magnetic Resonance Diagnostic Device 510(k) Application, US Food and Drug Administration, Silver Spring, MD, 1988.

175. National Health and Medical Research Council, Safety Guidelines for Magnetic Resonance Diagnostic Facilities: Radiation Health Series, Number 34, Australian Government Publishing Service, Canberra, 1991.

176. International Electrotechnical Commission (IEC), International Standard: Part 2 Particular Requirements for the Safety of Magnetic Resonance Equipment for Medical Diagnosis, CEI/IEC 601-2-33, International Electrotechnical Commission, Genève, Suisse, 1995.

177. Normile D. Race for stronger magnets turns into marathon. Science1998;281:164-165.

178. Service RF. NMR researchers look to next generation of machines. Science 1998;279:1127-1128.

179. Organization for Economic Cooperation and Development, Total Population. In: OECD Factbook 2010 Economic, Environmental and Social Statistics, OECD Publishing, 2010.

Chapter 3   Bioeffects of Gradient Magnetic Fields

Donald W. McRobbie, Ph.D.

Senior Lecturer in Imaging
Imperial College London
United Kingdom and
Chief Physicist
South Australia Medical Imaging
Adelaide, Australia

INTRODUCTION

During magnetic resonance imaging (MRI), the patient is exposed to the static magnetic field, which produces the nuclear magnetisation in tissues, radiofrequency (RF) pulses, which manipulate the magnetisation in order to detect an MR signal, and low frequency pulsed magnetic field gradients, which are used for localization of the signal in image formation. This chapter concerns the physiological effects of exposure to time-varying magnetic fields from the imaging gradients, hereafter simply referred to as "gradient magnetic fields."

The principal known biological effect from exposure to gradient magnetic fields is peripheral nerve stimulation (PNS). Other types of magnetically-induced stimulation (e.g., of the heart, retina or brain) do not occur at exposure levels currently encountered during MRI but will be considered briefly. Another important effect of the gradients is the generation of acoustic noise resulting from the Lorentz force. This is considered elsewhere in this textbook. In this chapter, the basic physical and physiological processes of magnetic stimulation, the properties of magnetic simulation, human PNS associated with MRI, models of induced electric fields, and the relevant patient exposure limits will be considered along with various issues requiring further research.

BASIC PHYSICS AND PHYSIOLOGY

Physics

The imaging gradients are defined as linear spatial variations in the z-component of the static magnetic field B_z, that is, along the axis of the MR system's bore, as follows:

$$G_x = dB_z/dx; \quad G_y = dB_z/dy; \quad G_z = dB_z/dz; \tag{1}$$

and are specified in millitesla per meter (mT/m). Within the imaging field of view, the gradients produce static magnetic fields whose z-axis components are additive to B_0:

$$B_z(x,y,z) = B_0 + x\,G_x + y\,G_y + z\,G_z \tag{2}$$

The gradients alter the Larmor frequency of the MR signal depending upon its source location. For example, with $G_x = 10$-mT/m at 0.2-m from the magnet isocenter, the field from the x-gradient is 2-mT. The maximum field experienced by the patient will depend upon the patient's size and the linearity of the gradients. However, the peak exposure may exceed the maximum specified value within the imaging field of view, or the specification volume because only the linear portion of the gradient field is utilized during MRI.

Gradient pulses are commonly applied as trapezoidal waveforms with durations of a few milliseconds, ramp times of typically 0.1 to 1.0-ms and amplitudes of up to, and in excess of, 50-mT/m (**Figure 1**). The gradient slew rate (SR), defined in T/m/sec., is given by:

$$SR = (G_+ + G_-)/t_{min} \tag{3}$$

Figure 1. Typical gradient waveform, showing amplitude and minimum ramp time. Slew rate is defined as $(G_+ + G_-)/t_{min}$.

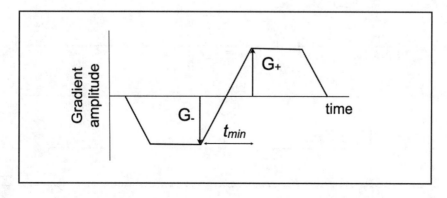

where G_+ and G_- are the maximum and minimum amplitudes and t_{min} is the minimum time to ramp between them. In modern scanners SR may reach 200-T/m/sec. for whole body gradient systems, and higher for head-only gradient inserts. In the example above, if the slew rate is 100-T/m/sec., the ramp time for one gradient lobe is 0.1-ms and the rate of change of field (dB/dt) is 20-T/sec.

In order to acquire an image, the gradient and RF pulses are arranged as a pulse sequence which is repeated with the repetition time (TR) (**Figure 2**). In the pulse sequence, the gradient pulses are denoted by their function in the image formation process (i.e., the slice selection, phase or frequency encoding). Depending on the anatomical orientation of the image section location, these may or may not correspond to the magnet axes x, y, and z, and thus, frequently the patient may be exposed to the simultaneous action of all three physical gradients G_x, G_y, G_z.

Faraday's law of induction forms the basis of the generation of induced fields in tissue:

$$\oint E_i \bullet dl = -\frac{d}{dt} \int_S B \times dS \qquad (4)$$

Figure 2. Example of a basic spin echo MRI pulse sequence, consisting of gradients (G_{SS}, G_{PE}, G_{FE}) and RF pulses with echo time (TE) and repetition time (TR).

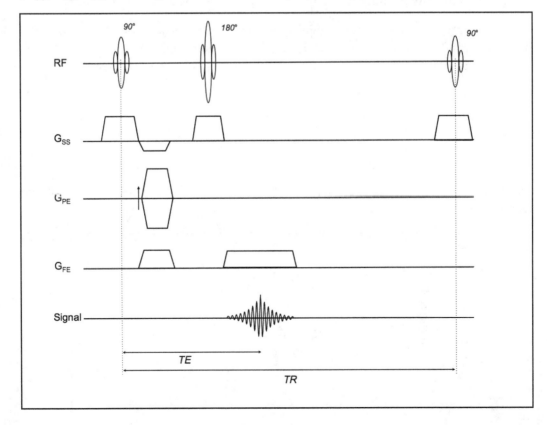

where E_i is the induced electric field around a closed path and dS is the differential area vector normal to the applied field. For a circular loop of radius r, in a uniform medium normal to the applied field (**Figure 3**) this simplifies to (1):

$$E_i = 0.5 \ r \ dB/dt \tag{5}$$

Thus, the largest induced electric field will occur in the patient's superficial tissues, and larger patients will experience higher induced fields. The induced electric field generates a current density J_i (A/m^2) in tissue:

$$J_i = \sigma \ E_i \tag{6}$$

where σ is the electrical conductivity of the tissue (S/m). Values in the range 0.1 to 0.2-S/m are often used for average body conductivity at low frequencies. For an elliptical body cross-section perpendicular to the magnetic field, the maximum current density is (2):

$$J_{max} = \frac{a^2 b}{a^2 + b^2} \sigma \ dB/dt \tag{7}$$

Figure 3. Induced electric field E, and current density J in a homogeneous medium arising from dB/dt from a typical gradient waveform.

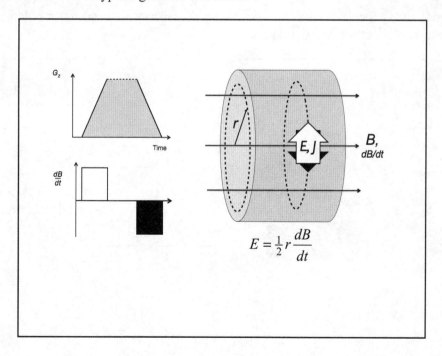

where *a* is the semi-major axial length and *b* is the semi-minor. As the gradients produce time-varying components of B_z, the orientation of the induced field and current will be generally orthogonal to the magnet axis but their distribution will depend upon the orientation of the applied gradient pulses.

The induced electric field and current density from a trapezoidal gradient pulse consists of two opposed polarity rectangular pulses separated by the gradient pulse plateau length (**Figure 3**). The induced current direction will therefore reverse as the gradient waveform returns to zero.

Physiology

Peripheral nerves are the portion of a spinal nerve distal to the root and plexus. They consist of bundles of nerve fibers of varying diameter from 0.3 to around 20-µm. The larger fibers convey motor, touch and proprioceptive impulses, while the smaller ones convey pain, temperature and autonomic impulses. The nerve fiber consists of the long axon surrounded by a myelin sheath that has periodic breaks, or Nodes of Ranvier. The axon electric potential is maintained, at rest, at around -70mV by the intra-extra cellular balance of sodium, potassium and chlorine ions (**Figure 4**). A change in the axon potential of +15-mV will result in the nerve firing, with the sodium channels opening to allow ingress of positive sodium ions, thus elevating the potential further, until the channels close. At this point the potassium channels open allowing egress of positive potassium ions until the resting potential of -70-mV is restored. Once stimulated, the impulse will be transmitted along the nerve. A refractory period inhibits further firing. Rapid repetitive stimulation may lead to accommodation, or a decrease in the magnitude of the response.

Figure 4. Ionic balance (sodium Na^+, Potassium K^+, chlorine Cl^-) and action potential for a peripheral nerve at rest and during excitation.

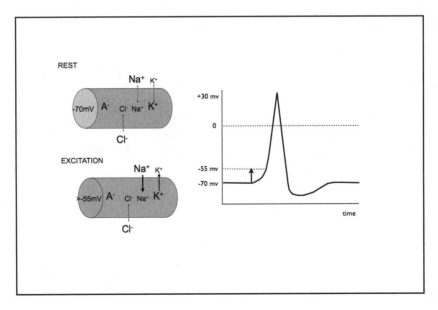

The physiology of electrical stimulation of nerves has been known for a very long time and is characterized by the strength-duration (SD) curve. Two basic forms of SD curves have been used: the earliest is the hyperbolic form of Weiss (3):

$$I_{thresh}(\tau) = I_{rheo} \left(1 + c/\tau \right) \tag{8}$$

where I_{thresh} is the threshold generator current (applied via electrodes) to cause stimulation and τ is the stimulus duration (for a rectangular pulse). The constant c is the chronaxie and is the stimulus duration required to double the threshold from its minimum value. This minimum value I_{rheo} is known as the rheobase and is asymptotic for long stimulus durations. The SD curve may also be described in terms of the more physiologically relevant electric field E in tissue or, in magnetic stimulation, by dB/dt (see dashed line in **Figure 5**).

The other common form of the SD curve is the exponential or Lapicque form (4):

$$I_{thresh}(\tau) = I_{rheo} / (1 - e^{-\tau/t_c}) \tag{9}$$

where t_c is the tissue time constant, shown for dB/dt as the solid line in **Figure 5**. Electrophysiologists have been arguing for years about the appropriate form of the SD curve. One theoretical advantage of the exponential form is that it produces the predicted response of a simple equivalent circuit of the nerve under the action of a rectangular current stimulus (**Figure 6**). Moreover, the tissue time constants can be theoretically derived from the fiber diameters (5). Time constants vary according to tissue type; peripheral motor nerves have time constants of the order of 0.1-ms, while cardiac muscle has t_c in the region 2- to 3-ms and synapses up to 25-ms. Based upon this equivalent circuit, the Spatially Extended Non-linear Node (SENN) model has been used extensively in electro-stimulation studies, and forms the theoretical basis for some patient exposure limits in MRI (6).

The specific agent of stimulation is usually considered to be the spatial gradient of the induced electric field. Nerve discontinuities such as bends or synaptic terminations (e.g., in muscle) effectively produce E-field spatial gradients, rendering them common stimulation sites.

In magnetic stimulation, the stimulus is usually considered to be dB/dt, which is directly proportional to the induced E_i in tissue. The exponential magnetic SD curve is (7):

$$(dB/dt)_{thresh}(\tau) = (dB/dt)_{rheo} / (1 - e^{-\tau/t_c}) \tag{10}$$

Figure 5. PNS strength-duration curve for magnetic stimulation redrawn from McRobbie and Foster (7). The dashed line is a fit to the hyperbolic SD curve, for which rheobase and chronaxie are shown. The solid line is a fit to the exponential form, resulting in a higher estimated rheobase. It is difficult to stimulate peripheral nerves for long pulse durations.

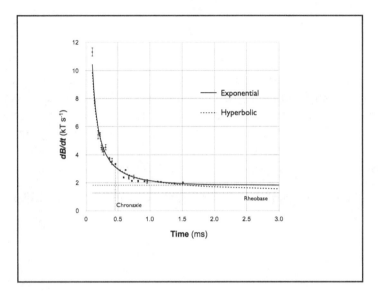

Figure 6. Simple electrical circuit representation of a myelinated nerve used in the SENN model (5, 6).

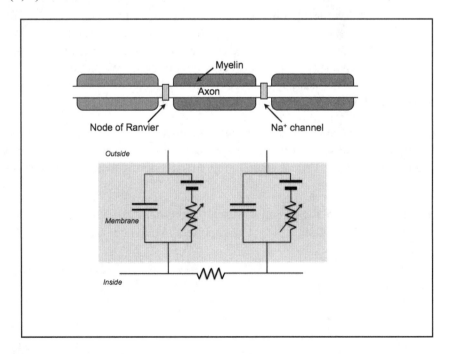

However, just as for electrical stimulation where the SD curve can be derived in terms of electrical charge Q (I = dQ/dt), one can consider the step change in magnetic field ΔB as the stimulus (8). The SD curve, now assuming its hyperbolic form, becomes linear for ΔB:

$$\Delta B(\tau) = \Delta B_{min}(1 + \tau/c) \tag{11}$$

where ΔB_{min} is the minimum change in magnetic field for an infinitely short stimulus, that is, an infinite dB/dt. Although not obviously intuitive, this latter formulation is instructive for comparing diverse physiological effects and stimuli. Glover (9) has also commented upon the role of ΔB for static field effects such as metallic taste and vertigo.

In a further development Chronik and Rutt (10) derived the law of stimulation in terms of the imaging gradient parameters:

$$\Delta G(\Delta t) = SR_{min} \, c + \Delta G_{min} \tag{12}$$

where SR_{min} is the smallest stimulating slew rate for infinitely long pulse durations, ΔG_{min} is the smallest stimulating gradient excursion for infinitely short pulse durations, and c is the chronaxie. This can be represented diagrammatically (**Figure 7**) where the gradient coil technical performance is shown in terms of its slew rate limitation and its amplitude limitation. The PNS threshold has a linear form and can easily be used to predict the PNS-limited region of the gradient's operation.

MAGNETIC STIMULATION

One of the most sensitive and earliest observed forms of magnetic stimulation was that of magneto-phosphenes, as reported in 1896 by d'Arsonval (11) (**Figure 8**), perceived by the subject as faint flashes of light, and which are thought to originate from stimulation of the retina or the optic nerve. Kavet, et al. (12) provided a review of the magneto-phosphene literature, but from these only two or three publications present sufficient dosimetric information to deduce accurate thresholds and frequency response. Losvund (13) conducted the most extensive of these studies, reporting a minimum threshold of 12-mT root mean square (RMS) in the frequency range 20- to 45-Hz, depending upon the ambient light conditions and dark-adaption of the subjects. **Figure 9** summarizes the available quantitative data on magneto-phosphenes.

Direct magnetic stimulation of nerves was first demonstrated *in vitro* by Oberg (14) in 1973, resulting in a measurable twitch of the gastrocnemius muscle of the frog suspended in Ringer's solution. In 1982, Polson, et al. (15) were the first to demonstrate human peripheral nerve stimulation *in vivo* using a small diameter topical solenoidal coil powered by a capacitance discharge system. They estimated an induced current density of 20-A/m²

Figure 7. Gradient performance and PNS limitations redrawn from Chronik and Rutt (10). The shaded region is where peripheral nerve stimulation is likely to occur.

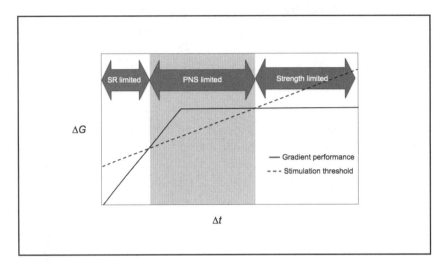

Figure 8. Magneto-phosphene experiments of Arsene d'Asonval, Paris 1896 (11).

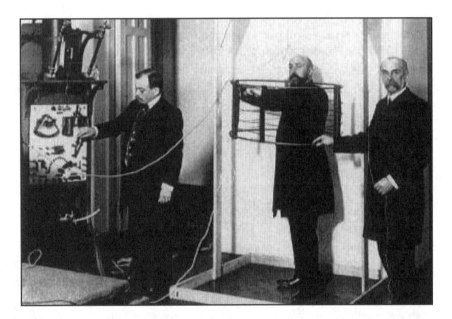

and demonstrated the stimulus-response curve from threshold to supra-maximal (when all the fibers in the bundle have been recruited). The topical magnetic stimulation technique was subsequently applied by Barker, et al. (16) to the motor cortex of the brain, and forms the basis of transcranial magnetic stimulation (TMS).

McRobbie and Foster (7) first demonstrated the strength-duration curve from topical stimulation of the median nerve in 1984 using electro-myography (EMG) to determine reproducible thresholds (**Figure 5**). They fitted an exponential form of the SD curve with a

Figure 9. Magneto-phosphene thresholds from the literature, derived from Kavet, et al. (12). The data from Barlow were assumed to be peak to peak. All stimuli were sinusoidal waveforms with results shown as rms.

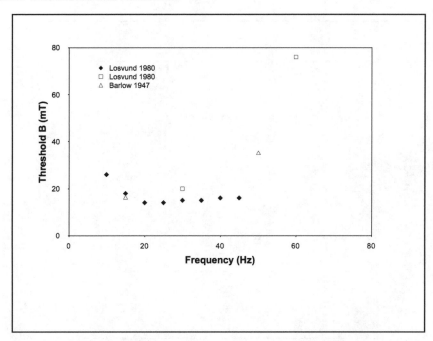

time constant of 0.47-ms and an estimated J rheobase of 3.6-A/m^2, corresponding to an estimated E_{rheo} of 12-V/m. McRobbie and Foster (7) also demonstrated that, contrary to expectations, the biphasic damped sinusoidal pulse produced by their capacitance discharge system was a more effective stimulus than mono-phasic pulses (**Figure 10**). Additionally, they showed an inverse correlation between threshold stimulus and limb diameter for stimulation of the forearm surrounded by a Helmholtz coil. Reilly (5) has further reviewed some of the early magnetic stimulation literature.

Magnetic stimulation of the phrenic nerve in humans, resulting in respiratory disruption, has been reported by Mouchwar, et al. (17) using a damped sinusoidal pulse from a topical coil with a frequency of 853-Hz. In later work, the median canine respiration threshold for a 0.53-ms pulse was shown to be around 900-T/sec. (18).

Direct cardiac stimulation is more difficult to achieve due to the longer time constants of cardiac muscle and the smaller induction paths around the organ. Early attempts with small coil systems produced violent muscular contractions and estimated current densities in the range 5 to 20-A/m^2 but without any detected cardiac arrhythmias in rats (19, 20). Nevertheless, Bourland, et al. (21) achieved trans-chest magnetic simulation of the dog heart, producing ectopic beats but not ventricular fibrillation, with an estimated induced electric field of 50-V/m and a median threshold dB/dt of 2,700-T/sec. for a 0.53-ms pulse. Using a tissue time constant of 3-ms, a rheobase of 400-T/sec. can be extrapolated. Yamaguchi, et al. (22) showed similar results with an estimated E_{rheo} of 55- to 340-V/m. Cohen, et al. (23) did not detect any changes in the electrocardiogram (ECG) of canines exposed to up to 66-T/sec. using a human whole body gradient system. The cardiac stimulation dB/dt

Figure 10. Pulse shape dependence. Bipolar damped sinusoidal pulses are shown to have lower dB/dt thresholds than unipolar pulses with a similar waveform. Adapted from reference 7.

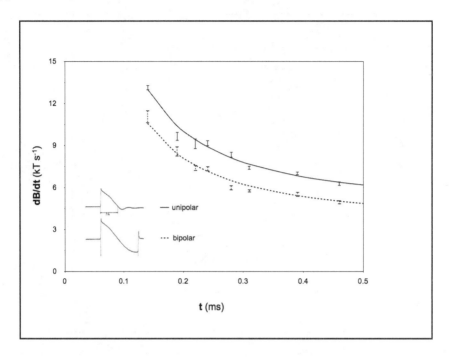

rheobase for the most sensitive percentile of the population has been theoretically estimated as 62-T/sec. (24). It is thought that at least 50 times the electrical stimulus for cardiac stimulation is required to cause ventricular fibrillation (25). Exposure of pregnant mice to dB/dt of up to 3,600-T/sec. at 2.2-kHz caused significant muscular contractions but showed no effect on the litter size or teratogenicity (2).

PERIPHERAL NERVE STIMULATION FROM THE MRI-RELATED GRADIENT MAGNETIC FIELDS

PNS associated with MRI gradient magnetic fields was first reported by Cohen, et al. (23) and Budinger, ct al. (26). Initially, the possibility of PNS was limited to high slew rate specialist gradient systems, based upon capacitance discharge technology, for echo planar imaging (EPI). The advent of improved linear amplifiers for the MRI gradients has resulted in a much greater likelihood of patients experiencing stimulation. For example, Vogt, et al. (27) exposed 210 patients to gradient slew rates of 120% of the International Electrotechnical Commission (IEC) limit for PNS (28) using a rapid gradient echo (FLASH) sequence. For this study group, 16.7% reported PNS with 2.9% reporting very uncomfortable stimulation. There are a number of excellent reviews of PNS and MRI-related gradient magnetic fields including those by Glover (9) and Schaefer, et al. (29).

The Purdue University group (18, 30) has published extensive studies of MRI gradient stimulation using y- (anatomically aligned anterior-posterior) and z-gradient coil systems

Figure 11. Individual SD curves from y- and z-gradients showing perception (score = 1), discomfort (score = 5) and intolerable stimulation (score = 10) from Nyenhuis, et al. (30). In this experiment the y-axis refers to the AP direction. The solid lines are fitted to the hyperbolic SD curve. Reproduced with permission.

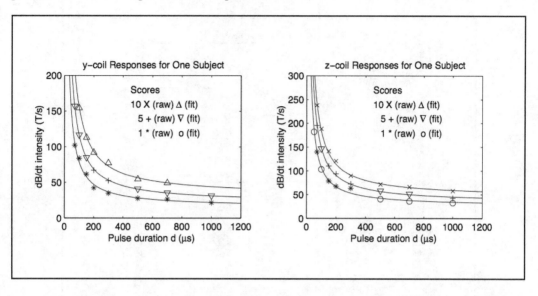

external to the bore of the MR system. **Figure 11** shows SD curves for an individual subject's subjective reporting of three levels of stimulation (1 = threshold, 5 = uncomfortable, 10 = intolerable) fitted to the hyperbolic form. The subjects (n = 84) reported uncomfortable stimulation at about 50% higher exposure than for the threshold, and about 100% higher than threshold for intolerable. Pooling these data, one can calculate a stimulus or dose response curve and a population SD curve (**Figure 12**). For perception the median dB/dt rheobases were 15-T/sec. for the y-gradient and 26-T/sec. for x with similar chronaxies (0.37-ms, 0.38-ms). The stimulus was a train of 64 trapezoidal gradient lobes, resulting in 128 rectangular dB/dt pulses of duration 0.05 to 1.0-ms. Using dB/dt pulse lengths of 0.2- and 0.5-ms, there was no correlation between subject height, sex or age on stimulation threshold. Limited correlation of girth and threshold for the z-gradient coil was observed but not evaluated statistically. Abart, et al. (31) also noted lack of correlation of stimulus threshold with age, body surface, and sex.

Many other authors have investigated peripheral nerve stimulation (PNS) perception thresholds for various combinations of axes on whole body MRI gradient systems (32-36). Rheobases and chronaxies from these studies are shown in **Table 1**. Given the range of combinations of waveforms, axes and coil designs, there is a striking consistency across these results. Taking the weighted mean from these studies, we arrive at an average dB/dt rheobase of 19.4-T/m/sec. and a chronaxie of 0.42-ms. Using equations (6), (7) and (11) with a=0.4-m, b=0.2-m and σ =0.2-S/m one can deduce the rheobase for E_i, and J to be in the region of 3.1-V/m and 0.62-A/m^2 with a ΔB_{min} of 8.1-mT.

Table 2 shows a summary of PNS studies using the alternative gradient formulation of the SD curve (33, 36-40). Excluding the results from Feldman, et al. (40) who used planar

Figure 12. Pooled results from a human PNS experiment (Nyenhuis, et al.). *Top.* The group stimulus-response curves for perception, discomfort and intolerable stimulation. *Bottom.* From the above, the median population SD curves may be derived, fitted to a hyperboic SD curve. Reproduced with permission.

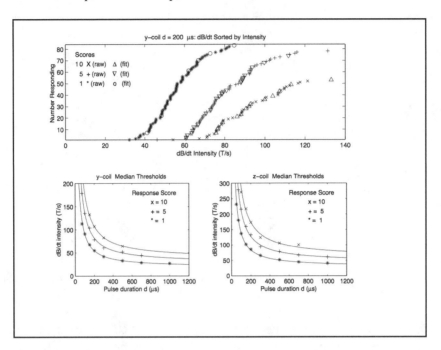

coils, the weighted average minimum stimulating slew rate was 59.3-T/m/s, the minimum gradient amplitude (at infinite slew rate) for stimulation was 35.4-mT/m with a mean chronaxie of 0.69-ms. A notable observation from Zhang, et al. (36) is that there appears to be a dependence of the chronaxie on the coil dimension. The results from Feldman, et al. (40) show that huge increases in gradient coil performance without causing PNS are achievable, and secondly, that the chronaxie appears to have some dependence upon the coil design, and not just physiologic factors. As with earlier experiments, the linear SD formulation found no convincing correlation with anatomical measurements, including weight, height, girth, and average body fat percentage (39) although a weak correlation between ΔG_{min} and the effective radius was reported (**Figure 13**).

Hoffman, et al. (37) used EMG to determine responses to gradient stimulation. They concluded that EMG thresholds and perception thresholds were equally reproducible with standard deviations of 2.1- and 2.0-mT/m, respectively, and a difference of only 0.45-mT/m, the subjective threshold being the lower. Weinberg, et al. (41) investigated ultra high dB/dt, high frequency (> 100 kHz) pulses, using a topical coil, and reported a significantly reduced probability for stimulation at these frequencies (**Figure 14**). They concluded that ultra-short pulses (were the technology available) in whole body gradient systems are unlikely to cause PNS despite very high dB/dt.

Table 1. Literature results for gradient coil PNS perception thresholds and chronaxies using the hyperbolic formulation of the SD curve. The mean values are weighted for number of subjects, N. The column ΔB is calculated from equation (11).

	Reference	Waveform	N	Axis	dB/dt (T/sec.)	ΔB (mT)	c (ms)
Irnich and Schmitt	8	Sinusoid	1	Z	18.0	9.9	0.55
Bourland	18	Trap 128	84	Y	14.9	5.4	0.37
			84	Z	26.2	9.9	0.38
Den Boer, et al.	34	Trap	153	Y	18.8	6.8	0.36
Hebrank, et al.	35	Trap 128	65	Y	16.3	8.6	0.52
			65	XY	18.6	8.7	0.47
			65	XYZ	20.1	10.2	0.51
Zhang, et al.	36	Trap 64	20	XY	24.7	11.1	0.53
MEAN					19.4	8.1	0.42

EXPOSURE LIMITS

Most standards for patient exposure during MRI utilize PNS SD data derived theoretically or from direct measurement in volunteers according to a defined protocol (28, 42, 43). The Normal Mode of Operation for an MR system is defined as 80% of the median perception threshold for PNS. The First Level Controlled Operating Mode is defined as 100% of the median perception threshold. Where MR system-specific experimental data is unavailable, theoretical data may be used. The International Electrotechnical Commission (IEC) standard 60601-2-33 3rd Edition uses a theoretical dB/dt rheobase (rb) of 20-T/sec. with a chronaxie of 0.36-ms for PNS, giving its normal mode (L01) and first level controlled mode (L12) limits:

$$L12 = 1.0 \times rb \ (1+0.36 \ / t_{eff}) \tag{13}$$

$$L01 = 0.8 \times rb \ (1+0.36 \ / t_{eff}) \tag{14}$$

where t_{eff} is the duration of the dB/dt pulse. Alternatively, an E-field rheobase of 2.2-V/m may be used. Gradient weighting-factors are applied to the scanner's stimulation pre-

Table 2. Literature results for gradient coil PNS perception thresholds and chronaxies using the Chronik and Rutt formulation of the SD curve as in equation (12). The results of Feldman, et al. (40) were for planar coils and are excluded from the weighted mean calculation. N is the number of subjects. The results for Zhang, et al. (36) were for 48[1], 40[2] and 35[3] cm DSV coils.

	Reference	Waveform	N	Axis	SR_{min} T(m/sec.)	G_{min} (T/m)	c (ms)
Ham, et al.	33	Sinusoid	4	Z	41.5	34	0.81
Zhang, et al.	36	Trap 64	20	XY [1]	66.8	24.7	0.37
			20	XY [2]	75.4	34.0	0.45
			20	XY [3]	77.0	40.5	0.53
Hoffman, et al.	37	Trap	14	Y	26.0	20.8	1.03
Chronik, et al.	38	Trap	20	XY	62.2	44.4	0.77
Chronik, et al.	39	Trap	18	XY	50.1	48.5	1.054
Feldman, et al.	40	Trap	14	X	252	218	0.87
			14	Y	222	147	0.66
			14	Z	210	133	0.63
MEAN					59.3	35.4	0.69

diction monitor to account for the different sensitivities of each axis: $W_{AP} = 1.0$, $W_{LR} = 0.8$, $W_{HF} = 0.7$ where AP, HF, and LR are the anatomical orientations of the gradient axes. This results in a modified limiting SD curve:

$$\sqrt{(\sum_i (w_i (dB/dt)_i)^2} < 20(1+0.36/t_{eff}) \tag{15}$$

For cardiac stimulation, the exponential form is used with a cardiac time constant of 3-ms and a dB/dt rheobase of 20-T/sec. or an induced electric field rheobase of 2-V/m. The IEC limits are shown in **Figure 15**. In the United States (U.S.) the Food and Drug Administration (FDA) does not specify numerical limits, but advocates that uncomfortable or painful PNS be avoided (44). Exposure limits are considered in greater detail in other chapters in this textbook.

Figure 13. Experimental values of ΔG_{min} and effective loop radius R_{ax} plotted for 37 subjects fitted to a power law function. Reproduced with permission from reference 39.

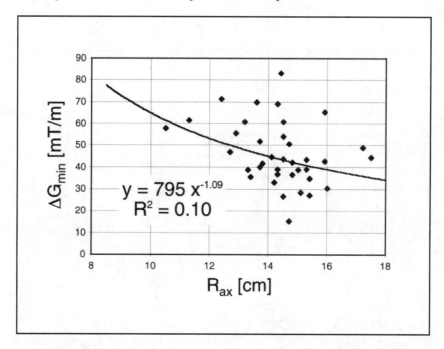

Figure 14. Probability of PNS sensation at various frequencies, at magnitude 0.4-T. Error bars correspond to exact confidence intervals with 95% power. Data points are labeled with frequency values. Reproduced with permission from reference 41.

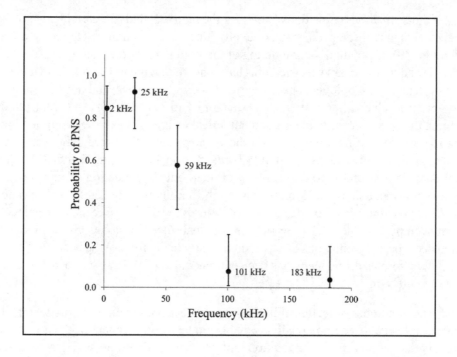

Figure 15. IEC limits for cardiac stimulation and normal mode (L01) and first level controlled mode (L12) for peripheral nerve stimulation. t_{eff} is the effective duration of the field change.

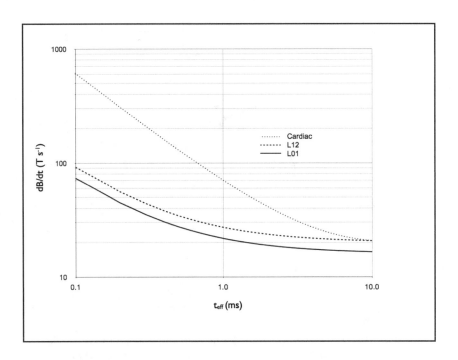

MODELING OF INDUCED CURRENT DENSITIES

The simple equations (Equations 5 to 7) for the induced field and current are only useful in idealized, but unrealistic geometries, or to provide an understanding of the basic principles of induction (39). Computational modeling of the field interactions using realistic anatomical models and gradient coil specifications have shown that the induced E-field and current densities are highly inhomogeneous for various body geometries, and not as strongly correlated with the induced field patterns as Equations 5 to 7 would suggest (45). Both quasi-static finite difference or finite integration numerical techniques have been applied (46-48). **Figure 16** reproduced from reference (47) shows the pattern of induced E-field arising from a planar y-gradient coil with dB/dt of 100-T/m/sec. So, et al. (48) used actual PNS experimental data from y- and z-gradient coils with theoretical calculation of induced electric fields in subcutaneous fat and skin, estimating the stimulation thresholds in the range 3.6 to 5.8-V/m, close the SENN model predicted value of 6.2-V/m. Recently, strong correlations between peak induced electric field in a human model in a head/neck gradient coil and subjects' reported stimulation sites, predominantly in the front of the head, in the vicinity of the sinuses, forehead, and teeth, has been demonstrated (49). Peak induced E-fields were estimated as 40-V/m.

There are a number of technical limitations to electromagnetic field modeling such as the proprietary details of commercially available gradient coil geometries, the use of a single sinusoidal gradient waveform, the requirement for computation time-saving strategies such

Figure 16. Results of computer simulation of the induced electric fields from whole body magnetic field gradients. Calculation of the induced electric fields inside the human whole-body model excited by a typical planar gradient y-coil with a slew rate of dB/dz/dt=100-T/m/sec., at a frequency of 1 kHz. Reproduced with permission from reference 47.

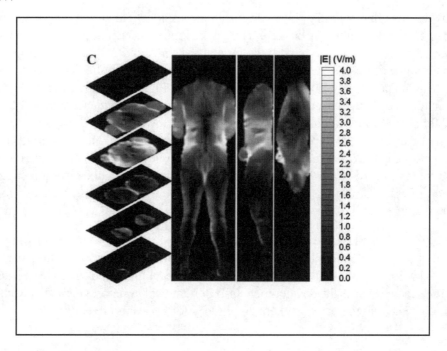

as frequency scaling, the spatial resolution of the model, and partial volume effects where tissues are mixed within a voxel. Notwithstanding these issues, computational modeling has provided various insights into the induced electric fields and current densities and their role in peripheral nerve stimulation.

REMAINING CONTROVERSIES

From the perspective of patient safety in the MRI setting, sufficient well-controlled experimental data exist to support appropriate safety standards and limits, and to alert MR system operators to the likelihood of stimulation arising from specific MRI acquisitions or techniques. Recently, the literature has raised or revisited a number of controversies, reviewed in this section.

The first issue is which form of the SD curve to use, with researchers apparently divided between the hyperbolic and exponential. When considering the available data, is it possible to determine once and for all which is the most appropriate form? Taking the exponential model, for very short stimulus durations, much less than the tissue time constant ($\tau < t_c$) we obtain:

$$\Delta B_{thresh} = \left(\frac{dB}{dt} \right)_{rheo} t_c \qquad\qquad (16)$$

This implies that for very short stimuli, the threshold field step to cause stimulation should be the product of the rheobase and the tissue time constant (i.e., the threshold is itself constant). By contrast, in the hyperbolic model, the threshold ΔB decreases linearly to a minimum value for $t = 0$. **Figure 5** presents fits to both hyperbolic and exponential SD curves using data re-analyzed under both models (7). **Figure 17** shows the linearized SD curve, in terms of B field excursion, where there appears to be evidence of a constant B of 0.17-T for short stimuli in this particular experiment. However, Havel, et al. (50) reported a slightly better fit for the hyperbolic SD curve using an effectively monopolar dB/dt stimulus. Whole-body gradient studies that favor the hyperbolic SD curve lack the short duration threshold data to distinguish between the forms. Studies of ultra short stimuli suggest an elevation of dB/dt thresholds, hence a breaking down of the SD characteristics for ultra high frequency stimuli (41) as shown in **Figure 14** and which is as yet unexplained.

The form of the SD curve matters for two reasons, one is that the estimation of rheobase is different for the two models, and therefore affects the determination of limits. The IEC limits for PNS are based on the hyperbolic and, therefore, more conservative rheobase for PNS. The second issue is the development of faster gradient systems, where the exponential SD curve would allow greater gradient amplitudes for very short rise times.

Figure 17. Adaption of data from reference 7 showing an arguably constant stimulating B for short pulse durations (filled symbols).

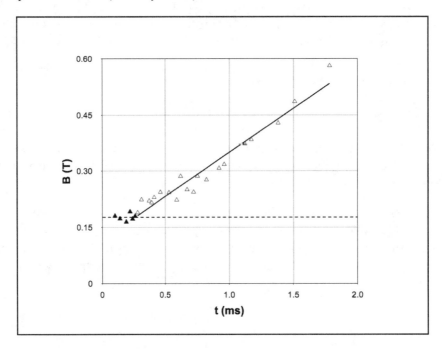

The second controversy surrounds the form of the stimulus waveform. It has been a constant prediction of the SENN model, used for electrical stimulation, that monophasic pulses are more effective stimuli than biphasic pulses (5, 6). This assertion of the SENN model is backed up experimentally in magnetic stimulation by some work by Irnich and Schmitt (8) but with limited data. Havel, et al. (50) varied the plateau length of a trapezoidal B waveform, effectively generating bi- and uni-polar dB/dt pulses and reported no difference in thresholds. However, there is also a considerable body of evidence from the earliest magneto-stimulation work (7), from the TMS literature (51, 52) and the recent ultra-high slew rate studies (53) that bipolar magnetic pulses from damped sinusoidal waveforms have lower stimulation thresholds than similarly shaped uni-polar pulses. A solution to this apparent contradiction is offered by the ΔB linear SD formulation, in which a biphasic pulse will have a greater ΔB excursion than a monophasic pulse, and therefore lower dB/dt thresholds.

The third controversy is over the reported values of chronaxies or nerve time constants. In the SENN model, a 20-um nerve fiber is shown to have a theoretical time constant of 0.12-ms (5). However, MRI-related gradient PNS chronaxies lie in the range of 0.37- to 1.05-ms, with a range of 0.3- to 0.65-ms reported for topical PNS. In carefully devised experiments, Rescoskie, et al. (54, 55) demonstrated large discrepancies in chronaxies from electrical and topical magnetic stimulation of the ulner nerve for both perception and EMG thresholds. Perception chronaxies were 0.024 ± 0.02-ms for electrical stimulation, against 0.67 ± 0.18-ms for magnetic stimulation. A confounding factor is the huge variation (thirty times) in reported electrical stimulation chronaxies. This raises issues about the validity of applying electrical stimulation data to formulate limits for time-varying magnetic fields.

An additional question arising from this is the possibility that there may be a non-Faradaic component to magnetic stimulation (56, 57). However, the fit of the data with the standard induction model is very good, and it is more likely that the discrepancy between magnetic and electrical stimulation arises because they are not the same. Notably, their methods of producing the required electric fields in tissue are physically different.

The final point is not really controversial, just misunderstood. Regulators and standard bodies have used magneto-phosphenes as the most sensitive reproducible sensory affect (58). Subsequently occupational and public limits have been anchored by magneto-phosphene data, which we have seen is sparse and mostly lacking rigorous dosimetry. The best data gives ΔB_{min} of around 30-mT (peak-to-peak) for magneto-phosphenes, while that for PNS from whole body gradient systems is around 8-mT. PNS, and not magneto-phosphenes, is the most sensitive sensory effect of time-varying magnetic fields. Regulators may need to modify their methodologies accordingly.

CONCLUSIONS

Despite the uncertainties outlined above, there is sufficient data from well-conducted human exposure studies with whole-body MRI gradient systems, to have a very high degree of confidence in the stimulation prediction algorithms of clinical MR scanners. These studies consistently show dB/dt rheobases for perception of around 20-T/sec., with a ΔB_{min} of around 8-mT. The y-gradient (anterior-posterior) is the most effective for stimulation with a rheobase in the range 15 to 19-T/sec. and measured chronaxies are remarkably similar across many different experiments. The threshold for discomfort or pain from PNS is about 50 to 100% higher than the perception threshold, and not generally achievable in clinical MR systems. The longer time constant for cardiac muscle and the smaller conduction loops around the heart make direct cardiac stimulation extremely unlikely.

The new understanding of the mechanism of PNS gained from the linearizing of the strength-duration curve offers the prospect of higher gradient performance with less stimulation, while further studies of ultra-short rise time pulses are also likely to aid the design of higher slew rate gradients in future MR systems. However, the issue of acoustic noise related to gradient magnetic fields remains.

ACKNOWLEDGEMENTS

Special thanks to John Nyenhuis, Joe Bourland and Alexander Kildishev of Purdue University, Lafayette, IN and Daniel (Joe) Schaefer of General Electric Medical Systems, Milwaukee, WI for assistance with certain figures used in this chapter.

REFERENCES

1.   Budinger TF. Thresholds for physiological effects due to RF and magnetic fields used in NMR imaging. IEEE Trans Nucl Sci 1979;NS-26:2821-2825.

2.   McRobbie D, Foster MA. Pulsed magnetic field exposure during pregnancy and implications for NMR foetal imaging: A study with mice. Magn Reson Imaging 1985; 3:231-234.

3.   Weiss G. Sur la possibility de rendre comparables entre eux les appareils servant a l'excitation electrique. Arch Ital Biol 1901;35: 413-46.

4.   Lapicque L. Recherches quantitatifs sur l'excitation electrique des nerfs traite comme un polarisation. J Physiol Paris 1907;9:622-35.

5.   Reilly JP. Peripheral nerve stimulation by induced electric current: Exposure to time-varying magnetic fields. Med. Bio Eng Comput 1989;27:101-110.

6.   Reilly JP, Diamant AM. Electrostimulation: Theory, Applications, and Computational Mode. Norwood, MA USA: Artech House; 2011.

7.   McRobbie D, Foster MA. Thresholds for biological effects of magnetic fields. Clin Phys Physiol Meas 1984;5:67-78.

8.   Irnich W, Schmitt F. Magnetostimulation in MRI. Magn Reson Med 1995;33:619-623.

9.   Glover PM. Interaction of MRI field gradients with the human body. Phys Med Biol 2009; 54:R99-R115.

10. Chronik BA, Rutt BK. Simple linear formulation for magnetostimulation specific to MRI gradient coils. Magn Reson Med 2001;45:916-919.

11. D'Arsonval A. Dispositifs pour la mesure des courants alternatifs de toutes frequences. Compt Rend Soc Biol 1896;3:450-451.

12. Kavet R, Hailey WH, Bracken TD, Patterson RM. Recent advances in research relevant to electric and magnetic field exposure guidelines. Bioelectromagnetics 2008;29:499-525.

13. Lovsund P, Oberg PA, Nilsson SEG. Magnetophosphenes: A quantitative analysis of thresholds. Med Biol Eng Comput 1980;18:326-334.

14. Oberg PA. Magnetic stimulation of nerve tissue. Med Biol Eng Comput 1973;55:64.

15. Polson MJ, Barker AT, Freeston IL. Stimulation of nerve trunks with time-varying magnetic fields. Med Bio Eng Comput 1982;20:243-244.

16. Barker AT, Freeston IL, Jalinous R, Jarratt JA. Magnetic stimulation of human brain and peripheral nervous system: an introduction and the results of an initial clinical evaluation. Neurosurgery 1987;20:100-109.

17. Mouchawar G, Bourland JD, Voorhees WD, Geddes LA. Stimulation of inspiratory motor nerves with a pulsed magnetic field. Med Biol Eng Comput 1990; 28:613.

18. Bourland JD, Nyenhuis JA, Schaefer DJ. Physiologic effects of intense MR imaging gradient fields. Neuroimaging Clin N Am 1999;9:363-377.

19. McRobbie D, Foster MA Cardiac response to pulsed magnetic fields with regard to safety in NMR imaging. Phys Med Biol 1985;30:695-702.

20. Polson MJR, Barker AT, Gardner S. The effect of rapid rise-time magnetic fields on the ECG of the rat. Clin Phys Physiol Meas 1982;3:231-234.

21. Bourland JD, Mouchawar, Geddes LA, et al. Trans chest magnetic (eddy current) stimulation of the dog heart. Med Biol Eng Comput 1990;28:196-198.

22. Yamaguchi M, Andoh T, Goto T, et al. Effects of strong pulsed magnetic field on the cardiac activity of an open chest dog. IEEE Trans BioMed Eng 1994;41:1188-1191.

23. Cohen MS, Weisskopf MR, Rzedian RR, et al. Sensory stimulation by time varying magnetic field. Magn Reson Med 1990;14:409-414.

24. Reilly JP. Peripheral nerve and cardiac excitation by time-varying magnetic fields: a comparison of thresholds. NY Acad of Sci 1992;649:96-117.

25. Reilly JP. Neuroelectric mechanisms applied to low frequency electric and magnetic field exposure guidelines – part 1: sinusoidal waveforms. Health Physics 2002;83:341-355.

26. Budinger TF, Fischer H, Hentschel D, et al. Physiologic effects of fast oscillating magnetic field gradients. J Comput Assist Tomogr 1991;15:609-614.

27. Vogt FM, Ladd ME, Hunold P, et al. Increased time rate of change of gradient fields: effect on peripheral nerve stimulation at clinical MR imaging. Radiology 2004;233:548-554.

28. International Electrotechnical Commission. Medical Electrical Equipment – Part 2-33: Particular Requirements for the Safety of Magnetic Resonance Equipment for Medical Diagnosis. IEC 60601-2-33 3rd Edition. Geneva: IEC, 2009.

29. Schaefer DJ, Bourland JD, Nyenhuis JA. Review of patient safety ion time-varying magnetic fields. J Mag Res Imaging 2000;12:20-29.

30. Nyenhuis JA, Bourland JD, Kildishec AV. Health Effects and Safety of Intense MRI Gradient Magnetic Fields. In: Shellock FG, Editor. Magnetic Resonance Procedures: Health Effects and Safety. Boca Raton, USA: CRC Press, 2001.

31. Abart J, Eberhardt K, Fischer H, et al. Pepripheral nerve stimulation by time-varying magnetic fields. J Comput Assist Tomogr 1997;21:523-538.

32. Ehrhardt JC, Lin CS, Magnotta VA, Fisher DJ, Yuh WT. Peripheral nerve stimulation in a whole-body echo-planar imaging system. J Magn Reson Imaging 1997;7:405-409.

33. Ham CL, Engels JM, van de Wiel GT, Machielsen A. Peripheral nerve stimulation during MRI: effects of high gradient amplitudes and switching rates. J Magn Reson Imaging 1997;7:933-937.

34. Den Boer JA, Bourland JD, Nyenhuis JA, et al. Comparison of the threshold for peripheral nerve stimulation during gradient switching in whole body MR systems. J Magn Reson Imaging 2002;15:520-525.

35. Hebrank FX, Gebhardt M. SAFE-Model – a new method for predicting peripheral nerve stimulation in MRI. In: Proceedings of the Joint Annual Meeting of the International Society for Magnetic Resonance in Medicine and the European Society for Magnetic Resonance in Medicine and Biology, 19-25 May 2007, Berlin. Berkeley CA, USA: 2007.

36. Zhang B, Yen YF, Chronik BA, et al. Peripheral nerve stimulation properties of head and body gradient coils of various sizes. Magn Reson Med 2003;50:50-58.

37. Hoffmann A, Faber SC, Werhahn KJ , Jager L, Reiser M. Electromyography in MRI - first recordings of peripheral nerve stimulation caused by fast magnetic field gradients. Magn Reson Med 2000;43:534-539.

38. Chronik BA, Rutt BK. A comparison between human magnetostimulation thresholds in whole-body and head/neck gradient coils. Magn Reson Med 2001;46:386-94

39. Chronik BA, Ramachandran MJ. Simple anatomical measurements do not correlate significantly to individual peripheral nerve stimulation thresholds as measured in MRI gradient coils. Magn Reson Imaging 2003;17:716-21.

40. Feldman RE, Hardy CJ, Aksel B, Schenck J, Chronik BA. Experimental determination of human peripheral nerve stimulation thresholds in a 3-axis planar gradient system. Magn Reson Med 2009;62:763-70.

41. Weinberg IN, Stepanov PY, Fricke S, et al. Increasing the oscillation frequency of strong magnetic fields above 101 kHz significantly raises peripheral nerve excitation thresholds. Med Phys 2012;39:2578-2583.

42. Health Protection Agency. Protection of patients and volunteers undergoing MRI procedures. Documents of the Health Protection Agency RCE-7, Chilton, UK: Health Protection Agency, 2008.

43. International Commission on Non-Ionizing Radiation Protection. Medical magnetic resonance (MR) procedures: protection of patients. Health Phys 2004;87 197-216.

44. Food and Drugs Administration. Criteria for significant risk investigations of magnetic resonance diagnostic devices. Rockville, MD: Center for Devices and Radiological Health, U.S. Food and Drug Administration, 2003.

45. Bencsik M, Bowtell R, Bowley R. Electric fields induced in the human body by time-varying magnetic field gradients in MRI: numerical calculations and correlation analysis. Phys Med Biol 2007;52:2337-53.

46. Zhao H, Crozier S, Lui F. Finite difference time domain (FDTD) method for modeling the effect of switched gradients on the human body in MRI. Magn Reson Med 2002;48:1037-42.

47. Liu F, Crozier S. A distributed equivalent magnetic current based FDTD method for the calculation of E-fields induced by gradient coils. J Magn Reson Imaging 2004;169:323-327.

48. So PP, Stuchly MA, Nyenhuis JA. Peripheral nerve stimulation by gradient switching fields in magnetic resonance imaging. IEEE Trans Biomed Eng 2004;51:1907-14.

49. Feldman RE, Odengaard J, Handler WR, Chronik BA. Simulation of head-gradient-coil induced electric fields in a human model. Magn Reson Med 2012;68:1973-82.

50. Havel WJ, Nyenhuis JA, Bourland DJ, et al. Comparison of rectangular and damped sinusoidal dB/dt waveforms in magnetic stimulation. IEEE Trans Magnetics 1997;33:4269-71.

51. Maccabee PJ, Amassian VE, Cracco RQ, Cadwell JA. An analysis of peripheral motor nerve stimulation in humans using the magnetic coil. Electroencephalogr Clin Neurophysiol 1988;70:524-3

52. Claus D, Murray NM, Spitzer A, Flugel D. The influence of stimulus type on the magnetic excitation of nerve structures. Electroencephalogr Clin Neurophysiol 1990;75:342-9.

53. Weinberg IN, Stepanov P, Glidden SC, et al. Threshold for peripheral nerve stimulation with ultra-fast gradients. Proceedings of the International Society for Magnetic Resonance in Medicine 2011;19:1787.

54. Recoskie BJ, Scholl TJ, Chronik BA. The discrepancy between human peripheral nerve chronaxie times as measured using magnetic and electric field stimuli: The relevance to MRI gradient coil safety. Phys Med Biol 2009;54:5965-79.

55. Recoskie BJ, Scholl TJ, Zinke-Allmang M, Chronik BA. Sensory and motor stimulation thresholds of the ulnar nerve from electrical and magnetic field stimuli: implications to gradient coil operation. Magn Reson Med 2010;64:1567-79.

56. Forbes LK, Crozier S. On a possible mechanism for peripheral nerve stimulation during magnetic resonance imaging scans. Phys Med Biol 2001;46:591-608.

57. Mao W, Chronik BA, Feldmman RE, et al. Consideration of magnetically-induced and conservative electric fields within a loaded gradient coil. Magn Reson Med 2006;55:1424-32.

58. International Commission on Non-Ionizing Radiation Protection. ICNIRP statement on the "Guidelines for limiting exposure to time-varying electric, magnetic, and electromagnetic fields (1 Hz to 100 kHz)". Health Physics 2009; 93:257-258.

Chapter 4 Acoustic Noise Associated With MRI Procedures

MARK McJURY, PH.D.

Department of Clinical Physics and Bio-Engineering
Beatson Cancer Centre
Glasgow, Scotland
United Kingdom

INTRODUCTION

During the operation of the magnetic resonance (MR) system, various types of acoustic noises are produced. The problems associated with acoustic noise for patients and healthcare workers are wide ranging, from simple annoyance and difficulties in verbal communication between staff and patients, to heightened anxiety or discomfort, and even potentially permanent hearing impairment (1-9). Acoustic noise may pose a particular problem for specific patient groups that may be at increased risk. For example, patients with head injuries or psychiatric disorders, the elderly, young children, and infants may be confused or suffer from heightened anxiety during MRI procedures (2). Patients taking medications may experience increased hearing sensitivity (3). Additionally, neonates with immature anatomical development may be at increased risk for adverse effects associated with acoustic noise. For example, significant fluctuations in vital signs of newborns have been reported during magnetic resonance imaging (MRI) examinations, which may partly be attributable to acoustic noise (4). High levels of acoustic noise may also impact the quality of the MRI procedure by causing distress in the patient.

Due to several of the issues listed above and the more specific issues discussed below, acoustic noise levels also pose a significant problem for one particular area of MRI: the increasing amount of research in functional MRI (fMRI) studies of brain activation. Typically, patients and volunteer subjects will be provided earplugs to wear during fMRI. However, these may impair vocal communication with staff members and also the perception of study stimuli. The acoustic noise associated with fMRI procedures can often be comparatively loud, as the use of fast acquisition sequences (e.g., echo planar imaging, EPI) are normally used. Acoustic noise can often lead to motion-related artifacts and degraded image quality. Furthermore, acoustic noise has been reported to interfere with auditory functional studies, and more broadly, with cross modal neural activity (10-14). A summary of the potential issues related to the acoustic noise that is associated with fMRI is shown in **Table 1**.

MR system-related acoustic noise will interfere with the communication of activation task instructions that often must be provided during scanning. One area of particular interest is the study of auditory and language function (13). In this work, the response to pure tone stimuli is analyzed. Therefore, any background levels of unwanted or uncontrolled acoustic noise can interfere with the delivery of these sound stimuli and affect experimental integrity. Solutions specific to controlling acoustic noise exposure during fMRI are generally sequence-related and a full discussion of this topic is presented later in this chapter.

Acoustic noise levels during echo planar imaging have been reported to significantly increase pure tone hearing thresholds in the optimal frequency hearing range (0- to 8-kHz) (15). These effects vary across the frequency range and the threshold changes depend on the characteristics of the sequence-generated acoustic noise. It may be possible to take into account, or adjust for, the MR system-induced auditory activation by using a control series

Table 1. A summary of potential issues with unwanted acoustic noise in fMRI (14). Reproduced by permission, Wiley - John Wiley & Son Publishers, NY

Mechanism		Characteristics
Direct confounding	Intra-acquisition response	Activation by scanner noise within same volume acquisition. Primarily interfering with auditory fMRI.
	Inter-acquisition response	Activation by scanner noise of preceding volume acquisition. Primarily interfering with auditory fMRI.
Indirect confounding	Attention	Increased activation in attention-related cortical areas.
	Distraction	Decreased activation in cortical areas by (inter-modal) distraction.
	Habituation	Slowly developing adaption-related loss of attention. May be advantageous in noisy environments.
	Motion artifacts	Not substantially related to scanner noise.
	Masking	Overlap of spectral components of scanner noise and auditory stimuli. Confined to auditory fMRI.
	Stapedial muscle reflex	Changes in cochlear perception of auditory stimuli (intensity and frequency). Confined to auditory fMRI.
	Temporary hearing loss	Changes in cochlear perception of auditory stimuli (intensity and frequency). Confined to auditory fMRI.

of scans during task paradigms. Results have been reported on mapping auditory activation induced by MR system-induced acoustic noise (16).

The problem of acoustic noise may also have implications for the operational costs of an MRI facility. Notably, there can be a potential decrease in image quality due to patient movement resulting from the patient being startled or uncomfortable in association with acoustic noise. This may add to the need to repeat scans or to interrupt studies that can adversely impact the efficiency of an MRI facility. For all the above reasons, it is important that the MRI-related acoustic noise is quantified and characterized as part of a safety and quality assurance program. Furthermore, any exposure to acoustic noise that is excessive must be controlled or alleviated.

Acoustic noise experienced during routine clinical MRI examinations can generally be confined to levels within permissible limits with relatively little effort by using passive hearing protection (e.g., disposable earplugs). Several more sophisticated methods are also under investigation by researchers, offering more comprehensive and elegant solutions without the disadvantages of passive methods. This chapter will discuss acoustic noise and hearing, describe the common characteristics of MRI-related acoustic noise, explain the current permissible levels for acoustic noise, and present the main methods used for measurement and control of this potential hazard.

ACOUSTIC NOISE AND HEARING

The ear is a highly sensitive wide-band receiver, with the typical frequency range of 2-Hz to 20-kHz for normal hearing (17). The arrival of sound waves at the ear sets up a fluctuating pressure just outside the entrance to the external auditory canal. These fluctuations are then transmitted as pressure waves along the auditory canal. Normally under slight tension, the eardrum, or tympanic membrane, is physically moved by these pressure waves.

On the other side of the membrane, three tiny bones known as the ossicles, transmit this movement across the middle ear cavity to another membrane, the oval window, which forms the end of the spiral-shaped, fluid-filled cochlea. The vibration of the membrane and hair cells in the cochlea is transformed, via the auditory nerve to give a sense of hearing. **Figure 1** shows the main components of the hearing mechanism.

At high sound intensities, the muscles that control the motion of the ossicles alter their tension creating the acoustic reflex to protect the ear from damage. However, this reflex occurs approximately 0.5-milliseconds after the insult, such that the ear is particularly vulnerable to impact noise of high intensity. The human ear does not tend to discern sound powers in absolute terms, but assesses how much greater one power is than another. Reflecting the very wide range of powers that exist, the logarithmic decibel scale, dB, is used when referring to sound power.

The sound level that is measured depends not only on the source, but also the environment (e.g., the proximity of surfaces that may reflect sound). Thus, sound levels are usually quoted in terms of sound pressure level (SPL), which accounts for the environment of the measurement. **Table 2** displays a range of sound pressure levels for some typical sources of acoustic noise.

Figure 1. The main components of the human hearing mechanism.

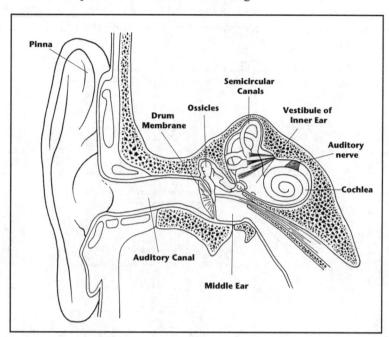

Table 2. Sound pressure level for some typical sources of acoustic noise.

Sound Pressure Level (dB)	Typical Sound Sources
140	Threshold of pain
130	Pneumatic drill
120	Chainsaw
110 -120	Car horn at 1-meter
80 - 90	Inside a bus
70 - 80	Traffic at street corner
60 - 70	Normal voice
50 - 60	Typical office
30	Whisper
0	Threshold of hearing

The sensitivity of the ear is also frequency dependent, as shown is **Figure 2** (18). Peak hearing sensitivity occurs in the region of 4-kHz. This is also the region where potential maximum hearing loss will occur, with damage spreading into neighboring frequencies. Since the ear is not equally sensitive to all frequencies, measured data may be weighted using the dB(A) measurement or "A-weighted" scale, which biases the meter to respond similarly to the human ear. The quality, or efficiency of hearing, is defined by the audible threshold, which is the SPL at which one can just begin to detect a sound. This is normally defined as 0 (zero) dB.

Figure 2. The frequency response of the human ear. The dashed line shows the relative frequency response of the human ear and the solid line shows the A-weighted filter approximation to this response (18). Reproduced by permission through the HMSO Open Government License.

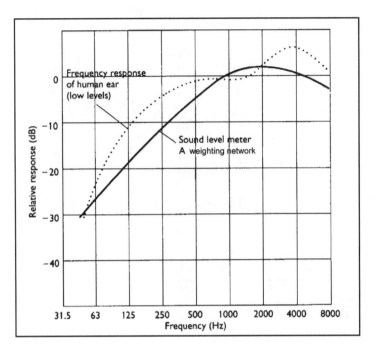

Acoustic noise is defined in terms of frequency spectrum (measured and indicated in Hz), intensity (indicated in decibels or dB), and duration (or time). Additionally, noise may be steady state, intermittent, impulsive, or explosive. Time-varying noise is reported in terms of L_{eq}, which is defined as the continuous SPL that contains the same sound energy as the time-varying sound over the measurement period. This can be considered as the average noise level. Stimulation of the ear by acoustic noise has three potential effects: (1) Adaptation, (2) Temporary threshold shift (TTS) (post-stimulation fatigue), and (3) Permanent threshold shift (PTS) (permanent impairment).

In hearing adaption, loud sounds cause a small muscle attached to one of the bones of the inner ear to contract. This attenuates the transmission of sound vibration to the inner ear, which is a protective mechanism that does not work well for short duration, very intense sounds. Transient hearing loss may occur following loud noise [>100-dB(A)], resulting in a temporary threshold shift (i.e., a shift in audible threshold). With a TTS, subjects may experience a dulling in hearing at the end of the noise and tinnitus in some cases. Recovery typically occurs quickly (1). However, full recovery can take up to several weeks if the noise insult is particularly severe. Intense impulsive noises at 650-Hz with cut-offs at 300- and 1-kHz have also been shown to generate substantial TTS (19). Noise above 100-dB(A) can cause disturbances of the microcirculation in the cortical organ and short impulsive noise at levels of 120- to 130-dB(A) can lead to mechanical damage in this organ.

If the noise is sufficiently severe, this may result in a permanent threshold shift at specific frequencies (20, 21). Hearing damage from steady-state noise usually takes the form of inner ear damage. That is, destruction of the hair cells that convert acoustic energy to electrical impulses transmitted via the nervous system to the brain. These cells cannot regenerate and, therefore, the damage is irreversible. This damage is similar to age-related hearing loss (presbycusis) in that it progresses slowly, with the affected hearing threshold rising. Mean hearing loss is a function of noise frequency and duration (20). Permanent damage is primarily a risk for prolonged daily exposure to loud (>85-dB) occupational noise or short impulsive noise around 140-dB. Excessive noise is known to be one of the most common causes of hearing loss (20). The risk of hearing damage increases with the noise level, duration of the noise, the number of exposures to the noise, and the susceptibility of the individual (20, 21). Along with sensitive groups, children have a lower threshold for hearing damage and, therefore, restricting exposure levels to around 120-dB or lower are recommended (22). It is generally accepted that exposure to noise levels up to a maximum of 75-dB(A) will not result in PTS irrespective of the duration of exposure (22). Over the years, several instances of noise-related incidents have been reported in the literature (see below).

Noise That Is Not Perceived Via the Ear Canal

The ear canal is not the only path for transmission of sound to the cochlea. Sound may be conducted via air and bone conduction, through the ear canal, head, and body. Protection of the ear canal via earplugs will, thus, never lead to silence, due to the remaining sound conduction via the other paths. Sound can be conducted directly to the cochlea, to the middle ear and then to the cochlea, or through the walls of the middle ear, along the ear canal to the middle ear, and then to the cochlea (23). When the ear canal is relatively unprotected, this path will be the dominant one for perception of sound. However, as noise is attenuated along the ear canal, the other paths become increasingly dominant and further hearing protection measures will have little effect on the residual noise. Using a helmet in addition to conventional earplugs and "defenders", Ravicz and Melcher (24) studied the impact of isolating the head and ear canal from sound. Isolating the head enabled the original noise attenuation of 39- to 41-dB to increase to 55- to 63-dB.

Fetal MR Imaging

By around the twentieth week of gestation, the outer, middle, and inner ear of the fetus appear to be fully formed. The fetus can then begin to detect sounds (25). Indeed, Hepper and Shahidullah (26) reported that the responsiveness of the fetus to audio stimuli occurs between 19 to 35 weeks, with initial responses being to sounds at low frequencies. They measured an initial response at 20 weeks to a 500-Hz pure tone. As the pregnancy progressed, there was a significant reduction (20- to 30-dB) in the intensity of sound required to elicit a response. Studies report that maternal tissues and fluid surrounding the fetal head act as efficient low-pass filters for sound (27-31).

MRI procedures may be performed during the first trimester of pregnancy. In a survey conducted by De Wilde, et al. (32), 83% of clinics responding suggested they would scan patients during the first trimester in cases of clinical need. While the mother may wear hearing protection, the fetus does not and, thus, noise has been reported to affect the fetus (33).

To minimize motion-related artifacts, fast imaging techniques are required for fetal MRI examinations, which results in the potential for exposures to comparatively high levels of acoustic noise. Glover, et al. (34) investigated acoustic noise absorption through the abdomen using a hydrophone in the stomach of a (male) volunteer. For scans performed at 0.5-T, these researchers reported a reduction of approximately 30-dB in acoustic noise levels. However, this study was a very limited approximation to scanning a pregnant patient and the associated sound absorption. The strength of the static magnetic field of the MR system, which directly affects acoustic noise levels generated, was also low (0.5-T) compared to the majority of clinical scanners in current use. Certain research has reported high frequency hearing loss, shortened gestation, and decreased birth weight following exposure to high levels of acoustic noise [>99-dB(A)] (35).

In a recent study, Reeves, et al. (36) investigated the rates of cochlear impairment for a cohort of second and third trimester neonates who had been exposed to acoustic noise during 1.5-T MRI examinations. Their data showed no association between exposure to noise and an increased risk of hearing impairment. General guidelines for managing exposure to acoustic noise produced by the United Kingdom (UK), Medicines and Healthcare products Regulatory Agency (MHRA) (37) and based on evidence in several reports (38-40) suggest that the data on the effects of noise on the health of the fetus is inconclusive.

CHARACTERISTICS OF MRI-RELATED ACOUSTIC NOISE

Early measurements of MRI-related acoustic noise offered little more than an assessment of intensity levels. Over time, researchers began to investigate the noise in more detail and to characterize it in terms of frequency components, variability with pulse sequences, and the contribution of individual gradients.

The gradient magnetic field of the MR system is the primary source of acoustic noise associated with MRI. This noise occurs during the rapid alterations of currents within the gradient coils. These currents, in the presence of the strong static magnetic field of the MR system, produce significant (Lorentz) forces that act upon the gradient coils. From basic physics, a conductor element dl carrying a current $\mathbf{I} = I\,\underline{i}$ placed into a magnetic uniform field $\mathbf{B} = B\,\underline{k}$, will experience a Lorentz force F per unit length given by,

$$\boldsymbol{F} = \boldsymbol{I} \times \boldsymbol{B} = jBI \sin\theta \tag{1}$$

where θ is the angle between the conductor and the field direction and $\underline{i}$, $\underline{j}$, $\underline{k}$ are unit vectors along the conductor, force, and magnetic field direction respectively. Therefore, acoustic noise is theoretically linear with static magnetic field of the MR system (41). The noise from these mechanical forces is then transferred into airborne acoustic noise or sound pressure, due to an acoustic noise transfer function (42). The sound pressure level (SPL) verses static magnetic field strength for various MR systems is presented in **Figure 3** (43).

Figure 3. Sound Pressure Level dB (A) verses static magnetic field strength for twenty-eight different MR systems (mean SPL is displayed for each static magnetic field strength). The MR systems were running a "clinical worse-case" noise protocol based on maximizing the gradient duty cycle (43). Measurements were performed by the MagNET research group at Imperial College London (1998-2006).

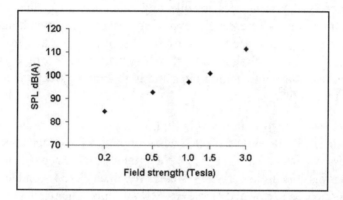

Acoustic noise, manifested as loud tapping, knocking, and other sounds is produced when the forces cause motion or vibration of the gradient coils as they impact against their mountings, which then also flex and vibrate. All structures have intrinsic resonance frequencies and these frequencies have their own modal shapes. In fact, there are several pathways of noise generation associated with MRI (44).

If the gradient coil modal shape due to deformation corresponds to the shape of the exciting Lorentz force distribution, then large gradient coil displacements occur and result in the generation of significant acoustic noise. Current designs of gradient coils are often manufactured to have a high stiffness, which minimizes coil motion and, thus, the structural resonances of the coils.

Various factors have been shown to affect the acoustic noise generated during MRI, including the strength of the static magnetic field (mentioned above) and alteration of the gradient output (i.e., rise time and amplitude). Interestingly, Price, et al. (43) reported that there is greater impact on acoustic noise levels generated from imaging parameters than the field strength. Acoustic noise is enhanced by decreases in section thickness, field of view, repetition time, and echo time. The physical features of the MR system and its environment as well as the material and construction of the gradient coils and support structures also affect the transmission of the acoustic noise and its perception by the patient and MR system operators.

Gradient magnetic field-induced noise levels have been measured during a variety of pulse sequences for clinical and research MR systems with static magnetic field strengths ranging from 0.35- to 4-T, with acoustic noise levels of over 130-dB reported (43-58). Obviously, since the gradient magnetic field is primarily responsible for acoustic noise, the ability of the MR system to produce noise is dependent upon the specifications for the gradients (amplitudes and slew rates) as well as the types of imaging parameters that are available on the scanner.

Not surprisingly, fast gradient echo pulse sequences produce, comparatively, louder noise during MRI than spin echo sequences. Three-dimensional pulse sequences, where multiple gradients are applied simultaneously, are among the loudest. Many studies have focused on assessing the maximum MR system acoustic noise, which is usually related to using EPI methods, due to the associated high gradient performance inherent in these ultra-fast sequences. Echo planar sequences, in collecting a complete image in one radiofrequency (RF) excitation of the spin system, require extremely fast gradient switching times and high gradient amplitudes. The increased interest in diffusion imaging and fMRI has meant a heightened interest in using high field strength MR systems (i.e., mostly 3-, 4-, and 7-Tesla) with fast gradient capability (switching rates and high amplitudes) to acquire multi-slice, EPI images of high quality.

Shellock, et al. (47) reported relatively high levels of acoustic noise, up to 102- 103-dB(A) on the two 1.5-T MR systems tested when running EPI sequences with parameters selected to represent a "worst-case" protocol. Nevertheless, these acoustic noise levels were within current permissible limits for MR systems. Miyati, et al. (54) conducted an extensive survey of EPI sequences performed on eleven MR systems. The results of the sound level measurements reported to be at levels within permissible limits.

Price, et al. (43) surveyed fifteen MR scanners, with static magnetic field strengths from 0.2-T to 3-T, reporting worst case noise levels in the range 82.5- to 118.3-dB(A), but for two-dimensional MRI techniques, only. They reported the lowest noise levels for the lowest static field strength scanner and the highest noise recorded for the highest field strength scanner, but noted low levels of acoustic noise recorded for a 1.5T scanner fitted with vac-uum-encased gradient coils. Higher acoustic noise levels have been reported by Ravicz, et al. (56) (up to 138-dB for 3-T) and More, et al. (57) (130-dB for 4-T).

Foster, et al. (58) reported EPI-related acoustic noise levels of 123- to 132-dB(A) for a 3-T research scanner. Since EPI sequences are significantly shorter in duration than con-ventional sequences, in terms of acoustic noise exposure, higher sound exposure levels are possible for the shorter times involved. However, these levels, when converted to eight hour equivalent values [L_{eq} = 108-dB(A)], are higher than the limits for occupational acoustic noise exposure used in the United Kingdom (UK) and in the United States (U.S.). Therefore, hearing protection must be used for patients undergoing MRI procedures under these cir-cumstances.

Measurements of sound pressure levels offer a limited amount of information with re-gard to the quality of the noise and its impact on hearing. In addition to measurements of noise level, several groups have recorded and analyzed the acoustic noise. Similar noise levels and characteristics are found when comparing different clinical MR systems. Fre-quency analysis of the noise shows that noise is pseudo-periodic, with variations in the de-gree of periodicity depending on the pulse sequence used and the vibrational characteristics of the gradient coils (50).

For conventional pulse sequences used for MRI, peak noise levels are found at the low frequency region of the spectra. **Figure 4** shows an example of the octave band spectra for a 1.0-T and 1.5-T MR systems (48,49). Spectral peaks in the sound levels were found in the range of 0.2- to 1.5-kHz (22). Cho, et al. (52) have also reported that pre-scan noise

Figure 4. Octave band spectra for two MR systems: 1-T Siemens Impact (black squares) and a 1.5-T Siemens Magnetom (open squares). Measurements obtained on these MR systems show that the peaks in noise intensity are at approximately 200-Hz (49).

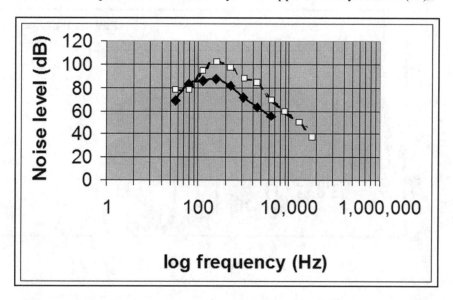

generated high levels (100-dB, C-weighted scale) across a wide spectral range up to 4-kHz with peaks around 2.4-kHz.

More, et al. (57) noted that repetition time (TR) had a minimal impact on overall SPL, while increasing the echo time (TE) increased attenuation, in agreement with Price, et al. (43). Unlike the use of conventional sequences, EPI-related sound levels have been reported to contain a larger fraction of high frequency noise (around 4-kHz) with most noise in the frequency range of 0.5- to 4-kHz (56), with the noise comprising the fundamental frequency and harmonics. For EPI sequences, More, et al. (57) also noted considerable non-harmonic noise flanking the harmonics. The acoustic noise was also noted to contain a higher proportion of broad frequency spectrum noise (**Figure 5**). For their pulse sequence, More, et al. (57) found the even harmonics to be associated with the phase-encoding gradient, the frequency encoding gradient generated the odd harmonics and non-harmonic acoustic noise, while the slice-selective gradients generated the broad spectrum noise (**Figure 6**).

In addition to the dependence on pulse sequence parameters, MR system hardware and construction, acoustic noise is dependent on the immediate environment. Additionally, noise characteristics have a spatial dependence. Spatially, the acoustic noise will vary along the bore of the scanner. However, how it varies will depend on the MR system's structure and design. Reports providing values of acoustic noise disagree, for example, on whether the maximum acoustic noise levels were measured at the isocenter of the bore or not (43, 51, 53). The noise distributions along radial and axial directions are also likely to be asymmetric, due to standing wave effects in the scanner's bore (57). Furthermore, noise levels have been found to vary by as much as 10-dB as a function of the patient's position inside the MR system (51) such that the presence and size of the patient affects the level of acoustic noise. For example, an increase of 1- to 3-dB has been measured with a patient present inside of

Figure 5. Measured acoustic noise for an EPI pulse sequence. Acoustic noise spectrum at the right ear (57). Reproduced by permission, Wiley - John Wiley & Son Publishers, NY.

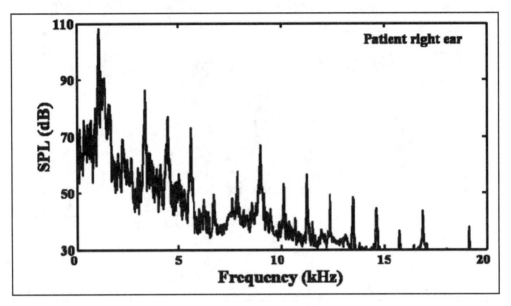

the MR system (51), which may be due to pressure doubling (i.e., the increase in sound pressure close to a solid object, caused when sound waves reflect and undergo in-phase enhancement).

Analysis, Simulation and Modeling of MR System Acoustic Noise

Hedeen and Edelstein (51) demonstrated the similarity between the gradient pulse spectrum and the acquired noise spectrum, which are affected by additional system acoustic resonances (**Figure 7**). There was a good qualitative match between the input signal and resulting acoustic noise spectrum. Hedeen and Edelstein (51) derived an acoustic transfer function that is independent of input, and which once determined, may be applied to any input impulse function and will then predict the generated acoustic noise.

Defining the scanner's frequency response function (FRF) as $H(f)$, the input signal represented in the frequency domain as $G(f)$, and the resulting acoustic noise, $P(f)$, the following may be expressed,

$$P(f) = H(f) \cdot G(f) \tag{2}$$

Hedeen and Edelstein (51) applied this analysis to a fast spin echo (FSE) pulse sequence and achieved an agreement between measured and predicted acoustic noise level to within 0.4-dB (**Figure 8**). Other authors, such as More, et al. (57) and Rizzo-Sierra, et al. (59) have used similar approaches in deriving simple acoustic transfer or impulse response functions

Figure 6. Relationship between the operating acoustic noise at the left ear and gradient pulse waveform for an EPI pulse sequence. Data is shown for each separate gradient and the associated noise spectral peaks (57). Reproduced by permission, Wiley - John Wiley & Son Publishers, NY.

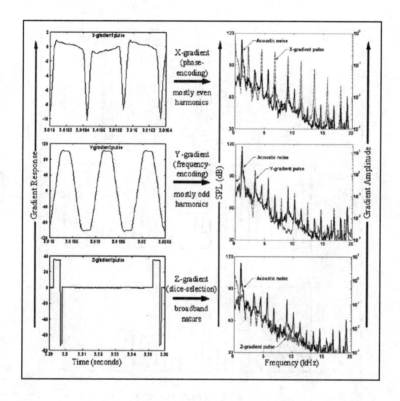

with considerable success in predicting the acoustic noise associated with the MR system's gradient behavior.

A number of groups have reported detailed acoustic analysis and modeling of the acoustic noise from commercial and purpose-built gradient coil systems. Investigators (60-67) have made a significant contribution to this field, reporting on a number of approaches to gradient modeling as well as conducting evaluations and testing on noise reduction techniques. In 2002, Mechefske, et al. (60) developed the simulation of a cylindrical whole-body gradient coil housed in a 4-T MR scanner and driven by triangular and trapezoidal gradient pulses. The simulation was based on finite element (FE) analysis. Acoustic frequency responses predicted by the simulation were compared to experimental measures, showing broad agreement. Further reports investigated experiments and simulation of purpose-built gradient coils, including vibration and acoustic noise measurements (61, 62). In their finite element model, Lorentz forces were used as the system load, with acoustic radiation modeled using the Kirchhoff-Helmholtz equation. These researchers performed the analysis for a small head geometry gradient coil and achieved reasonable agreement of theory and experiment (61, 62).

Figure 7. Gradient trapezoidal current excitation and acoustic noise response. (a) Trapezoidal current wave-form time series. The signal consisted of a series of simple trapezoidal gradient pulses. (b) Fourier transform of trapezoidal time series, and (c) measured acoustic response (51). Reproduced by permission, Wiley - John Wiley & Son Publishers, NY.

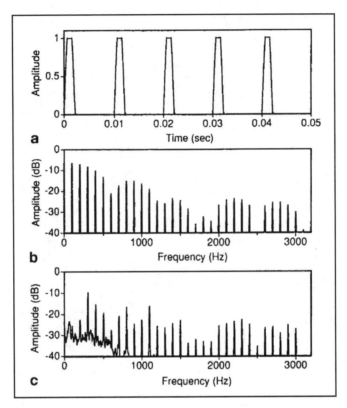

Further work in this field has been conducted by Kuijpers, et al. (68), who created a mathematical model of acoustic noise radiation in finite ducts. Shao and Mechefske (63) reported on the development of a predictive analytical model, allowing for inclusion of acoustic liners inside the gradient coil inner wall. They also compared analytic and boundary element models. The analytical model was comparative in terms of results, but computationally more efficient. Additional papers investigated the dynamic behavior of gradient coils of varying wall thickness (64-67) and by applying shell theory (69). Investigators have also investigated the coupling of gradient coils to other associated structures, reporting on structural analyses (70). Several other researchers reported on the use of gradient coil analysis with finite element modeling (71-73).

ACOUSTIC NOISE LEVELS AND PERMISSIBLE LIMITS

Several of the available guidance documents discussed below adopt a similar framework, referring back to the same source for action levels and permissible limits. Much of the international guidance is based on occupational exposure limits which assume chronic

Figure 8. Predicted (top) and measured (bottom) acoustic noise spectrums, SPL, for a fast spin echo (FSE) pulse sequence. Overall predicted and measured levels were 93.1- and 92.7-dB respectively. Good agreement over a broad spectral range is evident (51). Reproduced by permission, Wiley - John Wiley & Son Publishers, NY.

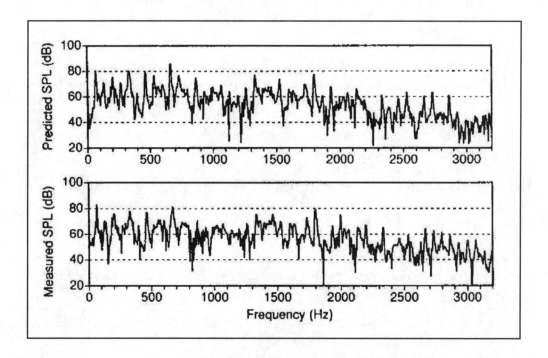

exposures. These are not entirely satisfactory for application to patient exposures associated with MRI, which can be short but with potentially intense noise, causing discomfort. When time-averaged, these types of exposures can fall below action levels but still present a hazard. For normal individuals, the typical threshold for discomfort related to acoustic noise is approximately 120-dB in the 1- to 5-kHz range (74), however, those with particular sensitivity can experience discomfort at much lower acoustic noise levels (75).

The United Kingdom (UK) has undoubtedly the most comprehensive guidance covering control of noise exposure. For acoustic noise exposure, the current UK occupational guidelines are based on the Control of Noise at Work legislation, published in 2005 (76). This document sets out the responsibilities of the employer and makes a number of recommendations based on a small set of action levels. Acoustic noise is graded to that which is below 80-dB(A), a lower action level at 80-dB(A) daily or weekly exposure [peak 135-dB(C)], and upper action level at 85-dB(A) daily or weekly exposure [peak 135-dB(C)]. It should be noted that values for lower and upper action levels have been reduced by 5-dB(A), compared to previous Noise at Work action levels published in 1989. This document also recommends that hearing protection should be available for all staff members, and that its use be mandatory for noise above the upper action level. The management of exposure to acoustic noise for the general public is covered by the Management of Health and Safety at Work (1999) (77), but, since the general public will not have access to the controlled area or MR system room, the risks are usually low.

In the United States (U.S.), occupational limits are mandated by the Occupational Safety and Health Authority (OSHA) (78) and have also been adopted by the Food and Drug Administration (FDA) (79). Now somewhat outdated, the OSHA guidelines apply to a slightly raised action level of 90-dB(A) (daily or eight-hour average) in line with the older UK guidance (80). McRobbie (81) has a recent review of occupational exposure in MRI. However, it is concerned mostly with EMF exposure and makes little mention of acoustic noise.

Current UK guidance on noise exposure limits for patients and volunteer subjects (including staff members) is presented in the MHRA guidelines (35), which are based on documents from the National Radiological Protection Board (NRPB) (82-84), and the International Commission on Non-Ionizing Radiation Protection (ICNIRP) (85, 86). For patients and volunteer subjects, it refers to the same action levels as the Control of Noise at Work (76), suggesting hearing protection should always be offered unless noise levels are proven to be below 80-dB(A). Hearing protection should reduce levels at the ear to below 85-dB(A). The recommended action levels are based on the noise at work regulations (76) and are shown in **Table 3**. The ICNIRP (85, 86) notes the range of guidance from the International Electrotechnical Commission (IEC) (87) and the German Commission on Radiological Protection (88), but accepts the need for a conservative approach to protect vulnerable patient groups, also recommending the MHRA action levels. The MHRA document shows the relationship between the acoustic noise level and time necessary to reach the daily action level (27) (**Table 3**). Recommendations for acoustic noise and hearing protection are, as follows (37):

- The use of hearing protection is highly recommended. Protection should be available and all patients and volunteers should be encouraged to use it. Protection should always be worn by vulnerable patients.

- Staff should be trained in the selection and fitting of hearing protection. Protection should be selected to match the noise frequency spectrum of the scanner. Implicitly, this must, therefore, be known.

- Staff should be offered hearing protection if acoustic noise levels are above the lower action level and use is mandatory for noise at the upper action level.

- Particular care should be taken with vulnerable patient groups, such as pediatric and unconscious patients.

- Pregnant staff members are advised not to remain in the MR system room during scanning. Sites should undertake a risk assessment to assess staff time and motion around the scanner in order to minimize exposure to the static magnetic field.

In the U.S., various patient exposure guidelines related to the MRI environment were initially recommended in a document issued by the American College of Radiology in 2002 (89). Notably, this document makes little mention of the risks associated with acoustic noise. However, it does recommend that all patients should be offered hearing protection and that this is mandatory for those undergoing MRI procedures using research pulse sequences.

While the acoustic noise levels suggested for patients exposed during MRI examinations on an infrequent and short-term temporal basis are considered to be highly conservative,

Table 3. Occupational noise action values and limits (adapted from reference 76). Reproduced by permission, HMSO (Open Government License).

Action Level	Daily or Weekly Personal Exposure dB(A) (average value)	Peak Sound Pressure, dB
Lower exposure value	80	135
Upper exposure value	85	137
Exposure limit values	87	140

they may not be appropriate for individuals with underlying health problems who may be sensitive to noise at certain levels or at particular frequencies.

Overall, the acoustic noise produced during MRI on a modern-day scanner should represent a minimal risk to patients if good quality hearing protection is used. However, the possibility exists that substantial gradient magnetic field-induced noise may represent a heightened risk in certain patients who are particularly susceptible to the damaging effects of loud noises or for those with poorly fitting hearing protection. In fact, there have been unconfirmed claims of permanent hearing loss associated with MRI examinations (9). Therefore, special care is essential when controlling noise levels associated with MR procedures.

Adverse Incidents Associated with Exposure to MRI-Related Acoustic Noise

(A) Temporary Threshold Shifts (TTS)

As mentioned above, short-term exposure to intense noise [>100-dB(A)] can induce a temporary shift in the hearing threshold. Brummett, et al. (1) reported temporary shifts in hearing thresholds in 43% of the patients scanned without hearing protection or with improperly fitted earplugs. Normal hearing returned after 15-minutes. Notably, noise levels during scanning were not measured as part of their study. However, Hurwitz, et al. (46) made measurements using the same scanner, reporting values for gradient echo sequences (likely to be some of the loudest sequences on this system) of around 93-dB(A). Of the 14 patients scanned without hearing protection in their study, six suffered TTS with threshold loss greater than 15-dB. For those using hearing protection, only one experienced a TTS. It should be noted that these data were associated with scans performed on a comparatively low field strength MR system (0.35-T). A study by Wagner, et al. (90), found conflicting results.

Ulmer, et al. (16) measured changes in pure tone thresholds in volunteer subjects wearing hearing protection exposed to EPI pulse sequences. Intense impulse noise at 0.65-kHz with cut-offs at 0.3-kHz and 1.0-kHz were also shown to generate substantial hearing threshold shifts. In 2011, Govindaraju, et al. (91) reported a possible incidence of TTS for a man scanned while wearing earplugs on a 3-T scanner. The patient experienced unilateral hearing loss and tinnitus immediately following the MRI examination. The hearing loss resolved completely within 24-hours but the tinnitus persisted. Acoustic noise levels were checked for the conventional sequences that were performed and found to be in the range of L_{eq} 101- to 112-dB(A) (L_{peak} 115- to 124-dB).

(B) Permanent Threshold Shifts (PTS)

If the noise exposure at intense levels is prolonged, or repeated in close time intervals, threshold shifts can be permanent. The threshold for permanent hearing damage is approximately 140-dB for short impulsive noise and around 85-dB for chronic exposure. Commercial MR systems that are designed to be compliant with IEC standards are not able to generate noise in excess of 140-dB (87). De Wilde, et al. (9) reported one case of excessive acoustic noise that occurred in the United Kingdom. The patient reported severe headaches, dizziness, and ear pain following the MRI examination. Importantly, this patient was not provided hearing protection because the manager of the MRI site was confident that the noise levels generated by the 0.5-T MR system were not at a level of concern.

ACOUSTIC NOISE CONTROL TECHNIQUES

Controlling acoustic noise is generally accomplished in one of three simple ways: control of noise at the receiver (e.g., using earplugs), control along the path of the noise, or control of the noise at the source (e.g., redesigned gradients). Once acoustic energy has been generated in the air, it can be difficult to control, so the control of noise at the source is considered to be the preferred method.

Passive Hearing Protection

The simplest, most convenient, and least expensive means of preventing problems associated with acoustic noise during MRI procedures is to use disposable earplugs and/or headphones. Earplugs, when properly fitted can abate noise by 10- to 30-dB (depending on the frequency), which is usually an adequate amount of sound attenuation for the MRI environment. **Figure 9** shows examples of the octave band spectra of some commercially available earplugs and other hearing protection devices, demonstrating typical noise attenuation values. The use of ear-muffs, headphones, or disposable earplugs has been shown to provide a sufficient decrease in acoustic noise that, in turn, would be capable of preventing the potential temporary hearing loss associated with MRI procedures (1).

The level and frequency range of noise attenuation will vary with the type and design of hearing protection that is utilized. If data is unavailable for the noise abatement device, the protector should be tested. Since the designs of hearing protectors do vary, care should be taken when offering these to patients. Additionally, proper fitting instructions must be provided. A patient who may be confused, young, or have difficulty in correctly fitting the hearing protection may need additional assistance to prevent poorly fitting the device and having compromised noise attenuation. If using earmuffs or headphones, these should be regularly assessed for wear to the seals and replaced, as needed. Current guidelines suggest staff members should have training in the selection and fitting of hearing protection (35).

Unfortunately, earplugs, earmuffs, and headphones suffer from a number of problems. These devices tend to hamper verbal communication with the patient during the operation of the MR system. In certain circumstances, these devices can also create discomfort or im-

Figure 9. Noise attenuation for several commercial ear plugs and ear defenders. Note the significant variability in attenuation at low frequencies. Reproduced by permission, the 3M Company. 3MTM, E.A.R.TM and PeltorTM are trademarks of the 3M Company.

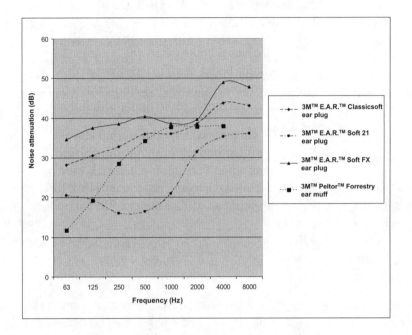

pair immobilization of the patient's head, which is problematic when optimal immobilization is required for certain studies that are particularly sensitive to patient movement (e.g., diffusion and phase-sensitive studies).

Standard earplugs are often too large for the ear canal of babies. Some small sizes are available (Carbot Safety Ltd., Slough, United Kingdom), although snug fit is essential if acoustic noise is to be efficiently attenuated. Neonates present a particular challenge when trying to use conventional earplugs or other similar devices. Nordell, et al. (92) reported on a patient-independent device constructed from absorbent padding, which can be placed over the neonate during the MRI examination. Reductions in peak noise levels of 16- to 22-dB(A) averaged over the hearing spectrum of 4 to 13-dB(A) were reported.

Passive devices used for hearing protection may attenuate noise non-uniformly over the hearing range. While high frequency sound may be well attenuated, attenuation can be poor at low frequency. This is unfortunate because the low frequency range is also where the peak in MRI-related acoustic noise is often generated, however, this may be balanced by the lower hearing sensitivity also in this frequency range (**Figure 2**).

Passive protection devices will also offer poor attenuation of noise transmitted to the patient through bone conduction (93). The effect of vibration being conducted during MRI and affecting noise has been reported by Glover, et al. (32). The presence of an insulating foam mattress on the patient couch has been found to reduce vibrational coupling to the patient and noise levels by around 10-dB. This underlying bone conduction transmission path puts a practical attenuation limit for passive protection at around 40-dB (94). As previously indicated, Ravicz and Melcher (24) studied the potential for isolating the body from the MR system using a helmet to minimize acoustic noise transmission via bone conduction. They used passive hearing protection in combination with the helmet system. Adding protection, they reported a total noise attenuation of 55- to 63-dB, by using a combination of earplugs (25- to 28-dB alone), "ear defenders" (39- to 41-dB alone), and an isolating helmet. While the use of a helmet may suit research studies with volunteer subjects, it may not be clinically acceptable for use in patients. However, in general, earplugs and defenders can also be used effectively in combination, offering added hearing protection. Wearing earplugs and defenders with individual attenuation ratings of 30-dB, when combined, will offer a total potential attenuation of around 33-dB.

Methods Using Anti-Phase Noise: Active Noise Control

A significant reduction in the level of acoustic noise caused by MRI procedures has been accomplished by implementing the use of a noise cancellation, or "anti-phase" noise technique (45, 82 95, 96). Unlike many other noise control solutions that result in compromised performance of the MRI examination or hardware, this technique should have no impact on the performance of the MR system. The principle is simply to generate noise, which will interfere destructively with the scanner noise incident at the patient's ear.

The loudspeaker producing this anti-phase noise can be built into the scanner bore or built into a pair of headphones for the patient (thus, harnessing passive protection as well). A major disadvantage of this technique is that, if it performs poorly at certain frequencies or in some spatial regions, noise levels may be enhanced rather than attenuated by the superposition of the additional anti-noise.

Controlling acoustic noise from a particular source by introducing anti-phase noise to interfere destructively with the noise source is by no means a new idea (97, 98) (**Figure 10**). For use in the MRI environment, conventional active-noise control (ANC) systems require some modification. Firstly, loudspeakers and microphones designed to be utilized in the MRI setting must be used to acquire scanner noise and to transmit control anti-noise and, secondly, the ANC controller must be optimized and synchronized to the scanner.

The initial results for the use of anti-noise applied to MRI achieved only modest noise attenuation. Goldman, et al. (45) acquired MR system noise with a microphone, performed a Fourier transform (FT) of the noise, and generated control noise by inverting the phase of the major components of the FT, and then transmitted this anti-noise through a loudspeaker built into a set of headphones (i.e., a combination active-passive system), achieving an average noise reduction of around 14-dB. The performance of this system was not much better than that of some standard passive headphones, alone, in the low frequency region of the hearing range. The control sound was delivered using long tubes, introducing a time delay, which limited control efficiency.

Advances in digital signal processing (DSP) technology permit efficient modern ANC systems to be realized at a modest cost (99). The essence of an anti-noise system involves either a continuous feed-forward or feedback loop with continuous sampling of the sounds in the noise environment so that the gradient magnetic field-induced noise is attenuated.

Figure 10. Principle of sound attenuation using anti-phase noise to create a zone of quiet. This diagram shows a noise (periodic) source and synthesized anti-phase noise interfering destructively in a specific region to produce a zone of quiet.

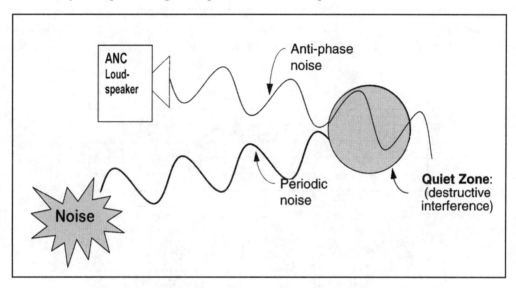

Thus, it is possible to attenuate the pseudo-periodic MR system-related noise while allowing the transmission of vocal communication or music to be maintained. The feedback loop uses a sampling microphone placed close to the ear, where noise reduction is required. It will attempt to attenuate all noise propagating into the ear. A feed-forward algorithm uses a sampling microphone close to the problematic noise source, offering a potentially more selective cancellation of noise source. Frequently, time limitations in anti-noise getting from the loudspeaker to the subject as well as stability requirements set a practical upper frequency limit for ANC systems. This problem of poorer high frequency attenuation performance is mitigated by building the systems into complementary passive ear defenders, resulting in a better broad frequency noise reduction.

Similar to Goldman, et al. (45), commercial manufacturers have offered ANC systems based on delivering anti-noise to patient headphones (46), however, the long tubing imposes a time delay in getting noise to the ear, limiting the performance of such a system. In 1995, Pla, et al. (100) reported improved results using a system based on an x-filtered least mean squares (LMS) algorithm, driving piezoelectric speakers near the patient's ears. These researchers achieved noise attenuation up to 25-dB for frequencies below 1.2-kHz and for the first few harmonics only. In 1997, McJury, et al. (95) reported on the performance of a multichannel filtered U-least mean squares algorithm for acoustic noise control. Acoustic noise was recorded digitally from a series of typical clinical MRI protocols performed on a 1.0-T Siemens Impact. This noise was then replayed through a bench-top adaptive real-time DSP ANC system (Motorola DSP 56001). A typical peak sound attenuation of approximately 30-dB was achieved over the frequency range from 0- to 700-Hz (**Figure 11**).

In 1999, Chen, et al. (96) published results using an ANC system based on a modified feedback method with a second order cascaded neural network architecture, with loud-

Figure 11. Results of noise cancellation for a typical clinical spin echo pulse sequence. Noise level spectra before (dotted line) and after cancellation (solid line) are shown for time and frequency domain spectra. A major disadvantage of this technique is that, if performed below optimal efficiency, at certain frequencies or in some spatial regions, noise levels may be enhanced rather than attenuated by the superposition of the additional anti-noise (95). Reproduced by permission, Elsevier, Philadelphia, PA.

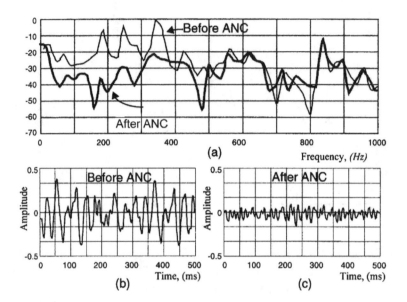

speaker mounted in a headset. For acoustic noise up to 3-kHz, they achieved an average attenuation of 19-dB. This study was also based on recorded scanner noise attenuated with a lab-based ANC system.

More recently, Chambers, et al. (101) demonstrated improved results over a wide frequency range using an ANC system that was based on an LMS feed-forward algorithm and built into a set of ear defenders. From 600-Hz to 4-kHz, peak attenuation of around 40-dB was measured for scanner noise. Importantly, the use of feed-forward methodology allows cancellation of scanner noise with less attenuation of any noise stimuli introduced during the use of fMRI protocols. However, this system did not acquire its reference noise in real-time, but required a recording phase to obtain reference data.

One of the most successful to date, are the results from Li, et al. (102). This group reported results with a patented, ANC system based on a feed-forward, x-LMS algorithm that uses multiple reference signals. The ANC system was built into a headset to also benefit from the passive attenuation of noise at higher frequencies. Impressive acoustic noise reductions of up to 55-dB at a harmonic frequency were achieved, with an average of 21-dB (30-dBA) over the entire spectrum. As for passive noise control, bone conduction remains a residual issue, limiting noise control.

Active Vibration Control (AVC)

Aeronautical engineers, amongst others, have an interest in noise reduction inside cylindrical shells. In their case, the cylindrical models represent airplane cabins. Results from their studies show that a significant amount of low frequency noise is associated with shell vibration (103,104), which is directly applicable to an MR system with a similar cylindrical geometry. Their methods of using active vibration control are also transferrable, however, until recently (105,106), they received little attention from the MRI community. These methods aim for global control of the entire gradient loudspeaker, not just the noise impacting on the ear canal, and would also control noise from bone conduction.

Qiu and Tani (107) devised an AVC system for use with a typical MRI-clamped, cylindrical gradient coil, which is based on distributed piezoelectric actuators. These attempt to suppress a limited set of vibrational modes of the gradient coil over a set frequency range. Their system, similarly to other aeronautical models, tries to reduce mainly low frequency (<1.2-kHz) noise, where passive hearing protection performs poorly. They achieved an average reduction in vibrational amplitudes of 20-dB with an optimized system (**Figure 12**). More recently, Roozen, et al. also designed an AVC system based on seismic mass piezoelectric actuators (106). However, for a gradient coil driven by FE-EPI, their system comprising only four actuators achieved a more modest averaged vibrational amplitude reduction of 3-dB over the frequency range 0.5- to 1.5-kHz.

Figure 12. Reduction in vibrational amplitudes with AVC. Results are shown for no control, case 1 (non-optimized control), and case 2 (optimized control)(107). Reproduced by permission, Institute of Physics Publishing.

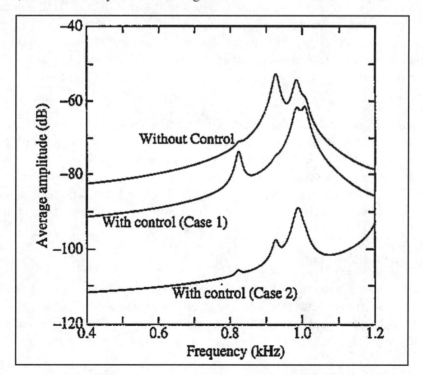

Quiet MRI Sequences

(A) Minimizing Conventional Gradient Levels

Because the dominant effect of acoustic noise levels lies with the signal details of a particular MRI protocol rather than the structure of the MR system (51), it follows that it should be possible to reduce the noise level by optimizing the choice of pulse sequence parameters. Simply using a spin echo (SE) sequence rather than a gradient echo (GE) pulse sequence and running the sequence with reduced gradient parameters (rise-time and amplitude) can significantly reduce the levels of acoustic noise. Skare, et al. (108) designed "quiet" sequences in this way and defined a simple "quietness factor" (QF) as,

$$QF = \frac{RT_m}{RT_s} \qquad \qquad (3)$$

where the RT_m is the rise-time of the modified sequence and RT_s , the original/default rise-time. On a 1.5-T MR system, a QF of 6 resulted in a noise attenuation of 20-dB. This procedure, however, lengthens the echo time (TE), reduces the number of acquisition slices, and results in a longer examination time.

(B) Minimizing the Number of Gradient Echoes

A reduction of acoustic noise levels may also be achieved by reducing the level of gradient pulsing in a pulse sequence (109, 110). A rapid, single-shot, multi-slice imaging technique (i.e., STEAM-Burst) is based on stimulated-echoes without the rapid gradient switching necessary in other single-shot techniques such as echo planar (110). The STEAM-Burst sequence uses a combination of the "Burst" technique (111), involving the application of multiple RF pulses under a constant gradient and subsequent refocusing of the resultant set of echoes, and the STEAM-stimulated echo acquisition mode (112). Limited data on acoustic noise measurements shows peak noise attenuation of 15-dB compared with a similar EPI sequence (110).

This pulse sequence offers the potential for rapid acquisition of MR images, but it is sensitive to artifacts due to static magnetic field inhomogeneities while generating reduced levels of acoustic noise. The sequence suffers from two main problems. First, the signal-to-noise ratio (SNR) is low compared with other rapid imaging techniques. Second, the images acquired at 3-Tesla have an SNR of approximately of 20:1. Thus, these pulse sequences remain more suited to specific research applications than routine use in the clinical MRI setting.

(C) Using Soft Gradient Pulses

An elegant solution has been suggested by Hennel (114), which may be applied to minimize the acoustic noise generated by a range of conventional MRI pulse sequences. As mentioned above, it has been shown that the acoustic response of the gradient system to current pulses is linear (51). Thus, the sound generated by a gradient waveform can be derived from a product of the FT of the source input and the frequency response function (FRF) of the gradient system (see equation 2). If gradient pulses are designed such that their current waveforms contain no frequencies for which the amplitude of the FRF is high, then resultant acoustic noise levels should be minimized (113). The FRF of the gradient system in a 3-Tesla MR system was measured and a very low response noted at low frequencies (below 200-Hz). Frequency components below this threshold should be attenuated in the acoustic spectrum of any pulse sequences.

In minimizing high frequency components in the gradient pulses, it is possible to avoid or reduce sharp transitions, such as step functions in the waveform, and to replace these with more slowly varying sinusoidal transitions. This may be accomplished by following three simple rules:

    (1)   Use sinusoidal ramping rather than trapezoidal ramping.

    (2)   Maximize ramp duration (keeps cut-off frequency low for efficient band limiting).

    (3)   Minimize the number of ramps (merge consecutive gradients on the same channel).

The use and efficiency of soft pulses are shown in **Figure 13**. With the sinusoidal ramping, high frequency acoustic components above 500-Hz are severely attenuated. Acoustic

Figure 13. The efficiency of soft gradient pulses. Magnitude spectra are shown (with an arbitrary linear scale) for the sound generated by the readout gradient of a FLASH (i.e., fast gradient echo) pulse sequence. Data was acquired with a linear ramp, 0.5-msec duration (top plot) and sinusoidal ramp duration 4-msec (lower plot). With the sinusoidal ramping, high frequency acoustic components above 500-Hz are severely attenuated (113). Reproduced by permission, Wiley - John Wiley & Son Publishers, NY.

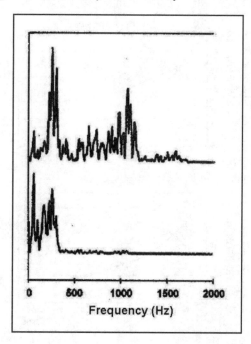

noise levels, (dB, A-weighted scale) averaged over 1-second, were measured for spin-echo and gradient-echo sequences as a function of echo time (**Figure 14**). Good quality MR images may be acquired with sound levels dropping as echo time (TE) increases. At echo times of 30- to 50-msec, good quality images are still possible and acoustic noise levels are below the ambient room noise [i.e., with the air-conditioning running, room sound levels approach 45-dB(A)]. Three main limitations were identified with the initial implementation of this technique, as follows: (1) there was an increased sensitivity of the pulse sequences to vascular flow, (2) the high-speed MRI pulse sequences tended to be unsuitable for clinical applications, and (3) increased voltages by factor of two were needed to produce sinusoidal ramps instead of linear ramps.

The pulse sequence strategy was extended to fast imaging sequences (FLASH and RARE) in 2001 (114). Noise reductions of 20- to 40-dB(A) were reported compared to standard sequences (**Figure 15**). However, acquisition time remained at around one second per slice, which is unsuitable for an fMRI examination. Loenneker, et al. (115) also extended the technique, by integrating into a "T_2*" pulse sequence, and improving the volume coverage by using simultaneous multi-slice excitation with SIMEX (i.e., a modem statistical technique that estimates bias by tracking measurement error as a function of added noise) pulses. This enabled the technique to be applied to fMRI. Oesterle, et al. (116) also reported

Figure 14. Acoustic noise levels for gradient-echo and spin-echo pulse sequences measured as a function of echo time (TE, milliseconds) at 3-Tesla. The top lines in the graphs correspond to sequences using soft (S) gradient pulses. The middle lines in the graphs show sequences with linear (L) ramps of maximum duration. The bottom lines in the graphs show standard sequence default settings. The dashed line is the level of ambient room noise from the air-conditioning system (113). Reproduced by permission, Wiley - John Wiley & Son Publishers, NY.

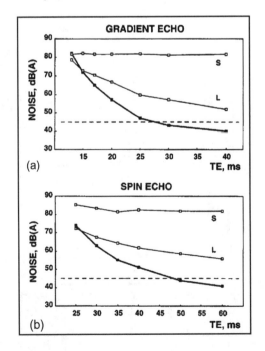

Figure 15. Optimized use of soft gradient pulses for two fast imaging sequences: (Top) FLASH sequence, (Bottom) RARE sequence. In each case, three types of gradient waveform are compared: (a) hard trapezoidal, (b) older style soft waveforms designed according to (113), and (c) new soft waveforms designed according to (114). Reproduced by permission, Wiley - John Wiley & Son Publishers, NY.

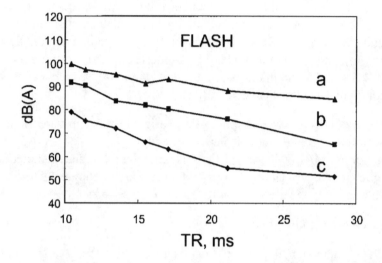

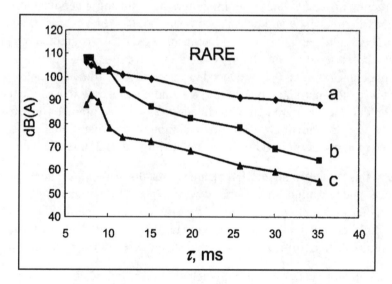

on an improved technique utilizing "soft" gradient pulses. In this case, the limitation due to long acquisition times was minimized using interleaved spiral gradient, read-out trajectories. Using this pulse sequence with optimized sampling scheme on a 2-T MR system, an average noise reduction of 22-dB(A) was achieved.

(D) Using Parallel Imaging

Similar to the slew rate reduction associated with a soft gradient pulse technique, De Zwart, et al. (117) used SENSE parallel imaging techniques to obtain significant reductions in gradient slew rates and achieved reductions in acoustic noise. The use of sensitivity encoding in combination with multi-channel detector arrays allows reduced gradient switching through reduced k-space sampling. Using anther type of MRI sequence (i.e., SENSE), a gradient slew rate reduction was achieved at constant image acquisition time and image spatial resolution. For two-fold SENSE under sampling, the gradient amplitude was reduced to 50% (13-mT/m), and ramp time doubled (360-microseconds), resulting in a slew rate of 37-T/m/sec (a 4-fold reduction in the maximum slew rate). SPL reductions for two scanners were reported: 14-dB(A) (1.5-T) and 12-dB(A)(3-T).

Moelker, et al. (118) reported an interesting variant of this approach. This group built a manual controller to reduce gradient slew rates and the associated acoustic noise for use during interventional MRI, where acoustic noise may be particularly unpleasant for staff members, while small degradations to image quality can be tolerated. Their controller allowed a 16-fold reduction in slew rate, with acoustic noise reduced by up to 21-dB(A).

(E) Using Hardware Optimization

Cho, et al. (119) developed a "quiet" MRI technique based on a variation of the projection reconstruction method that also minimizes gradient pulsing. In conventional projection reconstruction, the frequency and phase encoding gradients remain on simultaneously at a low level throughout the acquisition of a line of image data. Less gradient pulsing is done and gradient amplitudes are generally lower than in conventional two dimensional, Fourier transform imaging. Cho, et al. (119) reduced gradient pulsing with a projection reconstruction type of pulse sequence and replaced the two gradient pulses with a single mechanically rotating direct current (DC) gradient coil. In addition, the DC gradient remains on for the entirety of the image acquisition using this technique (in conventional projection reconstruction, the gradients are pulsed on for the acquisition of each line of image data).

The use of this "quiet "or silent MRI technique results in a 20.7-dB attenuation in sound level. However, the technique suffers from two important limitations. First, the slices may be selected in the z-axis only due to the readout gradient rotating around the z-axis (i.e., no acquisition of oblique slices is possible). Second, there is a loss of slice volume at each angle of rotation due to a tilting of the selected slice caused during gradient rotation.

At the meeting for the Radiological Society of North America in 2012, General Electric (GE) Healthcare unveiled a new solution to MRI-related acoustic noise (120). Based on GE Silent Scan Technology, it was suggested that the scanner can be operated with acoustic noise levels below standard ambient room conditions. Therefore, not just "quiet" MRI, but effectively silent. The Silent Scan Technology approach comprises the use of "Silenz", a new three-dimensional acquisition and reconstruction technique, in combination with a re-designed gradient system and RF hardware. Importantly, the Silenz protocol acquires k-space data radially rather than line-by-line, minimizing gradient switching. This product is not readily available on a commercial basis at the present time, so only limited information is available. However, this type of approach could have an enormous impact on future scanner design and the reduction in MRI-related acoustic noise.

(F) Adapting to the Scanner Acoustic Noise Response

For each separate gradient (x-, y-, and z-gradient), Tomasi, et al. (121) compared the current waveforms and resulting vibrational response. This group demonstrated, that by altering the read-out frequency of the EPI gradient (and, hence, the bandwidth) to avoid known vibrational resonances, significant reductions in acoustic noise could be achieved. Altering the read-out frequency from 720-Hz to 920-Hz resulted in a noise reduction of 12-dB.

A similar approach was reported by Schmitter, et al. in 2008 (122). These researchers devised the so-called "sEPI" technique, which is a low noise EPI pulse sequence for use with fMRI. This sequence produces a narrow acoustic frequency spectrum by using a sinusoidal read-out gradient waveform with smooth ramps and constant phase encode gradient. By varying the switching frequency of the read-out gradient, this narrow band can be shifted in frequency to match the minima of the scanner frequency response function, avoiding major resonance modes and minimizing acoustic noise. These researchers reported that the average SPL of the standard EPI, 82.5-dB(A), was reduced to 61.7-dB(A). This sequence did not include optimization of the slice selection gradient, and so this work was extended in 2010 with the introduction of noise-optimized "VERSE" pulses (123). Zapp et al. (124) further expanded sEPI with the use of parallel imaging.

(G) Using Noise Cancellation Gradient Pulses

Some researchers have proposed a technique involving additional "follow-up" gradient pulses, to cancel the initial pulses that would generate acoustic noise, which is a sort of an anti-noise approach using anti-gradients instead of anti-noise (125, 126). There is, in effect, a change to the gradient input function, such that initial impulsive forces generated by the gradients are cancelled by subsequent counter impulsive forces, minimizing the potential for the generation of acoustic noise. These ideas can be seen as an extension of the initial observations of the acoustic noise characteristics of trapezoidal gradient pulses as reported by Wu, et al. (127). Shou, et al. (126) demonstrated that follow-on trapezoidal gradient pulses can cancel two frequencies and their harmonics. The initial studies from this group showed that a significant noise reduction was possible (around 13-dB) when cancelling at least three of the dominant acoustic noise spectral peaks.

Segbers, et al. (128) have taken a hybrid approach to optimizing the gradient pulse sequence, based on using soft gradient pulses, cancellation pulses, and frequency shifting to avoid resonance modes. These researchers ran versions of EPI and turbo spin echo sequences with optimized gradient pulse sequences on a 3-Tesla MR system. The gradient coil had a maximum gradient strength of 21-mT/m and slew rate of 200-mT/m/ms. Using a combination of single and double follow-on trapezoidal gradient pulses, Segbers, et al. (128) managed to suppress several of the main acoustic noise spectral frequencies and achieved a maximum noise reduction of 12-dB.

(H) Functional MRI-Specific Methods

As mentioned above, MRI-related acoustic noise can interfere with the presentation and processing of functional stimuli and generate blood oxygen level dependent (BOLD)-related contrast in the auditory cortex. Passive hearing protection may not offer sufficiently quiet conditions for psychological studies of hearing (129). Unfortunately, residual noise can often be loud enough to mask the perception of experimental sound stimuli (11). The use of quiet MRI sequences employing shallow gradient ramps or soft gradient pulses frequently cannot be applied to fMRI due to its requirement for ultrafast image acquisition. It is possible to use "sparse" fMRI paradigms that modify the timing of image acquisition, restricting the image acquisition to the post-stimulus time interval and reducing any influence of the noise on brain activation (130, 131). However, these modifications tend to compromise the quality of the fMRI procedure, degrading either temporal resolution or data acquisition efficiency (132).

It is more common to manage these issues using two types of sequence-related solutions, as follows: (1) using silent gaps within fMRI sequences and (2) using event-related strategies (133). One is based on modifications to fMRI block design experiments and the other to event-related designs. Often in fMRI, the same stimuli are presented repeatedly for a block of time (typically 20- to 40-seconds). Then, two or more blocks with particular experimental conditions are alternated.

Modified Block Designs for fMRI. These sequences (also called clustered volume acquisition, flat car design, sparse, and behavior interleaved gradients), involve interleaving short (1- to 4-seconds) silent gaps within fMRI sequences. In the brain, the peak hemodynamic response to noise occurs after a time delay of around 5-seconds following stimulation. Knowing this, it is possible to present stimuli in these silent gaps where the scanner is silent and then to acquire the subsequent images when the peak response will occur. This cycle is then repeated for the entire block. The duration of the gap is dependent on the number of slices acquired and the repetition time (TR) used. Therefore, care is needed to avoid extending the sequence length, which can have penalties in terms of patient motion and image quality. An underlying assumption is also made with simple modified block designs, that any BOLD response to scanner noise during acquisition will apply equally when stimulus is on and when it is off. Optimization of the block design involves two additional criteria. If the silent gap is extended to 9- to 10-seconds, enough time will have elapsed to allow any hemodynamic response produced by the previous acquisition to return to baseline. Sampling of any BOLD signal relating to acoustic noise from the previous acquisition will then be minimized. Lastly, keeping the acquisition time under 2-seconds will prevent measurement of any hemodynamic response (HR) from the current acquisition.

Event-Related Designs for fMRI. This method involves sampling the peak of the stimulus HR, followed by a waiting period to avoid acquisition during scanner noise HR. When scanner HR has dissipated, baseline sampling then occurs. The speed of data collection directly determines study data quality and the repetition time should be kept to a minimum. This type of sequence typically allows one measurement every 20-seconds (134).

Methods Involving Optimized Gradient Hardware

The best, if not the most technically challenging, solution to address acoustic noise is to eliminate the noise at the source by designing a "quiet" gradient coil which generates no acoustic noise or vibration. Acoustic noise and vibration arises due to physical buckling and resonance of the gradient coil (and former), as well as coupling to other structures. Noise control may be achieved by special designs taking into consideration the construction and materials of the gradient coil formers, coupling with other structures, use of noise insulation materials, and finally the design of the coil windings themselves. This section discusses each of these aspects in more detail.

(A) Passive Insulation, Materials, and Structure

Stiffness and Damping. As suggested above, greater gradient coil stiffness should reduce mechanical vibration and associated noise. Stiffness is dependent on material properties and geometrical factors. Altering gradient coil dimensions or materials to increase Young's modulus will help reduce acoustic noise due to vibration. Lin, et al. (135) reported on the use of a variety of reinforcements to increase the gradient coil stiffness, reduce vibration, and the associated acoustic noise. These investigators found that increasing the stiffness of the gradient coil former reduced the amplitude of the forced vibration response of the gradient coil at low frequencies and the noise generated by the coil. In addition, the gradient coil demonstrated a reduced number of resonance modes in the low and medium frequency ranges, in turn, reducing the chance of the system being excited into resonance and generating high levels of acoustic noise.

Damping the gradient coil may also attenuate the mechanical vibration. This can be achieved by using particular materials for construction or by mounting the coil in such a way that an acoustic absorber surrounds it. Damping is most efficient at or near resonance and, unfortunately, will reduce the overall stiffness of the coil structure. Several commercial manufacturers use damping techniques for their gradient coil systems (50, 55). A reduction of around 3-dB(A) due to the use of acoustically damped commercial gradient systems have been reported (50). Mechefske, et al. (136) reported improved results by mounting an acoustic liner inside the bore of a 4-Tesla research scanner, with damping material applied to the back. The bore of this MR system was also fitted with an "endcap". Running an EPI sequence, acoustic attenuation of around 20-dB was possible, however the scanner did not have a body RF coil, *in situ*, at the time of the experiments, and the liner may be difficult to use in a commercial scanner.

In 2005, Shao, et al. (63) reported on the development of an analytic model that predicted the acoustic noise generated by an MRI gradient coil with finite acoustic impedance, which was based on initial work by Kuijpers, et al. (68). This group modeled the use of an absorptive liner inside the gradient coils and tested predictions with measurements made in a 4-Tesla MR system. They found that an acoustic noise reduction of the order of 10-dB at the low frequency end of the spectrum was possible, but the practicality of using thick materials in limited space is doubtful.

Isolation/Evacuation/Enclosure. Some groups have tried to isolate the gradient coil to prevent the transmission of vibrations to other structures (137-139). As acoustic waves can only travel in a medium, mounting or encasing the gradient coil in a vacuum should avoid transmission of any generated noise (137-140). Edelstein, et al. (139) controlled acoustic noise by using a combination of evacuating the gradient coil structure and using a magnet with a non-conducting inner cryostat bore. They achieved total reduction in acoustic noise of around 20-dB (peak). Their results showed that eddy currents caused by gradient shielding leakage can generate significant Lorentz forces on the inner cryostat bore. These forces contribute a significant level of the total scanner acoustic noise. Edelstein, et al. (139) reported that is it important to provide electromagnetic isolation. In 2005, based on finite element modeling, they redesigned standard active gradient shielding to include an additional passive copper layer (141). This added passive shield prevented power deposition in the warm bore, which resulted in an efficient hybrid active-passive shielding system. **Figure 16** shows examples of typical configurations for such a strategy. The modeled power reductions associated with the system predicted a reduction in acoustic noise of approximately 25-dB.

Katsunuma, et al. (137), evacuated the area surrounding the gradient coil system so that insulation would prevent propagation of sound and a separate mount (i.e., floor mounting the gradient coil former) that prevented transmission of vibration from other structures. Acoustic noise reduction levels of around 30-dB (peak) were possible, but this is an expensive solution and not suited for retrofit. "Enclosure" is a traditional technique used in noise

Figure 16. Examples of design configurations for active-passive gradient shielding systems (141). Reproduced by permission, Wiley - John Wiley & Son Publishers, NY.

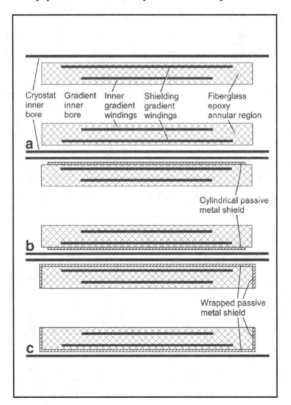

control, which involves enclosing the noise source in an airtight skin, damping the source side of the enclosure, and decoupling the enclosure from the source (55).

Perforating a noise-generating surface has been found to significantly reduce the levels of acoustic noise generated (142). Systems involving the use of micro-perforated panels (MPPs), first suggested by Maa (143), are typically used with an air-filled backing cavity and rigid back wall. These methods can also be difficult to implement efficiently in MR systems due to additional space requirements. More recently, Li and Mechefske (144) investigated the implementation of an MPP system for use in MRI. Their basic expansion modeling showed that the MPP systems can be particularly efficient at low frequencies. However, optimized parameters also allow good efficiency over a wider band. As with poorly designed ANC systems, noise levels have been found to increase with poorly designed perforation systems (144).

(B) Design of Gradient Coil Windings: Force-Balanced Coils (Active Acoustic Shielding)

In theory, it is possible to design gradient coil windings such that all Lorentz forces generated by current pulsing are balanced (i.e., each force is effectively cancelled by one of equal magnitude at a conjugate position relative to the coil center) (41,145-147). This is, in essence, similar to using anti-phase noise to cancel a noise source. For example, actively-shielded gradient coils are intrinsically force-balanced to a degree. They are designed to have a secondary coil operate in opposition to the main primary to minimize Lorentz forces on the primary. The combination of coil design and a consideration of construction methods and materials are essential for efficient results.

Rather than trying to mount a vibrating gradient coil to a heavy and immovable former or somehow damp the coil, if the coil is considered as a harmonic oscillator and coupled to another, back-to-back, and if masses and spring constants are equal, the center of mass of the system will be constant without the need for a heavy mount (146). This is the principle of active force balancing which may be applied to gradient coil design (**Figure 17**).

All solids have visco-elastic properties and this will result in residual movement of the conductors, limiting the ideal noise cancellation suggested above. These movements will result in compression waves propagating through the material with velocity,

$$v = \left(E \middle/ \rho \right)^{1/2} \tag{4}$$

Where, E, is Young's modulus and ρ is the density of the material. Knowing that wave velocity and frequency are related by $v = f\lambda$, a slow wave velocity will result in low frequency, above which progressive phase effects will be expected which will interfere with noise cancellation.

For optimal acoustic noise cancellation, strut material should have a large value for E and small value for ρ, resulting in a high compressional wave velocity. Thus, a light coupling

Figure 17. (a) Diagram representing two coupled line elements of conductor, dl, of equal mass, m, carrying equal and opposite currents. The center of mass of the system remains fixed if the spring constants, k, are equal. The system is placed in a magnetic field B, which gives rise to the forces, F, causing displacements. (b) Rectangular conductor loop carrying a current, I, placed in a magnetic field B, such that the loop plane is normal B. All forces F and F' are balanced, provided the plane of the coil is oriented perpendicular to the magnetic field direction. If these coils are coupled to similar others via non-compressive struts, then all forces in the system are balanced. If non-compressive materials are used, the conductors cannot move and no sound is generated (146). Reproduced by permission, Institute of Physics Publishing.

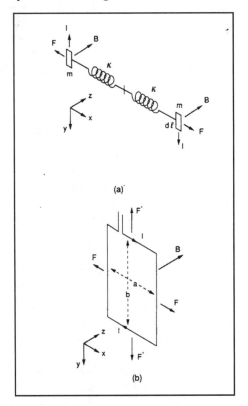

structure of high strength may perform as well as a heavier structure. Composite materials have been tested and found to perform well with a frequency response up to 20-kHz (single loop coil of dimensions 30-cm x 20-cm) (105). Using a bench-top prototype 2-coil system (a square coil design measuring 40-cm along each size, powered by a 10-A sinusoidal current), the reported noise attenuation, when powered in balanced mode, was approximately 40-dB at 100-Hz, dropping to 0-dB at 3.5-Hz (**Figure 18**). The results of attenuation levels agree reasonably well with a theoretical prediction (curve D) (146).

Designs have also been extended and tailored to include the capability of current balancing, acoustic screening and magnetic field screening in one coil (145). A head gradient coil has been designed analytically using co-axial return paths to minimize localized Lorentz forces and acoustic noise. When performing EPI (3-mm slice thickness, gradient switching

Figure 18. A plot showing SPL and attenuation A dB versus f for a test coil. Curve A corresponds to the radiated sound received when one coil only is powered. Curve B is the reduced level when two coils are powered in balanced mode. Curve C is the resultant sound attenuation (the difference between A and B) and curve D is the theoretical prediction. The results of attenuation levels agree reasonably well with a theoretical prediction (curve D)(146). Reproduced by permission, Institute of Physics Publishing.

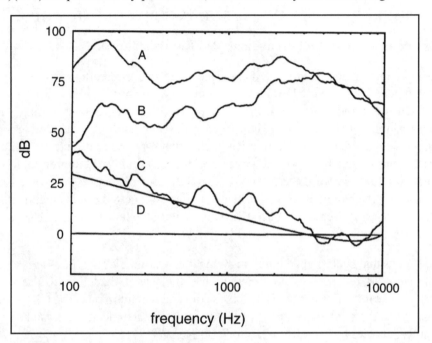

frequency 830-Hz, current 207-A) in a 3-Tesla MR system, noise levels of 102-dB (root mean square) have been reported (146).

The implications for gradient coil characteristics of the acoustic screening design mean a loss of gradient strength and an increase in coil inductance, thus, reducing high-speed performance. Estimates of the increase in inductance for a three-cylinder coil system (i.e., fully force shielded as well as acoustically and magnetically shielded) over a gradient coil with only active magnetic shielding is a factor of approximately eight.

To counteract this in keeping performance constant, an increase in driver current of the square root of 8 is required that will, in turn, increase the acoustic noise output of the coil. Throughout the data on sound generation in relatively simple gradient structures (41), the highest sound pressure levels were noted to come from spurious resonances, thought to be due to bending and buckling of the coil structures (Chladni resonances). Designing coil systems that completely cancel acoustic noise including contributions from these sources is a considerable challenge.

(C) Other Gradient Design Methods

Researchers have devised an analytical approach to the design of quiet gradient coils (148-150). This work, which is a form of target field approach, uses an inverse method for designing winding paths, explicitly accounting for finite coil length. It treats the Biot-Savart law as a first kind integral equation for the current density on the gradient coil, once the magnetic field has been specified, and uses Tikhonov regularization to handle the inherent non-unique aspect of the design problem. Researchers using this approach have achieved very modest acoustic attenuation levels.

OTHER SOURCES OF MR SYSTEM-RELATED ACOUSTIC NOISE

Auditory Perception of Radiofrequency (RF) Electromagnetic Fields

When the human head is subjected to pulsed RF radiation at certain frequencies, an audible sound perceived as a click or knocking noise may be heard (151-153). This acoustic phenomenon is referred to as "RF hearing", "RF sound" or "microwave hearing". Thermo-elastic expansion is believed to be the mechanism responsible for the production of RF hearing, whereby there is absorption of RF energy that produces a minute temperature elevation (i.e., approximately 1×10^{-6} °C) over a brief time period (i.e., approximately 10-microseconds) in the tissue of the head (151-153). Subsequently, a pressure wave is induced that is sensed by the hair cells of the cochlea via bone conduction. In this manner, the pulse of RF energy is transferred into an acoustic wave within the human head and sensed by the hearing organs.

The sounds that occur with RF hearing appear to originate from within or near the back of the human head, regardless of the orientation of the head in the RF field. The actual type of noise that is heard varies with the RF pulse width and repetition rate. The relative loudness is dependent on the total energy per pulse. RF energy-related acoustic noise has been observed at frequencies ranging from 216 to 7500-MHz (151-153).

RF hearing is mathematically predictable from classical physics and has been studied and characterized in laboratory animals and human subjects. Individuals involved with the use of microwaves in industrial and military settings commonly experience RF hearing. With specific reference to the operation of MR systems, RF hearing has been found to be associated with frequencies ranging from 2.4- to 170-MHz (151).

The gradient magnetic field-induced acoustic noise that occurs during MRI procedures is significantly louder than the sounds associated with RF hearing. Therefore, noises produced by the RF auditory phenomenon are effectively masked and not perceived by patients or MR system operators (151). Furthermore, there is no evidence of any detrimental health effects related to the presence of RF hearing. However, Roschmann, et al. (151) recommends an upper level limit of 30-kW applied peak pulse power of RF energy for head coils and 6-kW for surface coils used during MR imaging or spectroscopy to avoid RF-evoked sound pressure levels in the head increasing above the discomfort threshold of 110-dB.

Noise from Subsidiary Systems

Room air conditioners, fans for patient comfort, and cryogen reclamation systems associated with superconducting magnets are the main sources of ambient acoustic noise found in the MRI environment. Cryogen reclamation systems are devices that are effectively used to minimize the loss of cryogens and function on a continuous basis, producing sounds that are considerably less than those associated with the activation of the gradient magnetic fields during MRI procedures. Therefore, this acoustic noise may, at the very most, be a mild annoyance to patients or MR system operators in the MRI environment. Some authors have reported ambient room noise levels to be 60- to 70-dB (56,128).

SUMMARY AND CONCLUSIONS

MRI procedures can generate significant levels of acoustic noise under certain conditions (45, 58). This noise can be an annoyance, hinder communication with staff members and, at high levels, presents a possible safety hazard to patients and MRI healthcare workers that must be measured and controlled.

Many groups have measured and analyzed the acoustic noise associated with MRI. Acoustic noise levels increase with changes in imaging parameters including a decrease in section thickness, field-of-view, gradient ramp time, and an increase in the gradient amplitude. The environment, hardware design, and the presence of the patient in the MR system will also affect noise levels.

Although many options are available for noise control, the use of simple passive protection in the form of earplugs is sufficient to decrease noise to levels well within permissible limits for the great majority of patients. However, care must be taken to ensure passive protection is properly fitted (1).

Current documents regarding permissible limits vary, but a general consensus appears to set a permissible average noise level at the patients ear of 85-dB(A) (35, 76, 86). Noise levels outside the MR system's bore are lower and present reduced risks for an MRI healthcare worker present during the MRI examination.

Of course, passive methods have limitations and several more elegant solutions are possible and under investigation by researchers. These methods range from simply optimizing the MRI pulse sequences to be used in terms of gradient parameters (108-112), to the utilization of anti-noise systems, or redesigning the gradient coils, themselves.

As with many aspects of MRI, the specifications for achieving high noise attenuation often run counter to fast acquisition of high quality diagnostic images and compromises must be made. Optimizing procedures to lengthen gradient ramp times, lower amplitudes, or minimize pulsing can result in sequences with reduced performance (113-115). Designing gradient coils that are force-balanced to minimize acoustic resonances will compromise performance in terms of increasing inductance and loss of gradient strength (41, 145-147).

The solution that presents a minimal impact on the performance of the MR system is active noise control using anti-noise (95-102). This is a promising technique but an optimal system has yet to be fully investigated on clinical scanners. The new solution, Silent Scan Technology, from GE offers exciting potential (120). The ability to operate the scanner at or below ambient room noise levels is clearly quite impressive. The technique is not fully released at this time but a solution of this type could turn out to be a game-changer for controlling MRI-related acoustic noise.

Current trends in MRI include increasing static magnetic field strengths and improved gradient performance for rapid clinical imaging applications. The need for ultrafast sequences for fMRI continues. These developments will result in increases in MRI-generated acoustic noise levels. This will mean an increasing interest in acoustic noise control methods and warrants continued investigation, development, and commercial implementation of these techniques.

REFERENCES

1. Brummett RE, Talbot JM, Charuhas P. Potential hearing loss resulting from MR imaging. Radiology 1988;169:539-540.

2. Quirk ME, Letendre AJ, Ciottone RA, Lingley JF. Anxiety in patients undergoing MR imaging. Radiology 1989;170:463-466.

3. Laurell G. The combined effect of noise and cisplatin. Ann Otol Rhinol Laryngol 1992;1001:969-976.

4. Philbin MK, Taber KH, Hayman LA. Preliminary report: changes in vital signs of term newborns during MR. Am J Neurorad 1996;17:1033-6.

5. Kanal E, Shellock FG, Talagala L. Safety considerations in MR imaging. Radiology 1990;176:593-606.

6. Shellock FG, Kanal E. Policies, guidelines, and recommendations for MR imaging safety and patient management. J Magn Reson Imaging 1991;1:97-101.

7. Shellock FG, Litwer CA, Kanal E. Magnetic resonance imaging: bioeffects, safety, and patient management. Rev Magn Reson Med 1992;4:21.

8. Kanal E, Shellock FG, Sonnenblick D. MRI clinical site safety survey: phase I results and preliminary data. Magn Reson Imaging 1989;7(Suppl 1):IT-03.

9. De Wilde JP, Grainger D, Price DL, Renaud C. Magnetic resonance imaging safety issues including an analysis of recorded incidents within the UK. Prog Nucl Magn Reson Spectr 2007;51:37-48.

10. Zhang N, Zhu XH, Chen W. Influence of gradient acoustic noise on fMRI response in the human visual cortex. Magn Reson Med 2005;54:258-283.

11. Shah NJ, Jancke L, Grosse-Ruken ML, Muller-Gartner HW. Influence of acoustic masking noise in fMRI of the auditory cortex during phonetic discrimination. J Magn Reson Imaging 1999;9:19-25.

12. Ravicz ME, Melcher JR, Kiang NY. Acoustic noise during functional magnetic resonance imaging. J Acoust Soc Am 2001;108:1683-1696.

13. Hall DA, Haggard MP, et al. Functional magnetic resonance imaging measurements of sound-level encoding in the absence of background scanner noise. Acoust Soc Am 2000;109:1559-1570.

14. Moelker A, Pattynama MT. Acoustic noise concerns in functional magnetic resonance imaging. Human Brain Mapping 2003;20:123-141.

15. Strainer JC, Ulmer JL, et al. Functional MR of the primary auditory cortex: an analysis of pure tone activation and tone discrimination. Am J Neuroradiol 1997;18:601-610.

16. Ulmer JL, Biswal BB, et al. Acoustic echo-planar scanner noise and pure tone hearing thresholds: the effects of sequence repetition times and acoustic noise rates. J Comp Assist Tomog 1998;22:480-486.

17. Bess FH, Humes LE. Audiology, The Fundamentals, 4th Edition. Baltimore: Williams and Wilkins;1995.

18. Department of Health. Acoustics: design considerations, HTM 2045. London: HMSO;1996.

19. Hetu R, Laroche C, Quoc HT, LePage B, St Vincent J. The Spectrum of Impulse Noise and the Human Ear Response. In: Dancer AL, Henderson D, Salvi RJ, Hamernik RP, Editors. Noise-Induced Hearing Loss. St. Louis: Mosby Press;1992. pp. 361.

20. Alberti P. Noise and the Ear. In: Stephens D, Editor. Adult Audiology. UK: Butterworths;1987.

21. Mills JH. Effects of Noise on Auditory Sensitivity, Psychophysical Tuning Curves and Suppression. In: Hamernik RP, Henderson D, Salvi R, Editors. New Perspectives on Noise Induced Hearing Loss. New York: Raven Press;1982.

22. Prasher D. Estimation of Hearing Damage From Noise Exposure. Report From the Technical Meeting on Exposure-Response Relationships of Noise on Health, Bonn, Germany. Geneva: World Health Organisation;2003. pp. 82-97.

23. Khanna SM, Tonndorf J, Queller J. Mechanical parameters of hearing by bone conduction. J Acoust Soc Am 1976;60:139-154.

24. Ravicz ME, Melcher JR. Isolating the auditory system from acoustic noise during fMRI: noise conduction through the ear canal, head and body. J Acoust Soc Am 2001;1:216-231.

25. Pujol R, Lavigne-Rebillard M, Uziel A. Physiological correlates of development of the human cochlea. Semin Perinatol 1990;14:275-280.

26. Shepper PG, Shahidullah BS. Development of fetal hearing. Arch Dis Child 1994;71:81-87.

27. Richards DS, Frenzen B, Gerhardt KJ, McCann ME, Abrams RM. Sound levels in the human uterus. Obster Gynecol 1992;80:186-190.

28. Shepper PG, Shahidullah BS. Noise and the fetus: a critical review of the literature. Sudbury: HSE Books;1994.

29. Gerhardt KJ, Abrams RM. Fetal hearing: characterization of the stimulus and response. Semin Perinatol 1996;20:11-20.

30. Gerhardt KJ, Abrams RM. Fetal exposures to sound and vibroacoustic stimulation. J Perinatol 2000;20(8 Pt.2):S21-S30.

31. Lecanuet JP, Gautheron B, et al. What sounds reach fetuses: biological and non-biological modeling of the transmission of pure tones. Dev Psychobiol 1998;33:203-219.

32. De Wilde JP, Rivers AW, Price DL. A review of the current use of magnetic resonance imaging in pregnancy and safety implications for the fetus. Progr Biophys and Mol Biol 2005;87:335-353.

33. Brezinka C, Lechner T, Stephens K. The fetus and noise. Gynal-geburt Runds 1997;37:119-129.

34. Glover P, Hykin J, Gowland P, Wright J, Johnson J, Mansfield PM. An assessment of the intrauterine sound intensity level during obstetric echo-planar magnetic resonance imaging. Brit J Rad 1995;68:1090-4.

35. Etzel RA, Balk SJ, Bearer CF, Miller MD, Shea KM, Simon PR. Noise: a hazard for the fetus and newborn. Paediatrics 1997;100;724-727.

36. Reeves MJ, Brandreth M, et al. Neonatal cochlear function: measurement after exposure to acoustic noise during in utero MR imaging. Radiology 2010;257:802-9.

37. Medicines and Healthcare Products Regulatory Authority (MHRA) Guidelines, DB2007;2007.

38. Health and Safety Executive. Noise and the Fetus: A Critical Review of the Literature. Sudbury: HSE Books;1994.

39. Health and Safety Executive. Non-Auditory Effects of Noise at Work: A Critical Review of the Literature Post 1998. Sudbury: HSE Books;1999.

40. American Academy of Paediatrics: Committee on environmental health. Noise: a hazard for the fetus and newborn. Paediatrics 1997;100:724-727.

41. Mansfield P, Glover PM, Beaumont J. Sound generation in gradient coil structures for MRI. Magn Reson Ned 1998;39:539-550.

42. Moelker A, Wielopolski PA, Pattynama PMT. Relationship between magnetic field strength and magnetic resonance-related acoustic noise. Magn Reson Mater Phys Biol 2003;16:52-55.

43. Price DL, De Wilde JP, Papadaki AM, Curran JS, Kitney RI. Investigation of acoustic noise on 15 MRI scanners from 0.2 to 3 T. J Magn Reson Imaging 2001;13:288-293.

44. Roozen NB, Koevoets AH, den Hamer AJ. Active vibration control of gradient coils to reduce acoustic noise of MRI systems. IEEE Trans Mechatronics 2008;13: 325-334.

45. Goldman AM, Gossman WE, Friedlander PC. Reduction of sound levels with antinoise in MR imaging. Radiology 1989;173:549-550.

46. Hurwitz R, Lane SR, Bell RA, Brant-Zawadzki MN. Acoustic analysis of gradient-coil noise in MR imaging. Radiology 1989;173:545-48.

47. Shellock FG, Morisoli SM, Ziarati M. Measurement of acoustic noise during MR imaging: Evaluation of six "worst-case" pulse sequences. Radiology 1994;191:91-93.

48. McJury M, Blug A, Joerger C, Condon B, Wyper D. Acoustic noise levels during magnetic resonance imaging scanning at 1.5 T. Brit J Radiol 1994;64:413-5.

49. McJury MJ. Acoustic noise levels generated during high field MR imaging. Clin Radiol 1995;50:331-333.

50. Counter SA, Olofsson A, Grahn HF, Borg E. MRI acoustic noise: sound pressure and frequency analysis. J Magn Reson Imaging 1997;7:606-611.

51. Hedeen RA, Edelstein WA. Characteristics and prediction of gradient acoustic noise in MR imagers. Magn Reson Med 1997;37:7-10.

52. Cho ZH, Park SH, Kim JH, et al. Analysis of acoustic noise in MRI. Mag Res Imaging 1997;15:815-822.

53. Shellock FG, Ziarati M, Atkinson D, Chen DY. Determination of gradient magnetic field-induced acoustic noise associated with the use of echo planar and three-dimensional fast spin echo techniques. J Magn Reson Imaging 1998;8:1154-7.

54. Miyati T, Banno T, Fujita H, et al. Acoustic noise analysis in echo planar imaging: multi-center trial and comparison with other pulse sequences. IEEE Trans Med Imag 1999;18:773-6.

55. Sellers MB, Pavlids JD, Carlberger T. MRI acoustic noise. Int J Neuroradiol 1996;2:549.

56. Ravicz ME, Melcher JR, Kiang NYS. Acoustic noise during functional MRI. J Acoust Soc Am 2000;108:1683-96.

57. More SR, Lim TC, Li M, Holland CK, Boyce SE, Lee JH. Acoustic noise characteristics of a 4T MRI scanner. J Magn Reson Imag 2006;23:388-397.

58. Foster JR, Hall DA, Summerfield AQ, Palmer AR, Bowtell RW. Sound level measurements and calculations of safe noise dosage during EPI at 3 T. J Magn Reson Imaging 2000;12:157-163.

59. Rizzo-Sierra CV, Verslius MJ, Hoogduin JM, Duifhuis H. Acoustic fMRI noise: linear time-invariant system model. IEEE Trans Biomed Eng 2008;55:2115-2123.

60. Mechefske CK, Wu Y, Rutt BK. Characterization of acoustic noise and magnetic field fluctuations in a 4 T whole-body MRI scanner. Mech Systems and Sign Proc 2002;16(2-3):459-473.

61. Yao GZ, Mechefske CK, Rutt BK. Characterization of vibration and acoustic noise in a gradient coil insert. MAGMA 2004;17:12-27.

62. Yao GZ, Mechefske CK, Rutt BK. Acoustic noise simulation and measurement of a gradient insert in a 4T MRI. Appl Acoust 2005;66:957-973.

63. Shao W, Mechsfske CK. Acoustic analysis of a gradient coil winding in an MRI scanner. Concepts in Magn Reson Part B 2004;24B:15-27.

64. Wang F, Mechefske CK. Modal analysis and testing of a thin-walled gradient coil cylinder model. Concepts in Magn Reson Part B 2004;27B:34-50.

65. Mechefske CK, Wang F. Theoretical, numerical, and experimental modal analysis of a single-winding gradient coil insert cylinder. Magn Reson Mater Phys Biol 2006;19:152-166.

66. Wang F, Mechefske CK. Modal analysis of a multilayered gradient coil insert in a 4T MRI scanner. Concepts in Magn Reson Part B 2007;31B:237-254.

67. Wang FL. Dynamic modeling of gradient coils in a MRI scanner. Doctoral thesis, 2006. Queen's University, Kingston, Ontario, Canada.

68. Kuijpers AHW, Rienstra SW, Verbeek G, Verheeij JW. The acoustic radiation of baffled finite ducts with vibrating walls. J Sound and Vibr 1998;216:461-493.

69. Sodel W. Vibrations of Shells and Plates, 3rd Edition. New York: Dekker;2004.

70. Li G, Mechefkse CK. Structural-acoustic modal analysis of cylindrical shells: application to MRI scanner systems. Magn Reson Mater Phys Biol 2009;22:353-364.

71. Rausch M, Gebbardt M, Kaltenbacher M, Landes H. CAD of clinical MRI scanners by coupled magneto-mechanical-acoustic modeling. IEEE Trans on Magnetics 2005;41:72-81.

72. Singhal RK, Guan W, Williams K. Modal analysis of a thick walled circular cylinder. Mech Syst Signal Proc 2002;16:141-153.

73. Singal RK, Williams K. Theoretical and experimental study of vibrations of thick circular cylindrical shells and rings. ASME J Vib Acoust Stress Rehab Des 1998; 110:533-537.

74. Findell IH. Fundamentals of Human Response to Sound. Fahy FJ and Walker JG, Editors. Fundamentals of Noise and Vibration. London: Spon; 1998. pp.145.

75. Anari M, Axelsson A, Eliasson A, Magnusson L. Hypersensitivity to sound- questionnaire data, audiometry, and classification. Scand Audiol 1999;28:219-230.

76. Control of Noise at Work. London: HMSO;2005.

77. The Management of Health and Safety at Work Regulations. Statutory Instrument No. 3242;1999.

78. Occupational Safety and Health Administration (OSHA). Occupational noise exposure. 29 C.F.R., pt. 1910.95;1988.

79. Food and Drug Administration. Magnetic resonance diagnostic device panel recommendation and report on petitions for MR reclassification. Fed Regist 1998;53:7575-9.

80. Department of Health, Guidelines for Magnetic Resonance diagnostic equipment in clinical use. London: HMSO;1993.

81. McRobbie DW. Occupational exposure in MRI. Brit J Radiol 2012;85:293-312.

82. National Radiological Protection Board. Principles for the protection of patients and volunteers during clinical magnetic resonance diagnostic procedures. Documents of the NRPB;1991;2.

83. National Radiological Protection Board. Review of the scientific evidence for limiting exposure to electromagnetic fields (0-300GHz). Documents of the NRPB;2004;15.

84. National Radiological Protection Board. Electromagnetic fields and the risk of cancer: Report of an advisory group on non-ionizing radiation. Documents of the NRPB;1992;3.

85. International Commission on Non-Ionizing Radiation (ICNIRP). Guidelines on limits of static magnetic fields. Health Physics 1994;66:100-106.

86. International Commission on Non-Ionizing Radiation (ICNIRP). Statement on MR procedures: protection of patients. Health Physics 2004;87:197-216.

87. International Electrotechnical Commission (IEC). Particular requirements for the safety of magnetic resonance equipment for medical diagnosis. Geneva: IEC; 60601-2-33;2001.

88. German Commission on Radiological Protection. Recommendations on the safe application of magnetic resonance in medical diagnostic. Recommendation of the German Commission on Radiological Protection (SSK), approved in the 180 Session of the SSK on 19/20 September 2002. Munich: Urban and Fischer; Reports of the SSK, Vol. 36; Available at: www.ssk.de;2003.

89. Kanal E, Borgstede JP, Barkovich AJ, et al. American College of Radiology white paper on MR Safety. Amer J Radiol 2002; 178:1335-1347.

90. Wagner W, Staud I, et al. Noise in magnetic resonance imaging: no risk for sensorineural function but increased amplitude variability of otoacoustic emissions. Laryngoscope 2003;113:1216-23.

91. Govindaraju R, Omar R, Rajagopalan R, Norlisah R, Kwan-Hoong N. Hearing loss after noise exposure. Auris Nasus Larynx 2011;38:319-322.

92. Nordell A, Lundh M, Horsch S, Hallberg B, Aden U, Nordell B, Blennow M. The acoustic hood: a patient-independent device for improving acoustic noise protection during neonatal magnetic resonance imaging. Acta Paed 2009;98:1278-1283.

93. Naughton RF. The Measurement of Hearing by Bone Conduction. In: Jerger J, Editor. Modern Developments in Audiology. New York: Academic Press; 1963.

94. Berger EH. Hearing protection: surpassing the limitations to attenuation imposed by the bone conduction pathways. J Acoust Soc Am 2003;114:1955–67.

95. McJury M, Stewart RW, Crawford D, Toma E. The use of active noise control (ANC) to reduce acoustic noise generated during MRI scanning: some initial results, Mag Res Imaging 1997;15:319-322.

96. Chen CK, Chiueh TD, Chen JH. Active cancellation system of acoustic noise in MR imaging. IEEE Trans Biomed Eng 1999;46:186-191.

97. Lueg P. Process of silencing sound oscillations, U.S. Patent, 2043416,1936.

98. Chaplain GBB. Anti-noise: the Essex breakthrough. Chart Mech Eng 1983;30:41.

99. Elliott SJ, Nelson PA. The acoustic control of sound. Electr Comm Eng 1990;2:127.

100. Pla FG, Sommerfeldt SD, Hedeen RA. Active noise control in magnetic resonance imaging. Proc of Active 95, Newport Beach, CA 2005;P573-582.

101. Chambers J, Akeroyd MA, Sumerfield Q, Palmer AR. Active control of the volume acquisition noise in functional magnetic resonance imaging: method and psychoacoustical evaluation. J Acoust Soc Am 2001;110:3014-54.

102. Li M, Rudd B, Lim TC, Lee JH. In situ active control of noise in a 4T MRI scanner. J Magn Reson Imaging 2011;34:662-669.

103. Fuller CR. Noise control characteristics of synchrophasing: Part 1. Am Inst Aeron Astron J 1986;24:1063-8.

104. Jones JD, Fuller CR. Noise control characteristics of synchrophasing: Part 2. Am Inst Aeron Astron J 1986;24:1271-6.

105. Nestorovic-Trajkov T, Koppe H, Gabbert U. Active vibration control using optimal LQ tracking system with additional elements. Int J Control 2005;78:1182-1197.

106. Roozen NB, Koevoets AH, den Hamer AJ. Active vibration control of gradient coils to reduce acoustic noise of MRI systems. IEEE Trans Mech 2008;13:325-334.

107. Qiu J, Tani J. Vibration control of a cylindrical shell used in MRI equipment. Smart Mater Struct 1995;4:A75-A81.

108. Skare S, Nordell B, et al. An incubator and "quiet" pulse sequences for MRI examination of premature neonates. Proc Soc Magn Reson 1996;1727.

109. Jakob P, Schlaug MG, et al. Functional burst imaging. Magn Res Med 1998;40:614-621.

110. Cremillieux Y, Wheeler-Kingshott CA, Briguet A, Doran SJ, STEAM-BURST: a single-shot multi-slice imaging sequence without rapid gradient switching. Mag Res Med 1997;38:645-652.

111. Hennig J, Hodapp M. Burst imaging. MAGMA 1993;1:39-48.

112. Frahm J, Merboldt K, Hanicke W, Haase A. Stimulated echo imaging. J Magn Reson 1985;64:81-93.

113. Hennel F, Giard F, Loenneker T. Silent MRI with soft gradient pulses. Mag Res Med 1999;42:6-10.

114. Hennel F. Fast spin echo and fast gradient echo MRI with low acoustic noise. J Magn Reson Imaging 2001;13:960-966.

115. Loenneker T, Hennel F, Ludwig U, Hennig J. Silent BOLD imaging. Magn Reson Mater Phys Biol Med 2001;13:76-81.

116. Osterle C, Hennel F, Hennig J. Quiet imaging with interleaved spiral read-out. Magn Reson Imaging 2001;19:1333-1337.

117. de Zwart JA, Van Gelderen P, Kellman P, Duyn JH. Reduction of gradient acoustic noise in MRI using SENSE-EPI. Neuroimage 2001;16:1151-1155.

118. Moelker A, Vogel MW, Pattynama PMT. Real-time modulation of acoustic gradient noise in interventional MRI. Concepts in Magn Reson Part B 2003;20B:34-39.

119. Cho ZH, Chung ST, et al. A new silent magnetic resonance imaging using a rotating DC gradient. Magn Reson Med 1998;39:317-321.

120 Medical Physics Website. Available at: http://medicalphysicsweb.org/cws/article/newsfeed/51679 Accessed June 2013.

121. Tomasi DG, Ernst T. Echo planar imaging at 4 Tesla with minimum acoustic noise. J Magn Reson Imaging 2003;18:128-130.

122. Schmitter S, Diesch E, Amann M, Kroll A, Moayer M, Schad LR. Silent echo-planar imaging for auditory fMRI. Magn Reson Mater Phys 2008;21:317-325.

123. Schmitter S, Bock M. Acoustic noise-optimized VERSE pulses. Magn Reson in Med 2010;64:1447-1453.

124. Zapp J, Schmitter S, Schad LR. Sinusoidal echo-planar imaging with parallel acquisition technique for reduced acoustic noise in auditory fMRI. J Magn Reson Imaging 2012;36:581-588.

125. Eagan T, Baig TN, Derakhshan JJ, Duerk JL, Brown RW. Acoustic noise suppression: gradient self-help? Proc. of the 15th Annual Meeting of ISMRM, Berlin, Germany 2007. p. 1101.

126. Shou X, Chen X, Derakhshan J, et al. The suppression of selected acoustic frequencies in MRI. Appl Acoustics 2010;71:191-200.

127. Wu Y, Chronik BA, Bowen C, Mechefske CK, Rutt BK. Gradient-induced acoustic and magnetic field fluctuations a 4-T whole-body MR imager. Magn Reson Med 2000;44:532-536.

128. Segbers M, Rizzo-Sierra CV, Duifhuis H, Hoogduin JM. Shaping and timing gradient pulses to reduce MRI acoustic noise. Magn Reson Med 2010;64:546-553.

129. Savoy RL, Ravicz ME, Gollub R. The Psychological Laboratory in the Magnet: Stimulus Delivery, Response Recording and Safety. In: Moonen C, Bandettini P, Editors. Medical Radiology, Diagnostic Imaging and Radiation Oncology: Functional MRI. Berlin: Springer; 1999. pp. 347-365.

130. Scheffler K, Bileen D, Schmid N, Tschopp K, Seelig J. Auditory cortical responses to hearing subjects and unilateraldeaf patients as detected by functional magnetic resonance imaging. Cereb Cortex 1998;8:156-163.

131. Hall DA, Haggard MP, Akeroyd MA, et al. "Sparse" temporal sampling in auditory fMRI. Human Brain Mapping 1999;7:213-223.

132. Melcher JR, Talavage TM, Harms MP. Functional MRI of the Auditory System. In: Moonen C, Bandettini P, Editors. Medical Radiology, Diagnostic Imaging and Radiation Oncology: Functional MRI. Berlin: Springer; 1999. pp. 393-406.

133. Amaro E, Williams SCR, Shergill SS, et al. Acoustic noise and functional MRI: current strategies and future prospects. J Magn Reson Imaging 2002;16:497-510.

134. Yang Y, Engelien A, Engelien W, Xu S, Stern E, Silbersweig DA. A silent event-related functional MRI technique for brain activation without interference of scanner acoustic noise. Magn Reson Med 2000;43:185-190.

135. Lin TR, O'Shea P, Mechefske CK. Reducing MRI gradient coil vibration with rib stiffeners. Concepts in Magn Reson Part B 2009;35B:198-209.

136. Mechefske CK, Geris R, Gati JS, Rutt BK. Acoustic noise reduction in a 4T MRI scanner. Magn Reson Mater Phys Med Biol 2002;13:172-176.

137. Katsunuma A, Takamori H, et al. Quiet MRI with novel acoustic noise reduction. Magn Reson Mater Phys Med Biol 2002;13:139-144.

138. Kabushiki Kaisha Toshiba. MRI system having mechanically decoupled field generators to reduce ambient acoustic noise. US patent 6043653, 2000.

139. Edelstein WA, Hedeen RA, Mallozzi RP, et al. Making MR quieter Magn Reson Imaging 2002;20:155-161.

140. Yoshida T, Takamori H, Katsunuma HA. EXCELART MRI system with revolutionary Pianissimo noise reduction technology. Medical Review No. 71;2000.

141. Edelstein WA, Kidane TK, et al. Active-passive gradient shielding for MRI acoustic noise reduction. Magn Reson Med 2005;53:1013-1017.

142. Mulholland KA. Noise Control. In: Tempest W, Editor. The Noise Handbook. New York: Academic Press;1985. p. 282.

143. Maa DY. Theory and design of microperforated panel sound absorbing constructions. Sci Sin 1975;18:155-170.

144. Li G, Mechefske CK. A comprehensive experimental study of micro-perforated panel acoustic absorbers in MRI scanners. Magn Reson Mater Phys Biol Med 2010;23:177-185.

145. Bowtell RW, Peters A. Analytic approach to the design of transverse gradient coils with co-axial return paths. Magn Reson Med 1999;41:600-608.

146. Mansfield P, Glover PM, Bowtell RW. Active acoustic screening: design principles for quiet gradient coils in MRI. Meas Sci Technol 1994;5:1021-25.

147. Bowtell RW, Mansfield PM. Quiet transverse gradient coils: Lorentz force balancing designs using geometric similitude. Magn Reson Med 1995;34:494-7.

148. Jackson JM, Brideson MA, Forbes LK, Crozier S. Tikhonov regularization approach for acoustic noise reduction in an asymmetric, self-shielded MRI gradient coil. Concepts in Magn Reson 2010;37B:167-179.

149. Forbes LK, Brideson MA, Crozier S, While PT. An analytical approach to the design of quiet cylindrical asymmetric gradient coils in MRI. Concepts in Mag Reson Part B 2007;31B:218-236.

150. Forbes LK, Crozier S. Novel target field method for designing shielded bi-planar shim and gradient coils. IEEE Trans on Magnetics 2004;40:1929-1938.

151. Roschmann P. Human auditory system responses to radio frequency energy in RF coils for magnetic resonance at 2.4 to 170 MHz. Magn Reson Med 1991;21:197-215.

152. Elder JA. Special senses. In: Biological Effects of Radio frequency Radiation, United States Environmental Protection Agency, Health Effects Research Laboratory, EPA-600/8-83-026F, Research Triangle Park 1984. p. 570.

153. Postow E, Swicord ML. Modulated fields and "window" effects. In: Polk C, Postow E, Editors. CRC Handbook of Biological Effects of Electromagnetic Fields. Boca Raton: CRC Press Inc.;1989. pp. 425.

Chapter 5   Bioeffects of Radiofrequency Power Deposition Associated With MRI

DANIEL J. SCHAEFER, PH.D.

Retired, Formerly Principal Safety Engineer
MR Systems Engineering
General Electric Healthcare
Waukesha, WI

INTRODUCTION

Radiofrequency (RF) energy is defined as nonionizing electromagnetic radiation in the frequency range of 3-kHz to 300-GHz, as distinguished from the very high photon energies and frequencies associated with ionizing electromagnetic radiation (e.g., gamma and X-rays). The RF spectrum includes radar, ultra high frequency (UHF), and very high frequency (VHF) television, AM and FM radio, and microwave communication frequencies. Resonant radiofrequency (RF) magnetic fields are used in magnetic resonance (MR) for imaging and spectroscopy procedures (1).

This chapter will present and discuss various important aspects of RF power deposition associated with magnetic resonance imaging (MRI) procedures with an emphasis on non-clinical, physical factors, calculations, and measurements used to characterize this electro-magnetic field.

RADIO FREQUENCY MAGNETIC FIELDS AND MRI PROCEDURES

During an MRI procedure, the patient absorbs a portion of the transmitted RF energy, which may result in tissue heating (2-16). Thus, whole-body and localized heating are the primary safety concerns associated with the absorption of RF energy. Notably, the elevation of core body temperatures to sufficiently high levels may be life-threatening (2, 17, 18). With local transmit RF coils, the primary safety concern is to prevent burns by limiting localized heating.

The specific absorption rate, or SAR, is the RF power absorbed per unit mass of tissue and is the metric for RF power deposition typically reported in W/kg. SAR is believed to serve as a crude measure of heating potential. It is essential for patient safety to limit whole-body-averaged and localized temperatures to appropriate SAR levels (2, 18-23). Therefore, national and international safety standards (2, 19-21) appropriately limit or recommend SAR levels for clinical MRI procedures. Heating experienced by the patient during an MRI examination depends on the RF power deposited per unit mass (or SAR), ambient temperature, relative humidity, airflow rate, blood flow, sweating rate, and patient insulation.

Resonant frequency scales with the static magnetic field strength and nuclei of interest. For hydrogen protons, the resonant RF frequency is 42-MHz/Tesla (1). The tip angle is proportional to the area under the envelope of the RF waveform. Typically, the amplitude of the RF pulse (i.e., the tip angle) is adjusted to maximize the received signal. For a given waveform, RF energy is proportional to the square of the tip angle. Only the magnetic component of the RF field is useful in MRI. Designs usually reduce electric field coupling to patients. Since RF power deposition is mostly through magnetic induction, the distribution of the RF power deposition associated with an MRI procedure tends to be mostly peripheral or on the surface of the subject's body (9-11). Plane wave exposures (in non-MRI applications) may lead to greater heating at greater depths (18, 24).

The average RF power (and SAR) is proportional to the number of images per unit time and peak RF power. Peak RF power depends on patient dimensions, the RF waveform, tip angle, and whether the MR system's transmit RF coil is operating in a linear or quadrature (i.e., has a circularly polarized magnetic field vector) mode during the transmission of RF energy. It should be noted that quadrature excitation lowers RF peak power requirements and SAR by a factor of two and "stirs" any field inhomogeneities (10). For a given static magnetic field strength and RF waveform, SAR is independent of the type of nucleus.

MR SAFETY STANDARDS

The United States, Food and Drug Administration (FDA) published "Non-Significant Risk Criteria" for MRI devices (22). These criteria state that clinical MRI examinations need Investigational Device Exemption (IDE) if the SAR exceeds the following levels:

a)   4-W/kg (averaged over the whole body over any 15-min. period); or
b)   3-W/kg (averaged over the head over in 10-min. period); or
c)   8-W/kg in any gram (head or torso, averaged over any 5-min. period), or
d)   12-W/kg in any gram (extremities, averaged over any 5-min. period).

Notably, the FDA's significant risk criteria also include limits that are not related to RF power deposition.

The International Electrotechnical Commission (IEC) developed the international MRI safety standard IEC 60601-2-33 (23). The IEC MRI safety standard is three-tiered. The first tier is referred to as the *Normal Operating Mode* and is for routine scanning of patients. The second tier is designated as the *First Level Controlled Operating Mode*. The MR system operator must take a deliberate action (usually using an "accept" button on the MR system console) to enter the *First Level Controlled Operating Mode*. This mode provides higher MR system performance, but requires the MRI healthcare worker to closely monitor the patient during the MRI procedure. Finally, the third tier is the *Second Level Controlled Op–*

erating Mode, which is used only for research purposes under limits controlled by an Investigational Review Board (IRB).

When the environmental temperature is $\leq 25°C$, the current IEC MRI safety standard for RF energy during an MRI procedure permits (assuming SAR averaged over any 10-second period ≤ 2 times the 6-min. average SAR limit) the following limits for volume transmit RF coils:

a) Whole-body SAR (averaged over any 6-min period):
   1) The Normal Operating Mode - SAR $\leq$ 2-W/kg;
   2) The First Level Controlled Operating Mode - SAR $\leq$ 4-W/kg;
   3) The Second Level Controlled Operating Mode - SAR < IRB limit.
b) Partial Body SAR (averaged over any 6-min. period):
   1) The Normal Operating Mode - SAR $\leq$ 10 W/kg - (8-W/kg * exposed patient mass / patient mass);
   2) The First Level Controlled Operating Mode - SAR $\leq$ 10-W/kg - (6-W/kg * exposed patient mass / patient mass);
   3) The Second Level Controlled Operating Mode - SAR < IRB limit.
c) Head SAR (averaged over any 6-min. period):
   1) The Normal Operating Mode - SAR $\leq$ 3.2-W/kg;
   2) The First Level Controlled Operating Mode - SAR $\leq$ 3.2-W/kg;
   3) The Second Level Controlled Operating Mode - SAR < IRB limit.
d) The specific energy limit is 14400-Joules/kg (equivalent to 4-W/kg for one hour).

Whole-body SAR limits are de-rated by 0.25-W/kg for each degree C that the environmental temperature exceeds 25°C for the First Level Controlled Operating Mode, only.

For local transmit RF coils, local SAR limits (averaged over the worst-case 10-grams for 6- min.) are:

a) The Normal Operating Mode
   1) SAR $\leq$ 10-W/kg in the head or trunk (provided local temperature rise in the orbits is limited to a 1°C).
   2) SAR $\leq$ 20-W/kg in the extremities;
b) The First Level Controlled Operating Mode- SAR $\leq$ 3.2-W/kg;
   1) SAR $\leq$ 20-W/kg in the head or trunk (provided local temperature rise in the orbits is limited to a 1°C).
   2) SAR $\leq$ 40-W/kg in the extremities;
c) The Second Level Controlled Operating Mode - SAR < IRB limit.

Note that the third edition of IEC 60601-2-33 is current as this is written. Work is continuing on improving the scientific basis for local SAR limits or some equivalent criterion.

IEC 60601-2-33 does not require local SAR limits for volume transmit RF coils, but does require local SAR limits for local transmit RF coils that may produce inhomogeneous RF magnetic fields. For 3-Tesla MR systems and higher, MR image shading can be a concern. This concern apparently arises from standing waves interfering at field strengths where electrical lengths in the body become significant. There are now efforts (known as dual drive, parallel transmit, elliptical drive, or RF shimming; parallel transmit will be used here to represent these techniques) to minimize shading by adjusting excitations on two or more RF channels to improve the quadrature uniformity in the body (not necessarily in air).

These techniques are intended to improve quadrature uniformity in the body and reduce or at least not increase the local SAR over that caused by conventional quadrature (in air) excitation. The local SAR level could increase if the excitation is not properly controlled. Since there is a long safety record associated with conventional quadrature excitation, there generally is no concern provided that parallel transmit does not generate a local SAR higher than conventional quadrature imaging for similar tissues.

Another IEC safety standard, IEC 60601-1, establishes additional safety criteria for medical devices including electrical, mechanical, and thermal safety (25). Surface contact temperatures are limited to 41.0 °C (25). Note that during an MRI procedure using a high SAR, the average skin temperature of a human subject approaches 37.0 °C (for a 4.0°C margin for temperature rise). During an MRI examination using very low SAR, the average skin temperature is typically 33.0°C (for a temperature rise margin of 8.0°C).

The American College of Radiology published a useful paper for MRI safety guidance (26). This paper is not a regulatory document but, instead, it has many recommendations for safety procedures for MRI facilities, some of which pertain to the topic of this chapter.

The Technical Specification, ISO/TS 10974:2011 (27), is a trial standard available for active medical implants to aid in determining whether they are MR conditional devices. MR conditional devices are acceptable for MRI examinations only if certain conditions apply. There are also several American Society of Testing and Materials (ASTM) International test standards used to determine safe conditions for use for MR Conditional devices (28-33). Note that the ASTM International heating test implicitly assumes quadrature excitation. Importantly, parallel transmit excitation might produce different heating results.

CALCULATION OF MAGNETIC AND ELECTRIC FIELDS ASSOCIATED WITH THE SPECIFIC ABSORPTION RATE (SAR)

The patient's RF power absorption during an MRI procedure can be approximated from quasi-static analysis for homogeneous objects, assuming that electric field coupling to the patient can be neglected as well as the RF phase (34, 35). In practice, quasi-static approximations for whole-body SAR in homogeneous spheres appear to be adequate for MR systems operating up to 1.5-T/64-MHz. Calculation of actual SAR levels at 3-T/128-MHz and above, and for local SAR at all static magnetic field strengths, requires numerical techniques. Many commercially available packages exist at this time. Quasi-static methods will usually overestimate whole-body and local SARs (under homogeneous conditions and for certain shapes) when conductor dimensions approach a wavelength.

Assume a line segment of length, dl, carries current, I, and is located a vector, r', from the origin, O, (**Figure 1**). The magnetic vector potential, A, at a point located a vector r (x_2, y_2, z_2) from the origin may be expressed as (24, 35, 36):

$$\vec{A}(\vec{r}) = \int \frac{\mu \vec{I}(\vec{r}') \bullet dl'}{4\pi |\vec{r} - \vec{r}'|} \tag{1}$$

Figure 1. Calculation of the magnetic vector potential, A.

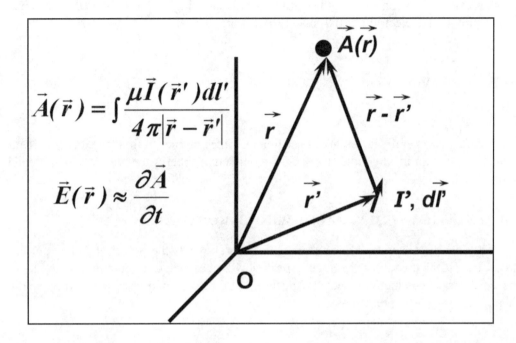

The radiofrequency magnetic field, B_1, may then be found from the magnetic vector potential:

$$\vec{B}_1 = \nabla \times \vec{A}$$

$$\Rightarrow B_{1x} = \frac{\partial A_z}{\partial y} - \frac{\partial A_y}{\partial z}, B_{1y} = \frac{\partial A_x}{\partial z} - \frac{\partial A_z}{\partial x}, and\, B_{1z} = \frac{\partial A_y}{\partial x} - \frac{\partial A_x}{\partial y}. \tag{2}$$

Note that B_1 scales with current. Coil current is scaled until the desired B_1 is produced at the appropriate site. Usually, the 180-degree pulse centers on the site resulting in the greatest total return signal. The signal distribution, S (x, y, z), might be approximated as:

$$S(x,y,z) = \left(\sin\left(\frac{\pi B_1(x,y,z)}{2B_{1\,max}} \right) \right)^3 \tag{3}$$

The total signal is the sum of the signal from all locations. Magnetic vector components are scaled by the coil current required to produce the 180-degree (or whatever is desired) tip angle.

Let ω be the radian frequency and let Φ be the electrostatic potential due to electric charges at electrical conductivity discontinuities. Neglecting currents induced from capacitive coupling, the electric field, E, may be expressed as:

$$E = -\frac{\partial A}{\partial t} - \nabla\Phi = -\omega A - \nabla\Phi \tag{4}$$

While it is generally necessary to use numerical techniques to find the electrostatic potential, for certain ideal geometries such as conductive spheres the electrostatic potential term vanishes.

QUAI-STATIC ESTIMATION OF WHOLE-BODY SAR

The specific absorption rate, SAR, is defined above as the power absorbed per unit mass. Let DC be the ratio of average to peak power over the pulse repetition period. Let σ be the electrical conductivity and ρ be the density of the surrounding tissue. SAR at a point in a sphere may be expressed as:

$$SAR = \frac{\sigma DC |E|^2}{2\rho} = \frac{\sigma DC |\omega A|^2}{2\rho} \tag{5}$$

For RF coils that produce homogeneous B_1 fields, it is possible to investigate the whole body average and peak SARs theoretically for certain object shapes. The patient's RF power absorption during an MRI procedure can be approximated from quasi-static analysis assuming electric field coupling to patients can be neglected (15, 35). Consider a homogeneous, tissue sphere of radius R. Assume that this sphere is placed in a uniform RF magnetic field of strength B_1. The total average RF power, P_{total}, deposited in the sphere may be expressed as:

$$P_{total} = \frac{\sigma DC \pi \omega^2 B_1^2 R^5}{15} \tag{6}$$

The average Specific Absorption Rate, SAR_{ave}, may be expressed as:

$$SAR = \frac{P_{total}}{\rho \left(\frac{4}{3} \pi R^3 \right)} = \frac{\sigma DC \omega^2 B_1^2 R^2}{20\rho} \tag{7}$$

The highest spatial peak SAR, SAR_{peak}, for a homogeneous sphere may be found, as follows:

$$SAR_{peak} = \frac{\sigma DC\omega^2 B_1^2 R^2}{8\rho} = 2.5\, SAR_{ave} \tag{8}$$

RF energy-induced heating during an MRI procedure is by magnetic induction. Power deposition in homogeneous spheres immersed in uniform RF magnetic fields, increases with the fifth power of the radius, R [see equation (6)]. Because heating is largely peripheral and little deep body heating occurs in a human subject, the body may more easily dissipate the additional heat load. The RF power, P, deposited between a smaller radius, $r = \alpha * R$ (where $\alpha < 1$), and the outer radius, R, normalized to the total power deposited is n:

$$n = \frac{P(R) - P(r)}{P(R)} = \frac{R^5 - r^5}{R^5} = 1 - \alpha^5 \tag{9}$$

Equation (8) shows that peak power deposition for homogeneous spheres is 2.5 times the average (15), consistent with the peripheral nature of RF deposition during the MRI procedure. From equation (9) it is clear that, at least for homogeneous spheres, 87% of the total RF power deposition is in the outer third of the sphere.

RF pulses are used in MRI examinations to flip the macroscopic magnetization vectors through desired angles. Recall that nuclei with magnetic moments precess about the static magnetic field vector in accordance with the right hand rule. Linearly polarized waves may be treated as the superposition of left and right handed circularly polarized waves. Only that portion of the RF that is circularly polarized in the same sense as the nuclear precession influences the nuclei (**Figure 2**). The other RF component contributes noise and increases RF power requirements. During the MRI procedure, transmit RF coils may be driven linearly (linearly polarized RF magnetic vector) or they may be driven in quadrature (circularly polarized RF magnetic vector). Quadrature RF transmit systems reduce patient heating during the MRI procedure by a factor of two, and spatially stir any RF "hot-spots" (9).

Let γ be the magnetogyric ratio for a given type of nucleus. Note that the energy, W, deposited per pulse depends on the square of the RF tip angle, θ, the square of the static field strength, B_0, and inversely on RF pulse width, τ, and a waveform factor, η:

$$\theta = \int \omega dt = \eta\gamma B_{1p}\tau \quad \Rightarrow \quad SAR \propto W \propto \tau\omega^2 B_{1p}^2 = \frac{\gamma^2 B_0^2 \theta^2 \tau}{(\eta\gamma\tau)^2} = \frac{B_0^2 \theta^2}{\eta^2 \tau} \tag{10}$$

Figure 2. Comparison of quadrature and linear RF excitation of spins. Note that linear excitation wastes half the applied power.

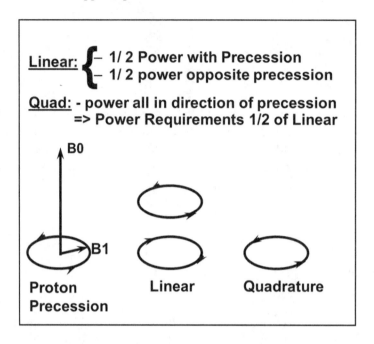

It is important to note that, for a given field strength and RF waveform, SAR is independent of the nucleus species.

SAR "HOT-SPOTS"

Next, consider localized regions of RF power deposition that might lead to heating, commonly referred to as SAR "hot-spots". Inhomogeneties in the electrical properties of tissue may result in high local SAR levels. RF-induced biological effects appear to depend upon temperature rather than on RF power deposition. A region of high local SAR may not be a region of high temperature due to blood flow or diffusion or other cooling mechanisms. The distinction between temperature hot-spots and SAR hot-spots is often ignored or misunderstood.

What effect do inhomogeneities have on the distribution of RF power deposition? Using spherical models, Schenck and Hussain (37) demonstrated that production of power deposition "hot-spots" depends upon both the dielectric constants and the conductivities of the media. The model was later reformulated and used to investigate several problems involving worst-case conditions and magnitudes of local power deposition (10). Assume that there is a small, homogeneous sphere (sphere 1) with permittivity ε_1 and conductivity σ_1 (**Figure 3**). Let sphere 2 be a much larger, homogeneous sphere of "standard tissue" representing the body. Sphere 2 has a permittivity ε_2 and conductivity σ_2. Sphere 1 may be placed outside sphere 2 at the pole (tangential electric field location) or at the equator (normal electric field location). In addition, sphere 1 may be placed inside sphere 2. When sphere 1 is placed near

Figure 3. Effect of inhomogeneities on RF power deposition. To model the effect, a small, homogeneous sphere is placed either inside a larger tissue sphere or at the pole or equator of the larger tissue sphere (with respect to the RF electric field vector).

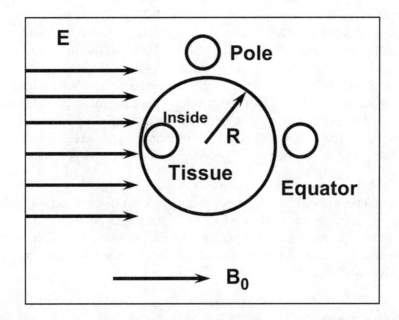

the pole of sphere 2, the local power deposition is amplified by a factor, A_p, which may be expressed as:

$$A_p = \frac{9(\sigma_1^2 + \omega^2 \varepsilon_1^2)}{(\sigma_1 + 2\sigma_2)^2 + \omega^2(\varepsilon_1 + 2\varepsilon_2)^2} \tag{11}$$

When sphere 1 is placed near the equator of sphere 2, the local power deposition amplification factor, A_e, may be expressed as:

$$A_e = \frac{9(\sigma_2^2 + \omega^2 \varepsilon_2^2)}{(\sigma_1 + 2\sigma_2)^2 + \omega^2(\varepsilon_1 + 2\varepsilon_2)^2}. \tag{12}$$

Finally, if sphere 1 is placed inside sphere 2, the local power deposition amplification factor, A_s, may be represented as:

$$A_s = \frac{9\sigma_1(\sigma_2^2 + \omega^2 \varepsilon_2^2)}{\sigma_2((\sigma_1 + 2\sigma_2)^2 + \omega^2(\varepsilon_1 + 2\varepsilon_2)^2)} = \left(\frac{\sigma_1}{\sigma_2}\right) A_e \tag{13}$$

All the terms in equations (11), (12), and (13) are positive. The electrical properties of sphere 1 are treated as variables so conditions for maximum amplification of local power deposition may be determined.

When sphere 1 is near the pole, amplification of local power deposition, A_p, is greatest when sphere 1 is a perfect conductor ($\sigma_1 \approx \infty$). A perfectly conducting small sphere at the pole will result in a local amplification factor of $A_p = 9$. Recall that the spatial peak SAR in a homogeneous sphere is already 2.5 times average SAR for the sphere. Combining these results, the peak SAR at the pole is $= 22.5$ times the SAR averaged over sphere 2. Conductive leads (e.g., used with electrocardiogram monitoring equipment) placed in contact with the skin of patients may simulate this situation. Note that there is almost no amplification of local power deposition if sphere 1 is a radius or more from sphere 2. Spacing conductors well away from patients can dramatically reduce the local heating potential.

Assume sphere 1 is placed near the equator of sphere 2. Then the greatest amplification of local power deposition takes place when sphere 1 electrical properties are minimal; i.e., $\sigma_1 = 0$ and $\varepsilon_1 = \varepsilon_0$ (free space value). So for a void, such as an air bubble, $A_e = 2.25$. Fat or bone at the equator produces slightly smaller amplifications (10, 37). When a low conductivity sphere is located near the outer edge of the equator of a larger (conductive) sphere, the local SAR is highest and is limited to 5.625 times the average SAR.

Finally, assume sphere 1 is placed inside the large sphere. This situation may simulate an implanted prostheses. While local SAR is amplified the most when $\sigma_1 = 2\sigma_2$ and $\varepsilon_1 = 2\varepsilon_2$ (not a likely situation), the amplification factor is only $A_s = 1.125$. The highest local SAR works out to 2.8125 times the local average SAR.

The analyses above assume linearly polarized RF magnetic fields. Notably, if the transmit RF coil produces quadrature excitation, then the amplification of local power deposition is reduced. The reduction in local power deposition results from rotating eddy current loops during quadrature excitation. Sphere 1 alternates between the equator and the pole of the larger sphere during quadrature excitation. So, worst-case quadrature local SAR amplification (assuming inhomogeneous biology) is $0.5 * (2.5 + 2.8125) = 2.66$. For maximum SAR amplification at the equator, the electrical properties of sphere 1 approach those of a void.

Similarly, for an infinitely conducting sphere 1, during quadrature RF excitation, the worst-case local power deposition amplification would be $0.5 * (2.5 + 22.5) = 12.5$. However, the presence of a conductor may complicate the production of a perfect quadrature RF field by setting up difficult boundary conditions.

Currently, many useful electromagnetic simulation packages are commercially available that can calculate whole-body average, head average, partial body average, and local SAR (averaged over the worst-case contiguous 10-grams). As mentioned under the MRI safety standards section above, it turns out that, in the transmit body RF coil, the ratio of peak local SAR to the whole-body average SAR may be high (as high as about 13 times) (38).

Transmit RF body coils induce electric fields in patients during MRI procedures. RF-induced electric fields are largest near RF coil conductors (**Figure 4**). Transmit RF coils may have high electric fields near capacitors on the coil as well. During high SAR MRI ex-

Figure 4. Electric fields inside a low-pass, RF birdcage coil. Note that the electric fields reach their maximum magnitude at the coil and fall to zero along the coil axis. Capacitors along the coil wall may also give rise to high electric fields, locally. Any conductors should be routed along regions of the low electric field or orthogonal to the electric field.

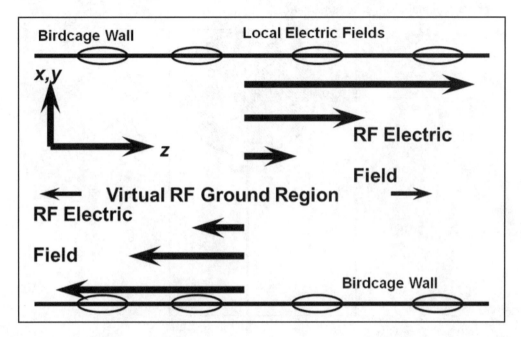

aminations, placing patients well away from transmit body RF coil conductors may reduce local power deposition and heating. The axis of birdcage RF coils is nearly a virtual ground. Conductors that must be introduced into the bore will minimally affect local SAR if they are placed along this virtual ground.

Receive-only RF coils, including most surface coils, typically use transmit body RF coils to transmit RF excitation pulses. Receive-only coils are resonant during RF reception. However, if these RF coils were resonant during transmission of RF energy, then large currents may be produced in the receive-only coils. These large currents would, by Lenz's law, induce opposing RF magnetic fields. Flip angle profiles could be altered by the opposing RF magnetic fields, degrading image quality. The opposing RF magnetic fields may induce large electric fields in the body leading to large local SAR levels. Manufacturers use high impedance blocking networks to detune surface coils and limit surface coil current during body coil transmit (**Figure 5**).

If conductive loops (e.g., associated with the use of monitoring equipment or even a coiled transmission line) are introduced into the MR system, high local SAR levels may result (39, 40) (**Figure 6**). Even straight conductors may increase local SAR significantly (41-44) (**Figure 7**). Therefore, for patient safety, fiber optic-based devices should be used instead of conductors, when possible.

Local temperature rise typically does not correlate well with local power deposition in a human subject. Thermal diffusion, blood flow, thermal radiation, sweating, and airflow

Figure 5. Receive-only RF surface coil with blocking network. During body RF coil transmission, the blocking network, Z, becomes a high impedance to prevent high-induced currents from flowing in the coil. Such currents could lead to very high local SAR levels. During surface coil receive, the blocking network becomes a very low impedance to improve the image signal to noise ratio.

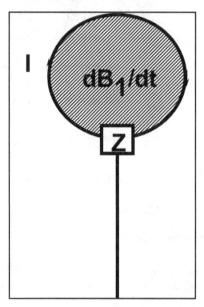

Figure 6. Any loop whose axis is parallel to the RF magnetic field may produce high currents and voltages by Faraday induction. Conductive loops should be avoided in the scanner.

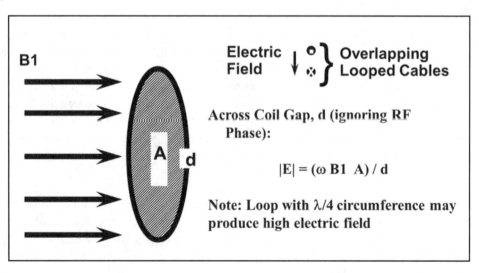

Figure 7. Even straight conductors may act as antennas and couple to the RF electric field (which is highest near the wall of the body RF coil). Loops may also short out a mode of quadrature coils, resulting in linear excitation.

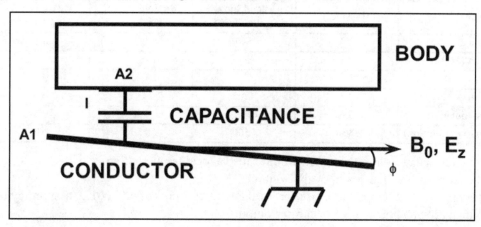

may influence the local temperature rise. Consider a region with a small mass, m, cooled by blood flowing from a cooler, more massive region. Under steady-state conditions, the SAR that is dumped to the more massive region depends upon an energy constant, K, the specific heat, C, the temperature difference between the massive and small region, ΔT, and the mass rate of blood flow, dM/dt, and may be expressed as:

$$SAR = \frac{K\,C\,\Delta T}{m}\left(\frac{dM}{dt}\right) \tag{14}$$

The SAR required for a 1°C temperature rise in various organs may be estimated using equation (14). Blood flow rates per unit mass vary from 128-ml/kg/min for normal skin to 4200-ml/kg/min for the kidneys. **Table 1** lists local SAR levels required to produce a local temperature rise of one degree C for various organs (23). **Table 1** demonstrates the homogenizing property of blood flow to limit temperature "hot-spots" in the body. Resulting steady-state (maximum) temperature rises for each organ exposed locally to 4-W/kg is also presented in **Table 1**. Athey (45) has shown similar theoretical results demonstrating that significant thermal "hot spots" are not probable for typical head exposures.

RF POWER DEPOSTION IN BIRDCAGE COILS AND NEAR CONDUCTORS

Ideally, birdcage coils would produce uniform B_1 fields. Perfectly uniform B_1 requires an infinitely long birdcage coil (or a spherical current density). Components of A (and thus E) must be parallel to the current density on the conductors that produced them. The B_1 field is related to magnetic vector potential:

Table 1. Maximum local SAR level for local temperature rise of 1°Celsius for various perfused organs (data calculated from Ganong, reference 60).

Organ	Mass (kg)	Blood Flow (ml/kg/min)	Maximum SAR (W/kg)*	Maximum DT (°C)**
Brain	1.4	540	31	0.13
Heart (Muscle)	0.3	840	48.3	0.08
Liver	2.6	577	33.4	0.12
Kidneys	0.3	4200	243.2	0.02
Skin (normal)	3.6	128	7.4	0.54
Skin (vasodilation)	3.6	1500	86.9	0.05

*Maximum local SAR level which would cause a local temperature rise of 1°C, ignoring vasodilatation and changes in cardiac output.
**Maximum local temperature rise for local SAR exposures of 4.0-W/Kg, assuming no vasodilatation and no change in cardiac output.

$$B_1 = \nabla \times A = \hat{a}_x \left[\left(\frac{\partial A_x}{\partial y} \right) - \left(\frac{\partial A_y}{\partial x} \right) \right] + \hat{a}_y \left[\left(\frac{\partial A_x}{\partial z} \right) - \left(\frac{\partial A_z}{\partial x} \right) \right] + \hat{a}_z \left[\left(\frac{\partial A_y}{\partial x} \right) - \left(\frac{\partial A_x}{\partial y} \right) \right] \quad (15)$$

Assume that (at the moment of time we look) $B_1 = B_{1x}$ ($B_{1y} = B_{1z} = 0$). Assume that RF coil conductors lie only along the z direction, then $Ay = Ax = 0$ (remember that B_1 is constant):

Let "a" be the radius of the birdcage coil. Without significant coupling, equation (16) becomes:

$$\vec{B}_{1x} - \frac{\partial \vec{A}_z}{\partial y} ; \quad \Rightarrow \quad \vec{A}_z = \vec{B}_1 y ; \quad \Rightarrow \quad \vec{E}_z = -\omega \vec{B}_1 y \quad (16)$$

$$E_{max} = -\omega B_1 a \quad (at \ (0,a,0)) \quad (17)$$

Note that the z-component of the RF electric field inside an ideal birdcage coil depends linearly on the radial position. Suppose, for example, that at $\omega = 2\pi$ (63.86-MHz), $a = 0.3$-m, and $B_1 = 14.7$-µT, then $E_z = (-5898$-v/m²) y and $E_{max} = 1,769$-v/m.

Equation (16) predicts that the electric fields (and currents) in a birdcage coil of radius, a, need to be sinusoidal to produce a uniform magnetic field:

$$E_z(\theta) = -\omega B_1 a \sin(\theta) \tag{18}$$

Assume that the "duty cycle" (ratio of average to peak RF power), DC, is 5%. Assume the RF coil length, h, is 0.6-m. Then a conductor of length, L, (where $L \le h$) making an angle ϕ with the z-axis, will (ignoring RF electrical length and matching issues) experience a voltage, V, induced on it in the birdcage coil:

$$V = -\omega B_1 \, y \, L \cos(\phi) \tag{19}$$

If the conductor, whose impedance is Z, contacts a patient through a cross section of area, α, the current density, J, may be expressed as:

$$J = \frac{V}{\alpha Z} = \frac{-\omega B_1 L \cos(\phi)}{\alpha Z} \tag{20}$$

If the patient conductivity is σ, then the local electric field, E', in the patient (at the point of conductor contact) is $E' = J/\sigma$. Assume the patient density is ρ. Then the local SAR at the point of contact may be written as:

$$SAR = \frac{\sigma DC \left| E' \right|^2}{2\rho} = \frac{DC \left| \omega B_1 L \cos(\phi) \right|^2}{2\sigma \rho \alpha^2 Z^2} \tag{21}$$

Therefore, the SAR from conductors in the bore of an MR system may be limited by making the impedance to the body large ($Z = \infty$). SAR from conductors may also be limited by keeping conductors very short ($L = 0$). Additionally, the SAR from conductors may be minimized by routing the conductors down the center of the bore ($y = 0$) or by routing them along $\phi = \pi/2$. Note that the analysis above was for a linear coil in the homogeneous region (away from coil conductors) for simplicity.

WHOLE-BODY SAR MEASUREMENTS

By measuring the RF peak forward, reflected, and (possibly) dummy load power levels required for 180-degree pulses (**Figure 8**) with a known waveform, it is possible to measure the energy absorbed per pulse by the patient. Note that these measurements may be made while exposing human subjects to very low SAR levels. This information may be used to

Figure 8. Experimental measurement of whole-body-averaged specific absorption rate (SAR).

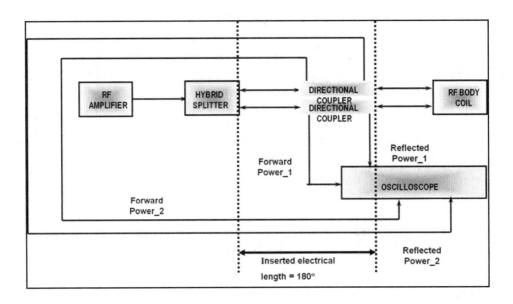

calculate whole-body SAR for any pulse with that patient in the same location. Details are in a National Electrical Manufacturers Association (NEMA) Standard (46).

TRANSMIT/RECEIVE SURFACE COILS AND LOCAL SAR

Planar, surface transmit RF coils are often used in MR spectroscopy studies. The primary safety concern with transmit/receive surface coils involves local SAR issues. While it is straightforward to calculate local RF power deposition in volume transmit RF coils, estimation of spatial peak specific absorption rate (SAR) for planar transmit surface coils is complex. To prevent excessive local RF power deposition, it is imperative to at least estimate an upper bound for the local SAR. The local SAR is highest near the coil conductors. For such cases, simplifying assumptions may be made to calculate appropriate design limits (47). Assume there is an anti-parallel pair of infinitely long conductors of width, d, with a return a distance $2 * a_1$ apart. Schenck, et al. (48) showed that the in-plane magnetic vector potential at a distance r from one conductor for the case where $d << a_1$ (and where quasi-static conditions apply) may be expressed as:

$$A_z = \frac{\mu_0 I}{4\pi d}\left[4\pi(a_1-r)+4r\tan^{-1}\left(\frac{2r}{d}\right)-4(2a_1-r)\tan^{-1}\left(\frac{2(2a_1-r)}{d}\right)+d\ln\left(\frac{4(2a_1-r)^2+d^2}{4r^2+d^2}\right)\right] \quad (22)$$

The local SAR may be calculated by inserting A_z from equation (22) into equation (5). It is necessary to scale current to levels that produce the desired B_1 at the desired location. Equations (2) and (22) may be used to find B_1:

$$B_1 = \frac{-\mu I}{\pi d}[\tan^{-1}\left(\frac{-2(dr+2a_1-r)}{r^2+d^2-2a_1 r}\right)-\pi]$$
(23)

Note that the local SAR falls off much faster than B_1 (or signal) with distance to the patient. In **Figure 9**, normalized B_1 and normalized local SAR are plotted against the normalized distance from a planar, circular coil. A seven-fold reduction in local SAR may be achieved at the expense of a 5% reduction in B_1. Equations (5), (22), and (23) should permit coil designers to theoretically estimate the local SAR. Quasi-static calculations could also be done using equations (1) through (5).

MEASUREMENT OF LOCAL SAR IN PHANTOMS

It is possible to experimentally measure local SAR in phantoms using materials with electrical properties and density similar to muscle (24, 49-51). To accomplish this, it is useful to use fiber-optic (non-conductive) temperature probes under the transmit RF coil conductors in contact with the tissue-phantom and thermally isolated from the coil. The local SAR may be calculated from the early (linear) portion of the heating curve:

$$SAR = C\frac{dT}{dt}$$
(24)

Figure 9. Normalized local SAR and B_1 versus distance for a circular RF coil. B_1 is calculated along the coil axis. The local SAR is calculated from under the coil conductor.

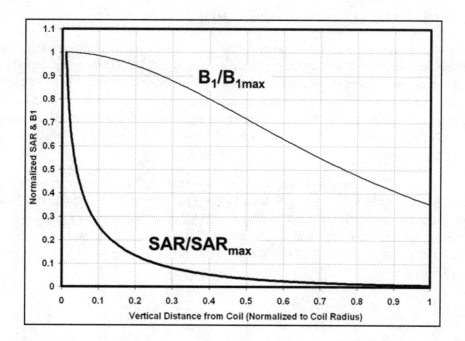

In the equation above, C is the specific heat of the tissue and T is the temperature. Equation (24) is expressed in MKS units. Other loss mechanisms (convection, radiation, and conduction) must be minimized during the experiment. Convection may be limited by using a gel-filled phantom (49). Conduction losses may be minimized by keeping materials insulated and by starting with the coil and the "tissue/phantom" at room temperature.

SAFETY CONSIDERATION OF RECEIVE-ONLY RF SURFACE COILS

Very large surface coil currents may flow if receive-only RF surface coils were resonant while RF excitation pulses are played out on the transmit body RF coil (51-53). These currents may result in extremely high local SAR levels near the surface coil. In addition, the surface coil reaction currents would destroy B_1 homogeneity, by generating opposing magnetic fields. To prevent such problems, a blocking network in the surface coil presents a high impedance to limit surface coil currents during RF excitation (**Figure 5**). The blocking impedance required depends on the area of the RF coil, frequency, and how large an opposing field is to be allowed. Typical blocking impedances are a few hundred ohms. Note that in the case of phased array receive coils, special care must be exercised to avoid the development of high local electric fields from differential voltages on adjacent conductors.

Unfortunately, surface coil blocking networks may become warm. IEC 60601-1 (25) sets a surface temperature limit ($T_{limit} = 41°C$) for objects that may touch human subjects. Skin temperature under normal, non-MRI or low SAR conditions is approximately 33.0°C. However, during an MRI procedure involving a high SAR level, skin blood vessels dilate and skin temperatures may approach the level of the core temperature. In tests with phantoms initially at ambient temperature, a 4.0°C rise should be the limit for systems capable of high SAR. For low SAR systems, the surface coil temperature rise may be limited to 8.0°C above ambient temperature.

POTENTIAL MECHANISMS FOR RF BIOEFFECTS

Thermal effects arise from the temperature dependence of most biological functions. Chemical reaction rates approximately double with each 10°C rise in temperature (54). Protein denaturation takes place at temperatures of approximately 45°C (18). The fluidity of cell membranes is also affected by temperature. Thermal effects may be caused by whole body heating of the organism or by localized heating of tissues. During an MRI procedure, while only the body parts inside of the transmit RF coil are exposed to RF power deposition, the entire body may be affected by thermal reactions.

The mechanisms behind non-thermal effects are unclear. The energy of a single photon at 85-MHz or 2-Tesla is 5.304×10^{-26} Joules (55). The energy of chemical bonds is much larger. In fact, even relatively weak hydrogen bonds between groups in protein structures have energies of 3.125×10^{-20} Joules (54). Notably, thermal energy at body temperature is 4.28×10^{-21} Joules, five orders of magnitude greater than the energy of RF photons at 2-Tesla (85-MHz).

LITERATURE REVIEW: THERMAL PHYSICS AND PHYSIOLOGY

RF fields are too high in frequency to electrically stimulate excitable tissues (56). Thus, as previously mentioned, the only well-established mechanism for RF energy-related bioeffects is heating (18). Guy, et al. (57) showed that the SAR threshold for cataractogenesis is 100-W/kg. The highest safe core temperature for workers is considered to be 39.4°C (24, 58, 59). The threshold core temperature for teratogenic effects in pregnant women is 38.9°C (60). During the day, core temperature fluctuates approximately 1°C or more (17, 60). Skin temperature fluctuates over a range of 15°C (17). The skin pain threshold is 43°C (61). Finally, the resting metabolic rate is 1.3-W/kg, while during vigorous exercise, in highly trained athletes, may be as high as 18-W/kg (24).

Consider an insulated tissue section. In one hour, the insulated tissue will, when exposed to an SAR of 1.0-W/kg, rise approximately 1.0°C. Insulated tissue would rise to infinite temperature in infinite time at any finite SAR. In use, physiologic heat dissipation mechanisms of the human body limit temperature rise to a steady-state value. A body, whose outer surface temperature, T_{sk}, is warmer than the ambient temperature, T_a, will radiate to the surroundings (17). When exposed to RF power deposition, the body temperature will increase until steady-state conditions prevail. In a steady state, the body dissipates energy to the environment at the same rate that it gains energy from RF power deposition. Temperature increases initially, and then asymptotically approaches the final steady state value. The temperature time course may be expressed as:

$$\Delta T = \Delta T_0 (1 - \exp^{(\frac{-t}{\tau})})$$

(25)

In equation (25), τ is a constant, ΔT, is the temperature rise at any time, t, and ΔT_0 is the steady state temperature rise. Note that an infinite duration RF exposure results in a finite, non-linear temperature rise. If σ_s is taken as the Stefan-Boltzmann constant, and A is the surface area of the body, then the radiated power, P, may be expressed as:

$$P = \sigma_s A (T_{sk}^4 - T_a^4) \approx 4 \sigma_s A T_a^3 \Delta T$$

(26)

Consider a hypothetical, uninsulated human subject (70-kg) who is constrained to lose energy to the environment only by radiation. Assume that the ambient temperature is 25°C and the thermal neutral (steady state) temperature of the skin is 33 °C. In a steady state, the hypothetical human would radiate about 1.4-W/kg, which is replaced by his own metabolic energy at the same rate. The result is no change in deep body or core temperature.

Next consider the same hypothetical human, but this time the skin temperature has risen to 38°C (vasodilatation of skin blood vessels may permit the skin to reach core temperature). Now the hypothetical human radiates energy at a rate of 2.4-W/kg, 1-W/kg above his meta-

Figure 10. Effects of specific absorption rate (SAR, W/kg) and ambient temperature on human core temperature during 60-minute MRI procedures. Based on Adair thermal model assuming a relative humidity of 50%, clothing = 0.2 clo, and a 40% impairment of blood flow at various SAR levels and ambient temperatures.

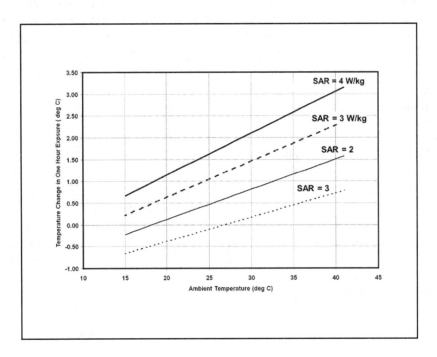

bolic rate. This hypothetical human might experience a 1.0°C rise in temperature in one hour when exposed to 2-W/kg, demonstrating the importance of ambient temperature to the core temperature rise.

Adair and Bergulund (62, 63) utilized a mathematical thermal model of the body, based on the Gagge model (64), to predict the effects of SAR, ambient temperature, impairment of blood flow, relative humidity, clothing, and scan time on core temperature rise. Their summarized results can be approximated with a simple program (63). The Adair program was used to predict the effect of ambient temperature on core temperature rise (10) (**Figure 10**). For the plot, it was assumed that clothing = 0.2 clo, relative humidity was 50%, blood flow impairment was 40%, and the scan duration was 60 minutes. A 40% reduction in cardiac output is life threatening (65). From the plot, it is evident that an exposure to 4-W/kg for an hour should result in only a 1°C core temperature rise when T_a = 19°C. However, if T_a = 25°C, then 3-W/kg is needed. A one hour exposure to 1 W/kg even at T_a = 27°C should result in no temperature rise. Ambient temperature plays an important role in core temperature rise.

SUMMARY AND CONCLUSIONS

A variety of physical factors affect the manner in which the RF fields used for MRI procedures impact patients. Both whole body and localized depositions of RF energy may result in tissue heating. In consideration of this primary safety concern of RF fields, regulatory agencies have provided guidelines based on whole body averaged and/or peak SARs to ensure the safe operation of MR systems. In this chapter, various techniques of calculating and estimating SARs associated with MRI procedures have been described. Additionally, there has been a discussion of the possible mechanisms responsible for observed RF bioeffects and a review of the thermal physics and mathematical models used to predict human thermal responses to absorption of RF energy. This work has served as the basis for characterizing the RF fields used during MRI procedures and helps to estimate the thermophysiologic alterations in patients.

REFERENCES

1.   Mansfield P, Morris PG. Advances in Magnetic Resonance. In: Waugh JS, Editor. NMR Imaging in Biomedicine. Academic Press, New York, 1982. pp. 310-314.

2.   Athey TW. Current FDA guidance for MR patient exposure and considerations for the future. Ann New York Acad Sci 1992;649:242-257.

3.   Bernhardt JH. Non-ionizing radiation safety: radio-frequency radiation, electric and magnetic fields. Phys Med Biol 1992;4:807-844.

4.   Budinger TF, Cullander C. Health Effects of In-vivo Nuclear Magnetic Resonance. In: Margulis AR, Higgins CB, Kaufman L, Crooks LE, Editors. Clinical Magnetic Resonance Imaging. Radiological Research and Education Foundation, San Francisco, 1983.

5.   Budinger TF. Emerging nuclear magnetic resonance technologies: Health and safety. Ann New York Acad Sci 1992;649:1-18.

6.   Kanal E. An overview of electromagnetic safety considerations associated with magnetic resonance imaging. Ann New York Acad Sci 1992;649:204-224.

7.   Persson BRR, Stahlberg F. Seminars on Biomedical Applications of Nuclear Magnetic Resonance. In: Potential Health Hazards and Safety Aspects of Clinical NMR Examinations. Sweden: Radiation Physics Department. 1984. pp. 178.

8.   Saunders RD, Smith H. Safety aspects of NMR clinical imaging. Br Med Bull 1984;40:148-154.

9.   Schaefer DJ. Safety aspects of magnetic resonance imaging. In: Wehrli FW, Shaw D, Kneeland JB, Editors. Biomedical Magnetic Resonance Imaging: Principles, Methodology and Applications. VCH Publishers, New York. 1988. pp. 553-578.

10. Schaefer DJ. Dosimetry and effects of MR exposure to RF and switched magnetic fields. Ann New York Acad Sci 1992;649:225-236.

11. Schaefer DJ. Bioeffects of MRI and patient safety. Amer Assoc Phys Med 1993;649:607-647.

12. Shellock FG. Biological effects and safety aspects of magnetic resonance imaging. Magn Reson Quarterly 1989;5:243-261.

13. Tenforde TS, Budinger TF. Biological effects and physical safety aspects of NMR imaging and in-vivo spectroscopy. In: Thomas SR, Dixon RL, Editors. NMR in Medicine: Instrumentation and Clinical Applications, Medical Monograph. No. 14. Amer Assoc Phys Med; 1986. pp. 493-548.

14. Schaefer DJ. Safety aspects of radio frequency power deposition in magnetic resonance. Magn Reson Imaging Clin N Am 1998;6:775-789.

15. Bottomley PA, Andrew ER. RF magnetic field penetration, phase shift and power dissipation in biological tissue: implications for NMR imaging. Phys Med Biol 1978;23:630-643.

16. Shellock FG, Kanal E. Bioeffects of Radiofrequency Electromagnetic Fields. In: Magnetic Resonance: Bioeffects, Safety, and Patient Management. 2nd Edition. Lippincott-Raven Press, New York, 1996. pp. 25-48.

17. Carlson LD, Hsieh ACL. Control of Energy Exchange. Macmillan, London. 1982. pp. 85.

18. Elder JE. Special Senses. In: Elder JE, Cahill DF, Editors. Biological Effects of Radio-Frequency Radiation. North Carolina: US Environmental Protection Agency; 1984. pp. 64-78.

19. U.S. Department of Health and Human Services, Food and Drug Administration. Magnetic resonance diagnostic device. Panel recommendation and report on petitions for MR reclassification. Fed Reg 1988;53:7575-7579.

20. U.S. Department of Health and Human Services, Food and Drug Administration. Recommendation and report on petitions for magnetic resonance reclassification and codification of reclassification, final rule, 21 CFR Part 892. Fed Reg 1989;54:5077-5088.

21. U.S. Department of Health and Human Services, Food and Drug Administration, Center for Devices and Radiological Health, Radiological Devices Branch, Division of Reproductive, Abdominal, and Radiological Devices, Office of Device Evaluation, Guidance for Industry and FDA Staff: Criteria for Significant Risk Investigations of Magnetic Resonance Diagnostic Devices. Issued July 14, 2003.

22. U.S. Department of Health and Human Services, Food and Drug Administration, Magnetic resonance diagnostic devices criteria for significant risk investigations. 1997. Available at http://www.fda.gov/cdrh/ode/magdev.html.

23. IEC 60601-2-33, Medical electrical equipment - part 2: particular requirements for the safety of magnetic resonance equipment for medical diagnosis. International Electrotechnical Commission (IEC), 2010.

24. Durney CH, Johnson CC, Barber PW, et al. Radiofrequency Radiation Dosimetry Handbook. 2nd Edition. 1978; pp. 8-126.

25. IEC 60601-1-1, Medical electrical equipment - art 1: general requirements for safety; safety requirements for medical electrical systems, 2005-12, International Electrotechnical Commission (IEC), 2005.

26. Kanal E, Barkovich AJ, Bell C. et al. ACR guidance document on MR safe practices: 2013. J Magn Reson Imaging 2013;37:501-530.

27. ISO/TS 10974:2011(E), Assessment of the safety of magnetic resonance imaging for patients with an active implantable medical device. ISO, Case postale 56 CH-1211 Geneva 20, 2011.

28. American Society for Testing and Materials (ASTM) International, F1542 Specification for the requirements and disclosure of self-closing aneurysm clips, 1995.

29. American Society for Testing and Materials (ASTM) International, F2052 Test method for measurement of magnetically induced displacement force on medical devices in the magnetic resonance environment, 2006.

30. American Society for Testing and Materials (ASTM) International, F2119 Test method for evaluation of MR image artifacts from passive implants, 2007.

31. American Society for Testing and Materials (ASTM) International, F2182 Measurement of radio frequency induced heating near passive implants during magnetic resonance imaging, 2011.

32. American Society for Testing and Materials (ASTM) International, F2213 Measurement of Magnetically Induced Torque on Medical Devices in the Magnetic Resonance Environment, 2006.

33. American Society for Testing and Materials (ASTM) International, F2503 Practice for marking medical devices and other items for safety in the magnetic resonance environment, 2007.

34. Bottomley PA, Roemer PB. Homogeneous tissue model estimates of RF power deposition in human NMR studies. Local elevations predicted in surface coil decoupling. Ann N Y Acad Sci 1992;649:144-59.

35. Ramo S, Whinnery JR, Van Duzer T. Fields and Waves in Communication Electronics. 3rd Edition. New York: J Wiley & Sons; 1965. pp. 108-124.

36. Plonus MA. Applied Electromagnetics. New York: McGraw-Hill; 1984. pp. 208,290-299, 453.

37. Schenck JF, Hussain MA. Power deposition during magnetic resonance: the effects of local electrical in-homogeneities and field exclusion. General Electric Corporate Research and Development Labs. 1984.

38. Collins CM, Mao W, Liu W, Smith MB. Calculated local and average SAR in comparison with regulatory limits. Proc Intl So Mag Reson Med 2006;14:2044.

39. Davis PL, Crooks L, Arakawa M, et al. Potential hazards in NMR imaging: heating effects of changing magnetic fields and RF fields on small metallic implants. Am J Roentgenol 1981;137:857-860.

40. Chou CK, McDougall JA, Chan KW. RF heating of implanted spinal fusion stimulator during magnetic resonance imaging. IEEE Trans Biomed Eng 1997;44:367-373.

41. Lemieux L, Allen PJ, Franconi F, et al. Recording of EEG during fMRI experiments: patient safety. Magn Reson Med 1997;38:943-952.

42. Hofman MB, de Cock CC, van der Linden JC, et al. Transesophageal cardiac pacing during magnetic resonance imaging: feasibility and safety considerations. Magn Reson Med 1996;35:413-422.

43. Hess T, Stepanow B, Knopp MV. Safety of intrauterine contraceptive devices during MR imaging. Eur Radiol 1996;6:66-68.

44. Shellock FG. Reference Manual for Magnetic Resonance Safety, Implants, and Devices: 2013 Edition. Biomedical Research Publishing Group, Los Angeles, CA, 2013.

45. Athey TW. A model of the temperature rise in the head due to magnetic resonance imaging procedures. Magn Reson in Med, 1989:177-184.

46. NEMA MS 8-1993. Characterization of the specific absorption rate for magnetic resonance imaging systems. National Electrical Manufacturers Association 2008.

47. Schaefer DJ. Estimation of current limits for RF power deposition from planar, transmit surface coils. New York: Abstracts of the Society of Magnetic Resonance Imaging; 1996. pp. 1446.

48. Schenck JF, Boskamp EB, Schaefer DJ, Barber WD, Vander Heiden RH. Estimating local SAR produced by RF transmitter coils: examples using the birdcage coil. Berkeley: Abstracts of the International Society of Magnetic Resonance in Medicine; 1998. pp. 649.

49. Chou CK, Chen GW, Guy AW, Luk KH. Formulas for preparing phantom muscle tissue at various radiofrequencies. Bioelectromagnetics 1984;5:435-441.

50. Gandhi OP, Chien, JY. Absorption and distribution patterns of RF fields. Ann New York Acad Sci 1992;649:131-143.

51. Grandolfo M, Polichetti A, Vecchia P, Gandhi OP. Spatial distribution of RF power in critical organs during magnetic resonance imaging. Ann New York Acad Sci 1992;649:178.

52. Buchli R, Saner M, Meier D, Boskamp EB, Boesiger P. Increased RF power absorption in MR imaging due to RF coupling between body coil and surface coil. Magn Reson Med 1989;9:105-112.

53. Boesigner P, Buchli R, Saner M, Meier D. An overview of electromagnetic safety considerations associated with magnetic resonance imaging. Ann New York Acad Sci 1992;649:160-165.

54. Lehninger AL. Biochemistry. New York: Worth; 1972. pp. 153.

55. Halliday D, Resnick R. Physics. New York: John Wiley; 1966. pp. 873.

56. Kennelly AE, Alexanderson EFW. The physiological tolerance of alternating-current strengths up to frequencies of 100,000 cycles per second. Electrical World 1910;56:154-156.

57. Guy AW, Lin JC, Kramer PO, Emery AF. Effect of 2450 MHz radiation on the rabbit eye. IEEE Trans Microwave Theory Tech 1975;23:492-498.

58. Goldman RF, Green EB, Iampietro PF. Tolerance of hot wet environments by resting men. J Appl Physiol 1965;20:271-277.

59. Smith DA, Clarren SK, Harvey MAS. Hyperthermia as a possible teratogenic agent. Pediatrics 1978;92:878-883.

60. Ganong WF. Review of Medical Physiology. 6th Edition. Los Altos: Lange Medical Publications; 1973. pp. 193-197, pp. 474-476.

61. Benjamin FB. Pain reaction to locally applied heat. J Appl Physiol 1952;52:250-263.

62. Adair ER, Berglund LG. On the thermoregulatory consequences of NMR imaging. Magn Reson Imaging 1986;4:321-333.

63. Adair ER, Berglund LG. Thermoregulatory consequences of cardiovascular impairment during NMR imaging in warm/humid environments. Magn Reson Imaging 1989;7:25.

64. Gagge AP. The New Effective Temperature (ET) - An Index of Human Adaptation to Warm Environments. In: Horvath S, Yousef M, Editors. Environmental Physiology: Aging, Heat, and Altitude. 1980. pp. 9-77.

65. Hurst J, Willis ED. The Heart. McGraw-Hill; 1978.

Chapter 6 Radiofrequency-Energy Induced Heating During MRI: Laboratory and Clinical Experiences

FRANK G. SHELLOCK, PH.D.

Adjunct Clinical Professor of Radiology and Medicine
Keck School of Medicine, University of Southern California

Adjunct Professor of Clinical Physical Therapy
Division of Biokinesiology and Physical Therapy
School of Dentistry, University of Southern California

Director for MRI Studies of Biomimetic MicroElectronic Systems
National Science Foundation, Engineering Research Center
University of Southern California

Institute for Magnetic Resonance Safety, Education, and Research
President, Shellock R & D Services, Inc.
Los Angeles, CA

INTRODUCTION

Radiofrequency (RF) energy is nonionizing, electromagnetic radiation in the frequency range of 3-kHz to 300-GHz (1– 4). The RF spectrum includes radar, ultra high frequency (UHF), and very high frequency (VHF) television, AM and FM radio, and microwave communication frequencies. During magnetic resonance imaging (MRI) procedures, most of the transmitted radiofrequency (RF) power is transformed into heat within the patient's tissue as a result the induction of eddy currents due to the nonzero conductivity of tissue via Faraday's law. Not surprisingly, the primary health effects and safety concerns associated with the RF energy-induced heating are directly related to the thermogenic qualities of this electromagnetic field (1-30). The deposition of thermalizing energy deep in the human body by exposure to RF fields provides a unique exception to the energy flows normally encountered by humans (2).

Research studies conducted over the last several decades have indicated that exposure to RF radiation may produce various physiologic effects including those associated with alterations in visual, auditory, endocrine, neural, cardiovascular, immune, reproductive, and developmental function (1-30). In general, these biological changes are believed to occur due to RF-induced heating of tissues.

Exposure to RF energy may also cause athermal, field-specific changes in biological systems that are produced without an increase in temperature (2, 5, 6, 22). However, athermal effects associated with RF radiation are not well understood and, to date, have not been systematically studied in association with the use of MRI. Those interested in thorough discussions of this topic are referred to the comprehensive reviews written by Adey (6) and Beers (22).

Prior to 1985, there were no published reports pertaining to the effects of exposing human subjects to RF energy during MRI examinations. In fact, there was a general lack of quantitative data on thermal and other physiological responses of human subjects exposed to RF radiation from any source. The previous investigations that were conducted on this topic typically examined responses to therapeutic applications of diathermy or thermal sensations related to exposure to RF radiation (2-5, 23, 24). Unfortunately, these localized or limited exposures to RF energy do not relate to the exposure conditions that occur during MRI.

Therefore, in order to properly characterize the thermophysiological aspects of RF energy, several investigations have been conducted using laboratory animals, volunteer subjects, and patients. This resulting research has yielded extremely useful and important data with regard to thermoregulatory responses to RF radiation-induced heating associated with MRI.

This chapter will review and discuss the various aspects of RF energy-induced heating during MRI with an emphasis on the studies performed in human subjects to assess thermal and other physiologic responses.

MRI PROCEDURES AND SPECIFIC ABSORPTION RATE

The thermoregulatory and other physiologic changes that a laboratory animal or human subject display in response to exposure to RF radiation are dependent on the amount of energy that is absorbed (3). The dosimetric term used to describe the absorption of RF radiation is the specific absorption rate, or SAR (2, 3, 5, 19, 20). The SAR is the mass normalized rate at which RF power is coupled to biological tissue and is typically indicated in units of watts per kilogram (W/kg).

The relative amount of RF radiation that an organism encounters during an MRI procedure is usually characterized with respect to the whole-body-averaged and peak SAR levels (i.e., the SAR averaged in one-gram of tissue). Importantly, SAR information is used by regulatory agencies with regard to safety guidelines for the exposure to RF energy during MRI.

Notably, measurements or estimates of SAR are not trivial, particularly in human subjects. There are several methods of determining this parameter for the purpose of RF energy dosimetry in association with the use of MRI. The SAR that is produced during MRI is a complex function of numerous variables including the frequency (i.e., determined by the strength of the static magnetic field of the MR system, with resonant frequencies producing the greatest effects), the type of RF pulse used (e.g., 90° vs. 180° pulse), the repetition time, the type of transmit RF coil used (e.g., linear vs. quadrature transmission, whole body vs. local RF coil, etc.), the volume of tissue contained within the RF coil, the shape of the anatomical region exposed, the orientation of the body to the field vectors, as well as other factors (1, 19, 20). Therefore, SAR, being an important parameter used to help ensure safety aspects of exposure to RF energy, may be difficult to calculate or estimate precisely for MRI procedures. Interestingly, MR system manufacturers appear to apply various safety or modeling factors to the SAR values reported by their scanners. Thus, manufacturers seem to err on the side of safety when estimating SAR values for clinical MRI examinations (20).

RF ENERGY-INDUCED HEATING AND MRI: EVALUATION OF LABORATORY ANIMALS

Although there have been several studies performed using laboratory animals to assess thermoregulatory reactions to tissue heating associated with exposure to RF radiation, these experiments do not directly apply to the specific conditions that occur with MRI. Furthermore, the results of these investigations cannot be easily extrapolated to provide useful information for human subjects (2-5, 7, 8, 25). For example, the pattern of RF coupling and resulting absorption of RF energy to biological tissues is primarily dependent on the organism's size, anatomical features, the duration of exposure, the sensitivity of the involved tissues, and a myriad of other variables (2-5, 7, 8, 25).

Importantly, there is no laboratory animal that sufficiently mimics or simulates the thermoregulatory responses with respect to the dimensions and specific responses that occur in a human subject. Therefore, experimental results obtained in laboratory animals cannot be simply "scaled" or extrapolated to predict thermoregulatory or other physiologic changes in human subjects exposed to RF radiation-induced heating during MRI. Nevertheless, experiments have been conducted in the MRI environment using laboratory animals as an initial step to determine the effects of RF energy-induced heating associated with exposures to high SAR levels.

Shuman, et al. (29) studied laboratory dogs undergoing MRI examinations at relatively high levels of RF energy. Superficial- and deep-tissue temperatures were measured in five laboratory dogs before, during, and after exposure to RF energy in order to determine whether significant temperature changes could be produced in association with operation of a 1.5-T/64-MHz MR system (29). The RF power output that was applied in this investigation was 6.3 times that required for routine MRI procedures, with calculated SARs that averaged 7.9-W/kg for the five dogs (29).

Shuman, et al. (29) reported that there was a linear temperature increase of several degrees, with a maximal average temperature change of 4.6 °C that was measured in the urinary bladder (i.e., a "deep" body site). Overall, the temperature elevations were slightly greater in deeper tissues compared to those recorded in superficial tissues. Shuman, et al. (29) stated that these findings suggested continued caution in the design and operation of MR systems that are capable of depositing high SAR levels, particularly when the scanners are used to image infants or patients with altered thermoregulatory capabilities.

While the results of Shuman, et al. (29) are intriguing, it should be noted that this study was conducted using anesthetized laboratory animals. As such, the findings are unlikely to pertain to conscious, adult human subjects because of the previously discussed factors related to the physical dimensions of the animals and the fact that an anesthetic agent was used that may substantially impact thermoregulation. Additionally, the thermoregulatory systems of these two species are quite dissimilar (e.g., the dog pants to dissipate heat while human subjects sweat). Nevertheless, data obtained by Shuman, et al. (29) may have important implications for the use of MRI in pediatric patients because this patient population is typically sedated or anesthetized for MRI examinations and the physical dimensions of the laboratory dog are somewhat comparable to a pediatric patient. Obviously, additional research is required to further examine this issue.

Barber, et al. (30) also conducted a study to determine the effects of heating related to MRI. The objective of this investigation was to provide a worst-case estimate of the thermal effects of MRI by subjecting anesthetized, unshorn sheep to RF power deposition at SAR levels well above approved standards for periods of time in excess of normal clinical imaging protocols (30). The sheep underwent MRI procedures using a 1.5-Tesla, 64-MHz MR system. A control period with no RF power was followed by experiments using 20- to 105-minutes of RF power applications. Afterward, there was a 20-minute or longer recovery period with no RF power applied to the sheep. Eight sheep were scanned at whole-body-averaged SARs that ranged from 1.5- to 4.0-W/kg while rectal and skin temperatures were monitored.

In addition to the whole body RF exposures, Barber, et al. (30) subjected four sheep to MRI procedures involving the head to determine the effects of RF energy-induced heating associated with MRI of the brain. The average scan time was 75-minutes and temperatures of the cornea, vitreous humor, head skin, jugular vein, and rectum were measured during this experiment.

In the whole body exposure experiments, elevation of rectal temperature was correlated with RF energy deposition. Deep body temperature rises in excess of 2°C were attained for the whole-body-averaged SAR level of 4.0-W/kg during exposure periods greater than 82-minutes. In the head scanning experiments, skin and eye temperatures increased approximately 1.5°C. Additionally, jugular vein temperature increased a maximum of 0.4°C after an average exposure time of 75-minutes. Animals exposed for 40-minutes to an SAR of 4.0-W/kg in either the transmit body RF coil (three sheep) or transmit head RF coil (two sheep) were recovered and observed to be in good health for 10-weeks. Importantly, no cataracts were found in these sheep (30).

Thus, using this animal model, Barber, et al. (30) concluded that RF power deposition at SAR levels well above typical clinical MRI protocols caused various tissue temperatures to increase. Furthermore, for exposure periods in excess of standard clinical MRI protocols, the temperature increase was insufficient to cause adverse thermal effects (30).

CHARACTERISTICS OF RF ENERGY-INDUCED HEATING: IMPLICATIONS FOR HUMAN SUBJECTS

The physical dimensions and anatomic configurations of biologic tissues in relation to the incident wavelength are important factors that determine the relative amount and pattern of RF energy that is absorbed by the human body (1-4, 20). For example, if the size of the tissue is large in relation to the incident wavelength, RF energy is predominantly absorbed on the surface (1-4). If it is small relative to the wavelength, there is little absorption of RF power and, thus, the effects of heating are minimized (1-6, 19, 20).

Tissue heating that results from the RF energy used during MRI is primarily caused by magnetic induction, with a negligible contribution from the electric fields (1, 19, 20). This ohmic heating of tissue is greatest at the surface or periphery and minimal at the center of a human subject's body. Predictive calculations and measurements obtained in phantoms, laboratory animals, and human subjects exposed to various MRI conditions support this pattern of temperature distribution (1, 19, 20).

Notably, the actual increase in tissue temperature caused by exposure to RF energy is dependent on a variety of factors related to the thermoregulatory system of the individual and the surrounding environment (1-4, 7, 8, 10, 11, 14-20, 21, 25). In regards to the thermoregulatory system, when subjected to a thermal challenge, the human body loses heat by means of convection, conduction, radiation, and evaporation. Each mechanism is responsible to a varying degree for heat dissipation, as the body attempts to maintain thermal homeostasis. If the thermoregulatory effectors are not capable of totally dissipating the heat load, heat accumulates and is stored, resulting in an elevation in local and/or overall tissue temperatures.

Various underlying health conditions may impact an individual's ability to tolerate a thermal challenge. These conditions include cardiovascular disease, hypertension, diabetes, fever, old age, and obesity (31-35). Various medications (e.g., diuretics, beta-blockers, calcium blockers, amphetamines, muscle relaxers, sedatives, etc.) can also greatly alter thermoregulatory responses to a heat load (36, 37). In fact, certain medications may have a synergistic effect with respect to tissue heating if the heating is specifically caused by exposure to RF radiation (36).

The environmental conditions that exist in and around the MR system will also affect the tissue temperature elevations associated with RF energy-induced heating. During MRI, the amount of tissue heating that occurs is dependent upon environmental factors that include the ambient temperature, relative humidity, and airflow within the bore of the MR system.

With further regard to the environmental conditions of the MR system, it has been proposed that, in order to counter-balance excessive tissue heating that may occur during exposure to high levels of RF energy, patients should be "pre-cooled" before MRI. However, the subjective perception to the environmental temperature depends on the gradient of temperature that is sensed by the peripheral thermoreceptors. Therefore, patients going from a cooler (i.e., using a "pre-cooling" room) to a warmer environment (i.e., the MR system) would likely be more uncomfortable.

IMPORTANT CONSIDERATIONS FOR EVALUATION OF PHYSIOLOGICAL CHANGES DURING RF ENERGY-INDUCED HEATING

Acquiring measurements of temperature and other physiologic parameters in human subjects within the harsh electromagnetic environment of the MR system is not a simple task. The static magnetic field of the MR system can easily create missiles out of conventional monitoring devices because they usually contain ferromagnetic components (1, 14, 15, 17, 18, 21). In addition, the static, gradient, and RF electromagnetic fields may adversely interfere with the proper operation of monitoring equipment. In turn, the devices may produce subtle or substantial artifacts by generating electromagnetic interference that can distort the quality of the MR images. Therefore, temperature recording devices and physiologic monitors must be specially adapted or modified and then rigorously tested prior to use in the MRI environment. Otherwise, the data pertaining to thermal and other physiologic responses may be erroneous. Another solution to this important matter is to simply use MR Conditional monitoring equipment that has been thoroughly tested and demonstrated to work appropriately in the MRI setting.

Currently, MR Conditional temperature recording devices and physiologic monitors, as well as other patient support devices are commercially available for use in the MRI environment. Every physiologic parameter that is typically recorded in the critical care area or operating room setting may be obtained during MRI, including heart rate, oxygen saturation, end-tidal carbon dioxide, respiratory rate, blood pressure, cutaneous blood flow and, most importantly, body and skin temperatures (38-42).

For the assessment of thermal responses during MRI, volunteer subjects and patients have been monitored throughout the experimental procedures using several different types of devices (43-54). For example, sublingual pocket or tympanic membrane temperatures have been obtained immediately before and after MRI using sensitive electronic thermometry or infrared devices. Notably, there is a good relationship between temperatures measured in the sublingual pocket or tympanic membrane and esophageal temperature, which is an indicator of core or "deep" temperature.

Skin temperatures have been measured immediately before and after MRI procedures using highly sensitive and accurate infrared thermometry or digital thermographic equipment (48, 50. 54). Body and skin temperatures measured at multiple sites have been recorded before, during, and after MRI using a fluoroptic (i.e., fiber-optic) thermometry system that is unperturbed by electromagnetic radiation of all types, including static magnetic fields of up to 9.0-Tesla (42).

Heart rate, oxygen saturation, blood pressure, respiratory rate, and cutaneous blood flow, which are important physiologic variables that change in human subjects in response to a thermal load, have been monitored before, during, and after MRI to assess the reaction of the thermoregulatory system to exposures to RF energy-induced heating. All of these parameters may be obtained with devices that have been extensively tested and demonstrated to provide sensitive and accurate data in the MRI environment.

RF ENERGY-INDUCED HEATING AND MRI: ASSESSMENT OF VOLUNTEER SUBJECTS AND PATIENTS

As previously described in this chapter, the increase in tissue temperature caused by exposure to RF energy during MRI depends on multiple physiologic, physical, and environmental factors. These include the rate at which RF energy is deposited, the status of the patient's thermoregulatory system, the presence of an underlying health condition or medications, and the ambient conditions within the MR system.

Although the main cause of tissue heating associated with MRI is attributed to RF radiation, it should be noted that various reports have suggested that exposure to the powerful static magnetic fields used for MRI may also cause temperature changes (55, 56). The mechanism(s) responsible for such an effect remains unclear. Nevertheless, the results of these previously published studies warranted investigations in human subjects to determine the possible contribution of the static magnetic field to temperature changes that may be observed during MRI (57, 58).

Studies were performed in human subjects exposed to a 1.5-Tesla static magnetic field to evaluate thermal alterations produced in body and/or skin temperatures (57, 58). The data revealed that there were no statistically significant alterations in any of the recorded tissue temperatures or other physiologic parameter (57, 58). Furthermore, Tenforde (59) examined this phenomenon in laboratory rodents exposed to static magnetic fields of as high as 7.55-Tesla and also reported no thermal effect. As far as the potential for production of heat by gradient (i.e., time-varying) magnetic fields is concerned, this is not believed to occur in association with conventional imaging parameters used for clinical MRI (15, 19, 20, 22).

With regard to the effects of RF energy-induced heating, Schaefer, et al. (60) conducted the first study of human thermal responses associated with MRI in 1985 (60). Temperature changes and other physiologic parameters were assessed in volunteer subjects exposed to relatively high, whole-body-averaged SAR levels (approximately 4.0-W/kg). The data indicated that there were no excessive temperature elevations or other deleterious physiologic consequences related to exposure to RF radiation (60).

Several studies were subsequently conducted involving volunteer subjects and patients undergoing MRI with the intent of obtaining information that would be applicable to the patient population typically encountered in the MRI setting (43-50, 52-54, 61, 62). The whole-body-averaged SAR levels ranged from approximately 0.05-W/kg (e.g., for MRI procedures involving the use of a transmit/receive head RF coil) to 6.0-W/kg (e.g., for MRI procedures involving the imaging of the spine or abdomen with a transmit/receive body RF coil) (43-54, 61, 62). **Figure 1** shows an example of body and skin temperature changes related to MRI performed at 1.5-Tesla/64-MHz and a whole-body-averaged SAR of 2.8-W/kg.

To date, the studies performed in human subjects demonstrated that changes in body temperatures were relatively inconsequential (i.e., less than 0.6°C). While there was a tendency for statistically significant increases in skin temperatures to occur, these were not physiologically deleterious or otherwise problematic. Furthermore, there were no substantial alterations in the hemodynamic parameters that were assessed during these investigations (i.e., heart rate, blood pressure, and cutaneous blood flow).

Figure 1. Body (sublingual pocket) and multiple skin temperatures measured at one-minute intervals using a fluoroptic thermometry system before (baseline), during (MRI), and after (post-MRI) MRI performed at whole-body-averaged SAR of 2.8-W/kg. Note that there were little or no changes in body temperature, whereas there were slight to moderate changes in skin temperatures (depending on the site of measurement) during MRI. After MRI, some skin temperatures returned to the baseline level, whereas others remained elevated during the 20-min post-MRI evaluation period (see reference 50).

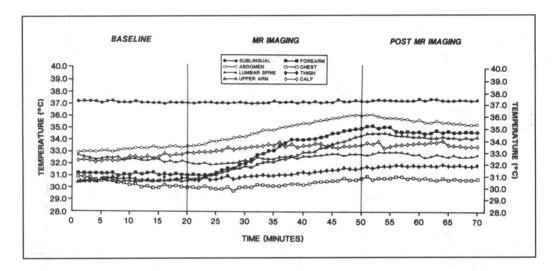

Notably, research has indicated that there is a poor correlation between changes in body and skin temperatures versus whole-body-averaged SARs for clinical MRI procedures (**Figure 2**). This finding is not surprising considering the previously mentioned myriad of variables that may alter thermal responses in a patient population. Therefore, the thermal responses to a given SAR may be quite variable depending on the individual's thermoregulatory system and the presence of one or more underlying condition(s) that can alter or impair the ability to dissipate heat.

At the present time, a whole-body-averaged SAR of 6.0-W/kg is the highest level of exposure to RF energy that has been reported for human subjects undergoing MRI (53). In this investigation, Shellock, et al. (53) performed experiments on volunteer subjects in cool (22.5°C) and warm (33°C) environments to characterize thermal and other physiologic responses to this high level of RF energy. The motivation for this study coincided with the advent of pulse sequences that had relatively high SAR levels associated with their use.

The temperature of the tympanic membrane (i.e., an index of deep body temperature) and seven different skin temperatures were monitored along with blood pressure, heart rate, oxygen saturation, and cutaneous blood flow (53). Measurements were obtained immediately before, during, and after exposure to RF energy.

In the cool environment, there were statistically significant increases in tympanic membrane, abdomen, upper arm, hand, and thigh temperatures as well as heart rate and skin blood flow. In the warm environment, there were statistically significant increases in tym-

Figure 2. (A) Changes in body temperature versus whole-body-averaged SARs during clinical MRI procedures. Note that there is a poor correlation between these two variables.

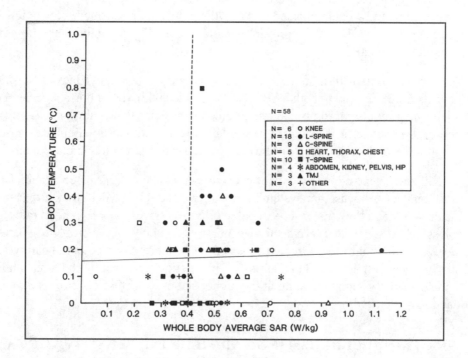

(B) Changes in skin temperature versus whole-body-averaged SARs during clinical MRI procedures. Note that there is a poor correlation between these two variables.

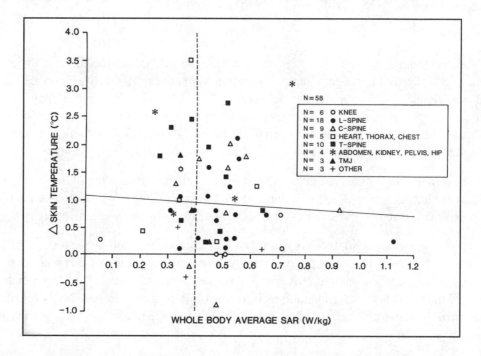

panic membrane, hand, and chest temperatures as well as systolic blood pressure and heart rate.

Importantly, the tissue temperature increases were within acceptable, safe levels. Of critical note is that these data indicated that an MRI procedure performed at a whole-body-averaged SAR of 6.0-W/kg can be physiologically tolerated by an individual with normal thermoregulatory function (53).

While the data obtained so far are encouraging regarding the relative lack of substantial health effects from exposure to high SAR levels associated with MRI it must be remembered that patients may have compromised thermoregulatory systems that could significantly alter their ability to handle a heat load. For example, patients with cardiovascular disease are known to poorly tolerate the effects of heating, which can lead to circulatory collapse.

Can RF power deposition in a patient with cardiovascular disease place potentially unsafe stress on the cardiovascular system? For example, could an MRI procedure cause an increase in skin blood flow that results in potentially excessive changes in heart rate and/or blood pressure? At some SAR levels, this thermal stress is likely to be a problem. Therefore, additional investigations are warranted to specifically address this potential safety issue, particularly since there is a need to address RF energy-induced heating in human subjects scanned using MR systems operating at the higher static magnetic field strengths (i.e., 3-, 4-, 7-, and 9.4-Tesla).

RF ENERGY INDUCED-HEATING AND THERMAL-SENSITIVE ORGANS

The testes and eyes of human subjects have reduced capabilities for heat dissipation and may be injured or damaged by elevated temperatures (6, 7). Therefore, the testes and eyes are primary sites of potentially harmful effects if exposure to RF radiation during MRI is excessive (6, 7, 11-15, 17, 18, 46, 48, 49, 63).

The Testes

Laboratory investigations have demonstrated that RF energy-induced heating may have detrimental effects on testicular function. If the exposure level to RF energy increases scrotal and/or testicular tissue temperatures between 38°C to 42°C (8), this heating may cause a reduction or cessation of spermatogenesis, impaired sperm motility, degeneration of seminiferous tubules, as well as other abnormal conditions (8, 64). Notably, there is a direct relationship between temperature and sperm motility and viability.

The temperature of the testes correlates directly with the temperature of the scrotal skin (64). This temperature level exists because the scrotum has little or no subcutaneous fat or connective tissue and, as such, there is no tissue mediated temperature gradient present (64).

In 1990, Shellock, et al. (48) conducted an investigation to examine the thermal effects of MRI performed on the scrotum to determine if excessive heating of this body part occurred. A non-contact infrared thermometer was used to measure scrotal skin temperatures (i.e., as a index to testicular temperatures) immediately before and after the MRI procedures performed at relatively high SAR levels (48). A statistically significant increase in scrotal skin temperature was associated with MRI and the highest scrotal skin temperature recorded was 34.2°C (48). Notably, these temperature alterations were below the threshold known to alter or adversely affect the function of the testes (8, 48).

Excessive heating of the scrotum associated with MRI could exacerbate a pre-existing disorder associated with increased testicular temperature (e.g., febrile illnesses, varicocele, etc.) in patients who are already oligospermic, leading to temporary or permanent sterility. Therefore, additional investigations designed to investigate these particular issues with regard to the testes are warranted, particularly if patients are subjected to MRI using RF energy levels (i.e., SARs) that are greater than those previously evaluated. This scenario is entirely possible considering the widespread use of pulse sequences that utilize high levels of RF energy (e.g., fast or turbo spin echo sequences) and MR systems operating at higher static magnetic field strengths that inherently have higher associated SAR levels.

The Eye

Dissipation of heat from the eye is a slow and inefficient process due to its relative lack of vascularization (7). Acute, near-field exposures of RF radiation to the eyes or heads of laboratory animals have been reported to be cataractogenic as a result of the thermal disruption of ocular tissue (7).

An investigation conducted by Sacks, et al. (63) revealed that there were no discernible effects on the eyes of rats caused by MRI performed at RF energy levels that far exceeded typical levels used in the clinical setting. However, as previously indicated, it may not be acceptable to extrapolate data from laboratory animals to human subjects. For example, the coupling of RF radiation to the eye of a laboratory rat is obviously quite different compared to the situation for a human subject, especially in consideration of the size, shape, tissue volume, and relative position of the eyes on the rat compared to man.

Shellock, et al. (46, 49) performed two separate clinical studies to evaluate the thermal effects of RF energy-induced heating of the eye associated with MRI. In both investigations, corneal temperatures were measured using a non-contact infrared thermometer immediately before and after MRI. Notably, corneal temperature is a representative site of the average temperature of the human eye (65).

In the first study, corneal temperatures were measured in patients undergoing MRI of the brain using a transmit/receive head coil at peak SARs ranged from 2.5- to 3.1-W/kg (46). The greatest change in corneal temperature change was 1.8°C and the highest temperature that was measured was 34.4°C.

The second study examined corneal temperatures in patients with suspected ocular pathology who underwent MRI using the body coil to transmit RF energy and a special eye coil for RF reception (49). Fast spin echo pulse sequences were used to examine the eye. The peak SARs for these sequences ranged from 3.3- to 8.4-W/kg. The greatest temperature change was 1.8°C and the highest corneal temperature that was measured was 35.1°C (49).

Thus, the findings from these two clinical investigations indicated that corneal temperatures did not exceed the upper limit of normal for the human cornea, which is 36°C (65). Of further note is that the temperature threshold for RF radiation-induced cataractogenesis in animal models has been reported to be 41 to 55°C for acute, near-field exposures (6). Therefore, it does not appear that clinical MRI under the conditions studied by Shellock, et al. (46, 49) have the potential to cause thermal damage to ocular tissue. However, with higher RF energy used for clinical MRI procedures, the thermal effects on ocular tissue may require further assessment.

MRI AND "HOT SPOTS"

Theoretically, during exposure to RF energy, "hot spots" (i.e., an excessive concentration of RF energy) may develop due to an uneven distribution of RF power in association with restrictive conductive patterns (12, 21, 44, 54). Obviously, an unwanted result of this would be if the RF energy-induced "hot spots" that occur during an MRI procedure generated thermal "hot spots".

Because RF radiation is mainly absorbed by peripheral tissues, surface thermography was used to study the heating pattern associated with MRI procedures that were performed in volunteer subjects exposed to relatively high whole-body-averaged SARs (44, 54). The findings of this research demonstrated that there was no evidence of surface thermal "hot spots" in the human subjects (44, 54). Apparently, the thermoregulatory system responds to any RF radiation-related "hot spot" by evenly distributing the thermal load utilizing the cutaneous circulation. Thus, thermal "hot spots" do not appear to occur in human subjects (44, 54).

There is the possibility, however, that thermal "hot spots" may develop internally during an MRI procedure. As previously-mentioned, Shuman, et al. (66) reported that significant temperature increases occur in the internal organs of laboratory dogs as a result of MRI performed using relatively high SAR levels. These findings suggest that internal thermal "hot spots" may occur in association with MRI. Therefore, the presence of possible internal "hot spots" needs to be thoroughly examined in human subjects undergoing MRI. This could likely be accomplished using one of the MRI thermometry techniques commonly used to guide therapeutic tissue heating and cooling (66, 67).

CONCLUSIONS

The characteristics of RF energy-induced heating associated with MRI have been presented with an emphasis on research pertaining to laboratory animals and human subjects. These investigations began in the mid-1980s and continued for approximately 10 years. The vast majority of these studies were conducted at 1.5-Tesla/64-MHz.

Because higher field strength MR systems (i.e., 3-Tesla or higher) and new clinical applications (e.g., advanced pulse sequences, specialized transmit RF coils, etc.) with associated higher levels of RF energy have become available over the years, additional work has been required to assess the effects of RF energy-induced heating to ensure patient safety. The vast majority of the studies performed after the mid-1990s involved attempts to predict or study the heating aspects of RF energy mainly by using modeling-based investigations, temperature measurements made in phantoms or, in a few instances, temperature measurements obtained in laboratory animals (68-82). Unfortunately, without validation in human subjects, the safety of high levels of RF energy exposures associated with the investigated MRI conditions remains unknown. Therefore, research is urgently needed to evaluate the thermoregulatory responses of human subjects to the potential thermogenic hazards of the higher field strength MR systems and the new clinical applications. Finally, additional investigations are needed to study patients with conditions that impair heat dissipation. As MRI technology continues to evolve, an on-going effort is required to characterize thermal and other physiologic responses in human subjects to ensure the safe use of MRI during procedures that require exposure to high levels of RF energy.

REFERENCES

1. Shellock FG, Kanal E. Chapter 3. Bioeffects of Radiofrequency Electromagnetic Fields, In: Magnetic Resonance: Bioeffects, Safety, and Patient Management. Second Edition. New York: Lippincott-Raven Publishers; 1996. pp. 25-48.

2. National Council on Radiation Protection and Measurements. Biological effects and exposure criteria for radiofrequency electromagnetic fields. Report No. 86. National Council on Radiation Protection and Measurements. Bethesda, MD; 1986.

3. Gordon CJ. Thermal Physiology. In: Biological Effects of Radiofrequency Radiation. Washington, DC: EPA-600/8-83-026A. 1984. pp. 1-28.

4. Gordon CJ. Effect of radiofrequency radiation exposure on thermoregulation. ISI Atlas Sci Plants Anim 1988;1:245-250.

5. Michaelson SM, Lin JC. Biological Effects and Health Implications of Radiofrequency Radiation. New York: Plenum; 1987.

6. Adey WR. Tissue interactions with nonionizing electromagnetic fields. Physiol Rev 1981;61:435-514.

7. Elder JA. Special Senses. In: Biological Effects of Radiofrequency Radiation, Washington, DC: EPA-600/8-83-026A.1984. pp. 5-78.

8. Berman E. Reproductive effects. In: Biological Effects of Radiofrequency Radiation, Washington, DC: EPA-600/8-83-026A. 1984. pp. 5-42.

9. U.S. Environmental Protection Agency. Evaluation of potential electromagnetic carcinogenicity. Office of Health and Environmental Assessment. U.S. Environmental Protection Agency, EPA-600/6 90 005A, 1990.

10. O'Conner ME. Mammalian teratogenesis and radio-frequency fields. Proceed IEEE 1980;68:56-60.

11. Lary JM, Conover DL. Teratogenic effects of radiofrequency radiation. IEEE Engineering in Medicine and Biology 1987;44:42-46.

12. Edelman RR, Shellock FG, Ahladis J. Practical MRI for the Technologist and Imaging Specialist. In: Edelman RR and Hesselink J, Editors. Clinical Magnetic Resonance. Philadelphia: Saunders; 1990.

13. Persson BRR, Stahlberg F. Health and Safety of Clinical NMR Examinations. Boca Raton, Florida: CRC Press; 1989.

14. Shellock FG. Biological effects and safety aspects of magnetic resonance imaging. Magn Res Q 1989;5:243-261.

15. Kanal E, Shellock FG, Talagala L. Safety considerations in MR imaging. Radiology 1990;176:593-606.

16. Morvan D, Leroy-Willig A, Jehenson P, Cuenod CA, Syrota A. Temperature changes induced in human muscle by radiofrequency H-1 coupling: measurement with an MR imaging diffusion technique. Radiology 1992;185:871-874.

17. Shellock FG. MRI Bioeffects and Safety. In: Atlas S, Editor. Magnetic Resonance Imaging of the Brain and Spine. New York: Raven Press; 1990.

18. Shellock FG. Thermal responses in human subjects exposed to magnetic resonance imaging. Annals of the New York Academy of Sciences 1992; 260-272.

19. Bottomley PA, Redington RW, Edelstein WA, et al. Estimating radiofrequency power deposition in body NMR imaging. Magn Reson Med 1985;2:336-349.

20. Bottomley PA. Turning up the heat on MRI. J Am Coll Radiol 2008;5:853-5.

21. Shellock FG, Litwer C, Kanal E. MRI bioeffects, safety, and patient management: a review. Reviews in Magnetic Resonance Imaging 1992;4:21-63.

22. Beers J. Biological effects of weak electromagnetic fields from 0 Hz to 200 MHz: A survey of the literature with special emphasis on possible magnetic resonance effects. Magn Reson Imaging 1989;7:309-331.

23. Coulter S, Osbourne SL. Short wave diathermy in heating of human tissues. Arch Phys Ther 1936;17:679-687.

24. Gersten JW, Wakim KG, Herrick JF, Krusen FH. The effect of microwave diathermy on the peripheral circulation and on tissue temperature in man. Arch Phys Med 1949;30:7-25.

25. Gordon CJ. Normalizing the thermal effects of radiofrequency radiation: Body mass versus total body surface area. Bioelectromagnetics 1987;8:111-118.

26. Athey TW. A model of the temperature rise in the head due to magnetic resonance imaging procedures. Magn Res Med 1989;9:177-184.

27. Adair ER, Berglund LG. On the thermoregulatory consequences of NMR imaging. Magn Reson Imaging 1986;4:321-333.

28. Adair ER, Berglund LG. Thermoregulatory consequences of cardiovascular impairment during NMR imaging in warm/humid environments. Magn Reson Imaging 1989;7:25-37.

29. Shuman WP, Haynor DR, Guy AW, et al. Superficial and deep-tissue increases in anesthetized dogs during exposure to high specific absorption rates in a 1.5-T MR imager. Radiology 1988;167:551-554.

30. Barber BJ, Schaefer DJ, Gordon CJ, Zawieja DC, Hecker J. Thermal effects of MR imaging: worst-case studies on sheep. Am J Roentgenol 1990;155:1105-1110.

31. Drinkwater BL, Horvath SM. Heat tolerance and aging. Med Sci Sport Exer 1979;11:49-55.

32. Fennel WH, Moore RE. Responses of aged men to passive heating. Amer J Physiol 1969;67:118-119.

33. Kenny WL. Physiological correlates of heat intolerance. Sports Med 1985;2:279-286.

34. Barany FR. Abnormal vascular reaction in diabetes mellitus. Acta Med Scand Suppl 1955;304:556-624.

35. Buskirk EF, Lundergren H, Magnussen L. Heat acclimation patterns in obese and lean individuals. Ann NY Acad Sci 1965;131:637-653.

36. Jauchem JR. Effects of drugs on thermal responses to microwaves. Gen Pharmacol 1985;16:307-310.

37. Shellock FG, Drury JK, Meerbaum S, et al. Possible hypothalamic thermostat increase produced by a calcium blocker. Clin Res 1983;31:64A.

38. Shellock FG, Myers SM, Kimble K. Monitoring heart rate and oxygen saturation during MRI with a fiber-optic pulse oximeter. Amer J Roentgenol 1992;158:663-664.

39. Shellock FG. Monitoring during MRI: An evaluation of the effect of high-field MRI on various patient monitors. Med Electron 1986;93-97.

40. Holshouser B, Hinshaw DB, Shellock FG. Sedation, anesthesia, and physiologic monitoring during MRI. J Magn Res Imaging 1993:3;553-8.

41. Kanal E, Shellock FG. Patient monitoring during clinical MR imaging. Radiology 1992;85:623-629.

42. Wickersheim KA, Sun MH. Fluoroptic thermometry. Med Electron 1987;84-91.

43. Shellock FG, Crues JV. Temperature, heart rate, and blood pressure changes associated with clinical MR imaging at 1.5-T. Radiology 1987;163:259-262.

44. Shellock FG, Schaefer DJ, Grundfest W, et al. Thermal effects of high-field (1.5 Tesla) magnetic resonance imaging of the spine: clinical experience above a specific absorption rate of 0.4 W/kg. Acta Radiol Suppl 1986;369:514-516.

45. Shellock FG, Gordon CJ, Schaefer DJ. Thermoregulatory response to clinical magnetic resonance imaging of the head at 1.5 Tesla: lack of evidence for direct effects on the hypothalamus. Acta Radiol Suppl 1986;369;512-513.

46. Shellock FG, Crues JV. Corneal temperature changes associated with high-field MR imaging using a head coil. Radiology 1988;167:809-811.

47. Shellock FG, Crues JV. Temperature changes caused by clinical MR imaging of the brain at 1.5 Tesla using a head coil. Am J Neuroradiol 1988;9:287-291.

48. Shellock FG, Rothman B, Sarti D. Heating of the scrotum by high-field-strength MR imaging. Am J Roentgenol 1990;154:1229-1232.

49. Shellock FG, Schatz CJ. Increases in corneal temperature caused by MR imaging of the eye with a dedicated local coil. Radiology 1992;185:697-699.

50. Shellock FG, Schaefer DJ, Crues JV. Alterations in body and skin temperatures caused by MR imaging: is the recommended exposure for radiofrequency radiation too conservative? Br J Radiol 1989;62:904-909.

51. Shellock FG, Rubin SA, Everest CE. Surface temperature measurement by IR. Med Electron 1986;86:81-83.

52. Shellock FG, Schaefer DJ, Crues JV. Evaluation of skin blood flow, body and skin temperatures in man during MR imaging at high levels of RF energy. Magn Reson Imaging 1989;7:335.

53. Shellock FG, Schaefer DJ, Kanal E. Physiologic responses to MR imaging performed at an SAR level of 6.0 W/kg. Radiology 1994;192:865-868.

54. Schaefer DJ, Shellock FG, Crues JV, Gordon CJ. Infrared thermographic studies of human surface temperature in magnetic resonance imaging. In: Proceedings of the Bioelectromagnetics Society, Eighth Annual Meeting.1986; p. 68.

55. Sperber D, Oldenbourg R, Dransfeld K. Magnetic field induced temperature change in mice. Naturwissenschaften 1984;71:100-101.

56. Gremmel H, Wendhausen H, Wunsch F. Biologische effeckte statischer magnetfelder bei NMR-tomographic am menshen. Wiss Mitt Univ Kiel Radiol Klinik 1983.

57. Shellock FG, Schaefer DJ, Gordon CJ. Effect of a 1.5 Tesla static magnetic field on body temperature of man. Magn Reson Med 1986;3:644-647.

58. Shellock FG, Schaefer DJ, Crues JV. Effect of a 1.5 Tesla static magnetic field on body and skin temperatures of man. Magn Reson Med 1989;10:371-375.

59. Tenforde TS. Thermoregulation in rodents exposed to high intensity stationary magnetic fields. Bioelectromagnetics 1986;7:341-346.

60. Schaefer DJ, Barber BJ, Gordon CJ, et al. Thermal effects of magnetic resonance imaging. In: Book of Abstracts, Society for Magnetic Resonance in Medicine. Berkeley, CA: Society for Magnetic Resonance in Medicine.1985;2:925.

61. Vogl T, Krimmel K, Fuchs A, et al. Influence of magnetic resonance imaging of human body core and intravascular temperature. Med Phys 1988;15:562-566.

62. Kido DK, Morris TW, Erickson JL, et al. Physiologic changes during high-field strength MR imaging. Am J Neuroradiol 1987;8:263-266.

63. Sacks E, Worgul BV, Merriam GR. The effects of nuclear magnetic resonance imaging on ocular tissues. Arch Ophthalmol 1986;104:890-893.

64. Kurz KR, Goldstein M. Scrotal temperature reflects intratesticular temperature and is lowered by shaving. J Urol 1986;135:290-292.

65. Mapstone R. Measurement of corneal temperature. Exp Eye Res 1968;7:233-243.

66. Le Bihan D, Delannoy J, Levin RL. Temperature mapping with MR imaging of molecular diffusion: application to hyperthermia. Radiology 1989;171:853-857.

67. Schwarzmaier HJ, Kahn T. Magnetic resonance imaging of microwave induced tissue heating. Magn Reson Med 1995;33:729-731.

68. Atkinson IC, Sonstegaard R, Pliskin NH, Thulborn KR. Vital signs and cognitive function are not affected by 23-sodium and 17-oxygen magnetic resonance imaging of the human brain at 9.4 T. J Magn Reson Imaging 2010;32:82-7.

69. Collins CM. Numerical field calculations considering the human subject for engineering and safety assurance in MRI. NMR Biomed 2009;22:919-26.

70. Collins CM, Wang Z. Calculation of radiofrequency electromagnetic fields and their effects in MRI of human subjects. Magn Reson Med 2011;65:1470-82.

71. de Greef M, Ipek O, Raaijmakers AJ, et al. Specific absorption rate inter-subject variability in 7-T parallel transmit MRI of the head. Magn Reson Med 2013;69;1476-85

72. Kangarlu A, Shellock FG, Chakeres D. 8.0-Tesla MR system: Temperature changes associated with radiofrequency-induced heating of a head phantom. J Magn Reson Imaging 2003;17:220-226.

73. Kangarlu A, Ibrahim TS, Shellock FG. Effects of coil dimensions and field polarization on RF heating inside a head phantom. Magn Reson Imaging 2005;23:53-60.

74. Neufeld E, et al. Analysis of the local worst-case SAR exposure caused by an MRI multi-transmit body coil in anatomical models of the human body. Phys Med Biol 2011;56:4649-59.

75. Shrivastava D, Hanson T, et al. Radiofrequency heating at 9.4T: *in vivo* temperature measurement results in swine. Magn Reson Med 2008;59:73-8.

76. Shrivastava D, Hanson T, Kulesa J, et al. Radio frequency heating at 9.4T (400.2 MHz): in vivo thermoregulatory temperature response in swine. Magn Reson Med 2009;62:888 95.

77. Shrivastava D, Hanson T, Kulesa J, et al. Radiofrequency heating in porcine models with a "large" 32 cm internal diameter, 7 T (296 MHz) head coil. Magn Reson Med 2011;66:255-63.

78. Voigt T, et al. Patient-individual local SAR determination: *In vivo* measurements and numerical validation. Magn Reson Med 2012;68:1117-26.

79. Wang Z, Lin JC, Vaughan JT, Collins CM. Consideration of physiological response in numerical models of temperature during MRI of the human head. J Magn Reson Imaging 2008;28:1303-1308.

80. Murbach M, Neufeld E, Kainz W, Pruessmann KP, Kuster N. Whole-body and local RF absorption in human models as a function of anatomy and position within 1.5T MR body coil. Magn Reson Med 2013, Feb 25. [Epub ahead of print].

81. Jin J, Liu F, Weber E, Crozier S. Improving SAR estimations in MRI using subject-specific models. Phys Med Biol 2012;57:8153-71.

82. Wolf S, Diehl D, Gebhardt M, et al. SAR simulations for high-field MRI: How much detail, effort, and accuracy is needed? Magn Reson Med 2013;69:1157-6.

Chapter 7   MRI Facility Design to Support MRI Safety

ROBERT JUNK, AIA, AHRA

President
JUNK Architects, PC and Radiology Planning
Kansas City, MO

INTRODUCTION

The majority of accidents associated with the magnetic resonance imaging (MRI) environment occur at the location with the highest magnetic field strength, which is at the bore of an MR system or scanner. Therefore, the majority of MRI safety research and prevention is focused around issues and operations that occur inside or near this area. This includes the testing of medical devices to determine their ability to be present in patients referred for MRI examinations without causing injury. While other chapters in this textbook focus on "inside the bore" issues, this chapter will focus on the built space within which the MR system is located and will outline how this physical environment can be configured to support the safe operation of an MR system and, more generally, the MRI facility. The siting issues outlined in this chapter are limited to issues that have a direct impact on MRI safety. Siting issues, which do not have a direct impact on MRI safety, while important, have been excluded for the sake of brevity. Non-MRI safety siting issues include everything from structural support, vibration, magnet delivery path, modality conflicts, electromagnetic interference, patient parking, and others. MRI providers should be aware that non-MRI safety related siting issues will have an impact on the overall operation and financial success of an MRI center and need to be integrated into an overall comprehensive facility layout.

To understand the impact of the physical environment on MRI safety, a wide range of components need to be considered. These components include, the following:

- MRI Facility Layout
- Building Systems and Materials
- MRI Facility and Suite Operation Protocols
- Building Codes and Standards
- Siting Information From MR System Vendors

While this chapter provides best practice recommendations and guidelines for the design and layout of an MRI facility to safely scan patients, it is important to point out that there is no single or ideal layout or plan. MRI facility safety cannot be boiled down to a "one size fits all" layout. While all MRI facilities share certain similarities, each facility is unique and is dependent upon the clinical needs of the patient population that it serves as well as the imaging services offered. It is important that each facility develop a layout that is tailored to meet its specific needs and unique conditions. In the United States (U.S.), building codes and state or municipal jurisdictions require that the construction documents for healthcare facilities be prepared by a registered design professional (1). This includes freestanding radiology and diagnostic imaging centers. This not only includes new construction, but also applies to renovations and/or equipment changes as well. The general recommendation is that any work that involves changing the layout of walls, doors, or room sizes should be reviewed by a registered design professional for conformance with the local building and life safety code. MRI facilities should engage the services of a registered professional that also understands MRI safety and has experience in implementing safe design practices.

MRI FACILITY LAYOUT
MRI Shielding

In order to understand the relationship between the MRI facility layout and MRI safety, it is also necessary to understand the basic underlying principals about how magnetic fields operate and how the different types of scanners, shielding, and construction methods impact the magnetic fields.

All whole-body MR systems use a wide variety of shielding methods, each with a specific purpose. The type and amount of shielding depends on the MR system manufacturer, the type of scanner and the static magnetic field strength. It is also important to understand that, unlike other forms of radiology that use ionizing radiation (e.g., computed tomography or X-ray), the magnetic field of an MR system is not contained by normal building construction materials, such as steel or concrete. A common misconception by individuals not familiar with MRI is that the 5-gauss field is stopped by the wall construction within the scanner room or that lead shielding can be used to contain it similar to X-ray, neither of which is true.

RF Shielding

All MR systems use radiofrequency (RF) shielding which completely encloses the room on all six sides. This includes the use of highly specialized RF doors, windows, wave guides and access panels. RF shielding prevents outside radio waves from entering into the room and interfering with the internal RF signals that are used during the acquisition of the MR image. The RF shield does not limit or reduce the extent of the magnetic field and, therefore, does not impede the spread of the magnetic field beyond the scan room.

Active Shielding

Most contemporary MR systems use a secondary shielding system built into the scanner known as "active shielding". Active shielding uses a series of secondary magnetic fields that have a canceling effect and limit the extent of the primary magnetic field, thereby shrinking the overall volume of the magnetic field and reducing the size of the 5-gauss exclusion zone. The introduction of active shielding has greatly reduced the need for passive magnetic shielding and has allowed MR systems to be placed in locations that were not previously possible. However, active shielding also increases the MRI safety risk by creating much stronger and steeper spatial magnetic gradients. The spatial magnetic gradient is the rate at which a magnetic field strength increases over a given distance. Prior to the use of active shielding, MR systems had long shallow spatial magnetic gradients that spread over a much greater distance. This typically meant that if a person carried a ferromagnetic object close to the magnetic field of the scanner, the object would begin to experience a slight tug, which was the danger sign that the object was unsafe, and this sensation allowed the individual time to react.

In today's MR system rooms with much higher static magnetic fields combined with active shielding, the spatial magnetic gradient is very steep in a much smaller foot print area around the scanner. This means that the distance that separates the range of magnetic influence on an object is relatively very small. As a result, the person carrying a ferromagnetic object will receive little or no warning during the approach to the scanner before the magnetic field "captures" the object and pulls it rapidly and with potentially uncontrollable force.

Passive Magnetic Shielding

The only way to contain the magnetic field outside of the MR system is with highly specialized shielding, which is typically comprised of layers of specialized silicon steel. Passive magnetic shielding is very expensive, difficult to install, extremely heavy and can distort the shape of the imaging field of view within the MR system. As a general rule, passive magnetic shielding should be used as the last resort to control the 5-gauss exclusion zone after the room size and layout options have been exhausted.

5-Gauss Exclusion Zone

It is widely accepted that exposure to a high strength magnetic field, by itself, does not cause any known persistent health risk (2). However, exposure to high field strength magnetic fields can interfere with the use and operation of medical implants and devices and, if the magnetic field is strong enough and depending upon the type and location of the medical device, it can cause injury or death (2). Therefore, the U.S. Food and Drug Administration (FDA) and other similar agencies has determined that the general public should be excluded from static magnetic field strengths of 5-gauss and above. Only individuals that have been properly screened to be free of devices with magnetic contraindications should be allowed to enter into magnetic fields higher then 5-gauss.

Most contemporary MR systems used in MRI today have a maximum static field strength that ranges from 0.2-Tesla to 3-Tesla, (1-Tesla = 10,000-gauss). To put this into perspective, the Earth's natural ambient magnetic field strength is generally considered to be around 0.5-gauss, depending upon proximity to the Earth's magnetic poles. All FDA approved MR system manufacturers provide what is known as a gauss plot map for each of their scanners. These gauss plots indicate the distances at which different gauss field strengths occur from the isocenter of the MR system. **Figure 1** shows an example. A review

Figure 1. Diagram showing an example of a gauss plot map associated with an MR system.

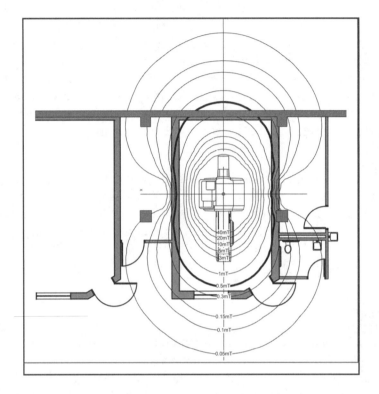

Figure 2. Diagram of a typical vendor siting plan showing the MR system room, control room and equipment room.

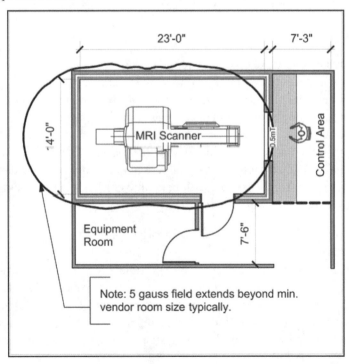

Figure 3. Diagram of typical cross section through a horizontal bore MR system, showing the extent of the 5-gauss field.

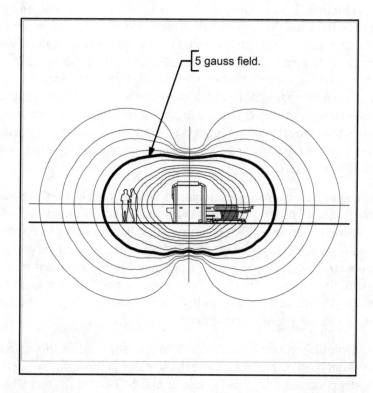

Figure 4. Diagram of typical cross section through vertical bore MR system, showing the extent of the 5-gauss field.

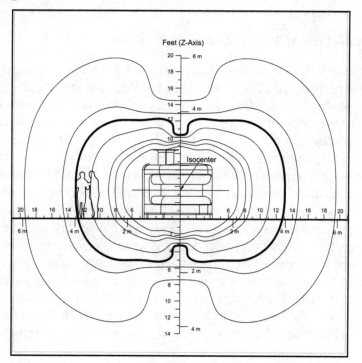

of most vendors 1-Tesla to 3-Tesla scanners will show that the 5-gauss field extends outside of the footprint of the minimum scan room size required by the vendor and spreads into the adjacent spaces (**Figure 2**). The extent of the 5-gauss field will depend on the strength of the static magnetic field and the type of MR system. Because the fringe field for different MR systems varies greatly, this is an important distinction to keep in mind when facilities are considering an equipment upgrade or replacement. An MRI facility should never assume that the 5-gauss exclusion zone that was appropriate for one MR system will be the same for any future equipment upgrades. It is also important to note that the 5-gauss field is a 3-dimensional volume and not only extends along the horizontal x-axis and y-axis of the MR system but also in the vertical z-axis (**Figure 3**). This applies to all MR system types, however it is more of a concern with vertical bore scanners where the major axis of the magnetic field is vertical (**Figure 4**).

This is critical in understanding the required 5-gauss containment area when the MR system is located in a multi-story building with spaces below and/or above the scanner room. In this situation, care must be taken to assure that not only the typical day-to-day building occupants are protected from the 5-gauss field, but also maintenance personal must be excluded from entering the 5-gauss area which may encroach into service areas adjacent to an MR system, until these individuals have been successfully screened for MRI contraindications. The fringe field areas include the ceiling access area on the floor below an MR system in a multi-story building (**Figure 5**).

Therefore, the initial primary goal for the layout of any MRI facility is to prevent individuals that have not been screened for contraindications to powerful magnetic fields from entering into a static magnetic field of 5-gauss or higher. This means that all MRI facilities should use physical barriers (e.g., walls and locked doors) and danger signage that will prevent anyone from inadvertently entering into a static magnetic field of 5-gauss or higher, until they have been successfully screened.

Implementation of the ACR Four Zone Areas

In 2002, the American College of Radiology (ACR) published a document pertaining to MRI safety in response to accidents involving the MRI environment (3). The goal of this publication was to begin to develop standardized guidelines and recommendations for the safe practice of MRI. While the majority of the publication focused on clinical and procedural issues, this document also introduced the concept that the physical layout of an MRI facility influences patient safety. The concept has become known as the ACR four zone areas and proposes the principal that the physical layout of an MRI facility be divided into four incremental zones. Everyone (i.e., patient, staff, and support personnel) is required to pass through each of these zones and successfully complete an MRI safety screening protocol before being allowed to enter into the next higher zone. The primary intent of this screening protocol is to identify medical device contradictions that could be adversely effected by the high static magnetic field and to eliminate ferromagnetic objects from being worn, carried, or brought into the scanner room and consequently pulled into the bore of the MR system. The later is often referred to as the missile effect in reference to the fact that objects caught by the strong magnetic field will fly across the room (4). These ferromagnetic items can be anything including chairs, oxygen cylinders, scissors, and wheel-

Figure 5. Diagram of typical building cross section for an MR system showing projection of 5-gauss field into adjacent floors. Top, Horizontal bore MR system. Bottom, Vertical bore MR system.

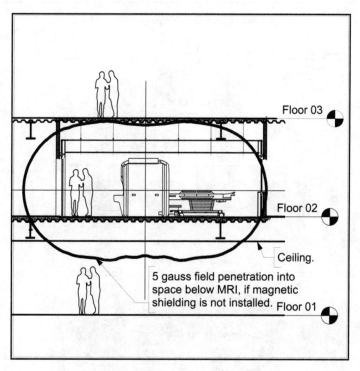

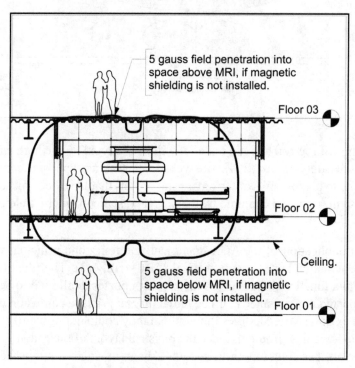

Figure 6. MRI diagram showing the four zones as described by the American College of Radiology (ACR).

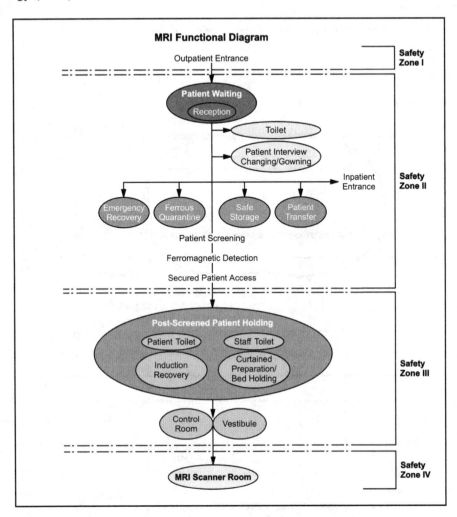

chairs. Anything with ferromagnetic material will be attracted by the high strength magnet and be a potential safety hazard (2, 4). The website, www.simplyphysics.com, has an entire section dedicated to photographs of ferromagnetic objects that have been mistakenly brought into an MR system room and captured by the powerful static magnetic field of the MR system (4).

In the first publication of the ACR document, the four zone principal was illustrated via a simple schematic plan of a hypothetical MRI facility (3). The illustration has since been changed to a functional diagram in subsequent updates to allow it to be more universally understood and implemented (5). The initial diagram caused confusion when first published because existing MRI facilities thought that they could not implement the principals of the four zone screening protocols since the physical layout of their facility did not match the illustrated plan. The contemporary functional diagram which is published in the current ACR document (5) is based on a version developed by the author for the Department of

Figure 7. Diagram showing combined MRI screening and changing room areas sized for multiple occupants.

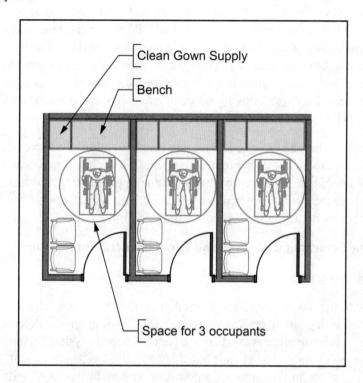

Clean Gown Supply

Bench

Space for 3 occupants

Veterans Affairs, Design Guide series for MRI (6) (**Figure 6**). The intent of the diagram is to illustrate a minimum of two intervening spaces between the entrance to the MRI facility (Zone I) and the MR system room (Zone IV), without limiting the implementation to a specific layout or plan. Everyone including patients, hospital staff, visitors, support personnel and MRI facility staff, must be screened for MRI contraindications in Zone II before being allowed to enter into Zone III. Zone III and Zone IV are secured areas and contain locations where the magnetic field strength exceeds 5-gauss and falls under the 5-gauss exclusion criteria. Patients, visitors and support staff (this includes transport, maintenance, and housekeeping staff) should not be allowed to enter these areas without an MRI staff member present and only after being successfully screened.

The ACR document also includes recommended screening protocols and forms for facilities to use as a basis of design for their own MRI safety protocols and screening forms, which is an operational issue and not a facility layout issue.

MRI Screening and the Health Insurance Portability and Accountability Act

As noted above, all personnel are to be screened within Zone II. Therefore, the facility layout needs to provide adequate spaces within Zone II to properly screen patients, visitors, and staff. The MRI screening process requires patients to divulge personal medical information and, if necessary, allow MRI staff to perform minor examinations of patients to check for possible contraindications to MRI.

With the implementation of the Health Insurance Portability and Accountability Act of 1996 (HIPAA)(7), patient privacy rules need to be adhered to by all healthcare providers. Therefore, it is recommended that MRI screening and interview rooms be private spaces that allow patients to share information with the MRI staff personnel without the risk of being over heard by other patients. Rather then having separate interview and change rooms, many facilities combine the patient screening area with the change room (**Figure 7**). This allows staff to interview the patient in a private room that also serves as a private changing room for the patient. This also helps support and streamline an operational policy of gowning all patients prior to performing an MRI procedure.

Slightly over-sizing the interview/changing rooms to allow for two or three occupants will make the space more comfortable. Enlarged interview/changing rooms are highly recommended for imaging facilities with a high volume of pediatric, geriatric, or other patient populations where the patient is often accompanied by a parent, spouse, or caregiver that may need to be present during the screening and gowning process.

Ferromagnetic Screening, Labeling, and Ferromagnetic Quarantine

Ferromagnetic Screening

In addition to the physical screening protocol performed by properly trained MRI staff, the ACR guidance document recommends the use of ferromagnetic detection systems to supplement the screening process (5). Ferromagnetic detection systems should never replace physical screening by trained MRI staff but should be used as a supplement. Recent developments and advances in ferromagnetic detection systems offer MRI staff members the ability to locate very small and/or hidden ferromagnetic objects within a patients clothing or hair. The type and style of ferromagnetic detection systems to use will depend on the type of patient population that a facility serves and how a facility plans to integrate the system into its screening protocol. The use of ferromagnetic detection portals or pillar systems (**Figure 8**) that "scan" patients and staff as they pass by may indicate the item's general location, but the use of a handheld ferromagnetic detection device may be better suited for determining the object's exact location. Based on this, the author's personal recommendation is that the use of a combination of a portal or pillar-type system along with a handheld style device offers the best overall detection flexibility, particularly in facilities where not all patients or their guests are required to change into a gown to enter the MR system room. This recommended strategy is similar to the dual system employed for security screening, where the portal is used for general screening and if the portal alarms, a handheld device is used to confirm the presence and exact location of the object.

It is also worth pointing out that ferromagnetic detection systems are not the same as conventional metal detectors used for airport and building security screening. Metal detectors are not designed or intended for use in MRI screening, as metal detectors will alarm on all metals, including metals which have no ferromagnetic mass and therefore pose no hazard in the MRI environment.

Figure 8. An example of a "pillar-type" ferromagnetic detection system.

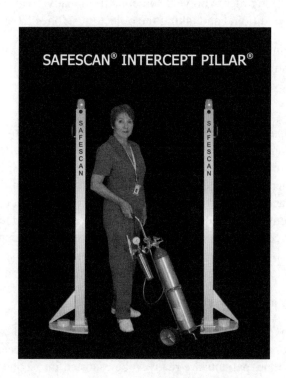

MRI Labeling

The labeling terminology used by the FDA which was developed by the American Society of Testing and Materials (ASTM) International for implants and devices as well as to assist MRI facilities in designating portable objects that can be used or not used within a MRI environment is, as follows:

MR Safe. This term is used for all objects that contain no ferromagnetic, electrically conductive and RF reactive materials and can be used safely in all MRI environments.

MR Conditional. This term is used for conditional objects, meaning that under certain conditions the object can be used safely inside of specific MRI environments. MRI facilities need to clearly understand the conditions of use for these objects.

MR Unsafe. This term is used for an object that is unsafe in all MRI environments and, thus, should never be brought into Zones III or IV.

Ferromagnetic Quarantine

In order to prevent unsafe objects from entering into Zones III and IV, MRI facility plans should include secure storage areas, where ferromagnetic objects can be safely quarantined (**Figure 9**). MR Unsafe objects are identified in the safety screening process and these objects should be placed into a locked quarantine room to prevent them from accidentally being brought into the scan room. Many of these objects are brought to the facility by patients and/or visitors and include items such as, portable oxygen cylinders, wheelchairs, canes, walkers, etc. The objects are placed in the secure quarantine area, rather then just leaving them in Zone II in order to prevent someone from inadvertently mistaking the object as MR Safe or MR Conditional and taking the object into Zones III and IV.

The facility design and layout needs to provide adequate space within Zone II to allow for the transfer of patients from unsafe transport devices to MR Safe or MR Conditional wheelchairs or gurneys. This needs to include storage of MR Safe and MR Conditional items when not in use.

Facilities with inpatient populations need additional space to allow the MRI staff members to safely screen and transfer these patients. Each facility needs to develop a protocol for how and where inpatients are screened for MR contraindications. Even if a facility has a protocol that inpatients are screened for MRI contraindications in the patient's room or on the patient floor, according to the ACR document (5) the final screening must be done by the MRI technologist at the MRI suite in Zone II. Therefore, the facility layout needs to provide sufficient space within Zone II to allow for the proper screening of inpatients, keeping in mind that the space also needs to be HIPAA compliant. This space can also be used to transfer inpatients to MR Safe or MR Conditional gurneys (**Figure 10**).

Patient Preparation and Recovery Areas

After patients have been gowned, properly screened, provided with attention to MR Safe or MR Conditional devices and all MR Unsafe objects have been secured inside the ferromagnetic quarantine, patients are ready to be escorted into Zone III by the MR staff. Zone III needs to contain adequate space for patient holding and recovery. Once again the facility layout needs to provide adequate space for these activities which will depend upon the clinical needs of the patient population that is served. Facilities that only serve outpatient populations will have substantially different space requirements than facilities that also serve inpatient populations and/or facilities with high volumes of patients that require sedation.

Typically facilities prefer to segregate outpatient and inpatient populations. This is done for a variety of reasons, but primarily to improve patient privacy. From a facility layout perspective, this allows inpatient areas, which require more space, staffing and support functions then outpatient holding areas to be more appropriately designed. The amount of preparation and recovery space needed will depend upon a wide range of elements, such as the number of scanners in operation, the patient acuity level and the type of imaging services provided (**Figure 11**).

MRI Technologists Situational awareness

Zone III requires that all patients, both outpatients and inpatients, are under the direct supervision of the MRI technologist on duty. The layout and design of the facility needs to support and enhance the MRI technologist's ability to maintain situational awareness of the patients within Zone III. Not only is the MRI technologist responsible for the patient inside the bore of the scanner, but also for the patients in the holding and recovery areas as well. Ideally, the MRI technologist should have direct visual observation of the following areas:

Figure 9. Diagram showing example of ferromagnetic quarantine area within the MRI environment.

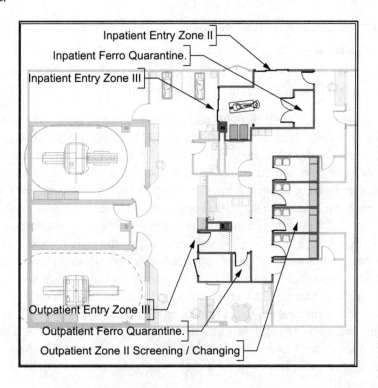

Figure 10. Example of Zone II inpatient transfer area within the MRI suite layout.

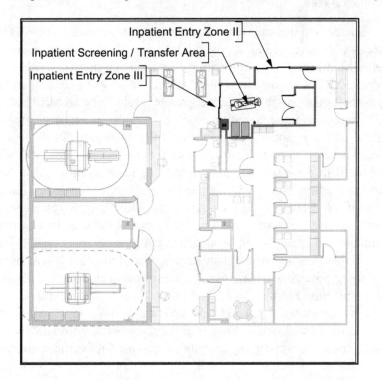

- MR system room interior, including the bore of the scanner
- Approach to the MR system room door
- Patient holding area within Zone III
- Patient recovery area within Zone III

If direct visual observation is not achievable, patient video monitoring systems can be used, but this should be limited and used as a last resort.

Facility designs which place the MRI technologist inside an enclosed control room with only a window to the MR system room, limit the MRI technologist's ability to maintain situational awareness for the other areas within Zone III. Control rooms that do not allow for a direct line of sight from the control counter to the scanner room door approach prevent the MRI technologist from being able to observe and possibly intercept MR Unsafe objects before they are brought into the scanner room. If the MRI technologist's only view of the MR system's room door is through the control room window (i.e., one of the most valuable means of MRI accident prevention), the responsibility of the technologist is compromised. The MRI technologist is the final gate keeper between Zone III and IV. A graphic example of the MRI technologist's ability to have 360-degrees situational awareness is shown in the attached sample plan (**Figure 12**). In this example, the technologist has direct visual observation of the scan room Zone IV, the approach path to the Zone IV scan room door, the inpatient holding/recovery area and the outpatient access to Zone III. It should be pointed out that with this open control room plan, care must be taken to ensure HIPAA compliance of patient information that is present on the monitors or work counters when patients are passing through Zone III.

Zone III Support Areas

Zone III also needs to include support spaces for both patients and staff. Once a patient has been successfully screened and moved into Zone III, the patient should not need to return to Zone II until the MRI examination is complete, otherwise MRI screening may need to be repeated. Allowing screened patients to move between Zone III and Zone II prior to scanning increases the possibility that the patient might bring an MR Unsafe object into Zone III or IV. Screening patients multiple times slows the overall patient throughput, requires additional staff time, and increases the possibility of an MR Unsafe item being missed or overlooked. The same logic holds true for staff as well. Each time MRI staff members move from Zone II to Zone III, they may need to be re-checked for MR Unsafe objects. Granted, personal medical history will not need to be rechecked each time but confirmation that an MR Unsafe object has not been inadvertently placed in a pocket or elsewhere should be confirmed. Likewise, items that have been identified or detected by a ferromagnetic detection system, but had been cleared by an MRI staff member, may need to be reassessed. The risk of multiple screenings of the same patient or staff member is screening fatigue and facilities need to but protocols in place to reduce re-screening as much as possible. Frequent and redundant screenings run the risk of the MRI staff becoming complacent about screening. Therefore, having staff toilets and break areas inside of Zone III will limit the amount of staff re-screening. In addition, having staff support spaces inside of Zone III, for staff working inside Zone III, reduces the amount of non-productive time going to and from break areas outside of Zone III.

Figure 11. Example of Zone III inpatient holding area within the MRI suite layout.

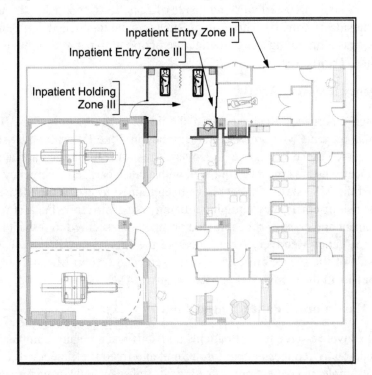

Figure 12. Example of situational awareness for the MRI technologist.

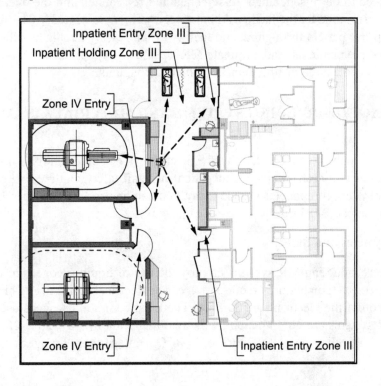

It is also recommended to have storage and supply areas within Zone III that can be stocked with consumable items that are typically used during clinical scanning operations. Again, this allows the MRI staff working inside of Zone III to re-stock as required without having to go outside of Zone III. These supply areas can be re-stocked during non-scanning days or times, thus eliminating any potential interaction with patients or having anyone inside the scanner (**Figure 13**).

MRI Emergency Recovery Area

A dedicated Emergency Recovery Area should be located within Zone III or Zone II. Any patient that presents with a medical emergency in Zone IV or Zone III should be immediately evacuated to the Emergency Recovery Area for resuscitation and appropriate patient management. The area must be equipped with a crash cart and emergency resuscitation equipment that the MRI staff members have been trained to use in the MRI environment. To reduce the risk of emergency equipment being taken into Zone IV, it is recommended that the equipment and crash cart be tethered or otherwise secured to restrict its movement to only the Emergency Recovery Area. Locating the Emergency Recovery Space within Zone II, outside of the secure area, allows non-screened or non-MR staff from other departments to assist in the recovery if needed (**Figure 14**).

MRI Safety May Improve Patient Throughput

As noted above, re-screening of patients and staff has a negative impact on scanning operations and greatly reduces patient throughput and overall efficiency of a facilities operations. For example, if a patient presents for a clinical scan, and during the scan an artifact is identified from a metallic object that was overlooked, the initial scan is wasted. The patient may need to be re-scheduled, re-screened and re-scanned and the overall operation generates zero revenue for the facility. Alternatively, well implemented MRI safety protocols actually improve patient throughput and facility efficiency, by having an efficient method to screen and prep patients, and eliminate MR Unsafe objects or patient contraindications before they become an issue and interrupt patient throughput.

THE IMPACT OF BUILDING SYSTEMS AND MATERIALS ON MRI SAFETY

In addition to the layout of a facility, the mechanical, electrical, and finish systems used within an MRI facility can greatly impact patient and staff safety. Outlined below is a review of the major system components used in today's contemporary MRI facilities and how each of these may impact MRI safety.

Cryogen Systems and Safety

All superconducting MR systems employ the use of liquid cryogens to maintain the near absolute zero temperatures required to reduce electrical resistance, which facilitates the generation of the electromagnetic field. The most common cryogens used in today's clinical MR systems are liquid helium, with a boiling point of -452°F or -269°C or liquid nitrogen with a boiling point of -320°F or -196°C. Both of these cryogens are non-toxic,

Figure 13. Example of Zone III with patient and staff support areas.

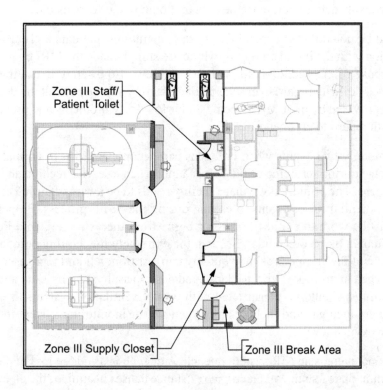

Figure 14. Example of Emergency Recovery Area within the MRI suite layout, Zone III.

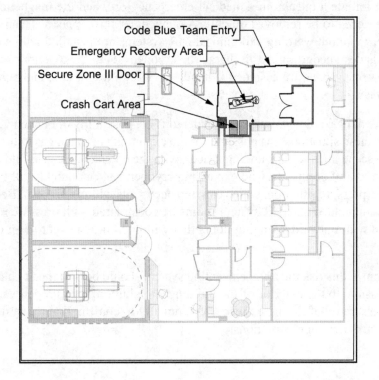

colorless, odorless and non-flammable, yet they pose a number of potential safety risks to building occupants due to their extreme cold and high rate of expansion.

It should be noted that in typical day-to-day operations, patients and staff never have any interaction with the liquid cryogens, which are stored inside the MRI containment vessel. The purpose of this section is to give an overview of the safety issues that MRI staff should be aware of with regard to cryogens. Each facility should consult the detailed safety information provided by their MR system vendor for safety protocols and procedures to be followed with regard to cryogen safety.

There are only two events when cryogens can become an issue in normal operations. The first occurs during servicing of the MR scanner when a service technician is replenishing the cryogens. The primary issue that a facility needs to be aware of during cryogen servicing is the potential for cryogens to escape during the re-fill process. Proper protective clothing must be worn to avoid frostbite or burns from the extremely cold liquid, which will freeze human tissue on contact. Second, the extremely low boiling point and the high expansion rate of the cryogens as they quickly convert from a liquid to a gaseous state can cause the oxygen in the room to be displaced and pose an asphyxiation risk to any occupants. All MRI facilities should be constructed with proper ventilation systems to quickly vent any escaped cryogen gas and include an oxygen sensor monitoring system to warn occupants of low oxygen levels.

The second event is an MR system quench. A quench is a sudden loss of superconductivity. The immediate rise in coil electrical resistance causes heating of the electromagnetic coils, leading to the rapid conversion of cryogens from a liquid to gaseous state and the subsequent venting of the cryogen gas from the MRI containment vessel. The MRI technologist can initiate a quench in a medical emergency or when the magnetic field of the MR scanner needs to be removed quickly. A quench, on rare occasions, can also spontaneously occur without warning. All clinical MR systems are installed with a quench vent system that is designed to safely discharge the cryogen gas to the exterior of the building. The quench vent systems are designed to handle both the extreme cold and rapidly expanding cryogen gas.

The potential hazard that must be considered is the possibility of quench vent failure or blockage. In these situations it is possible for the expanding cryogen gas to breach the vent system and escape into the surrounding spaces, with the potential to cause cold burns and/or asphyxiation to any occupants. The expanding cryogen gas can quickly fill the room and create an overpressure situation, which can trap occupants within the room. Because of this risk it is recommended that MR system rooms be constructed with pressure relief hatches and outfitted with outward swinging doors that will open in the event of an overpressure situation.

To minimize this risk the cryogen venting system should be designed to have the shortest route possible to the exterior of the building. In addition, the cryogen vents, exhaust, and over pressure relief should be inspected annually to confirm that the system is intact, operational, and clear of obstructions.

At the exterior of the building the cryogen vent discharge must terminate inside of a 25-foot exclusion zone that is clearly marked. In addition, the quench vent exclusion zone must be free of serviceable mechanical equipment, windows, doors, and air intake devices. If service personnel need to enter the cryogen exclusion zone, they should be properly trained, equipped and warned of the potential hazards.

Lighting Systems for MR System Rooms

MR system rooms require specialized lighting systems that will not interfere with the scanning process (**Figure 15**). Until recently these lighting systems were limited to the use of incandescent lamps. The typical life of an incandescent bulb in an MR system room is estimated at 1,500 hours. Assuming that a facility is operated 10-hours a day, 6-days a week, the lamps with in an MR system room will require changing every six months. The impact that this has on MRI safety is that it requires access to Zone IV by facility maintenance personnel every six months, increasing the potential risk of an accident from maintenance personnel unfamiliar with MRI safety or unaware of the risks of bringing MR Unsafe tools or ladders into the scan room.

In recent years the development of high quality light emitting diode (LED) lighting that is acceptable for use in MRI environments offers a safer solution for the MR system room. LED lighting has an estimated lamp life of 50,000 hours. Using the same 60-hours per week of room operation, LED lights would last 16-years before needing to be re-lamped. Since

Figure 15. Example of an MR system room with specialized lighting that does not interfere with the scanning process.

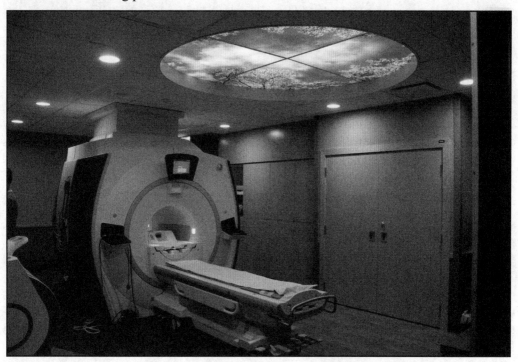

the average MR systems useful life is 7 to 10 years, the scanner will be replaced before the lighting system would require replacement.

MR System Room Finishes and Components

As noted above, anything that can reduce or eliminate the need for facility maintenance or housekeeping staff to enter into Zones III and IV helps to improve MRI safety. A quick search of the Internet will show hundreds of photos of floor polishers and vacuum cleaners sucked into the bore of MR systems, all brought in by well-intended cleaning staff (4). By designing spaces that can be easily cleaned, but don't require mechanical polishing, buffing or vacuuming, a facility can greatly reduce this risk. The simple principal is to select durable finishes that can be easily cleaned with a sponge or non-ferromagnetic mop. The following materials list, are suggestions that facilities should consider when planning or renovating an MRI suite:

Flooring - Seamless anti-static no wax flooring. It is also recommended to use a flooring system that allows for the integration of contrasting flooring patterns that can be used to highlight the major gauss fields within the MR system room.

Walls - Low maintenance wall coverings or panels should be used.

Cabinets - Use MR Safe or MR Conditional mobile RF coil and supply carts. Mobile carts provide the benefit that the carts can be repaired and re-stocked off-site, reducing activity in Zone IV.

MRI SUITE OPERATIONS

While operational protocols should be tailored to align with each facility's unique clinical needs, some universal operational elements that can be applied to all facilities are outlined below.

Multi-Modality Imaging Suites vs. MRI Safety

While multi-modality imaging suites can be successfully integrated with MRI safety, they do require special attention and operational protocols. The most critical issue is clearly defining the circulation path for each imaging modality. In order to implement the ACR's recommended four zone policy, the patient circulation system for MRI must be segregated from other imaging modalities.

The common mistake that arises with multi-modal suites is the combination of the MR system's control room with other control rooms, such as computed tomography (CT). The problem with sharing an MRI control room with other modalities is the breakdown in the four zone screening process at the most critical point in the process, within Zone III and Zone IV. To maintain the four zone process in a control room shared between MRI and another modality, everyone, including MRI patients and non-MRI patients, and staff members must be screened for possible contraindications. In addition, all support equipment, everything from gurneys to step stools, must be MR Safe or MR Conditional. For this reason MRI control rooms should not be designed to be shared with other modalities.

Access Control

As noted in the MRI facility layout section of this chapter, access control within an MRI facility is critical to the implementation of MRI safety. Access control, via locked doors and restricted access, is required at the following locations:

- Ferromagnetic quarantine area.
- Access point from Zone II to Zone III.
- Access point from Zone III to Zone IV

Suite Signage

MRI-related signage should be installed at the following locations:

- Each of the four zones should be clearly identified with signage, including signage at the access point between each zone.
- Zone IV should be clearly labeled with an illuminated sign with battery backup that clearly indicates that the "Magnet is Always On", even when power to the facility is off.
- "Danger" signage must be installed around the perimeter of the cryogen exclusion zone.

BUILDING CODES, STANDARDS AND REGULATIONS

In the U.S., the design and construction of healthcare facilities are closely regulated by national and regional agencies. While it is not necessary for radiologists, technologists or facility managers to understand these in detail, it is important that they be aware of the primary regulatory groups and their impact. It is also important to note that on a national level, there is no universally accepted code and many jurisdictions and municipalities follow multiple codes. Conflicts between the codes are left up to the interpretation of the local building official.

In additional to national model building codes there are a number of national healthcare regulatory bodies and agencies that offer recommendations and/or guidance with regard to MRI safety and operations as noted below:

The Joint Commission

The Joint Commission is well known to healthcare providers (9). The Joint Commission is an independent organization that accredits and certifies healthcare facilities. The Joint Commission does not develop its own building code or standards. Instead, it relies on and enforces standards and regulations developed by other nationally recognized bodies.

While the Joint Commission does not draft its own regulations it does issue Sentinel Alerts, which highlight specific health and safety issues. In 2008, the Joint Commission issued Sentinel Event Alert - 38: Preventing Accidents and Injuries in the MRI Suite (10). This alert noted a number of safety issues within the MRI environment and outlined several recommendations, including use of the four zone areas as indicated by the American College of Radiology (3, 5), danger signage, the use of ferromagnetic detectors, and improved access control, all of which have been addressed in this chapter. Various documents are referenced by the Joint Commission that impact MRI facilities.

American College of Radiology (ACR)

As noted elsewhere in this chapter, the ACR has issued a number of white papers and guidance documents related to MRI safety, the most current of which is the ACR guidance document published in 2013 (5).

International Building Code (IBC)

The International Code Council (ICC) (11) created the International Building Code (IBC) (12), which is a compilation of building codes and is the most common code used by municipalities on a national level. The IBC's goal is to protect the health, safety and welfare of building occupants, with a primary focus on fire prevention. The code outlines acceptable building materials, maximum building heights and areas and means of exit requirements. The IBC does not deal specifically with clinical issues in healthcare, but it does define general classifications of healthcare occupancies, from hospitals to medical office buildings, including the requirement that healthcare facilities be designed under the supervision of a registered design professional, licensed to practice in the state where the healthcare facility is located. The code is updated every three years.

National Fire Protection Association (NFPA)

National Fire Protection Association (NFPA) is a comprehensive code similar to the IBC, which also focuses primarily on fire protection (13). The NFPA is the most common building code used by federal agencies in the U.S. Similar to the IBC, the NFPA does not deal specifically with clinical issues in healthcare such as MRI safety, but it does define general healthcare classifications. The NFPA is also updated every three years.

Guidelines for Design and Construction of Healthcare Facilities

The only nationally recognized code for non-governmental healthcare organizations that offers recommendations with regard to MRI facilities is provided by the Facility Guidelines Institute (FGI)(14). The Guidelines for Design and Construction of Healthcare Facilities (15), as its name suggests, provides specific minimum standards and requirements for all aspects of healthcare facilities, and the 2010 edition addresses MRI design criteria. The guidelines are updated every four years. It should be noted that these guidelines establish the minimum requirements for healthcare facilities and all facilities must meet or exceed these minimum standards.

State Codes and Health Departments

A number of states develop and enforce independent state building and health codes. Most state codes are modifications of the model national codes that focus on specific geographic state issues, such as earthquake and hurricane resistance. Registered design professionals will be familiar with the codes and regulations that are used for a specific geographic region.

United States Governmental Healthcare Standards

The healthcare systems for the Department of Veterans Affairs (VA) (6) and the Department of Defense (DoD), have developed independent standards for their internal healthcare systems. Radiologists, technologists, and facility managers that work within with these agencies need to be aware of the requirements that are specific to their own organization.

MRI Safety and Documents From MR System Manufacturers

MR system manufacturers provide valuable and large amounts of information with regard to the installation and operation of their MR scanners, including recommended layouts and siting documents. While all parties involved in MRI desire to have the safest patient environment possible, it should be noted that even though the major vendors offer suggestions related to MRI safety, their siting and operation manuals clearly indicate that MRI safety systems and protocols are the responsibility of the medical facility where the MR scanner is located. Facilities are encouraged to engage the MR system manufacturer to offer assistance and recommendations with regard to MRI safety in context with the vendor's specific MR scanner, with the understanding that the final responsibility for implementation and execution of an MRI safety plan falls upon each individual facility.

CONCLUSIONS

Anyone that is involved in MRI understands the importance of safety and can appreciate the complexity for integrating clinical, operational, and facility requirements to provide the highest level of patient care possible. As this textbook illustrates, MRI safety is not limited to a single area or element and can only be achieved through a multi-disciplinary approach. Operations or protocols that have been successful in the past may not be appropriate for future systems. As more advanced MR systems are developed and introduced into clinical practice, including interventional and hybrid MR systems, MRI facility design and operations must continually evolve to address MRI safety within these new environments.

REFERENCES

1. Chapter 1, Section 107, A-107.1 General. 2012 International Building Code. Country Club Hills, IL: International Code Council: 2011.

2. Shellock FG. Reference Manual for Magnetic Resonance Safety, Implants, and Devices: 2013 Edition. Los Angeles, CA: Biomedical Research Publishing Group, 2013.

3. Kanal E, Barkovich AJ, Bell C, et al. American College of Radiology white paper on MR safety. AJR Am J Roentgenol. 2002;178:1335-47.

4. "DANGER! Flying Objects!" http://www.simplyphysics.com/flying_objects.html Accessed March, 2013

5. Kanal E, Barkovich AJ, Bell C, et al. ACR guidance document on MR safe practices: 2013. J Magn Reson Imaging 2013;37:501-530.

6. Veterans Administration (VA) Design Guide. Magnetic Resonance Imaging. April 2008; Department of Veterans Affairs; Veterans Health Administration; Office of Facilities Management, Standards Service. http://www.wbdg.org/ccb/VA/VADEGUID/mri.pdf

7. Health Insurance Portability and Accountability Act of 1996. www.hhs.gov/ocr/hipaa

8. American Society for Testing and Materials (ASTM) International, Designation: F2503-08, Standard practice for marking medical devices and other items for safety in the magnetic resonance environment. ASTM International, West Conshohocken, PA.

9. The Joint Commission. http://www.jointcommission.org Accessed March, 2013.

10. The Joint Commission. Preventing accidents and injuries in the MRI suite. Sentinel Event Alert, Issue 38, February 14, 2008.

11. ICC - International Code Council. International Code Council. http://www.iccsafe.org/

12. 2012 International Building Code. Country Club Hills, IL: International Code Council, 2011

13. National Fire Protection Association (NFPA), http://www.nfpa.org, Accessed March, 2013.

14. Guidelines for Design and Construction of Health Care Facilities. Chicago, IL: American Society for Healthcare Engineering of the American Hospital Association, ASHE, 2010.

15. 2.2-3.4.4 Magnetic Resonance Imaging (MRI). Guidelines for Design and Construction of Health Care Facilities. Chicago, IL: American Society for Healthcare Engineering of the American Hospital Association (ASHE), 2010. pp. 143-45.

Chapter 8   Claustrophobia, Anxiety, and Emotional Distress in the MRI Environment

Rosa Babbitt Spaeth, B.S.

Research Assistant
Laboratory of Pain, Placebo and Acupuncture Imaging
Department of Psychiatry
Massachusetts General Hospital
Charlestown, MA

Randy L. Gollub, M.D., Ph.D.

Professor of Psychiatry Associate Director of Psychiatric Neuroimaging
Massachusetts General Hospital
Charlestown, MA

INTRODUCTION

The increasing availability and capabilities of magnetic resonance imaging (MRI) to improve medical diagnosis and prognosis has dramatically increased the number of MRI procedures performed worldwide. Thus, many more first-time and repeat patients are undergoing these MRI examinations for an ever-widening spectrum of medical indications. Notably, increasing proportions of these procedures are performed on patients suffering from unstable medical and psychological illnesses. For many of the millions of patients who undergo MRI procedures every year, the experience may cause great emotional distress. The referring physicians, radiologists, and technologists are best prepared to manage affected patients if they understand the etiology of the problem and know the appropriate maneuver or intervention to implement for treatment of the condition (1).

This chapter will review the incidence of psychological distress in the MRI environment, discuss the impact of this distress for patients undergoing MRI examinations, characterize the sources and types of distress, and present specific measures documented to minimize dysphoric sensations.

INCIDENCE OF DISTRESS IN THE MRI ENVIRONMENT

In this chapter, we define psychological distress in the MRI environment to include all subjectively unpleasant experiences that are directly attributable to the MRI procedure. Distress for the patient undergoing an MRI procedure can range from mild anxiety that can be managed simply with minimal reassurance to a full-blown panic attack that requires psychiatric intervention. Severe psychological distress reactions to MRI examinations, namely severe anxiety and panic attacks, are typically characterized by the rapid onset of at least four of the following clinical signs: fear of losing control or dying, nausea, paresthesias, palpitations, chest pain, faintness, dyspnea, feeling of choking, sweating, trembling, vertigo, or depersonalization (2).

Many symptoms of panic attack mimic over activity of the sympathetic nervous system (3), prompting concern that catecholamine responses may precipitate cardiac arrhythmias and/or ischemia in susceptible patients during the MRI procedure (4). However, this has not been reported in a clinical MRI setting or any other similar situation. Nevertheless, it is advisable that, in a medically unstable patient, the use of physiologic monitoring be a routine component of the MRI examination. Pre-emptive efforts to minimize patient distress are the most important factors in preventing or containing a panic attack in susceptible patients.

In the mildest form, distress is the normal amount of anxiety any reasonable person will experience when undergoing a diagnostic procedure. Moderate distress severe enough to be described as a dysphoric psychological reaction has been reported by as many as 65% of the patients examined by MRI (5-8). The most severe forms of psychological distress described by patients are claustrophobia, panic attacks, and anxiety (3, 5-12), the latter of which occurs in moderate to severe forms in up to 37% of patients undergoing MRI procedures (13, 14).

Claustrophobia is a disorder characterized by the marked, persistent and excessive fear of enclosed spaces (2). In such affected individuals, exposure to enclosed spaces such as the MR system or MRI environment, but no other situations or stimuli, almost invariably provokes an immediate anxiety response that in it's most extreme form is indistinguishable from a panic attack as described above.

The reported incidence of distress in the MRI setting is highly variable across studies in part reflecting differences in outcome measures used to characterize distress. Some studies indicated that as many as 20% of individuals attempting to undergo MRI can't complete it secondary to serious distress such as claustrophobia or other similar sensation (15, 16). In contrast, others have reported that as few as 0.7% of individuals have incomplete or failed MRI procedures due to distress (8, 17). In a study of over 55,000 patients undergoing MRI, claustrophobia was present in 1.8% of cases, and a review of previous literature indicated that 2.3% of patients experienced claustrophobia requiring sedation or termination of the procedure (18). A reasonable estimate of the number of patients that experience distress that compromises either their own well-being or the diagnostic utility of the MRI procedure is 3 to 5% of all studies. For patients with pre-existing anxiety or claustrophobia, however, the termination rate can be as high as 39% (19, 20).

Notably, there are no perfect predictors of distress in the MRI environment. In fact, different studies cite opposing results such as which gender has greater difficulty tolerating MRI (17,18, 21). A cohort study of over 55,000 patients in an outpatient setting in Germany reported that females (2.3%) had a significantly higher rate of claustrophobia than males (1.3%) (18). This is in contrast to an earlier study conducted in Malaysia where the rate of MRI termination was found to be 0.54%, and of those, 67% of the patients who terminated their scan were male (17). Obviously, these differences may reflect cultural, socioeconomic or other influences.

THE IMPACT OF EMOTIONAL DISTRESS IN THE MRI ENVIRONMENT

Patient distress can contribute to adverse outcomes for the MRI procedure. These adverse outcomes include unintentional exacerbation of patient distress, a compromise in the diagnostic power of the MRI examination due to poor image quality, and decreased efficiency of the imaging facility due to delayed, cancelled or prematurely terminated studies. Patient compliance during an MRI procedure, such as the ability to remain in the MR system and hold still long enough to complete the study is of paramount importance to achieving a high quality, diagnostic examination.

If a good quality study can't be obtained, the patient may require an invasive diagnostic examination in place of the safer, less painful and risky MRI procedure. Thus, for the distressed patient unable to undergo MRI, there are potential clinical, medico-legal, and economic related considerations implications.

Patient distress due to MRI procedures may also impact regional brain activity as indicated by functional neuroimaging measurements. Elevated endocrine levels have been observed in association with scanning procedures compared to baseline, particularly in stress hormones such as cortisol (22-24). Studies have indicated that elevated salivary cortisol levels are associated with MRI procedures in both adolescents and healthy adults (23, 24). In contrast, Muehlhan, et al. (25) found changes in salivary alpha amalase but not in cortisol prior to MRI. This evidence, while inconclusive, points towards increased activity in the hypothalamic-pituitary-adrenal and the sympatho-adrenal-medullary axes which are, in turn, associated with regionally specific neural activation and deactivation (26, 27). Fluctuating endocrine levels have been implicated in the modulation of regional brain activity, a suggestion that has broad implications for interpreting functional neuroimaging results. Functional MRI (fMRI) has been at the forefront of neuroimaging research for nearly two decades. As fMRI is increasingly introduced into clinical practice, for example for pre-surgical mapping, the effects of hormone levels on brain activity could impact this diagnostic procedure.

Increasing pressure to use MR system time efficiently to cover the costs of this expensive diagnostic imaging equipment puts greater stress on both staff members and patients. The ability of referring physicians, radiologists, and technologists to detect patient distress at the earliest possible time, to discover the source of the distress, and then provide appropriate intervention can greatly improve patient comfort, the quality of the imaging studies, and the efficiency of the MRI facility (1).

Motion artifact disrupting image quality is frequently the result of patient distress. That is, the distressed patient becomes agitated and finds it difficult to remain motionless during MRI. Obviously, motion artifacts can compromise the diagnostic power of an MRI procedure. One investigation in 297 first-time outpatients undergoing MRI indicated that approximately 13% of the MRI studies showed motion artifacts (i.e., unrelated to normal body pulsations) and about half of these impaired the diagnostic quality of the examination (8). Subsequent studies have confirmed these estimates (20, 28). One of these investigations reported an even higher proportion of scans with motion artifacts (18%) in a sample of patients with pre-existing anxiety conditions and non-anxious controls (20).

Excessive anxiety with accompanying tremors, trembling, jaw clenching and other related body movements have been presumed to contribute to motion artifacts in MR images. Dantendorfer, et al. (8) attempted to investigate this directly and found that, while specific measures of anxiety do not predict motion artifacts, reported concerns about the MR system did predict motion artifacts. In a more recent study, Tournquist, et al. (28) designed an experiment to test whether increased awareness about the procedure prior to initiating the scan would reduce motion related artifacts. The investigators found nearly a three-fold reduction in the number of scans with artifacts in the intervention group (4%) compared to the control condition (15.4%). The patients in the intervention group received additional written information that included details about what the procedure would entail, as well as sensory and temporal information related to the procedure (28). These results support the interpretation that adequate patient education about the MRI procedure is one of the most important aspects of minimizing distress and the associated adverse outcomes.

FACTORS THAT CONTRIBUTE TO DISTRESS IN THE MRI ENVIRONMENT

Many factors contribute to distress experienced by certain patients undergoing MRI procedures. Most commonly cited are concerns about the physical environment of the MR system. Also well documented are the anxieties associated with the underlying medical problem necessitating the MRI examination. Notably, certain individuals, such as those with psychiatric illnesses, may be predisposed to suffer greater distress due to MRI.

The physical environment of the MR system is clearly one important source of distress to patients. Sensations of apprehension, tension, worry, claustrophobia, anxiety, fear, and even panic attacks have been directly attributed to the confining dimensions of the interior of the MR system. For example, for certain types of scanners, the patient's face may be three to ten inches from the inner portion of the MR system, prompting feelings of uncontrolled confinement and detachment (3, 5-12, 15, 16, 29-34). In one study, confinement was reported by 22.9% of patients as the most unpleasant feature of the MRI experience (34). This factor, combined with other physical aspects of the MRI environment may contribute to the high levels of distress observed in patients undergoing MRI.

Similar distressing sensations have been attributed to the other aspects of the MRI environment including the prolonged duration of the MRI examination, the gradient magnetic field-induced acoustic noise, the temperature and humidity within the MR system, and the distress related to the restriction of movement (3-12, 15, 16, 29-33, 35, 36). Other studies have reported stress related to the administration of an intravenous MRI contrast agent (3, 5-7, 9-12, 15, 16, 29-33, 35-37). Additionally, the MR system may produce feelings of sensory deprivation restriction, and suffocation, which are also known to be precursors of severe anxiety states (10, 38). Investigations have indicated that phobias related to specific aspects of the MRI environment can predict claustrophobic fears and psychological outcomes in the scanner (14, 34, 39, 40). Using pre-scan questionnaires, clinicians may be able to identify patients who are at risk for terminating the scan due to claustrophobia (20, 34, 39, 40).

One of the more overwhelming features of the MRI procedure is the acoustic noise generated by the MR system. Gradient field induced noise may be sufficiently intense to cause transient hearing threshold shifts in as many as 43% of patients undergoing MRI (41). Obviously, noise in and of itself can be a source of stress and, thus, particularly troublesome to certain patients in association with MRI. In one study, noise alone was considered the most unpleasant feature of MRI by 19.5% of patients (34). This result suggests that the noise reduction achieved in the new generation of scanners may be an important factor in reducing distress. The use of newer scanners demonstrated up to a 97% reduction in acoustic noise compared to older MR systems. Dewey, et al. (18) observed a three-fold reduction in reports of claustrophobia using the newer short- and wide-bore scanners that have noise emission levels below 99-dB compared to conventional, older scanners.

MR systems that have an architecture that utilizes a vertical magnetic field offer a more open design that is presumed to reduce the frequency of distress associated with MRI procedures. The latest versions of these so-called "open" MR systems, despite having static magnetic field strengths of 0.35-Tesla or lower have improved technology (i.e., faster gradient fields, optimized surface coils, etc.) that permit acceptable image quality for virtually all types of standard, diagnostic imaging procedures. Also, the latest generation of high-field-strength (1.5-Tesla and 3-Tesla) MR systems have shorter and wider bore configurations such that these newly designed systems may be more acceptable to patients with feelings of distress (**Figure 1**).

After the release of the first commercially available open MR systems, Datendorfer, et al. (8) designed a study to compare the new open system to the standard MR system. This report indicated that there was no difference between a standard 1.5-T MR system (Siemens Magnetom SP-65,Siemens Medical Solutions) and a more open 0.5-Tesla scanner (Philips Gyroscan P-5, Philips Medical Systems, Shelton, CT) with regard to the incidence of adverse reactions (i.e., pre or post scan anxiety, claustrophobia, aborted studies or motion artifacts).

More than a decade later, Enders, et al. (19) designed a study to compare the newest generation of short- and wide-bore MR systems to the equally state-of-the-art open, vertical, panoramic scanner in patients with self-reported feelings of MRI-induced claustrophobia. In this randomized study, Enders, et al. (19) also did not observe a significant difference in rate of claustrophobic events in the short- and wide-bore 1.5-Tesla system (Magnetome Avanto, Siemens Medical Solutions) compared to the open 1-Tesla scanner (Panorama, Philips Medical Systems).

In contrast to these studies, two non-randomized studies of claustrophobic patients demonstrated a decreased rate of claustrophobic events in open MR systems compared to

Figure 1. Examples of various types of MR system configurations that represent more open, shorter, and/or wider designs that may be more acceptable to patients with psychological distress. (A) Low-field-strength, "open" MR system (0.35 Tesla, MAGNETOM C!, Siemens Medical Solutions USA, Inc. Malvern, PA).

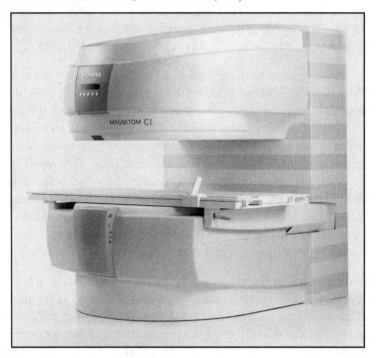

Figure 1. (Continued) (B) High-field, "open" MR system: (1.2-Tesla, Oasis, Hitachi Medical Systems America, Inc., Twinsburg, OH)

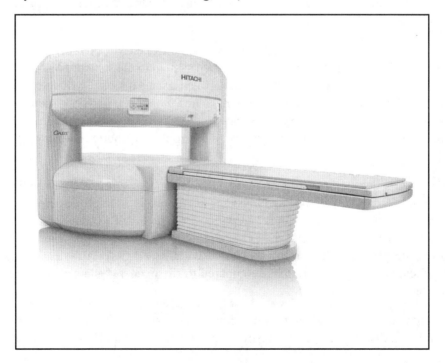

Figure 1. (Continued) (C) High-field-strength MR system with oval bore (1.5-T, Echelon Oval, Hitachi Medical Systems America, Inc., Twinsburg, OH)

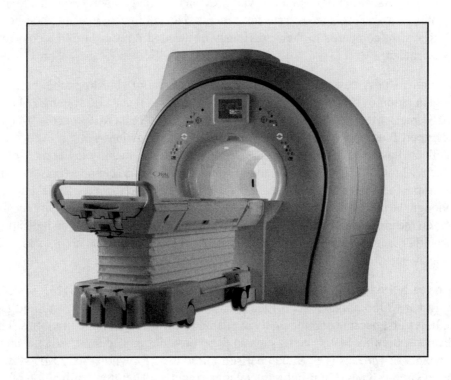

Figure 1. (Continued) (D) High-field-strength MR system with short- and wide-bore (1.5 Tesla, Signa HDxt MR System, General Electric Medical Systems, Milwaukee, WI).

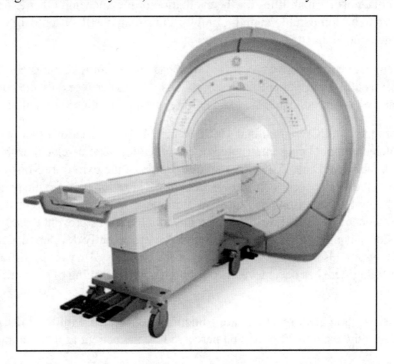

closed scanners (42, 43). Decreases of similar magnitude have been observed in newer generations of short- and wide-bore MR systems compared to conventional MR systems (44). In one study of claustrophobic patients who previously failed an MRI procedure, Hunt, et al. (44) observed an 89% success rate for patients scanned in a short- and wide-bore 1.5-Tesla MR system compared to their previously unsuccessful procedure in a conventional 1.5-Tesla scanner.

In another study, Dewey, et al. (18) compared the rate of claustrophobia between the current generation of short- and wide-bore configured 1.5-Tesla MR systems (Magnetom Avanto, Siemens Medical Solutions) and conventional 1.0-Tesla MR systems (Magnetom Impact Expert Plus, Siemens Medical Solutions) in an outpatient setting. Data from this study collected over the course of 8 years demonstrated significantly lower rates of claustrophobic reactions among patients scanned on newer 1.5-Tesla scanners (0.7%) compared to conventional 1.0-Tesla MR systems (2.1%) (18). Considered together, these data suggest that although the patient-centered design of MR systems has evolved in the past decade and a half, even the most state-of-the-art systems do not prevent claustrophobia, indicating that there are other factors besides the physical aspects of the scanner that are related to claustrophobic events.

In the early 1990s, a specially-designed, low-field-strength (0.2-Tesla) MR system (Artoscan, Lunar Corporation/General Electric Medical Systems, Madison, WI and Esaote, Genoa, Italy) first became commercially available for MR imaging of extremities. The use of dedicated extremity MR systems such as these provides an accurate, reliable, and relatively inexpensive means (i.e., in comparison to the use of a whole-body MR system) of evaluating various types of musculoskeletal abnormalities. Therefore, utilization of the extremity scanner to assess musculoskeletal pathology is a viable and acceptable alternative to the use of whole-body MR systems (45). This is particularly the case since the image quality and diagnostic capabilities for the evaluation of the knee and other extremities has been reported to be comparable to mid- or high-field strength MR systems for certain musculoskeletal applications (45).

The architecture of the extremity MR system has no confining features or other aspects that would typically create patient-related problems. This is because only the body part that requires imaging is placed inside the magnet bore during the MR examination.

A preliminary study reported that 100% of the MRI examinations that were initiated were completed without being interrupted or cancelled for patient-related problems (Shellock FG, Unpublished Data, 2011). The unique design of the extremity MR system likely contributed to the totally successful completion of MRI examinations in the patients of this study. Furthermore, these findings represent a dramatic improvement compared with the published incidence of patient distress that tends to interrupt or prevent the completion of MRI procedures using whole-body MR systems. A more recently developed, dedicated extremity MR system also permits MR imaging of the shoulder. A newer high-field-strength (1.5-Tesla) MR system has been developed for high quality imaging of extremities (**Figure 2**).

Adverse psychological reactions are sometimes associated with the MRI procedures simply because the examination may be perceived by the patient as a "dramatic" medical

Figure 2. Examples of dedicated extremity MR systems that have no substantial confining features and, therefore, may be more acceptable to patients with psychological distress. (A) Dedicated extremity, MR system, O-scan (0.31-Tesla Esaote North America, Inc., Indianapolis, IN)

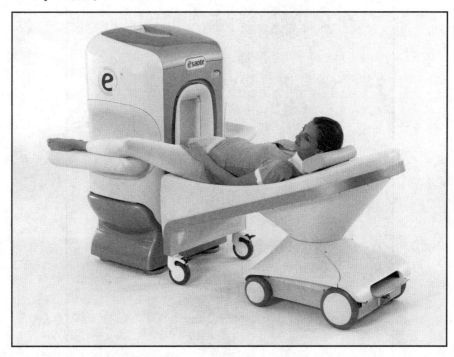

Figure 2. (Continued) (B) Dedicated extremity, MR system, S-scan (0.31-Tesla Esaote North America, Inc., Indianapolis, IN)

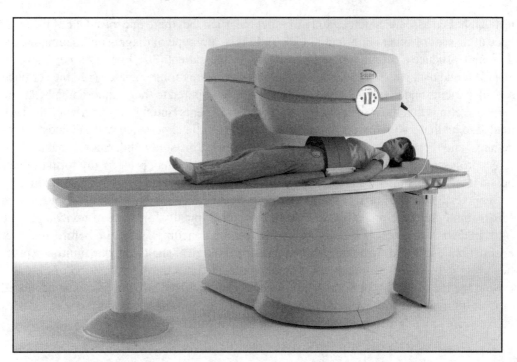

Figure 2. (Continued) (C) Dedicated extremity, MR system, MSK Extreme (1.5-Tesla, General Electric Medical Systems, Milwaukee, WI).

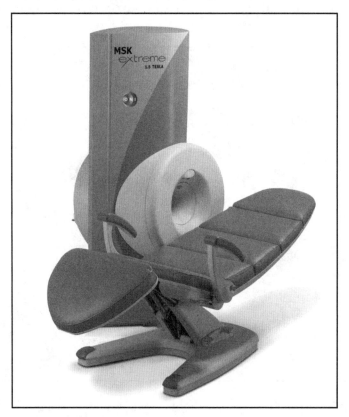

test that has an associated uncertainty of outcome, such that there may be a fear of the presence of disease or other abnormality (5, 10). In fact, any type of diagnostic imaging procedure may produce a certain amount of anxiety for the patient (30). For example, Thorp, et al. (16) found that, with the exception of the MR system environment issue (i.e., the confined space), patients undergoing computed tomography compared to those undergoing MRI had similar feelings that the procedure was unpleasant. Patients finding the experience difficult tended to be those with high initial levels of anxiety, little experience with diagnostic procedures, and those that believed they had cancer (16). This study underscores the need for direct professional interaction to prepare and educate the patient prior to any form of diagnostic imaging examination. Improved patient compliance was reported in a study that directly investigated the impact of more detailed patient education on adverse outcomes from MR mammography, a procedure known to have an atypically high rate of noncompliance (46). Likewise, in a recent study designed to test the noncompliance rate before and after hospital radiology staff were trained in nonpharmacological analgesia, one multi-site practice observed a significant decrease in noncompliance rates during the period of time following the training. This particular training program involved two components: advanced rapport training and self-hypnotic relaxation, both highlighting the importance of individualized care and interpersonal interactions in patient care (47).

Patients with pre-existing psychiatric disorders may be at greater risk for experiencing distress in the MRI environment. One problem that arises more often in this population is the refusal of the prescribed MRI procedure by the patient. Frequently, the cause for refusal is an inadequate understanding of why the procedure was ordered and what the actual procedure involves.

For patients with pre-existing anxiety disorders who agree to undergo MRI, it is prudent for hospital radiology staff to use augmented methods to minimize additional anxiety or distress. Grey, et al. (48) reported the efficacy of an anxiety reduction protocol in patients with moderate to high trait anxiety. Prior to MRI, patients in the intervention group were given detailed information regarding scanning procedures including descriptions of the acoustic noise, equipment and the procedure room, the timing of scans and degree of interaction with the MRI technologist, as well as coping strategies for anxiety in the scanner such as increasing the audio volume and paying attention to a clock on the wall. Patients in the intervention group were significantly less anxious during the procedure and retrospectively when asked about the whole procedure compared to those patients in the control condition, indicating that the extra time and effort spent preparing the patients in the intervention group made a positive impact on patients with pre-existing anxiety (48).

In a small study of older adults with generalized anxiety disorder (GAD) the rate of unsuccessful MRI examinations in patients with pre-existing anxiety was assessed and compared to a control group. In this study, an unsuccessful scan was defined as one in which there was excessive movement or premature termination of the scan. There was no significant difference in the rate of successful MRI outcome in this group of GAD patients and non-anxious controls (20). To date, this study is the only report of the differential frequency of distress or adverse outcomes for MRI procedures in such patients compared to non-psychiatrically impaired patients. Although these findings fail to find a difference between cohorts, future studies are still warranted and specific inquiry should be made to identify patients with pre-existing anxiety disorders including claustrophobia, generalized anxiety disorder, post-traumatic stress disorder, and obsessive-compulsive disorder in order to increase anxiety minimizing efforts in these patients.

Patients with other psychiatric illnesses such as depression and any illness complicated by thought disorder such as schizophrenia and manic-depressive disorder may also be at increased risk for distress in the MRI environment. Patients with psychiatric illnesses may, under normal circumstances, be able to tolerate the MRI setting without a problem, as is clear from the thousands who participate in clinical neuroimaging research studies each year (49). However, the increased stress due to their medical illness or fear of medical illness may exacerbate their psychiatric symptoms to such an extent that they may have difficulty complying with MRI procedures. At the very least, patients with psychiatric illnesses may require more time and patience to provide the appropriate level of preparatory information.

TECHNIQUES TO MINIMIZE PATIENT DISTRESS IN THE MRI ENVIRONMENT

We outline here a stepwise set of procedures for minimizing subjective distress for patients undergoing MRI. Certain measures to alleviate distress should be employed for all

MRI examinations. A number of other measures will be required if the patient is experiencing significant distress due to factors as described above. Finally, other distress-alleviation techniques will only be necessary for patients with co-existing psychiatric illness or other special problems. Coordination of these efforts among the referring physician, the radiologist, the MRI technologist and the facility support staff is crucial. Many of these methods have been described in the literature and are summarized in **Table 1** (3-5, 7, 9, 11, 12, 21, 33, 35, 36, 46, 50-54).

For All Patients Undergoing MRI Procedures

Referring clinicians should take the time to explain the rationale for the MRI procedure and what he/she expects to learn from the results with respect to the implications for treatment and prognosis. Importantly, the clinician should schedule time with the patient to communicate the results of the MRI procedure.

The single most important step is to educate the patient about the specific aspects of the MRI examination that are known to be particularly difficult. This includes conveying in terms that are understandable to the patient the internal dimensions of the MR system, the level of gradient magnetic field-induced acoustic noise to expect, and the estimated time duration of the examination.

Studies have documented a decrease in the incidence of premature termination of MRI procedures when patients are provided with more detailed information regarding the examination (46-48). This may be effectively accomplished by means of providing the patient time to view an educational videotape or written brochure supplemented by a question and answer session with an MRI-trained healthcare worker prior to MRI.

Some authors have proposed adding a pre-scan "fear assessment" to help predict patients who will experience psychological problems related to the MRI procedure (15, 20, 29, 30, 34, 39, 40). Such a brief questionnaire could be used to help elicit questions and concerns from patients and to provide guidance to staff about which distress minimization strategies are most likely to be effective for the patient.

Upon entering the MRI facility, patients who are treated with respect and are welcomed into a calm environment will report less distress. Many details of patient positioning in the MR system can increase comfort and minimize distress. Taking time to ensure comfortable positioning with adequate padding and blankets to alleviate undue discomfort or pain from positioning is also important. Adequate hearing protection should be provided routinely to decrease acoustic noise generated by the MR system. Demonstration of the two-way intercom system to reassure to patients that the MRI staff members can hear them when they speak and can speak to them during the examination can also be reassuring.

For Mildly to Moderately Distressed Patients

If a patient that continues to experience distress after the afore-mentioned measures are implemented, additional interventions are required. Frequently, all that is necessary to successfully complete an MRI examination is to allow an appropriately-screened relative or friend to remain with the patient during the procedure. A familiar person in the MR system room often helps the patient who is anxious to develop an increased sense of security (12,

Table 1. Recommended techniques for managing patients with distress related to MRI procedures.

(1) Prepare and educate the patient concerning specific aspects of the MRI examination (e.g., MR system dimensions, gradient noise, intercom system, etc.).

(2) Allow an appropriately-screened relative or friend to remain with the patient during the MRI procedure.

(3) Maintain physical or verbal contact with the patient during the MRI procedure.

(4) Use MR conditional headphones to provide music to the patient and to minimize gradient magnetic field-induced noise.

(5) Use an MR conditional video monitor to provide a visual distraction to the patient.

(6) Use a virtual reality environment system to provide audio and visual distraction.

(7) Place the patient in a prone position inside the MR system.

(8) Position the patient feet-first instead of head-first into the MR system.

(9) Use special mirrors or prism glasses for the patient.

(10) Use a blindfold so that the patient is not aware of the close surroundings.

(11) Use bright lights inside and at either end of the MR system.

(12) Use a fan inside of the MR system to provide adequate air movement.

(13) Use lemon or vanilla scented oil or other similar aroma therapy so that the patient can comfortably experience olfactory stimulation.

(14) Use relaxation techniques such as controlled breathing or mental imagery.

(15) Use systematic desensitization.

(16) Use medical hypnosis.

(17) Use a sedative or other similar medication.

35). If a supportive companion is not present, then simply having an MRI staff member maintain verbal contact via the intercom system or physical contact by having a staff person remain in the MR system room with the patient during the examination will frequently decrease psychological distress (7, 12, 35).

Placing the patient in a prone position inside the MR system so that the patient can visualize the opening of the bore provides a sensation of being inside a device that is more spacious and alleviates the "closed-in" feeling associated with the supine position (35, 55). Prone positioning of the patient may not be a practical alternative if MRI requires the use of a flat radiofrequency (RF) coil or if the patient has underlying medical conditions (e.g., shortness of breath, the presence of chest tubes, etc.) that preclude lying in this position. Another method of positioning the patient that may help is to place the individual feet-first instead of head-first into the scanner.

MR system-mounted mirrors or prism glasses can be used to permit the patient to maintain a vertical view of the outside of the scanner in order to minimize phobic responses. Using a blindfold so that the patient is not aware of the close surroundings has also been suggested to be an effective technique for enabling anxious patients to successfully undergo MRI (12, 35).

The environment of the MR system may be changed to optimize the management of apprehensive patients (12). For example, the presence of higher lighting levels tends to make most individuals feel less anxious. Therefore, the use of bright lights at either end and inside of the MR system can produce a less imposing environment for the patient. In addition, using a fan inside of the scanner to provide more air movement will help reduce the sensation of confinement and lessen any tissue heating that may result when high levels of RF power absorption are used for MRI (12). Some MRI staff members have reported that placing a cotton pad moistened with a few drops of lemon, vanilla, cucumber oil or other similar form of aromatherapy in the MR system for the patient to receive olfactory stimulation can also reduce distress.

Electronic devices that utilize compressed air or other acceptable means to transmit music or audio communication through headphones have been developed specifically for use with MR systems (51, 52, 56, 57). MR conditional music/audio systems may be acquired from a commercial vendor (51, 57). This equipment can be used to provide calming music to the patient and, with the proper design, help to minimize exposure to gradient magnetic field-induced acoustic noise. Reports have indicated that the use of these devices has been successful in reducing symptoms of anxiety in patients during MRI (52, 56, 58). Furthermore, one study suggested that having a live musician play music that matches the rhythm of the gradient magnetic fields improves patient perceptions of the MRI procedure (58). This improved perception may also be due in part to the perceived increase in the social interaction that the patient has during MRI.

Additionally, it is possible to provide visual stimulation to the patient via special goggles (57). Use of visual stimuli to distract patients may also reduce distress. Finally, a new system has been developed to provide a virtual reality environment for the patient that may likewise serve as an acceptable means of audio and visual distraction from the MRI examination (**Figure 3**). A case study of two patients with claustrophobia demonstrated that virtual reality distraction also decreased subjective anxiety ratings when compared to no distraction (59).

For Severely Distressed or Claustrophobic Patients

Patients who are at high risk for severe distress in the MRI environment and can be identified as such by their referring clinician or by the scheduling MRI staff person could be offered the opportunity to have pre-MRI behavioral therapy. MRI procedures that were conducted in patients that previously refused or were unable to tolerate the MRI environment have been reported to be successful as a result of treatment with relaxation techniques (9, 54), systematic desensitization (11), and medical hypnosis (33, 36, 53). Quirk, et al. (9) reported that psychological preparation that included information about the examination and the use of relaxation strategies (i.e., breathing relaxation techniques, visualization of pleasant images, performance of mental exercises, etc.) was more effective for reducing anxiety in patients compared to providing information alone.

Klonoff, et al. (11) provided a detailed example of one successful systematic desensitization protocol. This was conducted prior to MRI and involved having the patient lie on the floor at home with her head in a box. The size of the box was incrementally decreased until it approximated the internal dimensions of the MR system. Additionally, the patient was required to gradually increase the amount of time that she could tolerate spending time with the box over her head, until it equaled 50 to 60 minutes, to approximate the maximum time needed for MRI. The patient also wore prism glasses that permitted her to have a direct view in the vertical plane during MRI. After four treatment sessions, the patient was able

Figure 3. CinemaVision (Resonance Technology Inc., Northridge, CA) is an MR conditional audiovisual system. (A) Wireless technology allows transmission of the audio and video signals (DVD, CD, and AM/FM input) from the control room to the MR system room.

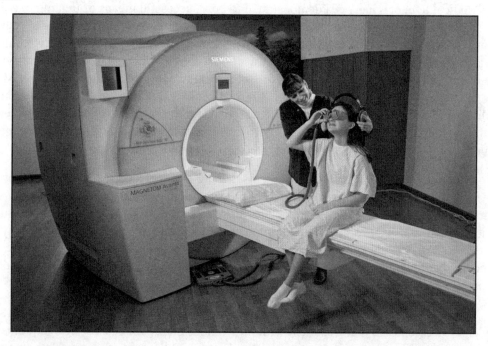

Figure 3. (Continued) (B) The digital audio headset system blocks 30-dB of acoustic noise, allows for two-way communication with MRI technologists and transmits audio signal from the console. This special equipment may be used during the MRI procedure to provide the patient with audio and visual distractions. The visor/goggles fits easily into all standard head coils.

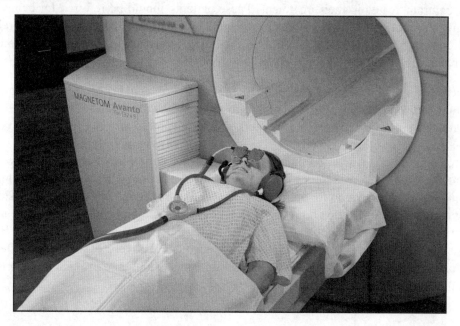

to successfully undergo MRI (11). Notably, because of the time involved with systematic desensitization, this technique of preparing the distressed patient for an MRI procedure may not be practical for most MRI facilities.

Medical hypnosis has been demonstrated to be a successful means of treating phobias (50) and, not surprisingly, has been used as an effective intervention to enable a claustrophobic or anxious patient to complete MRI (33, 36, 53). Successful hypnotherapy requires a trained medical hypnotist and a willing, trance-susceptible patient. Therefore, identifying the appropriate patient that would benefit from being hypnotized before and during MRI and having a hypnosis therapist available for treatment are prerequisites for instituting this technique of patient management. There is a secondary effect of using hypnosis for patients with psychological disorders undergoing MRI insofar as patients have reported feeling a general reduction in anxiety in their everyday lives after undergoing hypnosis for MRI (33).

In the majority of MRI facilities, patients that are severely affected by claustrophobia, anxiety, or panic attacks in response to MRI procedures are usually pharmacologically sedated when other attempts to counteract their distress fail. Using short-acting sedatives such as lorazepam, diazepam, alprazolam, or intranasal midazolam or one of the other anxiolytic medications may be the only means of managing patients with a high degree of anxiety related to MRI. Published reports of the rate of pharmacological sedation for patients undergoing MRI range from 2 to 14% (8, 21).

A study conducted by Avrahami (3) in patients with panic attacks who were unable to undergo MRI reported that treatment with intravenous diazepam caused the symptoms to disappear rapidly and permitted completion of the examination in every case. However, the use of sedatives in patients prior to and during MRI may not be required in all instances nor is it always practical (1).

Of special note is that anxious patients with a history of substance abuse who are in recovery programs may not be willing to take mind-altering medications because this is typically contraindicated in their treatment. These patients should be referred for behavioral therapy before MRI. In all cases, one or more of the recommended, non-medication-related techniques indicated in **Table 1** should be attempted before immediately electing to use a sedative in distressed patients in the MRI environment.

Performing sedation for the patient in the MRI environment is not a totally benign procedure. Confusion and respiratory compromise as well as other untoward reactions have been reported in response to relatively modest doses of commonly employed sedatives (6, 9). If a sedative or other similar drug is used in a patient in preparation for an MRI examination, it should be understood that the use of this medication involves several important patient management considerations (31). For example, the time when the patient should be administered the medication for optimal effect prior to the examination should be considered along with the possibility that there may be an adverse reaction to the drug (31). The use of proper physiologic monitoring equipment during the MRI examination is essential. Provisions should be available for an area to permit adequate recovery of the patient after the MRI procedure. The patient should also have someone available to provide transportation from the MRI facility after receiving medication.

For Pediatric Patients

Careful consideration of methods for reducing distress in pediatric patients is extremely important as the implications of imaging procedures have both short- and long-term effects in this population. In addition to the short-term effects of distress, anxiety and pain, resulting in crying and lack of cooperation, there may be long-term psychological effects into adulthood such as medical fears, less perceived control over health, and in some cases, posttraumatic stress responses and claustrophobic feelings (60, 61). Some of the methods for minimizing distress and discomfort in the scanner are similar to those used in adults, however, important differences should be highlighted. Similar to adults, pediatric patients can also benefit from preparation prior to the procedure, hypnosis, music and sedation. Other pediatric specific methods such as visual and audio distraction, positive reinforcement and parental involvement have also been shown to be effective (60).

Parental involvement can be a particularly useful technique as it engages the parents, which in turn reduces the parents' own anxiety and ensures that the child is in close proximity to them. Techniques with parental involvement include comforting and distracting the child while holding the child in a comforting position, educating and preparing the child for the procedure, and providing positive reinforcement. Parents must be careful in these interactions with their children, as any anxiety or stress they express can induce anxiety and stress in the child (60).

Educational materials and procedural preparation can be helpful for both the parents and the child. Parents and pediatric patients can watch educational videos together, practice positioning for the procedure, and observe other children modeling various coping skills. With the assistance of radiology staff members, parents can help their children practice breathing techniques and engage in positive imagery (60).

Some radiology teams also employ child-life specialists who are specifically trained to teach pediatric patients and their parents various coping skills that they can employ during MRI. These skills include visual, auditory and tactile distraction and breathing exercises (60). In addition to reducing stress and anxiety in pediatric patients, child-life specialists have been shown to contribute to the reduction of sedation rates associated with pediatric MRI procedures (62).

Just as there are risks associated with using sedatives in adult patients, there are risks for sedating pediatric patients. Unlike for adult patients, however, the process of inducing sedation can be equally as traumatizing to the child as the MRI procedure itself. Under certain circumstances, sedation is the only way to achieve the quality of scans required for diagnosis, particularly in young children under the age of eight (63). In this case, radiology teams should follow established sedation programs that are safe and effective (64).

ROLES AND RESPONSIBILITIES

As patient-centered medicine evolves, clinicians are increasingly empowering their patients to take an active role in managing their own healthcare. As a result, patient education has become an increasingly important aspect of healthcare. Over the past two decades there has been a rise in the presence of patient-centered educational materials, available through web-based portals and in the academic literature. Included in this are studies designed to investigate the impact on healthcare outcomes in patients who are given detailed information regarding their procedures.

With the increasing proportion of patients taking greater responsibility for their own health, there is a rise in the number of patients using these web-based portals for information on their own health as well as information about the procedures they will undergo. With more than 60% of patients using web-based systems (65) such as Medline Plus, WebMD, and other online sources to find healthcare information, it is important for hospital radiology teams to provide their patients with specific and up-to-date information regarding their procedures. An increased focus on patient-centered medicine and improved patient education has prompted hospitals and other medical imaging facilities to provide detailed information to patients and their families. Patients at hospitals such as the Massachusetts General Hospital and the Brigham and Women's Hospital can search for the name of the MRI facility plus the key term "MRI" and they will be directed to a set of education materials explaining the procedure. Resources such as these are available at many imaging facilities within academic institutions and other imaging center organizations. These websites provide useful information for patients and can serve as a model for other MRI facilities.

Just as patients are being recognized for their important role in their own healthcare, medical professionals should recognize the contributions of each member of the hospital radiology team who work together to provide the highest quality of care for patients undergoing MRI. It is important for the radiology team to define the roles and responsibilities of each member. Delineating a set of goals for the team and responsibilities for each member of the hospital radiology staff allows the team to be efficient while providing the patients with individualized support and education materials at each step in the process.

From the referring physicians and radiologists to the technologists and support staff, each member of the team has a specific role in providing care for their patients. Primary care physicians and specialists who order the procedures have a responsibility to engage their patients in the medical process and explain the rationale for the MRI procedure. The healthcare support staff that schedule, greet, and provide the patients with pamphlets of information are an extremely valuable resource for the patients as they are the most visible members of the team.

Patients entering the MRI facility should be welcomed into a calm environment. The radiology technologists who perform the diagnostic procedures have the most direct impact on the care of the patients during potentially distressing procedures. They are highly trained professionals who not only conduct a wide range of diagnostic tests but also provide educational information and prepare patients for the procedures prior to conducting tests. As always, the radiologists and physicians who interpret the results of the tests and discuss the diagnoses with their patients have the responsibility of establishing good lines of communication with the patients and understanding their mental state following potentially distressing procedures.

SUMMARY AND CONCLUSIONS

The advances in MRI technology coupled with the advances in clinical applications of MRI procedures to aid in the diagnosis and management of an ever-increasing number of medical conditions will ensure that the number of patients undergoing MRI continues to increase each year. Thus, the number of patients at risk for experiencing distress during MRI will continue to increase.

This chapter discussed the types of distress and potentially negative consequences that patients may experience in association with MRI. More importantly, simple and effective strategies for minimizing and perhaps eliminating this distress for patients have been presented. Patient education pertaining to the MRI examination is perhaps the single most important measure to reduce distress and the associated adverse outcomes. Importantly, adherence to the outlined measures will greatly improve patient comfort and, thereby, greatly decrease the number of aborted or poor quality studies.

REFERENCES

1. Shellock, FG. Claustrophobia, Anxiety, and Panic Disorders Associated with MR Procedures. In: Shellock FG, Kanal E, Editors. Magnetic Resonance: Bioeffects, Safety, and Patient Management. New York: Lippincott-Raven Press; 1996. pp. 65.

2. Diagnostic and Statistical Manual of Mental Disorders, 4th Edition. Washington, DC: American Psychiatric Press; 1994.

3. Avrahami E. Panic attacks during MR imaging: treatment with IV diazepam. Am J Neuroradiol 1990;11:833-835.

4. Brennan SC, Redd WH, Jacobsen PB, et al. Anxiety and panic during magnetic resonance scans. Lancet 1988;2:512.

5. Granet RB, Gelber LJ. Claustrophobia during MR imaging. New Jersey Medicine 1990;87:479-482.

6. Quirk ME, Letendre AJ, Ciottone RA, et al. Anxiety in patients undergoing MR imaging. Radiology 1989;170:463-466.

7. Shellock FG, Kanal E. Policies, guidelines, and recommendations for MR imaging and patient management. J Mag Reson Imaging 1991;1:97-101.

8. Dantendorfer K, Amering M, Bankier A, et al. A study of the effect of patient anxiety, perception and equipment on motion artifacts in magnetic resonance imaging. Magn Reson Imaging 1997;15:301-306.

9. Quirk ME, Letendre AJ, Ciottone RA, et al. Evaluation of three psychological interventions to reduce anxiety during MR imaging. Radiology 1989;173:759-762.

10. Flaherty JA, Hoskinson K. Emotional distress during magnetic resonance imaging. N Eng J Med 1989;320:467-468.

11. Klonoff EA, Janata JW, Kaufman B. The use of systematic desensitization to overcome resistance to magnetic resonance imaging (MRI) scanning. J Behav Ther Exp Psych 1986;17:189-192.

12. Weinreb J, Maravilla KR, Peshock R, et al. Magnetic resonance imaging: improving patient tolerance and safety. Am J Roentgen 1984;143:1285-1287.

13. Katz RC, Wilson L, Frazer N. Anxiety and its determinants in patients undergoing magnetic-resonance-imaging. J Behav Ther Exp Psychiatry 1994;25:131-134.

14. McIsaac HM, Thordarson DS, Shafran R, Rachman S, Poole G. Claustrophobia and the magnetic resonance imaging procedure. J Behav Med 1998;21:255-268.

15. Melendez C, McCrank E. Anxiety-related reactions associated with magnetic resonance imaging examinations. JAMA 1993;270:745-747.

16. Thorp D, Owens RG, Whitehouse G, et al. Subjective experiences of magnetic resonance imaging. Clin Radiol 1990;41:276-278.

17. Sarji SA, Abdullah BJ, Kumar G, Tan AH, Narayanan P. Failed magnetic resonance imaging examinations due to claustrophobia. Australas Radiol 1998;42:293-295.

18. Dewey M, Schink T, Dewey CF. Claustrophobia during magnetic resonance imaging: Cohort study in over 55,000 patients. J Mag Reson Imag 2007;26:1322-1327.

19. Enders J, Zimmermann E, Rief M, et al. Reduction of claustrophobia with short-bore versus open magnetic resonance imaging: a randomized controlled trial. PLoS One 2011;6:1-10.

20. Mohlman J, Eldreth DA, Price RB, Chazin D, Glover DA. Predictors of unsuccessful magnetic resonance imaging scanning in older generalized anxiety disorder patients and controls. J Behav Med 2012;35:19-26.

21. Murphy KJ, Brunberg JA. Adult claustrophobia, anxiety and sedation in MRI. Magn Reson Imag 1997;15:51-54.

22. Peters S, Cleare AJ, Papadopoulos A, Fu CHY. Cortisol responses to serial MRI scans in healthy adults and in depression. Psychoneuroendocrinology 2011;36:737-741.

23. Eatough EM, Shirtcliff EA, Hanson JL, Pollak SD. Hormonal reactivity to MRI scanning in adolescents. Psychoneuroendocrinology 2009;34:1242-1246.

24. Tessner KD, Walker EF, Hochman K, Hamann S. Cortisol responses of healthy volunteers undergoing magnetic resonance imaging. Hum Brain Mapp 2006;27:889-895.

25. Muehlhan M, Lueken U, Wittchen HU, Kirschbaum C. The scanner as a stressor: Evidence from subjective and neuroendocrine stress parameters in the time course of a functional magnetic resonance imaging session. Int J Psychophysiol 2011;79:118-126.

26. van Stegeren AH, Wolf OT, Everaerd W, et al. Endogenous cortisol level interacts with noradrenergic activation in the human amygdala. Neurobiol Learn Mem 2007;87:57-66.

27. Pruessner JC, Dedovic K, Khalili-Mahani N, et al. Deactivation of the limbic system during acute psychosocial stress: Evidence from positron emission tomography and functional magnetic resonance imaging studies. Biol Psychiatry 2008;63:234-240.

28. Tornqvist E, Mansson A, Larsson EM, Hallstrom I. Impact of extended written information on patient anxiety and image motion artifacts during magnetic resonance Imaging. Acta Radiol 2006;47:474-480.

29. Kilborn LC, Labbe EE. Magnetic resonance imaging scanning procedures: Development of phobic response during scan and at one-month follow-up. J Behav Med 1990;13:391-401.

30. MacKenzie R, Sims C, Owens RG, et al. Patient's perceptions of magnetic resonance imaging. Clin Radiol 1995;50:137-143.

31. Moss ML, Boungiorno PA, Clancy VA. Intranasal midazolam for claustrophobia in MRI. J Comp Assist Tomo 1993;17:991-992.

32. Deluca SA, Castronovo FP. Hazards of magnetic resonance imaging. Am Fam Phys 1990;41:145-146.

33. Friday PJ, Kubal WS. Magnetic resonance imaging: improved patient tolerance utilizing medical hypnosis. Am J Clin Hypnosis 1990;33:80-84.

34. Harris LM, Cumming SR, Menzies RG. Predicting anxiety in magnetic resonance imaging scans. Int J Beh Med 2004;11:1-7.

35. Hricak H, Amparo EG. Body MRI: Alleviation of claustrophobia by prone positioning. Radiology 1984;152:819.

36. Phelps LA. MRI and claustrophobia. Am Fam Phys 1991;42:930.

37. Thomsen HS. Frequency of acute adverse events to a non-ionic low-osmolar contrast medium: the effect of verbal interview. Pharmacol and Toxicol 1997;80:108-110.

38. Rachman S, Taylor S. Analyses of claustrophobia. J Anxiety Disord 1993;7:281-291.

39. Thorpe S, Salkovskis PM, Dittner A. Claustrophobia in MRI: The role of cognitions. Magn Reson Imag 2008;26:1081-1088.

40. Harris LM, Robinson J, Menzies RG. Predictors of panic symptoms during magnetic resonance imaging scans. Int J Behav Med 2001;8:80-87.

41. Brummett RE, Talbot JM, Charuhas P. Potential hearing loss resulting from MR imaging. Radiology 1988;169:539-540.

42. Bangard C, Paszek J, Berg F, et al. MR imaging of claustrophobic patients in an open 10T scanner: Motion artifacts and patient acceptability compared with closed bore magnets. Eur J Radiol 2007;64:152-157.

43. Spouse E, Gedroyc WM. MRI of the claustrophobic patient: Interventionally configured magnets. Br J Radiol 2000;73:146-151.

44. Hunt CH, Wood CP, Lane JI, et al. Wide, short bore magnetic resonance at 1.5 T. Clin Neuroradiol 2011;21:141-144.

45. Shellock FG, Stone KR, Resnick D, et al. Subjective perceptions of MRI examinations performed using an extremity MR system. Signals 2000;32:16-31.

46. Youssefzadeh S, Eibenberger K, Helbich T, et al. Reduction of adverse events in MRI of the breast by personal patient care. Clin Radiol 1997;52:862-864.

47. Lang EV, Ward C, Laser E. Effect of team training on patients' ability to complete MRI examinations. Acad Radiol 2010;17:18-23.

48. Grey SJ, Price G, Mathews A. Reduction of anxiety during MR imaging: A controlled trial. Magn Reson Imaging 2000;18:351-355.

49. Rauch SL, Renshaw PF. Clinical neuroimaging in psychiatry. Harv Rev Psychiatry 1995;2:297-312.

50. McGuinness TP. Hypnosis in the treatment of phobias: a review of the literature. Am J Clin Hypnosis 1984;26:261-272.

51. Axel L. Simpler music/audio system for patients having MR imaging. Am J Roentgenol 1988;151:1080.

52. Miyamoto AT, Kasson RT. Simple music/audio system for patients having MR imaging. Am J Roentgenol 1988;151:1060.

53. Simon EP. Hypnosis using a communication device to increase magnetic resonance imaging tolerance with a claustrophobic patient. Mil Med 1999;164:71-72.

54. Lukins R, Davan IG, Drummond PD. A cognitive behavioural approach to preventing anxiety during magnetic resonance imaging. J Behav Ther Exper Psych 1997;28:97-104.

55. Eshed I, Althoff CE, Hamm B, Hermann KGA. Claustrophobia and premature termination of magnetic resonance imaging examinations. J Mag Reson Imaging 2007;26:401-404.

56. Slifer KJ, Penn-Jones K, Cataldo MF, et al. Music enhances patient's comfort during MR imaging. Am J Roentgenol 1991;156:403.

57. Savoy RL, Ravicz ME, Gollub R. The Psychophysiological Laboratory in the Magnet: Stimulus Delivery, Response Recording, and Safety. In: Moonen CTW, Bandettini PA, Editors. Functional MRI. Berlin: Springer; 1999. pp. 347.

58. Walworth DD. Effect of live music therapy for patients undergoing magnetic resonance imaging. J Music Ther 2010;47:335-350.

59. Garcia-Palacios A, Hoffman HG, Richards TR, Seibel EJ, Sharar SR. Use of virtual reality distraction to reduce claustrophobia symptoms during a mock magnetic resonance imaging brain scan: A case report. Cyberpsychol Behav 2007;10:485-488.

60. Alexander M. Managing patient stress in pediatric radiology. Radiol Technol 2012;83:549-560.

61. Wood BS, McGlynn FD. Research on posttreatment return of claustrophobic fear, arousal, and avoidance using mock diagnostic imaging. Behav Modif 2000;24:379-394.

62. Khan JJ, Donnelly LF, Koch BL, et al. A program to decrease the need for pediatric sedation for CT and MRI. Applied Radiology 2007;36:30-33.

63. Hallowell, LM Stewart SE, Silva C, Ditchfield MR. Reviewing the process of preparing children for MRI. Pediatr Radiol 2008;38:271-279.

64. Keengwe IN, Hegde S, Dearlove O, et al. Structured sedation program for magnetic resonance imaging examination in children. Anaesthesia 1999;54:1069-1072.

65. D'Auria JP. In search of quality health information. J Pediatr Health Care 2010;24:137-140.

Chapter 9   MRI Procedures and Pregnancy

PATRICK M. COLLETTI, M.D.

Professor of Radiology
Professor of Medicine
Professor of Biokinesiology
Professor of Pharmacology and Pharmaceutical Sciences
Chief of MRI
Director Nuclear Medicine Fellowship
University of Southern California
LAC+USC Medical Center
Los Angeles, CA

INTRODUCTION

Medical imaging remains a common requirement in pregnant patients. Because of the increased scrutiny for possible radiation effects associated with pregnancy (1-4), it is not surprising that the question of whether a patient should undergo a magnetic resonance imaging (MRI) examination during pregnancy frequently arises. While a 1988 survey by Kanal, et al. (5) showed that 36% of sites did not perform MRI procedures in pregnant patients, a more recent survey by De Wilde, et al. (6) demonstrated that 91% of 352 MRI facilities in the United Kingdom performed MRI examinations in second and third trimester patients, and 8% had protocols for selective fetal imaging (6).

Although advice from regulatory agencies such as the United States Food and Drug Administration (FDA) is limited, the International Society of Magnetic Resonance Imaging (ISMRM), the American College of Radiology (ACR), and other organizations have provided useful clarifications, as follows (7-12):

- 1989, FDA: "The safety of MRI when used to image fetuses and infants has not been established" (7).

- 1991, Safety Committee for the Society of Magnetic Resonance Imaging (SMRI): "MR imaging may be used in pregnant women if other non-ionizing forms of diagnostic imaging are inadequate or if the examination provides important information that would otherwise require exposure to ionizing radiation...", and there is "... no indication that the use of clinical MR imaging during pregnancy has produce deleterious effects" (8). This policy adopted by the American College of Radiology was considered a "standard of care" (9) with reference to pregnant patients.

- 2002, the American College of Radiology (ACR) White Paper on MR Safety: "Pregnant patients can ... undergo MR scans at any stage of pregnancy if, in the determination of a Level Two MR Personnel–designated attending radiologist, the risk–benefit ratio to the patient warrants that the study be performed" (10).

- 2007, the ACR Guidance Document for Safe MR Practices: "Present data have not conclusively documented any deleterious effects of MR imaging exposure on the developing fetus", and; "... no special consideration is recommended for the first, versus any other, trimester in pregnancy" (11). It is, therefore, "prudent" to document pregnancy and consult with the patient and her physician regarding the clinical urgency for immediate MRI versus waiting for MRI until after delivery.

- 2013, the ACR updated the information for the use of MRI in pregnancy, as follows: "Present data have not conclusively documented any deleterious effects of MR imaging exposure on the developing fetus. Therefore, no special consideration is recommended for the first, versus any other, trimester in pregnancy. Nevertheless, as with all interventions during pregnancy, it is prudent to screen females of reproductive age for pregnancy before permitting them access to MR imaging environments. If pregnancy is established consideration should be given to reassessing the potential risks versus benefits of the pending study in determining whether the requested MR examination could safely wait to the end of the pregnancy before being performed.

  a. Pregnant patients can be accepted to undergo MR scans at any stage of pregnancy if, in the determination of a level 2 MR personnel-designated attending radiologist, the risk–benefit ratio to the patient warrants that the study be performed. The radiologist should confer with the referring physician and document the following in the radiology report or the patient's medical record:

      1. The information requested from the MR study cannot be acquired by means of nonionizing means (e.g., ultrasonography).

      2. The data is needed to potentially affect the care of the patient or fetus during the pregnancy.

      3. The referring physician believes that it is not prudent to wait until the patient is no longer pregnant to obtain this data.

  b. MR contrast agents should not be routinely provided to pregnant patients. This decision too, is one that must be made on a case-by-case basis by the covering level 2 MR personnel-designated attending radiologist who will assess the risk–benefit ratio for that particular patient." Notably, the 2013 document from the ACR does not indicate that there is a need for informed consent for the use of MRI in pregnant patients (12).

SAFETY

Basic Research and Animal Studies

MRI exposes the patient and fetus to a static magnetic field, rapidly changing, gradient magnetic fields, acoustic noise, and radiofrequency (RF) radiation. The effects of these electromagnetic fields on the human fetus are not easily determined. Consider the following:

- The strength of the static magnetic field is well known (e.g., 1.5-Tesla, 3-Tesla, etc.).

- The gradient amplitude (e.g., 20-mT/m) and slew rate, dB/dt (i.e., 3-T/s) can be determined at the location of the fetus for a given pulse sequence.

- RF energy power deposition or the specific absorption rate (SAR) level (e.g., whole body averaged SAR, 3.2-W/kg) will vary considerably with the type of transmit RF coil that is used and system configuration, as well as the pulse sequences that are selected for the procedure. Popular sequences for fast fetal imaging, such as fast spin echo, employ multiple rapid RF pulses, and would be expected to deposit more RF energy compared to gradient echo techniques.

- RF power deposition varies considerably with the body part undergoing MRI. While Schaefer (13) concluded that approximately 87% of the RF energy would likely be deposited in the outer 1/3 of the body (13), Hand, et al. (14) predicted that the fetus would be exposed to a peak of approximately 40 to 60% of the maternal peak value at 64-MHz (1.5-Tesla), increasing to approximately 50 to 70% at 128-MHz (3-Tesla). Thus, in most instances, the embryo or fetus would receive relatively small RF exposures (15-17).

- Heating is the only well established mechanism for RF bioeffects (18). The fetus might be somewhat heat energy tolerant due to a relatively large fetal surface area-to-volume ratio. In addition, amniotic fluid, with its relatively high heat capacity, would be expected to sufficiently absorb heat transferred by convection. Kikuchi S, et al. (19) used a thermal model to predict that 40-minutes of scanning at a whole-body averaged SAR of 2-W/kg might increase fetal temperature more than the 0.5°C, as recommended by the International Commission on Non-Ionizing Radiation Protection, but less than the proposed teratogenic cutoff value of 1.5 °C (19).

- The anatomically "deep" position of the fetus and the surrounding amniotic fluid could help to reduce the effects of gradient field-related, acoustic noise.

- In addition, the stage of pregnancy is important with regard to the potential risk to the embryo or fetus, and spontaneous adverse outcomes are very common (20) (**Table 1**).

A number of biological studies have assessed the effects of MRI in pregnancy. Most of these studies show no evidence for fetal harm (21-37) (**Tables 2** and **3**). However, there has been little clinical follow-up to humans exposed to MRI, *in-utero* (38-44) (**Table 4**). A survey of reproductive health among 280 pregnant MRI healthcare workers performed by Kanal, et al. (39), showed no substantial increase in common adverse reproductive out-

Table 1. Spontaneous adverse outcomes of pregnancy.

Period	Risk	Spontaneous Occurrence Rate
Day 1 to 10	Reabsorption	30%
Day 10 to 50	Abnormal Organogenesis	4 to 6%
>Day 50	Intra-uterine Growth Retardation	4%

Table 2. Safety of MRI in pregnancy: non-adverse outcomes in animals.

Study	Findings
McRobbie and Foster (21) 1985	No change in litter number or growth rate in mice exposed to gradients ranging from 3.5- to 12-kT/s.
Teskey, et al. (22) 1987	No change in stress reactivity or survivability in rats repeatedly exposed in-utero.
Heinrichs, et al. (23) 1988	No embryo toxicity or teratogenesis with prolonged exposure (BLB/c mice, midgestational, 0.35-T.
Kay, et al. (24) 1988	No adverse effects (*Xenopus laevis* embryo, long-term exposure, 1.5-T).
Tyndall (25) 1990	MRI exposure does not add to low level x-ray irradiation induced teratogenesis in C57B1/6J mice at 1.5-T.
Murkami, et al. (26) 1992	No change in pregnancy outcomes for mice exposed to 6.3-T for 1-hour per day from day 7 to 14.
Malko, et al. (27) 1994	No change in cell density (yeast cells grown at 1.5-T).
Yip, et al. (28) 1994 and Yip, et al. (29) 1995	No change in survival, migration, and proliferation and no effect on axonal growth in chick embryos exposed to simulated imaging conditions at 1.5-T.
Tablado, et al. (30) 2000	No testicular abnormalities in mice continually exposed in-utero from day 7 to birth at 0.7-T.
Ruckhaberle E, et al. (31) 2008	No significant amniotic fluid temperature or acoustic noise changes in pregnant ewes at 1.5-T. Intrauterine peak acoustic levels did not exceed 100.0-dB(L)

comes. Baker, et al. (40) showed no demonstrable increase in disease, disabilities, or hearing loss in 20 children examined *in-utero* with echo-planar MRI performed for suspected fetal compromise. Myers, et al. (41) showed no significant reduction in fetal growth vs. matched controls in 74 volunteers exposed *in-utero* to echo-planar MRI at 0.5-Tesla.

Use of MRI Contrast Agents in Pregnancy

While some moieties are transferred across the placenta by active transporters located on both the fetal and maternal side of the trophoblast layer, most substances administered during pregnancy will, to some degree, traverse the placenta and enter the fetus via passive diffusion. Transplacental passive diffusion is affected by molecular properties such as molecular weight, the acid dissociation constant (pKa), lipid solubility, and plasma protein binding (45-47). Polar molecules with a molecular weight of less than 500-D are more likely

Table 3. Safety of MRI in pregnancy: adverse outcomes in animals and human cultures.

Study	Findings
Tyndall and Sulik (32) 1991	At least two-fold increased incidence of eye malformations (C57B16J mice, 10% spontaneous eye malformations, gestational day 7, 1.5-T for 36-minutes).
Tyndall (33) 1993	Increased teratogenicity with reduced crown-rump length and craniofacial size in C57B1/6J mice exposed to clinically realistic MRI at 1.5-T.
Yip, et al. (34) 1994	"trend toward higher abnormality and mortality rates.." in chick embryos exposed simulated imaging conditions at 1.5-T.
Carnes, et al. (35) 1996	Fetal weight reduction (11%) in mice exposed to 8 hours in midgestation at 4.7-T
Narra, et al. (36) 1996	Reduced spermatogenesis and embryogenesis in Webster mice exposed in-utero to 1.5-T for 30-minutes
Lee JW, et al. (37) 2011	3-T MRI induces genotoxic effects (significant increase in the frequency of micronuclei and single-strand DNA breaks) in cultured human lymphocytes proportional to exposure time

Table 4. Safety of MRI in pregnancy: non-adverse outcomes in humans.

Study	Findings
Johnson, et al. (38) 1990	No change in fetal heart rate or Doppler-determined umbilical artery blood flow (humans, 10 to 20 weeks, 0.5-T).
Kanal, et al. (39) 1993	No increase in adverse reproductive outcomes (280 pregnant female MR imaging workers).
Baker, et al. (40) 1994	No increase in disease or disability, no hearing loss in 20 children at 3 years after in-utero exposure to echo-planar MRI at 0.5-T.
Myers, et al. (41) 1998	No significant decrease vs. matched controls in fetal growth in 74 volunteers exposed in-utero to echo-planar MRI up to 5 X at 0.5-T.
Vadeyar, et al. (42) 2000	No change in fetal heart rate in human volunteers at term (37 to 41 weeks), echo-planar MRI at 0.5-T.
Kok RD, et al. (43) 2004	No harmful effects of prenatal 1.5-T MR exposure in the third trimester of pregnancy were detected in 35 children at 1 to 3 years and in 9 children at 8-9 years.
Reeves MJ, et al. (44) 2010	2nd and 3rd trimester fetal exposure to 1.5-T MR imaging is not associated with an increased risk of substantial neonatal hearing impairment.

Table 5. Currently approved MRI contrast agents.

Agent	Molecular Weight	Charge	Relative Stability	Excess Free Ligand in Formulation
Gadolinium-based contrast agents				
Gadopentetate dimeglumine (Magnevist, Bayer Healthcare, Wayne, NJ) (48)	938	Linear-ionic	Moderate	0.4-mg/ml
Gadobenate (MultiHance, Gd-BOPTA, Bracco, Milan, Italy) (49)	1058	Linear-ionic	Moderate	0.4-mg/ml
Gadodiamide (Omniscan, Nycomed Amersham, Princeton, NJ) (50)	574	Linear-nonionic	Low	12-mg/ml
Gadovesetamide (OptiMARK, Mallinkrodt, St. Louis) (51)	661	Linear-nonionic	Low	28.4-mg/ml
Gadoteridol (ProHance, Bracco, Princeton, NJ) (52)	559	Macro-cyclic-nonionic	High	Not applicable
Gadobutrol Gd-BT-DO3A (Gadovist, Bayer Schering Pharma, Berlin, Germany) (53)	605	Macro-cyclic-nonionic	High	Not applicable
Gadoterate Gd-DOTA (Dotarem, Guerbet, Roissy, France) (54)	558	Macro-cyclic-nonionic	High	Not applicable
Gadofosveset trisodium (Ablavar, Lantheus Pharmaceuticals, Boston, MA) (55)	976	Linear-ionic; binds reversibly to serum albumin	High	Not applicable
Gadoxetic acid (Eovist, Bayer Healthcare, Wayne, NJ; Primovist, Bayer Healthcare, Berlin, Germany) (56)	725	Linear-ionic	High	Not applicable
Non-gadolinium-based contrast agents *FDA approved or discontinued				
Mangafodipar (Teslascan, Nycomed Amersham, Princeton, NJ) (57)	757	Manganese		fodipir, 0.25-mg/ml
Ferumoxide (Feridex IV, Berlex, Wayne, NJ) (58)	83, in 80 to 160-nm particles	Super-para-magnetic oxide particles		mannitol 61.3-mg, dextran 5.6– to 9.1-mg/ml

to traverse the placenta. Significant plasma protein binding favors maternal blood pool compartmentalization and placental blood pool localization without transplacental diffusion.

Most currently approved MRI contrast agents have a relatively low molecular weight and would be expected to readily cross the placental barrier (48-58) (**Table 5**). Massive doses of these agents have been shown to cause post-implantation fetal loss, delayed de-

Table 6. Safety of gadolinium-based MRI contrast agents in pregnancy*.

Retarded development without congenital abnormalities in rats (Magnevist, 2.5 X to 12.5 X human dose) and in rabbits (Magnevist, 7.5 to 12.5 X human dose for 12 days) (48).
Teratogenic in rabbits; microphthalmia/small eye and/or focal retinal fold in 3 fetuses from 3 litters (Multi-Hance, 6 X human dose during organogenesis, days 6 to 18) (49).
Increased intrauterine deaths in rabbits (MultiHance, 10 X human dose) (49).
No teratogenic effects or systemic toxicity or abnormal peri or post-natal birth, survival, growth, development or F1 generation fertility in rats (MultiHance, 3 X human dose) (49).
Skeletal and visceral abnormalities in rabbits (Omniscan, 5 X human dose) (50).
Reduced dam body weight and fetal "flexed" appendages and skeletal malformations (OmniScan, 0.6 X human dose for 13 days) (50).
No adverse effects in rats (OmniScan, 1.3 X human dose for 10 days) (50).
Maternal toxicity and reduced mean fetal weight, abnormal liver lobulation, delayed sternal ossification, and delayed behavioral development (startle reflex and air rights reflex) in rats (OptiMARK, 10 X human dose; gestation days 7 to 17). These effects were not observed at 1X human dose (51).
Forelimb flexures in rabbits (OptiMARK, 1 X human dose, gestation days 6 to 18) (51),
Malformed thoracic arteries, septal defect, and abnormal ventricle in rabbits (OptiMARK, 4 X human dose, gestation days 6 through 18) (51).
Postimplantation fetal loss doubled in rats (ProHance, 33 X human dose for 12 days) (52).
Increased spontaneous locomotor activity in rats (ProHance, 33 X human dose for 12 days) (52).
Increased spontaneous abortion and early delivery in rabbits (ProHance, 20 X human dose for 13 days) (52).
Radioactively labeled gadobutrol was detected in rabbit fetuses but not in rat fetuses (43).
No teratogenicity in rats, rabbits or cynomolgus monkeys (Gadovist, repeated doses) (53).
Delayed embryonal development in rats and rabbits and increased embryolethality in rats, rabbits and monkeys (Gadovist, repeated doses of 25 X to 50 X human dose) (53).
Fetal plasma level was 5% of maternal level in rats (Dotarem, gestation day 18) (54).
No evidence of embryotoxicity or teratogenicity in rats and rabbits (Dotarem, at 1.3 X (rats) or 2.4 X (rabbits) the human dose) (54).
Increased post-implantation loss, resorption, fetal death and maternal toxicity without fetal anomalies in rats and rabbits (Ablavar, at 11 X (rats) and 21.5 X (rabbits) the human dose) (55).
Embryotoxicity with increased post implantation loss and absorption and decreased litter size in rabbits (EOVIST, 26 X human dose) (56).
Maternal toxicity without teratogenicity in rats (EOVIST, 32 X human dose) (56).
Increased preimplantation loss in rats (EOVIST, 3.2 X human dose) (56).

* Data from package inserts of Magnevist, MultiHance, Omniscan, OptiMARK, ProHance, Gadovist, Dotarem, Ablavar, and EOVIST.

velopment, increased locomotive activity, and skeletal as well as visceral abnormalities in experimental animals [(48-56) (**Table 6**) and (57-58) (**Table 7**)]. Thus, the Food and Drug Administration generally lists MRI contrast agents as "PREGNANCY CATEGORY C". Statements such as "adequate and controlled studies in pregnant woman have not been conducted" and *this agent* "should only be used during pregnancy if the potential benefit jus-

Table 7. Safety of non-gadolinium-based MRI contrast agents in pregnancy (data from package inserts of Feridex and Teslascan).

Animal studies have shown that ^{54}Mn manganese crosses the placenta and locates in fetal liver and bones (57).
Increased skeletal malformations and decreased fetal body weight in rats (Teslascan, 2 to 8 X human dose gestation days 6 to 17 of gestation). No effects seen at 1 X human dose (57).
Increased post-implantation losses and resorption, and decreased fetal viability in rabbits, (Teslascan, 8 X to 10 X human dose days 6 to18 of gestation). No effects seen at 4 X human dose (57).
Teratogenicity in rabbits (Feridex, I.V, 6 X human dose) (58).

tifies the potential risk to the fetus" are typically noted in the package inserts for these products (48-58).

Because some of the effects described in animal experiments may be caused by the generic contrast agent, transmetallated gadolinium, or disassociated ligand moieties, for the purpose of this presentation, specific product names are presented rather than a generic contrast agent component, only for the adverse effects presented in **Table 6** and **Table 7**.

After intravenous administration of a gadolinium-based contrast agent, a portion of this substance will localize in the placental blood pool (59-62) (**Figure 1**). From there, a small portion will reach the fetus. If the fetal kidneys are developed (i.e., beyond seven weeks), the gadolinium chelate will be excreted into the fetal bladder (**Figure 2**), where it would be voided into the amniotic fluid. From there, the fetus would swallow some of the contrast material and it would pass through the fetal gut, eventually reentering the amniotic fluid (63-64). Based on postnatal animal studies that demonstrated less than 1% intestinal gadolinium chelate absorption (65-67), significant fetal intestinal absorption of gadolinium-based contrast agents might not be expected.

Conversely, fetal amniotic circulation may participate unpredictably in the breakdown and absorption of intact contrast agents and free gadolinium. Excess chelating ligand may be absorbed with potential fetotoxic effects as shown in **Table 6**. It is predictable that the dissociation of the gadolinium chelate bond will be greater with thermodynamically less stable MRI contrast agents (e.g., OmniScan, OptiMARK, and Magnevist) as compared to more stable agents (e.g., ProHance, MultiHance, and Doterem) and, thus, the latter three would be better choices for use when required in pregnant patients (69-70).

CLINICAL APPLICATIONS OF MRI PROCEDURES IN PREGNANT PATIENTS

Non-Pelvic Imaging

The pregnant patient is subject to most of the same brain, spine, body, and musculoskeletal conditions as the non-pregnant patient (71). In addition, abnormalities associated with pregnancy, such as toxemia and sagittal sinus thrombosis can occur. Furthermore, pituitary adenomas may show growth during pregnancy. Therefore, diagnostic imaging is frequently required with these conditions. Because MRI does not use ionizing radiation, it

Figure 1. Dynamic contrast enhancement of the placenta (arrows) in a 28-year-old pregnant woman at 30 weeks. Note the rapid, heterogeneous enhancement.

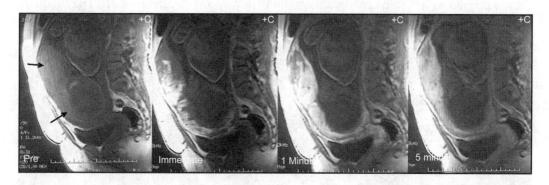

Figure 2. Contrast enhanced spoiled gradient echo MRI of the fetus at 32 weeks shows fetal renal enhancement, (arrows) (A, B, C) and fetal bladder (arrowheads) (D). Maternal kidney (k), bladder (b), placenta (p).

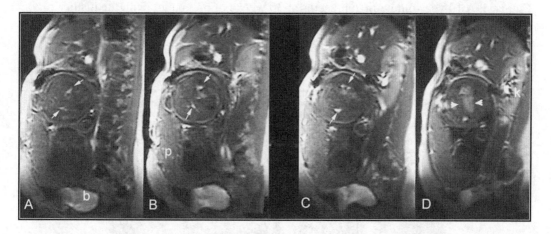

is particularly suited as an alternative to computed tomography (CT) in situations where ultrasound is either unsatisfactory and inappropriate.

Brain Imaging

Besides the specific brain conditions associated with pregnancy, other common cerebral abnormalities such as tumor, infarction, hemorrhage (**Figure 3**), demyelination, arteriovenous malformation, and aneurysm may occur during pregnancy (72). These are also best evaluated using MRI. MRI contrast agents should be reserved for patients in whom diagnosis (i.e., metastasis) or therapy (i.e., brain tumor therapy prior to surgery) is needed, immediately (**Figures 4** and **5**). Diffusion-weighted MR imaging is useful if acute cerebral infarction is suspected. MR angiography is helpful to screen for cerebral aneurysm in the pregnant patient with a family history of aneurysm in preparation for the stress of vaginal delivery.

Figure 3. A 23-year-old woman presents with severe headache and lethargy at 18 weeks of pregnancy. Axial T1 (A), T2 (B), FLAIR (C), and diffusion-weighted MR images (D) show a prominent left sided subdural hematoma (arrows) with midline shift. The subdural hematoma was evacuated and the patient improved. Non-traumatic subdural hematoma.

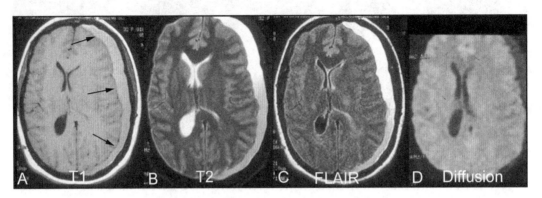

Figure 4. A 19-year-old woman presents at 30 weeks of pregnancy with the history of Chiari II congenital malformation. Sagittal TR-600, TE-20 images (A, B) demonstrate tonsillar herniation (arrows) and hydromyelia (arrowheads). Axial brain MRI (TR-2000, Effective TE-100) demonstrates hydrocephalus (C). Chiari II malformation.

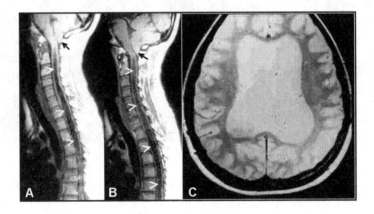

Spine Imaging

MRI should be reserved for specific cases of suspected disc extrusion in which surgery would be performed during the pregnancy. MRI is also appropriate for the evaluation of spinal tumor, unstable fracture, infection (73), syrinx (**Figure 4**), or vascular malformation, all of which may affect immediate therapy or mode of delivery (Caesarean section vs. vaginal).

Musculoskeletal Imaging

MRI is particularly useful in the evaluation of musculoskeletal abnormalities in selected patients in whom intervention is required during pregnancy. Routine knee and shoulder

Figure 5. This 24-year-old woman presents at 27 weeks of pregnancy with a right neck mass. Biopsy revealed low-grade lymphoma. Whole body ssFSE MRI shows extensive mediastinal adenopathy (arrows). No evidence of abdominal or pelvic disease. Gallstones and the fetus are seen. Lymphoma.

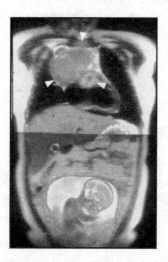

Figure 6. This 32 year-old woman presents with abdominal pain and elevated bilirubin at 12 weeks of pregnancy. Anterior and oblique MRCP projections (A to C) demonstrate innumerable gallstones (oval) and markedly dilated bile ducts, with one large obstruction common bile duct stone (circle). Incidentally noted are the fetal kidney and bladder (fb) and umbilical cord (uc). Choledocholithiasis.

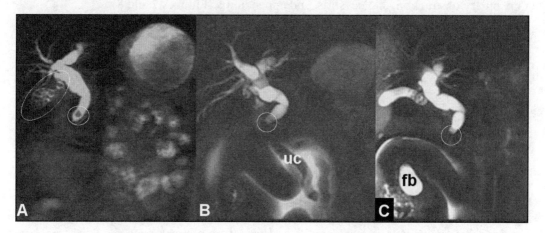

examinations can often be delayed until after delivery, but the evaluation of suspected infection or neoplasm must often be performed immediately (73).

Head and Neck Imaging

MRI of the head and neck may be advantageous as compared to CT because of its lack of ionizing radiation and lesser need for the use of contrast agents.

Chest and Cardiovascular Imaging

Hilar and mediastinal nodes can be shown easily with MRI without the use of ionizing radiation or contrast agents. Whole torso MRI examinations may be used to evaluate neoplasm staging in pregnancy (**Figure 5**). While echocardiography remains the standard non-invasive cardiac imaging modality of choice, particularly in the pregnant patient, MRI is ideal to demonstrate and confirm cardiovascular abnormalities such as coarctation of the aorta, aortitis, aortic dissection, and atrial myxoma (74-75). MRI may also be an alternative to CT pulmonary angiography for suspected pulmonary emboli in pregnancy (75).

Abdominal Imaging

Although sonography is the examination of choice for abdominal imaging in the pregnant patient, there has been considerable interest in the use of MRI for abdominal applications as an alternative to CT (76-84). The absence of ionizing radiation gives MRI an inherent advantage over CT, particularly to evaluate the liver, pancreas and retroperitonium. Large lesions such as tumors, pseudocysts, and abscesses are well shown with MRI. Fatty liver in pregnancy may also be evaluated with an MRI examination.

Masselli, et al. (82) demonstrated no significant difference between 61 MRI exams and 44 CT exams in comparable pregnant patients with acute abdominal symptoms (sensitivity 91% vs. 88%, specificity 85% vs. 90%, positive predictive value 81% vs. 91%, negative predictive value 94% vs. 85%, and diagnostic accuracy 88% vs. 88%, respectively) (82).

Specifically, MRI may be used effectively to evaluate the maternal urinary tract, biliary system (**Figure 6**), and appendix for suspected acute conditions including urinary obstruction, biliary obstruction, cholecystitis, and appendicitis (**Figures 7** and **8**).

Pelvic Imaging

Pregnancy can accelerate the growth of benign and malignant pelvic masses. A common diagnostic differential decision involves the separation of uterine abnormalities such as leiomyoma (**Figure 9**) from adnexal lesions, including ovarian cysts and neoplasms (**Figure 10**). Occasionally, ultrasound has difficulty with this distinction, particularly when larger lesions are present. MRI may better delineate and characterize these abnormalities (85-86). Breath-held images with relative T1- and T2-weighting are useful to localize and characterize lesions on MRI examinations.

MR angiography may be used to demonstrate pelvic arterial and venous vessels in the pregnant patient. An enlarged uterus may cause markedly reduced flow in the inferior vena cava and iliac veins with extensive collateral vessel formation during the third trimester. Two-dimensional, time-of-flight MR angiography with superior saturation shows these vessels exceptionally well. Normal fetal vessels may also be visualized with this technique.

Additionally, MRI may be useful to demonstrate pelvic abnormalities related specifically to pregnancy such as placenta previa, placenta acretea, abruptio placentae, chorioangioma, ectopic pregnancy, and abdominal pregnancy. MR-pelvimetry may be used as an alternative to radiographic or CT pelvimetry (87, 88).

Figure 7. This 27 year-old woman presented with right lower abdominal pain at 17 weeks of pregnancy. Coronal (A) ssFSE and sagittal (B) T2-weighted MR images demonstrate a dilated, fluid filled appendix with a thickened wall (arrows). The thickened, fluid filled appendix with surrounding inflammation (circled) is confirmed on axial FSPGR (C) and T2-weighted, FIESTA images (D). Acute appendicitis.

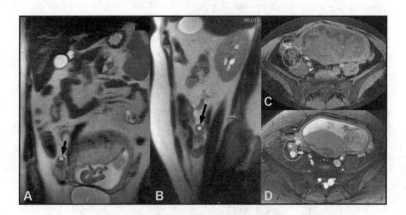

Figure 8. This 30 year-old woman presents at 6 weeks pregnancy with right lower abdominal pain and tenderness. Axial T2 ssFSE image demonstrates fluid within an intrauterine gestational sac (gs) and a fluid filled adjacent right lower quadrant appendiceal abscess (aa). Appendiceal abscess.

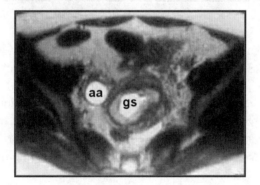

MRI of the Fetus

There have been a number of institutional review board approved, MRI investigations of fetal abnormalities (38, 89-133). Fetal sedation is no longer considered necessary to obtain good fetal MR images. While gross fetal motion may cause image degradation (**Figure 11**), much of the difficulty in fetal MRI is due to maternal respiration. Current techniques generally utilize breath-held MRI with single-shot, fast spin echo techniques (**Figure 12** and **Figure 13**) along with fast gradient refocused echo or fast spoiled gradient echo MRI techniques (101-133). Echo planar pulse sequences have also shown considerable success in fetal MRI (38).

Figure 9. This 34-year-old woman presented as "large for dates" at 12 weeks of pregnancy. Ultrasound showed a right mid abdominal complex mass. Coronal T1-weighted MR image demonstrates a relatively low signal pedunculated mass (*) connected to the gravid uterus (arrowheads) by a relatively narrow connection (arrows). Pedunculated leiomyoma.

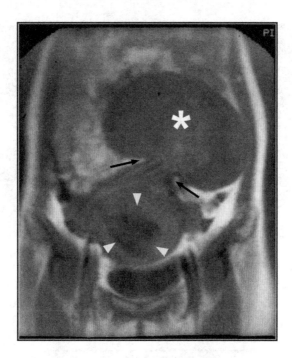

Because an abnormal fetus often has reduced fat due to growth retardation, MR images obtained in these fetuses may show relatively poor detail. Brain myelination *in-utero* may be demonstrated using T1- and T2-weighted MR images. Normal fetal structures such as the brain, face, spine, heart, liver, stomach, intestines, and bladder are seen routinely on MRI examinations. Frequently, the fetal genitalia are identified on MR images (**Figure 14**). Obviously, these structures are easier to evaluate in later pregnancy, although with higher quality, faster techniques, reasonable detail can be obtained by the mid-second trimester.

MRI can confirm most sonographically detected gross fetal abnormalities such as hydrocephalus, schizencephaly (**Figure 15**), anencephaly, meningocele, omphalocele, gastroschisis, and teratoma. Subtle anomalies, such as limb abnormalities are more difficult to detect, but even these are demonstrated occasionally with current imaging techniques. MRI provides information that is not readily apparent on sonography in approximately 10% of cases. This is most often seen in examination of the fetal brain but, again, with current techniques, occasionally fetal lungs, fetal diaphragm, fetal liver, and fetal kidneys may be better visualized using MRI.

It is particularly important to consider the added stress perceived by pregnant women undergoing MRI for the evaluation of possible fetal abnormalities. Ideally, comfortable po-

Figure 10. Pelvic ultrasound of this 25-year-old woman at 9 weeks of pregnancy demonstrated a 6 x 3 x 2-cm left adnexal mass. Axial TR-400, TE-20 (A) and TR-2200, TE-80 (B) images demonstrate a left adnexal mass (arrows) with fat signal on T1- and T2-weighted sequences. The gestational sac is noted (arrowheads). Dermoid.

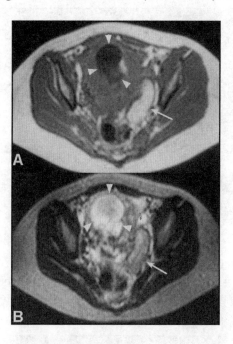

sitioning of pregnant patients should be individualized during the MRI examination. Noise protection should be optimized and rapid, efficient scanning should be carefully planned (134).

QUESTIONS TO CONSIDER PRIOR TO USING MRI IN A PREGNANT PATIENT

The decision to utilize MRI in the pregnant patient referred for diagnostic imaging involves answering a series of questions including, the following (71):

- Is imaging required?
- Is the patient pregnant?
- Is sonography satisfactory for diagnosis?
- Is MRI appropriate to address the clinical question?
- Can MRI be delayed until after delivery?
- Is obstetrical intervention prior to scanning a possibility?
- Is termination of pregnancy a consideration?
- Is early delivery a consideration?
- Is the use of an MRI contrast agent essential to diagnosis and treatment?

Figure 11. Thirty-two week fetus in a 22-year-old woman demonstrates gross fetal motion with marked positional changes seen in a repeat breath-held ssFSE coronal view at 30 minutes. Fetal movement.

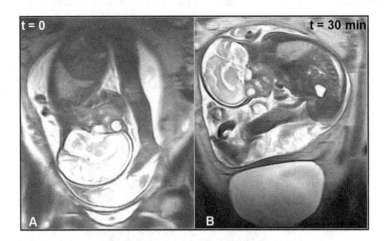

Figure 12. Twenty week twin gestation in a 30-year-old woman. Breath-held, 11-second ssFSE sagittal view shows demise of one twin with marked deformity (arrows). Incidentally noted are very large gallstones. Twins with demise of one fetus.

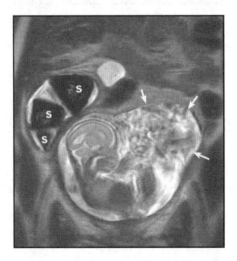

PREGNANT HEALTHCARE WORKERS IN THE MRI ENVIRONMENT

Pregnant healthcare workers occasional might find themselves within the MR system room during the performance of an MRI examination. Generally, there is little or no exposure to the time-varying and RF electromagnetic fields associated with MRI. The main exposure of the pregnant healthcare worker is to the powerful static magnetic field, with time and distance from the magnet being the major variations. The pregnant MRI technologist might be within a static magnetic field of several hundred gauss or more each working day

Figure 13. Axial breath-held 12-second ssFSE views show normal fetal anatomy at 28 weeks. Images at the level of the fetal midbrain (A), and pons (B) are seen.

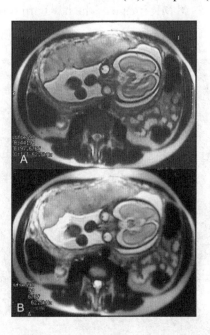

Figure 14. Fetal anatomy. Axial T1 weighted image (A) demonstrates the fetal heart; intraventricular septum (arrow), descending aorta (arrowhead), and right atrium (open arrow). Axial T1 weighted image (B) shows the fetal bladder (b) and high signal meconium filled rectum (r). Oblique reformatted ssFSE image (C) demonstrates low signal fetal liver and high signal meconium in the colon (c). Axial T2 FSE image demonstrates fetal testes and phallus (arrow).

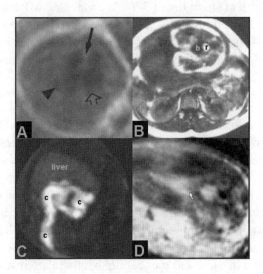

Figure 15. A coronal breath-held, 11-second ssFSE view (A, inverted for display) at 32 weeks of pregnancy shows agenesis of the corpus callosum and a large midline cleft (arrows). A sagittal TR-400, TE-18 MR image of the newborn on day 3 confirms these findings (B).

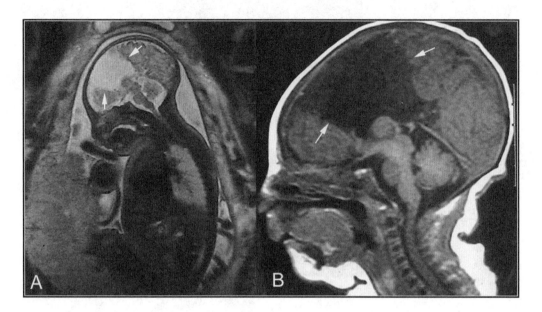

for prolonged periods of time. Although Kanal, et al. (39) reported that there is no increase in adverse outcomes of pregnancies in MRI workers, it may be reasonable to limit the amount of time spent by the pregnant worker within the MR system room. Thus, the pregnant physician or nurse anesthetist probably would be advised against monitoring the patient from within the scanner room or inside of the bore of the MR system during image acquisition. Particularly with field strengths of 3-Tesla or greater, MRI healthcare workers may experience vertigo-like sensations (135), especially when passing rapidly through spatial gradient magnetic fields near the magnet. While no evidence for injury has been demonstrated, it is reasonable to minimize such activities during pregnancy in consideration of taking a cautious approach to such situations.

Therefore, a policy is recommended that permits pregnant MRI technologists and other healthcare workers to perform MRI procedures, as well as to enter the MR system room, and attend to the patient during pregnancy, regardless of the trimester. Importantly, technologists and healthcare workers should not remain within the MR system room or magnet bore during the actual operation of the scanner. This later recommendation is especially important for those healthcare workers involved in patient management or interventional MRI-guided examinations and procedures, since it may be necessary for them to be directly exposed to the MR system's electromagnetic fields at levels similar to those used for patients. These recommendations are not based on indications of adverse effects, but rather, from a conservative point of view and the feeling that there are insufficient data pertaining to the effects of the other electromagnetic fields of the MR system to support or allow unnecessary exposures (12, 39).

CONCLUSIONS

MRI examinations should not be withheld from pregnant patients with the following conditions:

- With active brain or spine signs and symptoms requiring diagnostic imaging.
- With cancer requiring diagnostic imaging.
- With chest, abdomen, and pelvic signs and symptoms of active disease when sonography is non-diagnostic.
- In specific cases of suspected fetal anomaly, MRI may be helpful.

With regard to pregnant healthcare workers working in the MRI environment, especially the MR system room:

- These individuals have not been shown to be at increased risk of adverse outcomes from occupational exposures to static magnetic fields.
- Time in the scanner room should be minimized.

REFERENCES

1. Williams PM, Fletcher S. Health effects of prenatal radiation exposure. Am Fam Physician 2010;82:488–493.

2. Patel SJ, Reede DL, Katz DS, Subramaniam R, Amorosa JK. Imaging the pregnant patient for nonobstetric conditions: algorithms and radiation dose considerations. RadioGraphics 2007;27:1705–1722.

3. McCollough CH, Schueler BA, Atwell TD, et al. Radiation exposure and pregnancy: when should we be concerned? RadioGraphics 2007;27:909-917.

4. American College of Radiology. ACR practice guideline for imaging pregnant or potentially pregnant adolescents and women with ionizing radiation. Reston, VA: American College of Radiology, 2008.

5. Kanal E, Shellock FG, Sonnenblick D. MRI clinical site safety: Phase I results and preliminary data. Magn Reson Imaging 1988;1:106.

6. De Wilde JP, Rivers AW, Price DL. A review of the current use of magnetic resonance imaging in pregnancy and safety implications for the fetus. Prog Biophys Mol Biol 2005;87:335-353.

7. United States, Food and Drug Administration. Guidelines for Evaluating Electromagnetic Exposure Risk Trials of Clinical NMR Systems. Rockville, MD, Bureau of Radiological Health 1982.

8. Shellock FG, Kanal E. Policies, guidelines, and recommendations for MR imaging safety and patient management. J Magn Reson Imaging 1991;1:97-101.

9. Shellock FG, Kanal E. Magnetic Resonance Procedures and Pregnancy. In: Magnetic Resonance Bioeffects, Safety, and Patient Management, Second Edition. Philadelphia, New York: Lippincott-Ravin; 1996. Chapter 4.

10. Kanal E, Borgstede JP, Barkovich JA, et al. American College of Radiology white paper on MR safety. Amer J of Roentgenol 2002;178:1335–1347.

11. Kanal E, Barkovich JA, Bell C, et al. ACR guidance document for safe MR practices: 2007. Amer J of Roentgenol 2007;188:1447–1474.

12. Kanal E, Barkovich AJ, Bell C. et al. ACR guidance document on MR safe practices: 2013. J Magn Reson Imaging 2013;37:501-530.

13. Schaefer DJ. Safety aspects of radiofrequency power deposition in magnetic resonance. MRI Clin N Am 1998;6:775-789.

14. Hand JW, Li Y, Thomas EL, Rutherford MA, Hajnal JV. Numerical study of RF exposure and the resulting temperature rise in the foetus during a magnetic resonance procedure. Phys Med Biol 2010;55:913-930.

15. Nagaoka T, Togashi T, Saito K, et al. An anatomically realistic whole-body pregnant-woman model and specific absorption rates for pregnant-woman exposure to electromagnetic plane waves from 10 MHz to 2 GHz. Phys Med Biol 2007;52:6731–6745.

16. Dimbylow PJ, Nagaoka T, Xu XG. A comparison of foetal SAR in three sets of pregnant female models. Phys Med Biol 2009;54:2755–2767.

17. Hand JW, Li Y, Hajnal JV. Numerical study of RF exposure and the resulting temperature rise in the foetus during a magnetic resonance procedure. Phys Med Biol 2010;55:913–930.

18. Elder JE. Special senses. In: Elder JE, Cahill DP, Editors. Biological effects of radio-frequency radiation, 2nd Edition. US EPA, 1984. pp. 64-78.

19. Kikuchi S, Saito K, Takahashi M, Ito K. Temperature elevation in the fetus from electromagnetic exposure during magnetic resonance imaging. Phys Med Biol 2010;55:2411-2426.

20. Wilcox A, Weinberg C, O'Connor J, et al. Incidence of early loss of pregnancy. New Engl J Med 1988;319:189-194.

21. McRobbie D, Foster MA. Pulsed magnetic field exposure during pregnancy and implications for NMR foetal imaging: A study with mice. Magn Reson Imaging 1985;3:231-234.

22. Tesky GC, Ossenkopp KP, Prato FS, Sestini E. Survivability and long-term stress reactivity levels following repeated exposure to nuclear magnetic resonance imaging procedures in rats. Physiol Chem Phys Med NMR 1987;19:43-49.

23. Heinrichs WL, Fong P, Flannery M, et al. Midgestational exposure of pregnant BALB/c mice to magnetic resonance imaging conditions. Magn Reson Imaging 1988;6:305-313.

24. Kay HH, Herfkens RJ, Kay BK. Effect of magnetic resonance imaging on Xenopus laevis embryogenesis. Magn Reson Imaging 1988;6:501-506.

25. Tyndall DA. MRI effects on the teratogenicity of x-irradiation in the C57BL/6J mouse. Magn Reson Imaging 1990;8:423-433.

26. Murakami J, Toril Y, Masuda K: Fetal developmet of mice following intrauterine exposure to a static magnetic field of 6.3T. Magn Reson Imaging 1992;10:433-437.

27. Malko JA, Constatinidis I, Dillehay D, et al. Search for influence of 1.5T magnetic field on growth of yeast cells. Bioelectromagnetics 1987;15:495-501.

28. Yip YP, Capriotti C, Talagala SL, Yip JW. Effects of MR exposure at 1.5 T on early embryonic development of the chick. J Magn Reson Imaging 1994;4:742-748.

29. Yip YP, Capriotti C, Yip JW. Effects of MR exposure on axonal outgrowth in the sympathetic nervous system of the chick. J Magn Reson Imaging 1995;4:457 462.

30. Tablado L, Soler C, Nunez M, et al. Development of mouse testis and epididymis following intrauterine exposure to a static magnetic field. Bioelectromagnetics 2000;21: 19-24.

31. Ruckhäberle E, Nekolla SG, Ganter C, et al. In vivo intrauterine sound pressure and temperature measurements during magnetic resonance imaging (1.5 T) in pregnant ewes. Fetal Diagn Ther 2008;24:203-210.

32. Tyndall RJ, Sulik KK. Effects of magnetic resonance imaging on eye development in the C57BL/6J mouse. Teratology 1991;43:263-275.

33. Tyndall DA. MRI effects on craniofacial size and crown-rump length in C57BL/6J mice in 1.5T fields. Oral Surg Oral Med Oral Pathol 1993;76:655-660.

34. Yip YP, Capriotti C, Norbash SG, Talagala SL, Yip JW. Effects of MR exposure on cell proliferation and migration of chick motor neurons. J Magn Reson Imaging 1994;4:799-804.

35. Carnes KI, Magin RL. Effects of in utero exposure to 4.7T MR imaging conditions on fetal growth and testicular development in the mouse. Magn Reson Imaging 1996;14:263-274.

36. Nara VR, Howell RW, Goddu SM, et al. Effects of a 1.5T static magnetic field on spermatogenesis and embryogenesis in mice. Invest Radiol 1996;31:586-590.

37. Lee JW, Kim MS, Kim YJ, et al. Genotoxic effects of 3 T magnetic resonance imaging in cultured human lymphocytes. Bioelectromagnetics 2011;32:535-542.

38. Johnson IR, Stehling MK, Blamire A, et al. Study of the internal structure of the human fetus in utero by echo-planar magnetic resonance imaging. Am J Obstet Gynecol 1990;163:601-607.

39. Kanal E, Gillen J, Evans JA, et al. Survey of reproductive health among female MR workers. Radiology 1993;187:395-399.

40. Baker PN, Johnson IR, Harvey PR, et al. A three-year follow-up of children imaged in utero with echo-planar magnetic resonance. Am J Obstet Gynecol 170:32-33.

41. Myers C, Duncan KR, Gowland PA, et al. Failure to detect intrauterine growth restriction following in utero exposure to MRI. Br J Radiol 1998;71:549-551.

42. Vadeyar SH, Moore RJ, Strachan BK, et al. Effect of fetal magnetic resonance imaging on fetal heart rate patterns. Am J Obstet Gynecol 2000;182:666-669.

43. Kok RD, de Vries MM, Heerschap A, van den Berg PP. Absence of harmful effects of magnetic resonance exposure at 1.5 T in utero during the third trimester of pregnancy: a follow-up study. Magn Reson Imaging 2004;22:851-854.

44. Reeves MJ, Brandreth M, Whitby EH, et al. Neonatal cochlear function: measurement after exposure to acoustic noise during in utero MR imaging. Radiology 2010;257:802-809.

45. Syme MR, Paxton JW, Keelan JA. Drug transfer and metabolism by the human placenta. Clin Pharmacokinet 2004;43:487–514.

46. Pacifici GM, Nottoli R. Placental transfer of drugs administered to the mother. Clin Pharmacokinet 1995;28:235-269.

47. Ni Z, Mao Q. ATP-binding cassette efflux transporters in human placenta. Curr Pharm Biotechnol 2011;12:674–685.

48. Magnevist package insert: http://labeling.bayerhealthcare.com/html/products/pi/MagnevistPBP_PI.pdf

49. MultiHance package insert: http://www.multihanceusa.com/Shared%20Documents/MultiHance_Combined_PI.pdf

50. OmniScan package insert: http://www.fda.gov/downloads/AdvisoryCommittees/CommitteesMeetingMaterials/Drugs/DrugSafetyandRiskManagementAdvisoryCommittee/UCM192009.pdf

51. OptiMARK package insert: http://www.mallinckrodt.com/webforms/threecolumn.aspx?id=497&view=faq

52. ProHance package insert: http://www.multihanceusa.com/Shared%20Documents/ ProHance_Combined_PI.pdf.

53. Gadovist package insert: http://www.bayerresources.com.au/resources/uploads/PI/file9345.pdf

54. Dotarem package insert: http://www.medicines.org.au/files/aspdotar.pdf

55. ABLAVAR package insert: http://www.ablavar.com/docs/PI_ABLAVAR_US_515952-0211_(8.5x11)_v6_11Apr11.pdf

56. EOVIST package insert: http://labeling.bayerhealthcare.com/html/products/pi/Eovist_PI.pdf

57. Teslascan package insert: http://md.gehealthcare.com/shared/pdfs/pi/teslascan.pdf

58. Feridex IV package insert: http://www.drugs.com/pro/feridex.html

59. Salomon LJ, Siauve N, Balvay D, et al. Placental perfusion MR imaging with contrast agents in a mouse model. Radiology 2005;235:73–80.

60. Taillieu F, Salomon LJ, Siauve N, et al. Placental perfusion and permeability: simultaneous assessment with dual-echo contrast-enhanced MR imaging in mice. Radiology 2006;241:737–745.

61. Marcos HB, Semelka RC, Worawattanakul S. Normal placenta: gadolinium-enhanced dynamic MR imaging. Radiology 1997;205:493–496.

62. Tanaka YO, Sohda S, Shigemitsu S, Niitsu M, Itai Y. High temporal resolution dynamic contrast MRI in a high risk group for placenta accreta. Magn Reson Imaging 2001;19:635–642.

63. Novak Z, Thurmond AS, Ross PL, Jones MK, Thornburg KL, Katzberg RW. Gadolinium-DTPA transplacental transfer and distribution in fetal tissue in rabbits. Invest Radiol 1993;28:828–830.

64. Muhler MR, Clément O, Salomon LJ, et al. Maternofetal pharmacokinetics of a gadolinium chelate contrast agent in mice. Radiology 2011;258:455-460.

65. Weinmann HJ, Brasch RC, Press WR, Wesbey GE. Characteristics of gadolinium-DTPA complex: a potential NMR contrast agent. AJR Am J Roentgenol 1984;142:619-624.

66. Okazaki O, Murayama N, Masubuchi N, Nomura H, Hakusui H. Placental transfer and milk secretion of gadodiamide injection in rats. Arzneimittelforschung 1996;46:83–86.

67. Hylton NM. Suspension of breast-feeding following gadopentetate dimeglumine administration. Radiology 2000;216:325-326.

68. Junkermann H. Indications and contraindications for contrast-enhanced MRI and CT during pregnancy. Radiology 2007;47:774-777.

69. Garcia-Bournissen F, Shrim A, Koren G. Safety of gadolinium during pregnancy. Can Fam Physician 2006;52:309-310.

70. Webb JA, Thomsen HS, Morcos SK, et al. The use of iodinated and gadolinium contrast media during pregnancy and lactation. Eur Radiol 2005;15:1234-1240.

71. Colletti PM, Sylvestre PB. Magnetic resonance imaging in pregnancy. MRI Clin N Am 1994;2: 291-307.

72. Semere LG, McElrath TF, Klein AM. Neuroimaging in pregnancy: a review of clinical indications and obstetric outcomes. J Matern Fetal Neonatal Med 2012;1-31.

73. Wilbur AC, Langer BG, Spigos DG. Diagnosis of sacroiliac joint infection in pregnancy by magnetic resonance imaging. Magn Reson Imaging 1988;6:341-343.

74. Ain DL, Narula J, Sengupta PP. Cardiovascular imaging and diagnostic procedures in pregnancy. Cardiol Clin 2012;30:331-341.

75. Colletti PM, Lee KH, Elkayam U. Cardiovascular imaging of the pregnant patient. AJR Am J Roentgenol 2013;200:1–7.

76. Birchard KR, Brown MA, Hyslop WB, et al. MRI of acute abdominal and pelvic pain in pregnant patients. AJR Am J Roentgenol 2005;184:452-458.

77. Pedrosa I, Levine D, Eyvazzadeh AD, et al. MR imaging evaluation of acute appendicitis in pregnancy. Radiology 2006;238:891-899.

78. Oto A. MR imaging evaluation of acute abdominal pain during pregnancy. Magn Reson Imaging Clin N Am 2006;14:489-501.

79. Singh A, Danrad R, Hahn PF, Blake MA, et al. MR imaging of the acute abdomen and pelvis: acute appendicitis and beyond. Radiographics 2007;27:1419-1431.

80. Oto A, Ernst RD, Ghulmiyyah LM, Nishino TK, et al. MR imaging in the triage of pregnant patients with acute abdominal and pelvic pain. Abdom Imaging 2009;34:243-250.

81. Singh AK, Desai H, Novelline RA. Emergency MRI of acute pelvic pain: MR protocol with no oral contrast. Emerg Radiol. 2009;16:133-141.

82. Masselli G, Brunelli R, Casciani E, et al. Acute abdominal and pelvic pain in pregnancy: MR imaging as a valuable adjunct to ultrasound? Abdom Imaging 2011;36:596-603.

83. Long SS, Long C, Lai H, Macura KJ. Imaging strategies for right lower quadrant pain in pregnancy. AJR Am J Roentgenol 2011;196:4–12.

84. Baron KT, Arleo EK, Robinson C, Sanelli PC. Comparing the diagnostic performance of MRI versus CT in the evaluation of acute nontraumatic abdominal pain during pregnancy. Emerg Radiol 2012;19:519-25.

85. Weinreb JC, Brown CE, Lowe TW, et al. Pelvic masses in pregnant patients: MR and US imaging. Radiology 1986;159:717-724.

86. McCarthy SM, Stark DD, Filly RA, et al. Uterine neoplasms: MR imaging. Radiology 1989;170:125-128.

87. Stark DD, McCarthy SM, Filly RA, et al. Pelvimetry by magnetic resonance imaging. AJR Am J Roentgenol 1985;144:947-950.

88. Michel SC, Rake A, Götzmann L, et al. Pelvimetry and patient acceptability compared between open 0.5-T and closed 1.5-T MR systems. Eur Radiol 2002;12:2898–2905.

89. Angtuaco TL, Shah HR, Mattison DR, et al. MR imaging in high-risk obstetric patients: A valuable complement to US. Radiographics 1992;12:91-109.

90. Benson RC, Colletti PM, Platt LD, et al. MR imaging of fetal anomalies. AJR Am J Roentgenol 1991;156:1205-1207.

91. Brown CEL, Weinreb JC. Magnetic resonance imaging appearance of growth retardation in a twin pregnancy. Obstet Gynecol 1988;71:987.

92. Carswell H. Fast MRI of fetus yields considerable anatomic detail. Diag Imaging 1988:11-12.

93. Catizone FA, Gesmundo G, Montemagno R, et al. The non-invasive methods of prenatal diagnosis: the role of ultrasound and MRI. J Perinat Med 1991;19:42-49.

94. Colletti PM, Platt LD. When to use MRI in obstetrics. Diag Imaging 1989;11:84-88.

95. De Clyn K, Degryse H, Slangen T, et al. MRI in the prenatal diagnosis of bilateral renal agenesis. Fortschr Rontgenstr Ger 1989;150:104-105.

96. Deans HE, Smith FW, Lloyd DJ, et al. Fetal fat measurement by magnetic resonance imaging. Br J Radiol 1989;62:603-607.

97. Dinh DH, Wright RM, Hanigan WC. The use of magnetic resonance imaging for the diagnosis of fetal intracranial anomalies. Child Nerv Syst 1990;6:212-215.

98. Dunn RS, Weiner SN. Antenatal diagnosis of sacrococcygeal teratoma facilitated by combined use of Doppler sonography and MR imaging. AJR 1991;156:1115-1116.

99. Fitamorris-Glass R, Mattrey RF, Cantrell CJ. Magnetic resonance imaging as an adjunct to ultrasound in oligohydramnios. J Ultrasound Med 1989;8:159-162.

100. Fraser R. Magnetic resonance imaging of the fetus: Initial experience [letter]. Gynecol Obstet Invest 1990;29:255-258.

101. Gardens AS, Weindling AM, Griffiths RD, et al. Fast-scan magnetic resonance imagin of fetal anomalies. Br J Obstet Gynecol 1991;98:1217-1222.

102. Hill MC, Lande IM, Larsen JW Jr. Prenatal diagnosis of fetal anomalies using ultrasound and MRI. Radiol Clin North Am 1988;26:287-307.

103. Horvath L, Seeds JW. Temporary arrest of fetal movement with pancuronium bromide to enable antenatal magnetic resonance imagin of holosencephaly. AJR Am J Roentgenol 1989;6:418-420.

104. Lenke RR, Persutte WH, Nemes JM. Use of pancuronium bromide to inhibit fetal movement during magnetic resonance imaging. J Reprod Med 1989;34:315-317.

105. Mansfield P, Stehling MK, Ordidge RJ, et al. Study of internal structure of the human fetus in utero at 0.5T. Br J Radiol 1990;13:314-318.

106. Mattison DR, Angtuaco T, Miller FC, et al. Magnetic resonance imaging in maternal and fetal medicine. J Perinatol 1989;9:411-419.

107. Mattison DR, Angtuaco T. Magnetic resonance imaging in pernatal diagnosis. Clin Obstet Gynecol 1988;31:353-389.

108. Mattison DR, Kay HH, Miller RK, et al. Magnetic resonance imaging: A noninvasive tool for fetal and placental physiology. Biol Reprod 1988;38:39-49.

109. McCarthy SM, Filly RA, Stark DD, et al. Magnetic resonance imaging of fetal anomalies in utero: Early experience. AJR Am J Roentgenol 1985;145:677-682.

110. McCarthy SM, Filly RA, Stark DD, et al. Obstetrical magnetic resonance imaging: fetal anatomy. Radiology 1985;154:427-432.

111. Powell MC, Worthington BS, Buckley JM, et al. Magnetic resonance imaging (MRI) in obstetrics II. Fetal anatomy. Br J Obstet Gynaecol 1988;95:38-46.

112. Smith FW. Magnetic resonance tomography of the pelvis. Cardiovasc Intervent Radiol 1986;8:367-376.

113. Smith FW, Kent C, Abramovich DR, et al. Nuclear magnetic resonance imaging – a new look at the fetus. Br J Gynaecol 1985;92:1024-1033.

114. Smith FW, Sutherland HW: Magnetic resonance imaging: the use of the inversion recovery sequence to display fetal morphology. Br J Radiol 1988;61:338-341.

115. Stehling MK, Mansfield P, Ordidge RJ, et al. Echoplanar magnetic resonance imaging in abnormal pregnancies. Lancet 1989:157.

116. Toma P, Lucigrai G, Dodero P, et al. Prenatal detection of an abdominal mass by MR imaging performed while the fetus is immobilized with pancuronium bromide. AJR Am J Roentgenol 1990;154:1049-1050.

117. Toma P, Lucigrai G, Ravegnai M, et al. Hydrocephalus and porencephaly: prenatal diagnosis by ultrasonography and MR imaging. JCAT 1990;14:843-845.

118. Turner Rj, Hankins GVD, Weinreb JC, et al. Magnetic resonance imaging and ultrasonography in antenatal evaluation of cojoined twins. Am J Obstet Gynecol 1986;77:529-532.

119. Vila-Coro AA, Dominguez R. Intrauterine diagnosis of hydroencephaly by magnetic resonance imaging. Magn Reson Imaging 1989;7:105-107.

120. Weinreb JC, Lowe T, Cohen JM, et al. Human fetal anatomy: MR imaging. Radiology 1985;157:715-720.

121. Weinreb JC, Lowe T, Santos-Ramos R, et al. Magnetic resonance imaging in obstetric diagnosis. Radiology 1985;154:157-161.

122. Wenstrom KD, Williamson RA, Weiner CP, et al. Magnetic resonance imaging of fetuses with intracranial defects. Obstet Gynecol 1991;77:529-532.

123. Williamson RA, Weiner CP, Yuh WTC, et al. Magnetic resonance imaging of anomalous fetuses. Obstet Gynecol 1988;71:952-956.

124. Levine D, Hatabu H, Gan J, et al. Fetal anatomy revealed with fast MR sequences. AJR Am J Roentgenol 1996;167:905-908.

125. Garden AS, Griffiths RD, Weindling AM, et al. Fast-scan magnetic resonance imaging in fetal visualization. Am J Obstet Gynecol 1991;164:1190-1196.

126. Amin RS, Nikolaids P, Kawashima A, et al. Normal anatomy of the fetus at MR imaging. Radiographics 1999;19:S201-214.

127. Huppert BJ, Brandt KR, Ramin KD, et al. Single-shot fast spin echo MR imaging of the fetus: a pictorial essay. Radiographics 1999;19:S215-227.

128. Levine D, Barnes PD, Sher S, et al. Fetal fast MR imaging: reproducibility, technical quality, and conspicuity of anatomy. Radiology 1998;206:549-554.

129. Levine D, Barnes PD, Edelman RR. Obstetric MR imaging. Radiology 1999;211:609-617.

130. Yanashita Y, Namimoto T, Abe Y, et al. MR imaging of the fetus by HASTE sequence. AJR Am J Roentgenol 1997;168:513-519.

131. Colletti PM. Computer-assisted imaging of the fetus with magnetic resonance imaging. Comput Med Imaging Graph 1996;20:491-496.

132. Levine D. Obstetric MRI. J Magn Reson Imaging 2006;24:1–15.

133. Tsuchiya K, Katase S, Seki T, et al. Short communication: MR imaging of fetal brain abnormalities using HASTE sequence. Br J Radiol 1996;69: 668-670.

134. Leithner K, Pornbacher S, Assem-Hilger E, et al. Psychological reactions in women undergoing fetal magnetic resonance imaging. Obstet Gynecol 2008;111:396–402.

135. Glover PM, Cavin I, Qian W, Bowtell R, Gowland PA. Magnetic-field-induced vertigo: a theoretical and experimental investigation. Bioelectromagnetics 2007;28:349-361.

Chapter 10   Identification and Management of Acute Reactions to Gadolinium-Based Contrast Agents

ALBERTO SPINAZZI, M.D.

Senior Vice President
Global Medical and Regulatory Affairs
Bracco Group
Monroe, NJ

INTRODUCTION

The use of gadolinium-based contrast agents (GBCAs) in magnetic resonance imaging (MRI) has increased considerably over recent decades with the emergence of new clinical applications. Present estimates suggest that 15% to 35% of all MRI examinations use a GBCA agent (1). Currently, there are nine GBCAs approved for intravenous use in various countries throughout the world: Magnevist (gadopentetate dimeglumine), ProHance (gadoteridol), Omniscan (gadodiamide), OptiMARK (gadoversetamide), MultiHance (gadobenate dimeglumine), Eovist/Primovist (gadoxetic acid), Ablavar (gadofosveset), Gadavist/Gadovist (gadobutrol), and Dotarem (gadoterate meglumine). Although these agents are generally well-tolerated, adverse reactions can occur after their administration, particularly in patients with underlying risk factors.

"Adverse reactions" are defined by all regulatory authorities as noxious and unintended responses to a medicinal product (2). All medicinal products can produce an adverse reaction in someone who has been exposed to them. GBCAs, though generally safe and well tolerated, are no exception. Importantly, adverse reactions can occur after their administration, particularly in patients with underlying risk factors.

Acute reactions are defined as undesirable side effects that occur less than 60 minutes post-contrast agent exposure (3). They typically fall into the category of hypersensitivity reactions and are either allergic or allergy-like in nature (4). These latter two reactions are clinically indistinguishable due to their symptomatic similarities, however, they vastly differ mechanistically. Allergy-like reactions lack immunological specificity and do not require previous exposure to the triggering antigen to elicit a response. Conversely, allergic reactions are characterized by immunological specificity and transferability. In cases of allergic re-action, a patient's immune system is able to recognize and mount an immune response against an antigen, particularly due to subsequent exposures to the same antigen. Allergy-like reactions are not associated with immunological specificity but with direct release of histamine and other mediators from activated mast cells and circulating basophils and eosinophils, activation of the contact and complement systems, conversion of L-arginine into nitric oxide, and activation of the XII clotting system leading to the production of bradykinin (4). Current clinical evidence shows that most acute reactions to GBCAs are al-lergy-like in nature. However, cases of true allergic reactions to GBCAs have been published in the literature (4-6).

The symptoms that patients present with can vary in severity, as demonstrated by the categories shown in **Table 1**. According to the approved prescribing information of the com-mercially available GBCAs, the most frequent acute reactions that occur after administration are headache, nausea with or without vomiting, injection site reactions, dizziness, localized rash, and pruritus (incidence rate, 1 to 5%) (7-15). Most (i.e., greater than 75%) acute re-actions associated with GBCAs do not require specific treatment and are transient in nature. However, more severe and possibly life-threatening reactions may rarely occur (less than 1 in every 20,000 administered doses) (16-23). Serious adverse reactions may also have a fatal outcome, especially if they are not promptly and properly treated (4, 22). This chapter aims to provide information on the following: how to identify patients who may be at risk for developing serious acute reactions, how to properly assess the risks and benefits of using GBCAs in individual patients, the preventative measures that should be adopted and when; how to promptly recognize the type of reaction, and the treatments that are recommended for patients experiencing serious adverse reactions.

WHAT TO DO BEFORE THE EXAM

To prevent or minimize complications following administration of GBCAs, the follow-ing five steps should be followed before any exam: (1) be aware of possible complications; (2) know your patient; (3) assess risk/benefit of contrast administration; (4) adopt preven-tative measures, if and when necessary; and (5) be prepared to manage any adverse reac-tion.

(1) Be Aware of Possible Complications

Before using a GBCA, all personnel should be familiar with all the possible risk factors and be knowledgeable about all the possible adverse events that may occur after the admin-istration of the GBCA to be used. This can be achieved by carefully reading the prescribing information, being fluent with the relevant literature and, if needed, requesting specific safety information from the manufacturer.

(2) Know Your Patient

Before administering a GBCA, the healthcare professionals responsible for the proce-dure should be aware of the patient's conditions, including the main known/suspected dis-eases and any eventual co-morbidities. They should also identify any possible risk factors and ensure all medications the patient is taking have been identified. Patients at risk for de-

Table 1. Severity of acute adverse reactions to gadolinium-based contrast agents (adapted from references 3 and 4).

Mild
- Nausea, mild vomiting
- Urticaria
- Itching
- Cough
- Warmth
- Headache
- Dizziness
- Shaking
- Anxiety
- Altered taste
- Pallor
- Flushing
- Chills
- Sweats
- Rash
- Nasal stuffiness
- Swelling of eyes or face

Moderate
- Severe vomiting
- Marked urticaria
- Tachycardia/bradycardia
- Hypertension
- Generalized or diffuse erythema
- Dyspnea
- Mild hypotension
- Bronchospasm, wheezing
- Facial/laryngeal edema
- Vaso-vagal attack

Severe
- Hypotensive shock
- Respiratory arrest
- Cardiac arrest
- Convulsion
- Unresponsiveness
- Severe or rapidly progressing laryngeal edema
- Profound hypotension
- Clinically manifested arrhythmias

veloping acute reactions include those who have experienced prior reactions to a GBCA (3, 4, 20). These patients are eight-times more likely to experience subsequent reactions, the severity of which may be greater than that of previous reactions (4, 24). Patients with underlying asthma or allergic diatheses, including hypersensitivity to food, chemicals or other medications, are also considered to be at increased risk, with incidence rates reported as high as 3.7% (4, 24). Although there is no cross-reactivity, patients with known hypersensitivity to other types of medical imaging agents should be considered at higher risk for the development of hypersensitivity reactions to GBCAs.

Patients receiving treatment with beta-adrenergic blockers are also at increased risk for experiencing hypersensitivity reactions due to an increase in the release of mediators involved in anaphylaxis (25). Of note, in the event a severe hypersensitivity reaction occurs, beta-blocking agents may decrease the cardiovascular compensatory changes to the anaphylactic shock and epinephrine (adrenaline) may be ineffective or promote paradoxical reflex vagotonic effects when using epinephrine to resolve the reaction (25-29). As a preventative measure, a questionnaire may be developed and used to identify any possible risk factor and best assess risk of GBCA use in individual patients. Attention should be also given to the emotional state of patients (4). Anxiety may cause panic attacks with symptoms that may mimic anaphylaxis. Severe adverse effects to contrast media or to procedures can be mitigated at least in part by reducing anxiety (4).

(3) Assess Risk-Benefit

The benefits and risks of an MRI examination with the addition of a GBCA should be evaluated on an individual basis for each patient and possibly documented. Patients should be properly informed about those risks and benefits and provided with written informed consent.

(4) Adopt Preventative Measures, If And When Necessary

There are no widely accepted policies for dealing with patients who have experienced prior reactions to GBCAs and the need for subsequent exposure to the same or other GBCAs. However, the best approach to prevent any reaction is to avoid the trigger altogether. The prescribing information of each GBCA contraindicates their use in cases of known hypersensitivity to the active ingredient or any of its excipients. Therefore, in the event a patient who experiences an acute reaction to a GBCA requires a future MRI, every effort should be made to determine if a GBCA is absolutely necessary, and if so, identify the specific GBCA that elicited the initial reaction and a different agent be selected and used.

Premedication with corticosteroids and antihistamines should be considered for patients with history of previous hypersensitivity reactions to contrast agents, allergies or known hypersensitivity to drugs or chemicals (**Table 2**) (3, 4). Oral corticosteroids should be used with caution in patients with uncontrolled hypertension, diabetes, active tuberculosis, systemic fungal infections, active peptic ulcer, or diverticulitis. The relative risk for the use of corticosteroids compared to the likelihood of severe or fatal contrast reaction must be considered. Hypersensitivity to oral steroids is rare, but should always be ruled out. It is important to note that such regimens may reduce the frequency or severity of reactions but are not always effective as breakthrough reactions have been observed after GBCA administration in pre-medicated patients (20, 30).

(5) Be Prepared to Manage Any Adverse Reaction

Prerequisites to managing acute reactions include properly trained personnel and well-designed treatment plans. Personnel should be trained to rapidly recognize and assess reactions, and take all the necessary steps to initiate appropriate treatment. In addition, all MRI facilities should have available basic equipment and medications needed to treat acute re-

Table 2. Suitable pre-medication regimens (adapted from references 4 and 30).

Regimen	Drug and Timing	Adult Dose	Pediatric Dose
Option 1	Prednisone given at 13, 7, and 1 hour before GBCA, **plus**	50-mg PO	0.5 to 0.7-mg/kg PO (up to 50-mg)
	Diphenhydramine 1 hour before GBCA	50-mg PO	1.25-mg/kg PO (up to 50-mg)
Option 2	Methylprednisolone 12 and 2 hours before GBCA, **plus**	32-mg PO	N/A
	Diphenhydramine 1 hour before GBCA (optional)	50-mg PO	N/A

GBCA = gadolinium-based contrast agent; N/A = not applicable; PO = orally
Note: Suitable intravenous doses may be substituted for patients unable to take medication orally.

actions. As shown in **Table 3**, this list includes but is not limited to equipment such as a stethoscope, sphygmomanometer, blood pressure and pulse monitor, syringes and needles, as well as medications such as epinephrine, diphenhydramine, and beta-agonist inhalers (3, 4). MRI facilities should institute periodic monitoring programs to verify functionality of equipment and confirm all medications are within expiry date limits. It is also imperative to maintain up-to-date personnel training with documented review sessions and assessments.

WHAT TO DO DURING THE EXAM

During the exam, especially if a GBCA is administered to at-risk patients, use the minimum effective dose of contrast. Mild reactions, such as nausea and vomiting, are usually self-limiting and do not require treatment (3, 4). Patients who experience mild reactions should be monitored for approximately 30-minutes post-GBCA exposure, or longer if necessary, to ensure there is no progression of signs and symptoms (4). Moderate reactions can be more pronounced symptoms of reactions that fall under the mild category, or they can present as other clinically significant reactions that require specific treatment. Patients suspected of experiencing a moderate reaction should have their vital signs closely monitored to make certain that progression to a severe event is avoided. Severe reactions are rare but of utmost concern since they may be life-threatening. While they rarely occur, immediate recognition and treatment are necessary. In many cases, life-threatening events begin with mild signs and symptoms, and then rapidly evolve to a severe reaction. As a result, it is imperative that practitioners monitor all patients receiving a GBCA closely during the procedure.

Distinguishing between vagal reactions and hypersensitivity reactions, particularly those presenting as hypotension with tachycardia, is also critical since the approach to treatment is markedly different. Also known as neurally-mediated syncope, vagal reactions are char-

Table 3. Equipment and medications supply list for patient examination room or emergency carts (adapted from references 3 and 4).

Equipment	Medications
Oxygen	Epinephrine 1:1,000 (1-mL for SC/IM injection)
Suction (wall-mounted or portable), tubing and	or IM auto-injector
catheters	Epinephrine 1:10,000 (10-mL preloaded syringe for
Oral airways	IV injection)
"Ambu"-type bag	Atropine
Endotracheal tubes	Beta-agonist metered dose inhaler
Stethoscope, sphygmomanometer, tourniquets,	Diphenhydramine
tongue depressor	Nitroglycerin
One-way mouth breather apparatus	Aspirin
IV fluids (normal saline or Ringer's solution)	Anti-convulsive drugs
Syringes and needles of varying sizes	
Tracheostomy set, cut-down trays with sterile	
instruments	
On Emergency Cart or Immediately Available	
Defibrillator	Blood pressure/pulse monitor
Electrocardiogram	Pulse oximeter (optional)

IM = intramuscular; IV = intravenous; SC = subcutaneous

Table 4. Management of acute reactions to gadolinium-based contrast agents in adult patients (adapted from references 3 and 4).

Nausea/Vomiting

1. Transient: Supportive treatment
2. Severe, protracted: Appropriate antiemetic drugs should be considered

Urticaria

1. Discontinue injection if not completed
2. No treatment necessary in most cases
3. ACR guidelines:
   - Administer H_1-receptor blocker: Diphenhydramine PO/IM/IV 25 to 50-mg
   - If severe or widely disseminated: Give α-agonist (arteriolar and venous constriction): epinephrine SC (1:1,000) 0.1 to 0.3-mL (0.1 to 0.3-mg) (if no cardiac contraindications)
4. ESUR guidelines:
   - Scattered, transient: Supportive treatment including observation
   - Scattered, protracted: H_1-receptor blocker IM or IV should be considered
   - Generalized: H_1-receptor blocker IM or IV. Consider epinephrine IM (1:1,000) 0.1 to 0.3-mL (0.1 to 0.3-mg). Repeat as needed

Facial or Laryngeal Edema

1. Administer oxygen 6 to 10-L/min via mask
2. ACR guidelines:
   - Administer alpha-agonist (arteriolar and venous constriction): Epinephrine SC or IM (1:1,000) 0.1 to 0.3-mL (0.1 to 0.3-mg) or, especially if hypotension is evident, epinephrine (1:10,000) slowly IV – 3-mL (0.1 to 0.3-mg)
   - Repeat as needed to a maximum of 1-mg
   - If not responsive to therapy or if there is no obvious acute laryngeal edema, seek appropriate assistance (cardiopulmonary arrest response team)
3. ESUR guidelines (laryngeal edema):
   - Epinephrine IM (1:1,000) 0.5-mL (0.5-mg). Repeat as needed

Bronchospasm

1. Administer O_2 6 to 10-L/min via mask. Monitor: Electrocardiogram, O_2 saturation, and blood pressure
2. Administer beta-agonist inhalers (bronchiolar dilators such as metaproterenol, terbutaline, or albuterol) 2 to 3 puffs; repeat as necessary. If unresponsive to inhalers, use SC, IM, or IV epinephrine.
3. ACR guidelines:
   - Administer epinephrine SC or IM (1:1,000) 0.1 to 0.3-mL (0.1 to 0.3-mg) or, especially if hypotension is evident, epinephrine (1:10,000) slowly IV 1 to 3 mL (0.1 to 0.3-mg)
   - Repeat as needed to a maximum of 1-mg
   - Call for assistance (cardiopulmonary arrest response team) if severe bronchospasm or if O_2 saturation <88% persists
4. ESUR guidelines:
   - Normal blood pressure: Epinephrine IM (1:1,000) 0.1 to 0.3-mL (0.1 to 0.3-mg). Use smaller doses in patients with CAD or if elderly
   - Decreased blood pressure: Epinephrine IM (1:1,000) 0.5-mL (0.5-mg)

Hypotension with Tachycardia

1. Legs elevated 60-degrees or more (preferred) or Trendelenburg position
2. Monitor: Electrocardiogram, pulse oximeter, blood pressure
3. Administer O_2 6 to10-L/min (via mask)
4. Rapid IV administration of large volumes of Ringer's lactate or normal saline
5. ACR guidelines:

- If poorly responsive: Epinephrine (1:10,000) slowly IV 1-mL (0.1-mg)
- Repeat as needed to a maximum of 1-mg
- If still poorly responsive seek appropriate assistance (cardiopulmonary arrest response team)
6. ESUR guidelines (isolated hypotension):
   - If unresponsive: Epinephrine IM (1:1,000) 0.5-mL (0.5-mg). Repeat as needed

Hypotension with Bradycardia (Vagal Reaction)

1. Secure airway: give O_2 6 to 10-L/min (via mask)
2. Monitor vital signs
3. Legs elevated 60-degrees or more (preferred) or Trendelenburg position
4. Secure IV access: Rapid IV administration of Ringer's lactate or normal saline
5. Administer atropine 0.6 to 1-mg IV slowly if patient does not respond quickly to steps 2 to 4
6. Repeat atropine up to a total dose of 0.04-mg/kg (2 to 3-mg) in adult
7. Ensure complete resolution of hypotension and bradycardia prior to discharge

Hypertension, severe

1. Administer O_2 6 to 10-L/min via mask
2. Monitor: Electrocardiogram, pulse oximeter, blood pressure
3. Administer nitroglycerine 0.4-mg tablet, sublingual (may repeat x 3); or, topical 2% ointment, apply 1-inch strip
4. If no response, consider labetalol 20-mg IV, then 20 to 80-mg IV every 10 minutes up to 300-mg
5. Transfer to intensive care unit or emergency department
6. For pheochromocytoma: Phentolamine 5-mg IV (may use labetalol if phentolamine is not available)

Seizures or Convulsions

1. Administer O_2 6 to 10-L/min via mask
2. Consider diazepam 5-mg IV (or more, as appropriate) or midazolam 0.5 to 1-mg IV
3. If longer effect needed, obtain consultation; consider phenytoin infusion 15 to 18-mg/kg at 50 -mg/min
4. Careful monitoring of vital signs required, particularly of pO_2 because of risk to respiratory depression with benzodiazepine administration
5. Consider using cardiopulmonary arrest response team for intubation if needed

Pulmonary Edema

1. Administer O_2 6 to 10-L/min via mask
2. Elevate torso
3. Give diuretics: Furosemide 20 to 40-mg IV, slow push
4. Consider giving morphine (1 to 3-mg IV)
5. Transfer to intensive care unit or emergency department

Generalized Anaphylactoid Reaction

1. Call for resuscitation team
2. Suction airway as needed
3. Elevate legs if hypotensive
4. Oxygen by mask, 6 to 10-L/min
5. Epinephrine IM (1:1,000) 0.5 mL (0.5-mg). Repeat as needed
6. Intravenous fluids (e.g., normal saline, Ringer's solution)
7. H_1-blocker, e.g., diphenhydramine 25 to 50-mg intravenously

ACR = American College of Radiology; CAD = coronary artery disease; ESUR = European Society of Urogenital Radiology; IM = intramuscular; IV = intravenous; PO = orally; SC = subcutaneous

Table 5. Management of acute reactions to gadolinium-based contrast agents in pediatric patients (adapted from references 3 and 4).

Urticaria

1. No treatment necessary in most cases
2. For moderate itching, consider H_1-receptor blocker: Diphenhydramine PO/IM or slow IV 1 to 2-mg/kg, up to 50-mg
3. ACR guidelines:
   - If severe or widely disseminated: consider α-agonist: epinephrine IV (1:10,000) 0.1-mL/kg slow push over 2 to 5 minutes, up to-3 mL
4. ESUR guidelines:
   - Epinephrine IM (1:1,000):
     - 6 to 12 year old - 50% of adult dose
     - <6 years of age - 25% of adult dose
     - Repeat as needed

Facial Edema

1. Secure airway and administer O_2 6 to 10-L/min (via mask, face tent, or blow-by stream). Monitor: electrocardiogram, O_2 saturation, and blood pressure
2. Administer α-agonist: Epinephrine IV (1:10,000) 0.1-mL/kg slow push over 2 to 5 minutes, up to 3-mL/dose. Repeat in 5 to 30 minutes as needed
3. Consider H_1-receptor blocker: Diphenhydramine IM or slow IV push 1 to 2-mg/kg, up to 50-mg.
4. Note: If facial edema is mild and there is no reaction progression, observation alone may be appropriate
   - If not responsive to therapy, seek appropriate assistance (e.g., cardiopulmonary arrest response team)

Bronchospasm

1. Secure airway and administer oxygen 6 to 10-L/min (via mask, face tent, or blow-by stream). Monitor: electrocardiogram, O_2 saturation, and blood pressure
2. Administer beta-agonist (bronchiolar dilator such as albuterol) 2 to 3 puffs from metered dose inhaler; repeat as necessary.
3. ACR guidelines:
   - If bronchospasm progresses, administer epinephrine (1:10,000) IV 0.1-mL/kg slow push over 2 to 5 minutes, up to-3-mL/dose. Repeat in 5 to 30 minutes as needed
   - If not responsive to therapy, call for assistance (e.g., cardiopulmonary arrest response team) for severe bronchospasm or if O_2 saturation <88% persists
4. ESUR guidelines:
   - Epinephrine IM (1:1,000) when patient has normal blood pressure:
     - 6 to 12 year old – 50% of adult dose
     - <6 years of age – 25% of adult dose
     - Repeat as needed
   - Epinephrine IM (1:1,000) when patient has decreased blood pressure:
     - 6 to 12 year old – 0.3-mL (0.3-mg)
     - <6 years of age – 0.15-mL (0.15-mg)

Laryngeal Edema

1. Secure airway and administer oxygen 6 to 10-L/min (via mask, face tent, or blow-by stream). Monitor: electrocardiogram, O_2 saturation, and blood pressure
2. ACR guidelines:
   - Administer epinephrine (1:10,000) IV 0.1-mL/kg slow push over 2 to 5 minutes, up to-3-mL/dose. Repeat in 5 to 30 minutes as needed
   - If not promptly responsive to initial therapy, call for assistance (e.g., cardiopulmonary arrest response team)
3. ESUR guidelines:

- Epinephrine IM (1:1,000):
  - 6 to 12 years old – 0.3-mL (0.3-mg)
  - <6 years of age – 0.15-mL (0.15-mg)

Pulmonary Edema

1. Secure airway and administer oxygen 6 to 10-L/min (via mask, face tent, or blow-by stream). Monitor: electrocardiogram, O_2 saturation, and blood pressure
2. Administer diuretic: Furosemide IV 1 to 2-mg/kg
   - If not responsive to therapy, call for assistance (e.g., cardiopulmonary arrest response team)

Hypotension with Tachycardia (Anaphylactic Shock)

1. Secure airway and administer oxygen 6 to 10-L/min (via mask). Monitor: Electrocardiogram, O_2 saturation, and blood pressure
2. Legs elevated 60-degrees or more (preferred) or Trendelenburg position
3. Keep patient warm
4. Give rapid infusion of IV or IO normal saline or Ringer's lactate
5. ACR guidelines:
   - If severe, give α-agonist: Epinephrine IV (1:10,000) 0.1-mL/kg slow push over 2 to 5 minutes, up to 3-mL/dose. Repeat as needed 5 to 30 minutes as needed
   - If not responsive to therapy, seek appropriate assistance (e.g., cardiopulmonary arrest response team)
6. ESUR guidelines (isolated hypotension):
   - Epinephrine IM (1:1,000):
     - 6 to 12 year old – 0.3-mL (0.3-mg)
     - <6 years of age – 0.15-mL (0.15-mg)

Hypotension with Bradycardia (Vagal Reaction)

1. Secure airway and give oxygen 6 to 10-L/min (via mask). Monitor: Electrocardiogram, O_2 saturation, and blood pressure
2. Legs elevated 60-degrees or more (preferred) or Trendelenburg position
3. Keep patient warm
4. Rapid administration of IV or IO normal saline or Ringer's lactate. Caution should be used to avoid hypervolemia in children with myocardial dysfunction
5. Administer atropine IV 0.02-mg/kg if patient does not respond quickly to steps 2 to 4. Minimum initial dose of 0.1-mg.
   - ACR guidelines: Maximum initial dose of 0.5-mg (infant/child), 1.0-mg (adolescent). May repeat every 3 to 5 minutes up to a maximum dose of 1.0-mg (infant/child), 2.0-mg (adolescent). If not responsive to therapy, seek appropriate assistance (e.g., cardiopulmonary arrest response team)
   - ESUR guidelines: Maximum dose of 0.6-mg. Repeat if necessary to 2-mg total

Generalized Anaphylactoid Reaction

1. Call for resuscitation team
2. Suction airway as needed
3. Elevate legs if hypotensive
4. Oxygen by mask, 6 to 10-L/min
5. Epinephrine IM (1:1,000)
   - 6 to 12 year old - 0.3-mL (0.3-mg)
   - <6 years of age - 0.15-mL (0.15-mg)
6. Intravenous fluids (e.g., normal saline, Ringer's solution).
7. H_1-blocker, eg, diphenhydramine 25 to 50-mg intravenously

---

ACR = American College of Radiology; ESUR = European Society of Urogenital Radiology; IM= intramuscular; IO = intraosseous; IV = intravenous; PO = orally

acterized by abrupt peripheral vasodilation and hypotension, along with bradycardia. Patients can also experience pallor, nausea, and vomiting, but no cutaneous rash, bronchospasm, tachycardia, or angioedema is observed. The exact cause of vagal reactions is unknown, but triggers such as anxiety and fear are known to elicit the response (31, 32). Such reactions are effectively treated by elevating the patient's legs, increasing intravascular fluid volume, and administering atropine to reverse bradycardia.

In anaphylaxis, the most common areas affected include the skin (e.g., flushing, itching, urticaria, angioedema, etc.; 80 to 90%), respiratory tract (throat itching and tightness, dysphonia, hoarseness, stridor, dry staccato cough, wheezing/bronchospasm; 70%), gastrointestinal tract (abdominal pain, nausea, vomiting, diarrhea; 30 to 45%), heart and vasculature (e.g., hypotension, tachycardia, bradycardia, cardiac arrest; 10 to 45%), and central nervous system (altered mental status, dizziness, confusion, loss of consciousness; 10 to 15%) (33).

Anaphylaxis can sometimes be difficult to diagnose. Patients with concomitant impaired vision or hearing, neurologic disease, psychiatric illness, such as depression, substance abuse, autism spectrum disorder, attention deficit hyperactivity disorder, or cognitive disorders, might have diminished awareness of anaphylaxis triggers and symptoms (34). At any age, concurrent use of CNS-active medications such as sedatives, hypnotics, antidepressants, and first generation sedating H_1-antihistamines perhaps given to prevent reactions, can interfere with the recognition of anaphylaxis triggers and symptoms and with the ability to describe symptoms. In patients with concomitant medical conditions, for example, asthma, chronic obstructive pulmonary disease, congestive heart failure, pulmonary embolism, or pre-existing myocardial infarction, signs and symptoms of these diseases can also cause confusion in the differential diagnosis of anaphylaxis (34). Additionally, an anxiety or panic attack can cause diagnostic confusion because a sense of impending doom, breathlessness, flushing, tachycardia, and gastrointestinal symptoms can occur in both anxiety/panic attacks and in anaphylaxis. However, urticaria, angioedema, wheezing, and hypotension are unlikely to occur during an anxiety/panic attack (33).

Different from vagal reactions, anaphylactic or anaphylactic-like reactions are most effectively treated with rapid infusion of large volumes of fluids, along with epinephrine (3, 4). If administered properly and promptly, and the patient is not on a beta-adrenergic blocking agent, epinephrine can prevent or reverse the life-threatening symptoms of anaphylactic shock. Epinephrine is life saving because of its alpha-1 adrenergic vasoconstrictive effects in most body organ systems (skeletal muscle is an important exception), its ability to prevent and relieve airway obstruction caused by mucosal edema, and to prevent and relieve hypotension and shock (35-37). Other relevant properties in anaphylaxis include its beta-1 adrenergic agonist inotropic and chronotropic properties leading to an increase in the force and rate of cardiac contractions, and its beta-2 adrenergic agonist properties such as decreased mediator release, bronchodilation, and relief of urticaria. The evidence base for prompt epinephrine injection in the initial treatment of anaphylaxis is stronger than the evidence base for the use of antihistamines and glucocorticoids in anaphylaxis. Fatality studies provide the most compelling evidence for prompt epinephrine injection (38-40).

Unfortunately, epinephrine is under-used in anaphylaxis treatment. Failure to inject it promptly is potentially associated with fatality, encephalopathy because of hypoxia and/or ischemia, and biphasic anaphylaxis in which symptoms recur within 1 to 72 hours (usually within 8 to 10 hours) after the initial symptoms have resolved, despite no further exposure to the trigger (33, 41). Anaphylaxis guidelines published to date in indexed, peer-reviewed journals differ in their recommendations for administration of second-line medications such as antihistamines, beta-2 adrenergic agonists, and glucocorticoids. The evidence base for the use of these medications in the initial management of anaphylaxis, including doses and dose regimens, is extrapolated mainly from their use in treatment of other diseases such as urticaria (antihistamines) or acute asthma (beta-2 adrenergic agonists and glucocorticoids). Concerns have been raised that administering one or more second-line medications potentially delays prompt injection of epinephrine, the first-line treatment (33).

A small number of patients do not respond to timely, basic initial anaphylaxis treatment with epinephrine, positioning on the back with lower extremities elevated, supplemental oxygen, intravenous fluid resuscitation, and second-line medications. If possible, such patients should be transferred promptly to the care of a team specialized in emergency medicine, critical care medicine, or anesthesiology (33).

In order to identify the emergence of an acute reaction, the American College of Radiology (ACR) Manual on Contrast Media recommends five important assessments be made immediately, as follows (4): (1) How does the patient look? (2) Can the patient speak? How does the patient's voice sound?(3) How is the patient's breathing? (4) What is the patient's pulse strength and rate? (5) What is the patient's blood pressure? The severity of a reaction can be quickly determined by the patient's level of consciousness, skin appearance, voice quality, lung auscultation, blood pressure, and heart rate (4). The findings from these assessments can also aid in the differential diagnosis of anaphylaxis, vaso-vagal reactions and panic attacks. Once the type and severity of a reaction have been identified, the appropriate treatment should be initiated. In cases of severe reactions, such as cardiopulmonary arrest, it may be necessary to seek additional assistance to obtain access to specialized life-support equipment and the expertise of appropriately trained personnel. The ACR and the European Society of Urogenital Radiology (ESUR) both publish guidelines for practitioners to use as a reference. These guidelines, summarized in **Table 4** and **Table 5**, include information concerning the latest approaches to treatment for various signs and symptoms of acute reactions (3, 4).

WHAT TO DO AFTER THE EXAM

In all cases, patients should be held in the radiology department for 30-minutes post-GBCA administration (3, 4), and those at risk for reactions should be monitored for up to 2-hours.

FINAL RECOMMENDATIONS

GBCAs are, in general, very safe. Serious adverse reactions to GBCAs are fortunately rare and fatal reactions are extremely rare. Proper patient evaluation and adequate prophylactic measures can prevent some of these complications. Knowledge, training, and preparation are crucial for appropriate and effective management of these events. Prompt recognition and treatment are invaluable in attenuating an adverse response of a patient to

GBCAs, and may prevent a reaction from becoming severe or even life threatening. In any facility where GBCAs are injected, it is imperative that the equipment and medications be immediately available, but only used outside the MR system room so that none of the resuscitative equipment becomes an MRI hazard.

REFERENCES

1. AMR Procedural Data (2012). Arlington Medical Resources: Arlington VA, USA.

2. International Conference on Harmonisation of Technical Requirements For Registration of Pharmaceuticals For Human Use. ICH Harmonised Tripartite Guideline 2003. Post-Approval Safety Data Management: Definitions and Standards For Expedited Reporting E2D. Available at: http://www.ich.org/fileadmin/Public_Web_Site/ICH_Products/Guidelines/Efficacy/E2D/Step4/E2D_Guideline.pdf. Accessed February 2013.

3. European Society on Urogenital Radiology (ESUR). ESUR Guidelines on Contrast Media. Version 8.0. 2012. Available at: http://www.esur.org/guidelines/. Accessed February 2013.

4. American College of Radiology. Manual on Contrast Media. Version 8. 2010. Available at: http://www.acr.org. Accessed February 2013.

5. Hasdenteufel F, Luyasu S, Renaudin JM, et al. Anaphylactic shock after first exposure to gadoterate meglumine: two case reports documented by positive allergy assessment. J Allergy Clin Immunol 2008;121:527-528.

6. Schiavino D, Murzilli F, Del Ninno M, et al. Demonstration of an IgE-mediated immunological pathogenesis of a severe reaction to gadopentetate dimeglumine. J Invest Allergol Clin Immunol 2003;13:140-142.

7. MultiHance (gadobenate dimeglumine) injection (prescribing information). Monroe, NJ: Bracco Diagnostics Inc., July 2012.

8. ProHance (gadoteridol) Injection, 279.3 mg/mL (prescribing information). Monroe, NJ: Bracco Diagnostics Inc., July 2011.

9. Magnevist (brand of gadopentetate dimeglumine) injection (prescribing information). Wayne, NJ: Bayer Healthcare Pharmaceuticals, March 2012.

10. Gadavist (gadobutrol) injection (prescribing information). Wayne, NJ: Bayer Healthcare Pharmaceuticals, November 2011.

11. Dotarem (gadoterate meglumine) Injection (prescribing information). Bloomington, IN: Guerbet LLC, March 2013.

12. Omniscan (gadodiamide) injection (prescribing information). Princeton, NJ: Amersham Health Inc., December 2010.

13. OptiMARK (gadoversetamide injection) (prescribing information). St. Louis, MO: Mallinckrodt Inc., September 2010.

14. Eovist (gadoxetate disodium) (prescribing information). Wayne, NJ: Bayer Healthcare Pharmaceuticals, February 2013.

15. Ablavar (gadofosveset trisodium) (prescribing information). North Billerica, MA: Lantheus Medical Imaging, Inc., February 2011.

16. Abujudeh HH, Kosaraju VK, Kaewlai R. Acute adverse reactions to gadopentetate dimeglumine and gadobenate dimeglumine: experience with 21,659 injections. AJR Am J Roentgentol 2010;194:430-434.

17. Bruder O, Schneider S, Nothnagel D, et al. Acute adverse reactions to gadolinium-based contrast agents in CMR: multicenter experience with 17,767 patients from the EuroCMR Registry. JACC Cardiovasc Imaging 2011;4:1171-1176.

18. Dillman JR, Ellis JH, Cohan RH, Strouse PJ, Jan SC. Frequency and severity of acute allergic-like reactions to gadolinium-containing i.v. contrast media in children and adults. AJR Am J Roentgenol 2007;189:1533-1538.

19. Hunt CH, Hartman RP, Hesley GK. Frequency and severity of adverse effects of iodinated and gadolinium contrast materials: retrospective review of 456,930 doses. AJR Am J Roentgenol 2009;193:1124-1127.

20. Jung JW, Kang HR, Kim MH, et al. Immediate hypersensitivity reaction to gadolinium-based MR contrast media. Radiology 2012;264:414-422.

21. Li A, Wong CS, Wong MK, Lee CM, Au Yeung MC. Acute adverse reactions to magnetic resonance contrast media: gadolinium chelates. Br J Radiol 2006;79:368-371.

22. Murphy KP, Szopinski KT, Cohal RH, Mermillod B, Ellis JH. Occurrence of adverse reactions to gadolinium-based contrast material and management of patients at increased risk: a survey of the American Society of Neuroradiology Fellowship Directors. Acad Radiol 1999;6:656-664.

23. Prince MR, Zhang H, Zou Z, Staron RB, Brill PW. Incidence of immediate gadolinium contrast media reactions. AJR Am J Roentgenol 2011;196:W138-143.

24. Nelson KL, Gifford LM, Lauber-Huber C, Gross CA, Lasser TA. Clinical safety of gadopentetate dimeglumine. Radiology 1995;196:439-443.

25. Lang DM, Alpern MB, Visintainer PF, Smith ST. Elevated risk of anaphylactoid reaction from radiographic contrast media is associated with both beta-blocker exposure and cardiovascular disorders. Arch Intern Med 1993;153:2033-2040.

26. Javeed N, Javeed H, Javeed S, et al. Refractory anaphylactoid shock potentiated by beta-blockers. Cathet Cardiovasc Diagn 1996;39:383-384.

27. Lang DM. Anaphylactoid and anaphylactic reactions. Hazards of beta-blockers. Drug Safety 1995;12:299-304.

28. Lang DM, Alpern MB, Visintainer PF, Smith ST. Increased risk for anaphylactoid reaction from contrast media in patients on beta-adrenergic blockers or with asthma. Ann Intern Med 1991;115:270-276.

29. Greenberger PA, Meyers SN, Kramer BL, Kramer BL. Effects of beta-adrenergic and calcium antagonists on the development of anaphylactoid reactions from radiographic contrast media during cardiac angiography. J Allergy Clin Immunol 1987;80:698-702.

30. Dillman JR, Ellis JH, Cohan RH, Strouse PJ, Jan SC. Allergic-like breakthrough reactions to gadolinium contrast agents after corticosteroid and antihistamine premedication. AJR Am J Roentgenol 2008;190:187-190.

31. Bush WH, Swanson DP. Acute reactions to intravascular contrast media: types, risk factors, recognition, and specific treatment. AJR Am J Roentgenol 1991;157:1153-1161.

32. Lalli AF. Contrast media reactions: data analysis and hypothesis. Radiology. 1980;134:1-12.

33. Simons FE, World Allergy Organization. World Allergy Organization survey on global availability of essentials for the assessment and management of anaphylaxis by allergy-immunology specialists in health care settings. Ann Allergy Asthma Immunol 2010;104:405-412.

34. Simons FE. Anaphylaxis. J Allergy Clin Immunol. 2010;125:S161-S181. Erratum in: J Allergy Clin Immunol 2010;126:885.

35. Simons KJ, Simons FE. Epinephrine and its use in anaphylaxis: current issues. Curr Opin Allergy Clin Immunol 2010;10:354-361.

36. McLean-Tooke AP, Bethune CA, Fay AC, Spickett GP. Adrenaline in the treatment of anaphylaxis: what is the evidence? British Medical Journal 2003;327:1332-1335.

37. Kemp SF, Lockey RF, Simons FE, World Allergy Organization ad hoc Committee on Epinephrine in Anaphylaxis. Epinephrine: the drug of choice for anaphylaxis. A statement of the World Allergy Organization. Allergy 2008;63:1061-1070.

38. Bock SA, Munoz-Furlong A, Sampson HA. Further fatalities caused by anaphylactic reactions to food, 2001-2006. J Allergy Clin Immunol 2007;119:1016-1018.

39. Pumphrey RS, Gowland MH. Further fatal allergic reactions to food in the United Kingdom, 1999-2006. J Allergy Clin Immunol 2007;119:1018-1019

40. Greenberger PA, Rotskoff BD, Lifschultz B. Fatal anaphylaxis: postmortem findings and associated co-morbid diseases. Ann Allergy Asthma Immunol 2007;98:252-257.

41. Pumphrey RS. Lessons for management of anaphylaxis from a study of fatal reactions. Clin Exp Allergy 2000;30:1144-1150.

Chapter 11   MRI Contrast Agents and Nephrogenic Systemic Fibrosis

ALBERTO SPINAZZI, M.D.

Senior Vice President
Global Medical and Regulatory Affairs
Bracco Group
Monroe, NJ

INTRODUCTION

Nephrogenic systemic fibrosis (NSF) is a rare, systemic fibrosing disorder reminiscent, but distinct from scleroderma or scleromyxedema. Its most prominent and visible effects are observed in the skin, which led to the disease originally being named "nephrogenic fibrosing dermopathy", or NFD (1). "Nephrogenic" does not mean that the disease is caused by factors originating in the kidney, but that NSF has been observed only in patients with reduced kidney function. "Systemic" emphasizes the systemic nature of this fibrosing disorder. Along with involving nerves and skeletal muscles, it has also been linked with myocardial, pericardial, and pleural fibrosis (2). Even though the first cases of NSF were identified in 1997 and the first published report of 14 cases appeared in 2000 (3), this disease has received great attention only since 2006, when its high morbidity, absence of a specific treatment, and possible association with exposure to gadolinium based contrast agents (GBCAs), commonly and widely used in magnetic resonance imaging (MRI) for the past 25 years, became apparent.

NSF can be deadly, however, the disease by itself is not a cause of death. Rather, NSF may contribute to death by restricting effective ventilation, or by restricting mobility to the point of causing an accidental fall that may lead to fractures and clotting complications (4). As of October 2012, 335 cases of NSF were identified in the NSF Registry maintained by Yale University (4), whereas approximately 1,600 cases had been reported to the United States (U.S.) Food and Drug Administration (FDA), as well as other regulatory authorities. Many of these reports stemmed from multi-district litigation in the U.S., which explains why sixty hospitals in the U.S. account for 93% of these cases. Several spontaneous reports to regulatory authorities lack fundamental information to confirm a diagnosis of NSF. Therefore, this chapter will focus on 815 distinct cases reported in 200 articles in peer-reviewed literature from 2000 until December 2012 (5-204). These 200 papers were obtained by performing a literature search of the PubMed database using the following key words: "*nephrogenic systemic fibrosis*", "*nephrogenic fibrosing dermopathy*", "*scleromyxedema-like*", and "*scleroderma and gadolinium*". Cases from abstracts, letters-to-the-editor, or other correspondence were not included in this review if they lacked sufficient information. During the review, any additional publications reporting NSF cases, such as articles referenced by other articles being reviewed or articles that the authors obtained from other sources, including articles from peer-reviewed medical literature databases other than PubMed, were added to the literature pool for review. Cases were only counted the first time they appeared in the literature. When a case was presented in more than one article, that case was not considered an original case, although any additional information provided in subsequent articles was recorded and used for this review. In several cases, authors were contacted in order to obtain additional information or confirm existing information.

EPIDEMIOLOGY

Population Characteristics

The distribution and determinants of NSF are shown in **Table 1**. Of the 815 cases reported in peer-reviewed literature (5-204), age information was available for 493 patients. NSF occurred in patients from 8- to 87-years of age, with a peak between 50 and 69 years of age (48.6%). NSF affects males and females in approximately equal numbers and has been identified in patients from a variety of ethnic backgrounds and from 28 countries in North America, Europe and Asia. Overall, the majority of published NSF cases were observed in the U.S. [595/815 (73.0%)], with Denmark [46/815 (5.6%)], Germany [40/815 (4.9%)], the United Kingdom [38/815 (4.7%)], and Japan [19/815 (2.3%)] reporting the next highest number of cases.

All 815 published cases of NSF occurred in patients with acute or chronic renal insufficiency (807 cases), with acute renal insufficiency due to hepatorenal syndrome (four reports) or in the perioperative liver transplantation period (four cases). Most patients (616, 75.6%) had a history of dialysis. The type and degree of renal impairment prior to NSF onset was reported in 732 (90%) of the 815 published cases (**Table 2**). With the exception of one case, which reportedly occurred in a patient with Stage 3 chronic kidney disease (CKD; glomerular filtration rate, GFR, between 30- and 59- mL/min/1.73-m^2), all these cases (731/732, 99.9%) occurred in patients with acute renal failure (72 cases, 9.8%), severe CKD (Stage 4 CKD, GFR between 15 and 29- mL/min/1.73-m^2; 15 cases, 2.0%), or kidney failure (Stage 5 CKD, GFR < 15-mL/min/1.73-m^2; 644 cases, 88.1%).

Association with Exposure to Gadolinium-Based Contrast Agents

Despite considerable effort, no case of NSF has been identified before 1997 (205), and there are no published NSF cases with onset of symptoms after 2009 (5-204). This truly new disease entity should therefore result from exposure of patients with advanced renal failure to one or more new exogenous agents—that is, a new medication, toxin, or infectious agent —or to new ways of using previously existing medications (206). The first suspects

Table 1. Epidemiology of nephrogenic systemic fibrosis (5-204).

- Ages: 8 to 87 years, peak between 50 and 69 years of age
- No race predilection
- No sex predilection (Male = Female)
- Seen around the world (North America, South America, Asia, Europe, Australia)
- Always seen in patients with acute or chronic renal insufficiency
- Mostly seen in patients previously exposed to gadolinium-based contrast agents

Table 2. Number of cases of nephrogenic systemic fibrosis reported in the peer-reviewed literature, indicated by type and degree of renal impairment (5-204).

Severity of Renal Impairment	No. of Cases (%) (N = 815)
Not Reported	83 (10.2%)
Acute Renal Failure	72 (8.8%)
Chronic Kidney Disease (CKD)	**660 (81.0%)**
Stage 5 (eGFR <15-mL/min/1.73-m^2)	644 (79.0%)
Stage 4 (eGFR 15- to < 30-mL/min/1.73-m^2)	15 (1.8%)
Stage 3 (eGFR 30- to < 60-mL/min/1.73-m^2)	1 (0.14%)
Patients with History of Dialysis	**616 (75.6%)**
Hemodialysis	484 (72.7%)
Hemodialysis and peritoneal dialysis	25 (3.7%)
Peritoneal dialysis	67 (10.1%)
Dialysis, type not specified	40 (6.0%)

eGFR, estimated glomerular filtration rate.

were high-dose erythropoietin and lack of angiotensin-converting enzyme inhibitor therapy in the presence of co-factors such as hypercoagulable states, various forms of vascular injury, vascular surgical procedures, and liver failure (in particular, hepatorenal syndrome and liver transplantation) (207). Since 2006, multiple reports have correlated the development of NSF with exposure to GBCAs (36-88, 90-135, 137-141, 143-182, 184-204). GBCAs are now the prime suspects, even though they had been available for clinical use since the mid 1980s, that is, at least 10 years before the first cases of NSF were identified. As a matter of fact, in 1996 (i.e., one year before the occurrence of the first known case of NSF), the first of several articles was published suggesting that, unlike iodine-based contrast media, GBCAs were not nephrotoxic, even when administered at high doses (208). The perception that GBCAs were safer resulted in many institutions switching from computed tomography and angiography to MRI and magnetic resonance (MR) angiography in patients with renal impairment, and even to the use of GBCAs for radiographic examinations (209). Notably, the same U.S. medical center whose publication promoted the switch from iodinated contrast to GBCAs reported, twelve years later, 15 cases of NSF in patients with acute renal failure or severe CKD exposed to high GBCA doses (118).

With rare exceptions (89, 136, 142, 183), the published cases of NSF followed the administration of at least one dose of gadolinium-containing contrast material to patients with

Table 3. Time from last exposure to a gadolinium-based contrast agent (GBCA) and onset of symptoms of nephrogenic systemic fibrosis (NSF) (5-204).

GBCA to NSF onset	%	Cumulative %
< 1 week	6.8%	
< 2 weeks	6.0%	
< 1 month	22.8%	35.6
< 2 months	15.0%	
< 3 months	11.8%	
< 6 months	12.2%	74.6
< 1 year	10.0%	84.6
< 2 years	13.0%	97.6
> 2 years	1.8%	
> 4 years	0.4%	
> 6 years	0.2%	100.0

GBCA, gadolinium-based contrast agent; NSF, nephrogenic systemic fibrosis.

renal failure (36–88, 90–135, 137–141, 143–182, 184–204). The odds ratio (OR) for developing NSF in exposed versus unexposed patients with underlying kidney disease from four case control studies was greater than 20 (38, 62, 53, 67). This was borne out in a systematic review and meta-analysis that examined the risk for NSF with exposure to GBCAs; an OR of 26.7 was noted (210). Impaired renal function always pre-dated the administration of one or more GBCAs, and, in most cases, the onset of NSF symptoms occurred in the first 12 months after the last exposure to GBCAs (**Table 3**) (36–88, 90–135, 137–141, 143–182, 184–204).

It is estimated that more than 200 million doses of GBCAs have been administered to patients from 1997, when the first NSF case was detected, to 2009, when the last published NSF cases occurred. Recent large scale examinations have shown overall prevalence rates of 34.2 per 100,000 and 2.3 per 100,000 patients exposed to the two GBCAs associated with the highest number of NSF cases, Omniscan (active ingredient, gadodiamide) and Magnevist (active ingredient, gadopentetate dimeglumine), respectively (118, 126). Thus, using the total number of patients exposed to GBCAs as denominator, this condition is extraordinarily rare. However, the incidence of NSF in those with markedly reduced kidney function is substantially higher, especially with some GBCA products.

A recent study on 565 patients with moderate-to-severe renal insufficiency exposed to one or more GBCAs reported an overall prevalence of 3%, with the highest prevalence among CKD Stage 5 patients (195). In retrospective assessments of a total of 1,866 patient records, the prevalence rate has been reported to range between 1.5% and 4.4% among GBCA-exposed patients with end-stage renal disease, averaging 2.87 ± 1.01% (38, 52, 53, 61, 67, 123). Of note, significantly higher rates of 13% and 18% were reported from two centers that systematically and prospectively examined and interviewed patients with previously known exposures to gadopentetate dimeglumine and gadodiamide (75, 119).

The odds for NSF increase with repeated dosing over a relatively short period of time (days to six months) or higher single doses of GBCAs, although single standard doses of 0.1-mmol/kg had been clearly associated with the development of NSF (36–88, 90–135, 137–141, 143–182, 184–204).

It is clear that most patients with severe impairment of renal function or end-stage renal disease do not develop NSF even if exposed to high doses of GBCAs (67, 211). Other possible predisposing conditions have been suggested, such as a proinflammatory state, vascular surgery, hypercoagulability or thrombotic events, metabolic acidosis, and patient exposure to high doses of erythropoietin (207).

DIAGNOSIS

NSF is different from adverse events usually encountered by radiologists because it does not occur at the time of the imaging study. Instead, NSF typically occurs days to months later. Individually, the clinical and pathological features of NSF are not unique to that disease, so that no single test or other finding can be relied on to be 100% sensitive and specific for the diagnosis of NSF (1, 212). A confident diagnosis may be reached only through the combination of clinical history, a physical examination, and compelling histologic features of a biopsy specimen of involved skin (1, 212). A multidisciplinary team of highly experienced clinicians and dermatopathologists has recently completed a clinico-pathological definition of NSF (1). This definition relies upon a combination of clinical and pathological findings derived from the study of numerous patients, the relevant medical literature, and histological slides and data contained within the Yale NSF Registry to create a reproducible diagnostic and workup scheme for putative cases of NSF. As mentioned previously, to date, NSF has been observed only in patients either with acute or chronic renal insufficiency or, mostly end-stage renal disease. Therefore, the main elements that should guide physicians in the diagnostic process are clinical presentation and confirmatory cutaneous histopathologic findings in the setting of decreased or absent glomerular filtration, either acutely or chronically (1, 2, 207, 212).

Physical Examination

The skin changes caused by NSF can mimic progressive systemic sclerosis with a predilection for extremity involvement that can extend to the torso (2, 207, 212). Unlike scleroderma, NSF usually spares the face (2, 207, 212). Skin lesions typically begin with swelling, progressing to erythematous papules and coalescing violaceous to hyperpigmented, brawny plaques with follicular dimpling (peau d'orange) changes (**Figure 1**) (1, 2, 212). Peripheral irregular fingerlike or ameboid projections may be present along with islands of sparing (**Figure 2**) (1, 2). The involved skin and subcutis can become markedly thickened and hardened, unpinchable, with a wooden consistency to palpation (**Figure 3**) (1, 2, 212). The indurations characteristically involve the distal extremities first, gradually proceeding to involve the proximal extremities to the level of the mid-thigh and mid upper arms where they may show a pattern of bumpiness ("cobblestoning") (**Figure 4**)(1, 2, 212). Involvement of the skin and subcutaneous tissues overlying joints can cause a decrease in function of the hands and feet first and then of more proximal joints in the affected extremities, often leaving patients wheelchair-dependent (1, 2, 212). Joint contractures may be ac-

Figure 1. Affected areas showing follicular dimpling (peau d'orange) changes (major clinical criterion), usually present on the lower extremity above the knee, or upper extremity (1).

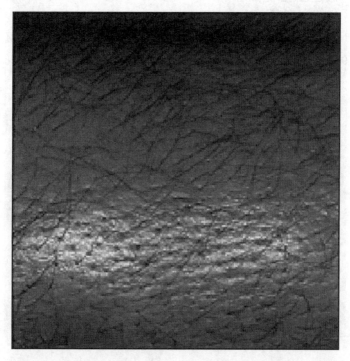

Figure 2. Red to violaceous, thin, fixed plaques showing polygonal, reticular, or "amoeboid" morphologies (patterned plaques, major clinical criterion) (1).

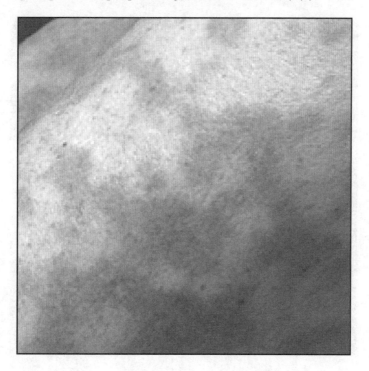

Figure 3. Unpinchable, firm, shiny, often hyperpigmented, bound-down skin over the extremities (marked induration, major clinical criterion) (1).

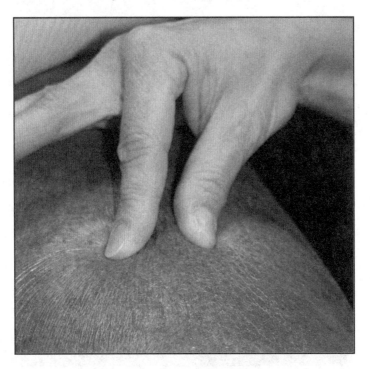

Figure 4. Bumpy, "pseudo-cellulite" pattern, formed by deep induration of the upper arms and/or thighs ("cobblestoning", major clinical criterion) (1).

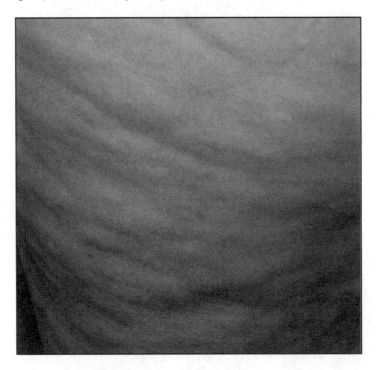

companied by edema of the fingers, wrists, toes, and ankles (**Figure 5**). In **Table 4**, more (major) and less (minor) frequent clinical findings are listed (1).

Patients with NSF may complain of itching and sharp pain that may be localized in the affected areas, in the rib cage, or the hips. Loss of appetite, paresthesia, and muscle weakness are also described (2, 207, 212). If these symptoms and these or other skin lesions are observed in a patient with reduced renal function and history of exposure to one or more GBCAs, a full-body skin examination should be performed on the patient by a dermatologist or rheumatologist who is familiar, not only with the clinical findings of NSF, but also with those of the other conditions within the differential diagnosis (1, 2). Of note, some patients (estimated at < 5%) develop rapidly progressive, fulminant NSF associated with an accelerated loss of mobility and severe pain (2, 207, 212, 213).

Histopathological Evaluation

If the signs and symptoms noted are observed in patients with severe renal insufficiency, a biopsy should be performed to obtain specimens of involved skin (1, 2, 207, 212). A deep punch biopsy of at least 4-mm in size and extending to the subcutaneous fat may reveal sufficient findings to make a more confident diagnosis in cases of superficial lesions. However, it is always better to obtain deeper biopsy specimens because the disease characteristically extends along fibrous septa into subcutaneous fat and fascia and sometimes into underlying skeletal muscle (1, 2, 207, 212). For lesions of differing morphologies and/or locations, multiple cutaneous biopsy specimens are recommended (1). Histologically, NSF is characterized by dermal fibrosis and may be indistinguishable from scleromyxedema (1). Preserved elastic tissue is a finding that allows dermatopathologists to distinguish NSF from morphea and scleroderma (1). In NSF, there is always an increased number of fibrocytes that are CD34-positive and procollagen I–positive when stained immunohistochemically (**Figure 6**). This dual positivity is characteristic of so-called "circulating fibrocytes," mes-

Figure 5. Edema of the fingers and wrists, with loss of range of motion of fingers and wrists (1).

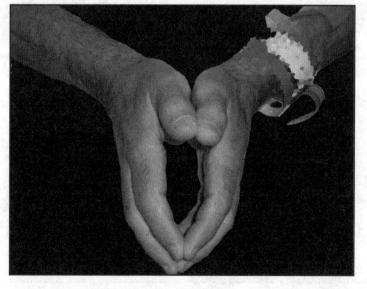

Table 4. Clinical findings for the diagnosis of NSF (1).

- Skin lesions
  - Lesion distribution: mostly upper and lower extremities with involvement of trunk in a minority of cases. Face is involved in approximately 3% of cases.
  - Lesion morphology: fixed plaques (polygonal, reticular, or amoeboid; red to violaceous to hyperpigmented); induration (unpinchable firm skin over the extremities with a wooden consistency to palpation and a pattern of bumpiness over the upper arms or thighs); papules, nodules, erythema, and swelling may be also present
- Major criteria for diagnosis
  - Patterned plaques
  - Joint contractures
  - "Cobblestoning"
  - Marked induration / Peau d'orange
- Minor criteria for diagnosis
  - Puckering/linear banding
  - Superficial plaque/patch
  - Dermal papules
  - Scleral plaques (age below 45 years old)

NSF, nephrogenic systemic fibrosis.

Figure 6. CD34+ spindle or epithelioid cells in a reticular or parallel arrangement with "tram-tracking" (CD34+ dendritic processes on either side of elastic fibers *) (1).

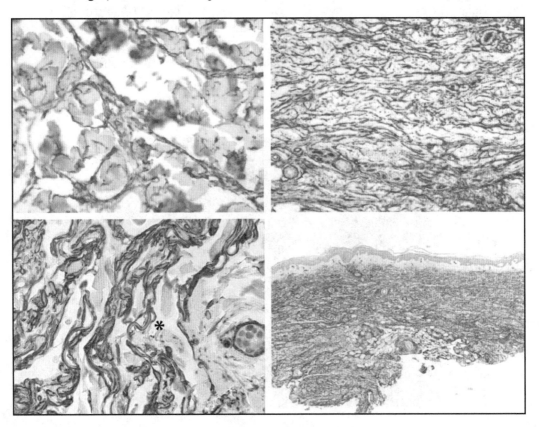

enchymal stem cells of bone marrow origin that participate in wound repair (214). Other features that, if present, help make a more confident diagnosis of NSF are: increased numbers of spindled and/or epithelioid cells (i.e., activated macrophages resembling epithelial cells) with few other inflammatory cells in the dermis; thin, especially in early lesions, and thick collagen bundles that generally maintain clefts of separation between their neighbors; involvement of subcutaneous septa which are markedly widened and collagenized as described above; osseous metaplasia, with foci of osteoid deposition, or calcified bone spicules around elastic fibers, which are considered a highly specific feature of NSF (1, 212).

Scoring and Reporting

The same multidisciplinary team of clinicians and dermatopathologists that completed the clinicopathological definition of NSF has also proposed a schematic and scoring system to assess putative cases of NSF (1). However, those NSF experts also warn healthcare professionals that accurate diagnosis of NSF requires judgment and interpretation, qualities that rely heavily on experience (1). If the signs and symptoms suggestive of NSF are observed in patients with severe renal insufficiency previously exposed to one or more gadolinium-based agents, a physical examination of those patients should be performed by experienced dermatologists or rheumatologists, and biopsy specimens should be examined by experienced dermatopathologists, bearing in mind that even experienced clinicians or pathologists may have personally examined only a limited number of patients with NSF (1).

HOW TO MINIMIZE THE RISK OF NSF

Because there is no consistently effective treatment for NSF, prevention is important. A prevention strategy implies sequential steps aimed at defining and identifying the population at risk in routine clinical practice, and at minimizing risk to that susceptible population.

Step 1. Identify Patients at Risk

Patients receiving any GBCA should be considered at risk of developing NSF if their GFR is equal to or below 40-mL/min/1.73-m². Patients with a GFR of 30- to 40-mL/min/1.73-m² should also be considered at risk because GFR levels may fluctuate (e.g., from the 30- to 40-mL/min/1.73-m² range one day to below 30-mL/min/1.73-m² on another day) (215). Therefore, all patients referred for a contrast-enhanced MRI examination, especially outpatients, should be screened for conditions and other factors that may be associated with renal function impairment. Many people with impaired renal function do not feel any symptoms (215). Therefore, the following is a suggested list of factors that warrants a pre-administration serum creatinine test and calculation of the level of GFR in individuals scheduled to receive any GBCA injection (215-219):

- Age over 60;
- Family history of CKD;
- Personal history of renal disease, including:
  - Glomerulonephritis,

- Proteinuria,

- Inherited diseases, such as polycystic kidney disease,

- Recurrent urinary infections,

- Kidney cancer,

- Dialysis,

- Kidney surgery;

- History of diabetes mellitus, hypertension, gout, and/or lupus and other autoimmune diseases; and

- History of recent exposure to nephrotoxic drugs (e.g., amphotericin B, cyclosporine, cisplatin, acyclovir, methotrexate, aminoglycoside antibiotics, iodinated contrast media, etc.).

The level of GFR should be estimated from validated prediction equations that take into account the serum creatinine concentration and some or all of the following variables: age, sex, race, and body size (217-219). The most widely used equations for adult patients are the Modification of Diet in Renal Disease (MDRD) Study equation (220) and the Cockcroft-Gault formula (221). Although both equations provide a marked improvement over serum creatinine alone (222), the MDRD Study equation may perform better than the Cockcroft-Gault formula, but the data are very limited (223–225). Both prediction equations assume that the amount of creatinine produced by the patient is equal to the amount being removed by the kidneys. Therefore, neither equation is suitable if renal function is in an unstable condition, that is, in patients with acute renal failure or on dialysis. Results may also deviate from true values in patients with exceptional dietary intake (e.g., vegetarian diet, high protein diet, creatine supplements), extremes of body composition (e.g., very lean, obese, paraplegia), or severe liver disease. In view of this latter limitation, patients with hepatorenal syndrome and those with reduced renal function who have had or are awaiting liver transplantation should be considered at risk of NSF if they have any level of GFR below 60-mL/min/1.73-m^2. In children, the Schwartz formula provides a clinically useful estimate of GFR (226). A number of websites and point of service tools are available that can calculate GFR values in adults and children using the equations above.

There is no evidence to guide the time interval within which GFR should be obtained prior to GBCA injection to patients identified by screening to have one or more risk factor for compromised renal function. However, it is recommended to measure renal function within two to seven days before the date of the contrast-enhanced procedure, independently of the GBCA used.

A single normal GFR measurement usually does not rule out acute renal insufficiency since there is a delay between a change in renal function and the corresponding change in serum creatinine (216). The patient's clinical condition should, therefore, also be assessed close to the time of the procedure and, if factors that could cause acute renal failure are detected, the renal function should be measured again before the GBCA is given (216). In practice all patients with suspected acute renal failure should be considered at risk of developing NSF, regardless of measured serum creatinine or calculated GFR values (215).

Step 2. Assess Risk–Benefit of Contrast-Enhanced MRI in Patients at Risk

A patient at risk of NSF should receive a GBCA only when no suitable diagnostic alternatives are available and a thorough risk–benefit assessment for that patient indicates that the benefit clearly outweighs the potential risk of NSF (215, 216). The risk–benefit evaluation should be made by the radiologist in conjunction with the referring physician and should be properly and prospectively documented. History of previous exposures to GBCAs, especially if recent, or if other factors that are thought to act as possible co-triggers of the disease, such as metabolic acidosis, vascular surgery, thrombotic events, and so on, should be taken into account during the risk–benefit assessment of each individual at-risk patient. Patients or parents or guardians (in the case of minors) should be properly informed of the benefits, risks, and diagnostic alternatives based on all the information available at that time and should provide their consent in writing (215).

Step 3. Perform Any Unenhanced MRI Sequence That May be Helpful Before Injecting the MRI Contrast Agent

Even after the decision is made to perform a contrast-enhanced MR examination, and the patient has consented to receive a GBCA, guidelines released by professional societies (215, 216) and prescribing information for individual GBCAs all indicate that the use of GBCAs should be avoided unless the diagnostic information from the use of contrast is essential and not available with unenhanced MRI. Therefore, all unenhanced MRI pulse sequences that may help to make a diagnosis should be performed and the MR images should be evaluated by an experienced radiologist to ensure that the administration of a GBCA is still deemed necessary.

Step 4. Choice of the GBCA and Dose

The working hypothesis in the development of NSF is that free gadolinium is released from the various chelates and stays for weeks, months, or even years in the skin and other tissues. In the skin of patients with advanced renal failure, the gadolinium ion, maybe as a precipitate engulfed in a macrophage, attracts or activates circulating fibrocytes, that is bone marrow–derived cells that participate in normal wound healing and fibrosis and which are believed to underlie aberrant fibrosis in NSF (2, 210, 215, 216).

This hypothesis is far from being proven. However, if free gadolinium triggers the disease, then the higher the amount of free gadolinium in the cutis, subcutis, and other tissues, the higher the risk of NSF. Two factors may favor gadolinium ion deposition in the body in patients with reduced kidney function: (a) the GBCA dose administered to at-risk patients (a single high dose or repeated doses), and (b) the stability of the GBCA molecule, that is, the ability of the chelating molecule to bind to and sequester the gadolinium ion.

In renal failure, the combination of low chelate stability, high GBCA dose, and absence of adequate GBCA clearance may lead to increased deposition of gadolinium in tissues, cutis and subcutis included. Therefore, besides the ability of the body to rapidly and effectively eliminate the exogenous GBCA, two physicochemical properties may play a role in the accumulation of gadolinium in the body. That is, the stability of the GBCA and its relaxivity. Consider the following: (a) The higher the stability of the active ingredient, the lower the possibility of releasing gadolinium in the body following its intravenous injection; and (b) The higher the relaxivity (i.e., the measure of the potency of GBCAs in altering T1-relaxation rates, corresponding to their contrasting efficacy in T1-weighted MR images), the lower the need to administer high single GBCA doses.

NSF cases occurring after the sole administration of one GBCA are defined as "single agent" or "unconfounded." If a case of NSF follows the administration of two or more agents, it is more difficult to determine which agent is associated with development of the disorder, and the case is reported as "confounded" (216). In the peer-reviewed literature (5-204), the majority of unconfounded, single-agent cases of NSF, approximately 78%, have been associated with Omniscan (active ingredient, gadodiamide), 20% with Magnevist (active ingredient, gadopentetate dimeglumine), and 1.3% with OptiMARK (active ingredient, gadoversetamide). Very few single-agent cases (0.7%) have been associated with Gadavist (active ingredient, gadobutrol) and Dotarem (active ingredient, gadoterate meglumine), while no unconfounded cases have ever been reported for MultiHance (active ingredient, gadobenate dimeglumine), Eovist (active ingredient, gadoxetate disodium), Ablavar (active ingredient, gadofoveset trisodium), or ProHance (active ingredient, gadoteridol)(**Table 5**). Of note is the following:

- Unconfounded NSF cases fulfilling the diagnostic criteria developed by a multidisciplinary team of experts (1) have been linked only with Omniscan, Magnevist and OptiMARK, never with any of the other GBCAs (5-204, 216); and

- GBCAs associated with the lowest number of putative cases of NSF, if any, are characterized either by high stability (Dotarem, Gadavist, ProHance) or high relaxivity (Ablavar, Eovist, MultiHance), or both.

In view of this clinical evidence, the FDA and many other regulatory authorities have requested that Omniscan, Magnevist, and OptiMARK be specifically contraindicated for use in patients at risk of NSF (227, 228). Therefore, if GBCA administration is still deemed

Table 5. Single-agent, unconfounded cases of nephrogenic systemic fibrosis (NSF) in peer-reviewed literature (5-204).

GBCA	Number of Cases	% Cases (N = 461)
Total number of single-agent, un-confounded cases of NSF	461	
Omniscan	363	78.7%
Magnevist	89	19.3%
OptiMARK	6	1.3%
Gadovist/Gadavist	2*	0.4%
Dotarem	1*	0.2%
Ablavar, Eovist, MultiHance, ProHance	0	0
* Cases not completely meeting NSF diagnostic criteria developed by a multidisciplinary team of clinicians and dermatopathologists		

GBCA, gadolinium-based contrast agent; NSF, nephrogenic systemic fibrosis.

necessary after unenhanced MRI, radiologists may select one of the high-stability and/or high-relaxivity agents (Ablavar, Dotarem, Eovist, Gadavist, MultiHance, or ProHance). Because the risk of NSF seems to increase with increasing doses, any of these GBCAs should be used at the lowest dose needed to reliably provide the diagnostic information sought, and it should generally not exceed the recommended single dose (215, 216). Importantly, doses lower than those approved have been investigated for high-relaxivity agents (229-243), but not for the high-stability GBCAs. Therefore, caution should be exercised so as not to administer a dose that is too low to provide the diagnostic information sought from the examination.

Step 5. What to Do After the MRI Examination

The GBCA and dose used should be accurately recorded. Patients at risk of NSF should be followed up for at least twelve months following the contrast-enhanced MRI examination in order to detect any sign or symptom suggestive of the disease. It is recommended to notify the local regulatory authorities immediately of any putative case of NSF and to keep them informed until the diagnosis of NSF is confirmed or ruled out. The usefulness of hemodialysis in the prevention of NSF is unknown. However, to enhance and speed up GBCA elimination, it is recommended that patients on dialysis undergo a hemodialysis session no later than two hours after the administration of the GBCA (215, 216). Because it may be difficult for a dialysis center to alter dialysis schedules at the request of imaging departments, it may be more feasible for elective imaging studies to be timed to precede a scheduled dialysis session (215). While it is possible that multiple dialysis sessions may be more protective than a single session, this possible incremental benefit remains speculative. Some experts recommend two or more hemodialysis sessions following GBCA administration, with use of prolonged dialysis times and increased flow rates and volumes to facilitate GBCA clearance (215). It has been estimated that three consecutive hemodialysis treatments over a six-day period would be needed to remove 97% of the administered extracellular GBCA (244). Peritoneal dialysis probably provides less potential NSF risk reduction compared to hemodialysis and should not be considered protective (215).

CONCLUSIONS AND FINAL THOUGHTS

NSF is a rare, serious, systemic, fibrosing disorder observed almost only in patients with acute or chronic severe renal insufficiency (GFR <30-mL/min/1.73-m^2), or with acute renal insufficiency of any severity due to hepatorenal syndrome, or in the perioperative liver transplantation period. Most patients with NSF had a GFR <15- mL/min/1.73-m^2 and were undergoing (or had undergone) either hemodialysis or peritoneal dialysis or both. It is unclear if GBCAs can trigger NSF. Nevertheless, it is appropriate to assume that a potential association might exist for all GBCAs. Use of the preventive measures discussed in this chapter may minimize the risk of developing NSF. Notably, altered patterns of use of GBCAs in susceptible populations in response to restrictive measures taken by regulatory authorities for some GBCAs and guidelines released by professional societies has resulted in the incidence of NSF dropping close to zero (245).

REFERENCES

1. Girardi M, Kay J, Elston DM, et al. Nephrogenic systemic fibrosis: clinicopathological definition and workup recommendations. J Am Acad Dermatol 2011;65:1095-1106.

2. Shellock FG, Spinazzi A. MRI Safety Update 2008: Part 1, MRI contrast agents and nephrogenic systemic fibrosis. Am J Roentgenol 2008;191:1-11.

3. Cowper SE, Robin HS, Steinberg SM, et al. Scleromyxedema-like cutaneous diseases in renal-dialysis patients. Lancet 2000;356:1000–1001.

4. Cowper SE. Nephrogenic Systemic Fibrosis [ICNSFR Website]. 2001-2012. Available at http://www.icnsfr.org. Accessed January, 2013.

5. Girardi M, Kay J, Elston DM, et al. Nephrogenic systemic fibrosis: clinicopathological definition and workup recommendations. J Am Acad Dermatol 2011;65:1095-1106.

6. Cowper SE, Su LD, Bhawan J, Robin HS, LeBoit PE. Nephrogenic fibrosing dermopathy. Am J Dermatopathol 2001;23:383-393.

7. McNeill AM, Barr RJ. Scleromyxedema-like fibromucinosis in a patient undergoing hemodialysis. Int J Dermatol 2002;41:364-367.

8. Baron PW, Cantos K, Hillebrand DJ, et al. Nephrogenic fibrosing dermopathy after liver transplantation successfully treated with plasmapheresis. Am J Dermatopathol 2003;25:204-209.

9. Swartz RD, Crofford LJ, Phan SH, et al. Nephrogenic fibrosing dermopathy: a novel cutaneous fibrosing disorder in patients with renal failure. Am J Med 2003;114:563-572.

10. Hubbard V, Davenport A, Jarmulowicz M, Rustin M. Scleromyxoedema-like changes in four renal dialysis patients. Br J Dermatol 2003;148:563-568.

11. Engelen JW, Kooistra MP, et al. Nephrogenic fibrosing dermopathy. Ned Tijdschr Geneeskd 2003;147:2435-2438.

12. Ishibe S, Perazella MA, Reilly RF. Nephrogenic fibrosing dermopathy: an unusual skin condition associated with kidney disease. Semin Dial 2003;16:276-280.

13. Jan F, Segal JM, Dyer J, et al. Nephrogenic fibrosing dermopathy: two pediatric cases. J Pediatr 2003;143:678-681.

14. Mackay-Wiggan JM, Cohen DJ, Hardy MA, Knobler EH, Grossman ME. Nephrogenic fibrosing dermopathy (scleromyxedema-like illness of renal disease). J Am Acad Dermatol 2003;48:55-60.

15. Streams BN, Liu V, Liegeois N, Moschella SM. Clinical and pathologic features of nephrogenic fibrosing dermopathy: a report of two cases. J Am Acad Dermatol 2003;48:42-47.

16. Ting WW, Stone MS, Madison KC, Kurtz K. Nephrogenic fibrosing dermopathy with systemic involvement. Arch Dermatol 2003;139:903-906.

17. Evenepoel P, Zeegers M, Segaert S, et al. Nephrogenic fibrosing dermopathy: a novel, disabling disorder in patients with renal failure. Nephrol Dial Transplant 2004;19:469-473.

18. Tan AW, Tan SH, Lian TY, Ng SK. A case of nephrogenic fibrosing dermopathy. Ann Acad Med Singapore 2004;33:527-529.

19. Jain SM, Wesson S, Hassanein A, et al. Nephrogenic fibrosing dermopathy in pediatric patients. Pediatr Nephrol 2004;19:467-470.

20. Chiu H, Wells G, Carag H, et al. Nephrogenic fibrosing dermopathy: a rare entity in patients awaiting liver transplantation. Liver Transpl 2004;10:465-466.

21. Chung HJ, Chung KY. Nephrogenic fibrosing dermopathy: response to high-dose intravenous immunoglobulin. Br J Dermatol 2004;150:596-597.

22. Edsall LC, English JC 3rd, Teague MW, Patterson JW. Calciphylaxis and metastatic calcification associated with nephrogenic fibrosing dermopathy. J Cutan Pathol 2004;31:247-253.

23. Jimenez SA, Artlett CM, Sandorfi N, et al. Dialysis-associated systemic fibrosis (nephrogenic fibrosing dermopathy): study of inflammatory cells and transforming growth factor beta1 expression in affected skin. Arthritis Rheum 2004;50:2660-2666.

24. Kafi R, Fisher GJ, Quan T, et al. UV-A1 phototherapy improves nephrogenic fibrosing dermopathy. Arch Dermatol 2004;140:1322-1324.

25. Lauchli S, Zortea-Caflisch C, Nestle FO, Burg G, Kempf W. Nephrogenic fibrosing dermopathy treated with extracorporeal photopheresis. Dermatology 2004;208:278-280.

26. Levine JM, Taylor RA, Elman LB, et al. Involvement of skeletal muscle in dialysis-associated systemic fibrosis (nephrogenic fibrosing dermopathy). Muscle Nerve 2004;30:569-577.

27. Moschella SL, Kay J, Mackool BT, Liu V. Case 35-2004. Nephrogenic fibrosing dermopathy. Authors reply. N Engl J Med 2004;352:1724.

28. Daram SR, Cortese CM, Bastani B. Nephrogenic fibrosing dermopathy/nephrogenic systemic fibrosis: report of a new case with literature review. Am J Kidney Dis 2005;46:754-759.

29. Dundova I, Treska V, Simanek V, Michal M. Nephrogenic fibrosing dermopathy: a case study. Transplant Proc 2005;37:4187-4190.

30. Dupont A, Majithia V, Ahmad S, McMurray R. Nephrogenic fibrosing dermopathy, a new mimicker of systemic sclerosis. Am J Med Sci 2005;330:192-194.

31. Kucher C, Xu X, Pasha T, Elenitsas R. Histopathologic comparison of nephrogenic fibrosing dermopathy and scleromyxedema. J Cutan Pathol 2005;32:484-490.

32. Markus JS, James AJ, Nunez-Gussman JK, et al. Nephrogenic fibrosing dermopathy. J Am Acad Dermatol 2005;52:166-167.

33. Neudecker BA, Stern R, Mark LA, Steinberg S. Scleromyxedema-like lesions of patients in renal failure contain hyaluronan: a possible pathophysiological mechanism. J Cutan Pathol 2005;32:612-615.

34. Ruiz-Genao DP, Pascual-Lopez MP, et al. Osseous metaplasia in the setting of nephrogenic fibrosing dermopathy. J Cutan Pathol 2005;32:172-175.

35. Schmook T, Budde K, Ulrich C, et al. Successful treatment of nephrogenic fibrosing dermopathy in a kidney transplant recipient with photodynamic therapy. Nephrol Dial Transplant 2005;20:220-222.

36. Grobner T. Gadolinium - a specific trigger for the development of nephrogenic fibrosing dermopathy and nephrogenic systemic fibrosis? Nephrol Dial Transplant 2006;21:1104-1108.

37. Boyd AS, Zic JA, Abraham JL. Gadolinium deposition in nephrogenic fibrosing dermopathy. J Am Acad Dermatol 2007;56:27-30.

38. Marckmann P, Skov L, Rossen K, et al. Nephrogenic systemic fibrosis: suspected causative role of gadodiamide used for contrast-enhanced magnetic resonance imaging. J Am Soc Nephrol 2006;17:2359-2362.

39. Nowack R, Wachtler P. Scleroderma-like syndrome triggered by gadolinium. Nephrol Dial Transplant 2006;21:3344.

40. Auron A, Shao L, Warady BA. Nephrogenic fibrosing dermopathy in children. Pediatr Nephrol 2006;21:1307-1311.

41. Cassis TB, Jackson JM, Sonnier GB, Callen JP. Nephrogenic fibrosing dermopathy in a patient with acute renal failure never requiring dialysis. Int J Dermatol 2006;45:56-59.

42. DiCarlo JB, Gupta EA, Solomon AR. A pediatric case of nephrogenic fibrosing dermopathy: improvement after combination therapy. J Am Acad Dermatol 2006;54:914-916.

43. Kim RH, Ma L, Hayat SQ, Ahmed MM. Nephrogenic fibrosing dermopathy/nephrogenic systemic fibrosis in 2 patients with end-stage renal disease on hemodialysis. J Clin Rheumatol 2006;12:134-136.

44. Kucher C, Steere J, Elenitsas R, Siegel DL, Xu X. Nephrogenic fibrosing dermopathy/nephrogenic systemic fibrosis with diaphragmatic involvement in a patient with respiratory failure. J Am Acad Dermatol 2006;54(2 Suppl):S31-S34.

45. Lewis KG, Lester BW, Pan TD, Robinson-Bostom L. Nephrogenic fibrosing dermopathy and calciphylaxis with pseudoxanthoma elasticum-like changes. J Cutan Pathol 2006;33:695-700.

46. Mendoza FA, Artlett CM, Sandorfi N, et al. Description of 12 cases of nephrogenic fibrosing dermopathy and review of the literature. Semin Arthritis Rheum 2006;35:238-249.

47. Panda S, Bandyopadhyay D, Tarafder A. Nephrogenic fibrosing dermopathy: a series in a non-Western population. J Am Acad Dermatol 2006;54:155-159.

48. Shelekhova KV, Kazakov DV, Michal M. Nephrogenic fibrosing dermopathy. Arkh Patol 2006;68:42-43.

49. Broome DR, Girguis MS, Baron PW, et al. Gadodiamide-associated nephrogenic systemic fibrosis: why radiologists should be concerned. AJR Am J Roentgenol 2007;188:586-592.

50. Cheung PP, Dorai Raj AK. Nephrogenic fibrosing dermopathy: a new clinical entity mimicking sclero-derma. Intern Med J 2007;37:139-141.

51. Clorius S, Technau K, Watter T, et al. Nephrogenic systemic fibrosis following exposure to gadolinium-containing contrast agent. Clin Nephrol 2007;68:249-252.

52. Collidge TA, Thomson PC, Mark PB, et al. Gadolinium-enhanced MR imaging and nephrogenic systemic fibrosis: retrospective study of a renal replacement therapy cohort. Radiology 2007;245:168-175.

53. Deo A, Fogel M, Cowper SE. Nephrogenic systemic fibrosis: a population study examining the relationship of disease development to gadolinium exposure. Clin J Am Soc Nephrol 2007;2:264-267.

54. Garovic VD, Helgen KE. Images in clinical medicine. Nephrogenic fibrosing dermopathy. N Engl J Med 2007;357:e2.

55. Hamilton-Persaud K, Ezell LD, Macklin JG. Nephrogenic fibrosing dermopathy/nephrogenic systemic fi-brosis. Nephrol Nurs J 2007;34:283-287.

56. Introcaso CE, Hivnor C, Cowper S, Werth VP. Nephrogenic fibrosing dermopathy/nephrogenic systemic fibrosis: a case series of nine patients and review of the literature. Int J Dermatol 2007;46:447-452.

57. Keyrouz S, Rudnicki SA. Neuromuscular involvement in nephrogenic systemic fibrosis. J Clin Neuromus-cul Dis 2007;9:297-302.

58. Khurram M, Skov L, Rossen K, Thomsen HS, Marckmann P. Nephrogenic systemic fibrosis: a serious ia-trogenic disease of renal failure patients. Scand J Urol Nephrol 2007;41:565-566.

59. Kintossou R, D'Incan M, Chauveau D, et al. Nephrogenic fibrosing dermopathy treated with extracorporeal photopheresis: role of gadolinium? Ann Dermatol Venereol 2007;134:667-671.

60. Krous HF, Breisch E, Chadwick AE, et al. Nephrogenic systemic fibrosis with multiorgan involvement in a teenage male after lymphoma, Ewing's sarcoma, end-stage renal disease, and hemodialysis. Pediatr Dev Pathol 2007;10:395-402.

61. Lauenstein TC, Salman K, Morreira R, et al. Nephrogenic systemic fibrosis: center case review. J Magn Reson Imaging 2007;26:1198-1203.

62. Martin DR. Nephrogenic systemic fibrosis. Pediatr Radiol 2008;38(Suppl 1):S125-S129.

63. Lim YL, Lee HY, Low SC, et al. Possible role of gadolinium in nephrogenic systemic fibrosis: report of two cases and review of the literature. Clin Exp Dermatol 2007;32:353-358.

64. Maloo M, Abt P, Kashyap R, et al. Nephrogenic systemic fibrosis among liver transplant recipients: a single institution experience and topic update. Am J Transplant 2006;6:2212-2217.

65. Marckmann P, Skov L, Rossen K, Heaf JG, Thomsen HS. Case-control study of gadodiamide-related nephrogenic systemic fibrosis. Nephrol Dial Transplant 2007;22:3174-3178.

66. Moreno-Romero JA, Segura S, Mascaro JM Jr, et al. Nephrogenic systemic fibrosis: a case series suggesting gadolinium as a possible aetiological factor. Br J Dermatol 2007;157:783-787.

67. Othersen JB, Maize JC, Woolson RF, Budisavljevic MN. Nephrogenic systemic fibrosis after exposure to gadolinium in patients with renal failure. Nephrol Dial Transplant 2007;22:3179-3185. Erratum in: Nephrol Dial Transplant 2007;22:3179-3185.

68. Pieringer H, Schmekal B, Janko O, Biesenbach G. Treatment with corticosteroids does not seem to benefit nephrogenic systemic fibrosis. Nephrol Dial Transplant 2007;22:3094.

69. Plamondon I, Samson C, Watters AK, et al. Nephrogenic systemic fibrosis: more hard times for renal failure patients. Nephrol Ther 2007;3:152-156.

70. Pryor JG, Scott GA. Nephrogenic systemic fibrosis: a clinicopathologic study of 6 cases. J Am Acad Dermatol 2007;57:902-903.

71. Richmond H, Zwerner J, Kim Y, Fiorentino D. Nephrogenic systemic fibrosis: relationship to gadolinium and response to photopheresis. Arch Dermatol 2007;143:1025-1030.

72. Sadowski EA, Bennett LK, Chan MR, et al. Nephrogenic systemic fibrosis: risk factors and incidence estimation. Radiology 2007;243:148-157.

73. Saussereau E, Lacroix C, Cattaneo A, Mahieu L, Goulle JP. Hair and fingernail gadolinium ICP-MS contents in an overdose case associated with nephrogenic systemic fibrosis. Forensic Sci Int 2008;176:54-57. Erratum in: Forensic Sci Int 2008;176:91-92.

74. Thakral C, Alhariri J, Abraham JL. Long-term retention of gadolinium in tissues from nephrogenic systemic fibrosis patient after multiple gadolinium-enhanced MRI scans: case report and implications. Contrast Media Mol Imaging 2007;2:199-205.

75. Todd DJ, Kagan A, Chibnik LB, Kay J. Cutaneous changes of nephrogenic systemic fibrosis: predictor of early mortality and association with gadolinium exposure. Arthritis Rheum 2007;56:3433-3441.

76. Tsai CW, Chao CC, Wu VC, Hsiao CH, Chen YM. Nephrogenic fibrosing dermopathy in a peritoneal dialysis patient. Kidney Int 2007;72:1294.

77. Weenig RH, Gibson LE, El-Azhary R. The role of the hospital dermatologist in the diagnosis and treatment of calciphylaxis and nephrogenic systemic fibrosis. Semin Cutan Med Surg 2007;26:163-167.

78. Yerram P, Saab G, Karuparthi PR, Hayden MR, Khanna R. Nephrogenic systemic fibrosis: a mysterious disease in patients with renal failure—role of gadolinium-based contrast media in causation and the beneficial effect of intravenous sodium thiosulfate. Clin J Am Soc Nephrol 2007;2:258-263.

79. Centers for Disease Control and Prevention (CDC). Nephrogenic fibrosing dermopathy associated with exposure to gadolinium-containing contrast agents—St. Louis, Missouri, 2002-2006. MMWR Morb Mortal Wkly Rep 2007;56:137-4.

80. Kallen AJ, Jhung MA, Cheng S, et al. Gadolinium-containing magnetic resonance imaging contrast and nephrogenic systemic fibrosis: a case-control study. Am J Kidney Dis 2008;51:966-975.

81. Swaminathan S, Horn TD, Pellowski D, et al. Nephrogenic systemic fibrosis, gadolinium, and iron mobilization. N Engl J Med 2007;357:720-722.

82. Khurana A, Runge VM, Narayanan M, Greene JF Jr, Nickel AE. Nephrogenic systemic fibrosis: a review of 6 cases temporally related to gadodiamide injection (omniscan). Invest Radiol 2007;42:139-145.

83. Khurana A, Greene JF Jr, High WA. Quantification of gadolinium in nephrogenic systemic fibrosis: re-examination of a reported cohort with analysis of clinical factors. J Am Acad Dermatol 2008;59:218-224.

84. Morris MF, MacGregor J, Zhang H, et al. Factors relating to development of nephrogenic systemic fibrosis following gadolinium. Proc Int Soc Magn Reson Med 2007;15:739.

85. Grebe SO, Haage P. Nephrogene systemische Fibrose (NSF) nach Applikation gadoliniumhaltiger Kontrastmittel bei Shuntpatienten. Gefasschirurgie 2007;12:449-454.

86. Edward M, Fitzgerald L, Thind C, Leman J, Burden AD. Cutaneous mucinosis associated with dermatomyositis and nephrogenic fibrosing dermopathy: fibroblast hyaluronan synthesis and the effect of patient serum. Br J Dermatol 2007;156:473-479.

87. Solomon GJ, Rosen PP, Wu E. The role of gadolinium in triggering nephrogenic systemic fibrosis/nephrogenic fibrosing dermopathy. Arch Pathol Lab Med 2007;131:1515-1516.

88. van der Meij N, Keur I, et al. Nephrogenic systemic fibrosis possibly caused by gadolinium-containing contrast agent. Ned Tijdschr Geneeskd 2007;151:2898-2903.

89. Wahba IM, Simpson EL, White K. Gadolinium is not the only trigger for nephrogenic systemic fibrosis: insights from two cases and review of the recent literature. Am J Transplant 2007;7:2425-2432.

90. Weiss AS, Lucia MS, Teitelbaum I. A case of nephrogenic fibrosing dermopathy/nephrogenic systemic fibrosis. Nat Clin Pract Nephrol 2007;3:111-115.

91. Swaminathan S, High WA, Ranville J, et al. Cardiac and vascular metal deposition with high mortality in nephrogenic systemic fibrosis. Kidney Int 2008;73:1413-1418.

92. Artunc F, Schanz S, Metze D, Heyne N. Nephrogenic systemic fibrosis. Dtsch Med Wochenschr 2008;133(Suppl:F1).

93. Bennett LK, Garrett AL. Nephrogenic systemic fibrosis: is gadolinium the missing piece to the puzzle? Cutis 2008;81:421-426.

94. Caccetta T, Chan JJ. Nephrogenic systemic fibrosis associated with liver transplantation, renal failure and gadolinium. Australas J Dermatol 2008;49:48-51.

95. Chan KH, Tang WY, Hau KC, et al. Nephrogenic systemic fibrosis in a Chinese renal-transplant recipient. Clin Exp Dermatol 2009;34:244-246.

96. Chandran S, Petersen J, Jacobs C, et al. Imatinib in the treatment of nephrogenic systemic fibrosis. Am J Kidney Dis 2009;53:129-132.

97. Chao CC, Yang CC, Hsiao CH, et al. Nephrogenic systemic fibrosis associated with gadolinium use. J Formos Med Assoc 2008;107:270-274.

98. Chen W, Huang SL, Huang CS, et al. Nephrogenic systemic fibrosis in advanced chronic kidney disease: a single hospital's experience in Taiwan. Eur J Dermatol 2009;19:44-49.

99. Dhungel A, Lattupalli R, Topf J. Nephrogenic fibrosing dermopathy. Scientific World Journal 2008;8:164-165.

100. Duffy KL, Green L, Harris R, Powell D. Treatment of nephrogenic systemic fibrosis with Re-PUVA. J Am Acad Dermatol 2008;59(2 Suppl 1):S39-S40.

101. Firoz BF, Hunzeker CM, Soldano AC, Franks AG Jr. Nephrogenic fibrosing dermopathy. Dermatol Online J 2008;14:11.

102. Golding LP, Provenzale JM. Nephrogenic systemic fibrosis: possible association with a predisposing infection. AJR Am J Roentgenol 2008;190:1069-1075.

103. Greloni G, Rosa Diez G, Hidalgo Parra I, et al. [Risk of using gadolinium in patients with renal insufficiency]. Medicina (B Aires) 2008;68:346-347. [Article in Spanish]

104. Gulati A, Harwood CA, Raftery M,et al. Magnetic resonance imaging with gadolinium enhancement in renal failure: a need for caution. Int J Dermatol 2008;47:947-949.

105. Hidalgo Parra I, Torre A, Galimberti G, et al. Nephrogenic fibrosing dermopathy. J Eur Acad Dermatol Venereol 2008;22:875-876.

106. Introcaso CE, Elenitsas R, Xu X, James WD. Periocular papules in nephrogenic systemic fibrosis. J Am Acad Dermatol 2008;59:536-537.

107. Kadiyala D, Roer DA, Perazella MA. Nephrogenic systemic fibrosis associated with gadoversetamide exposure: treatment with sodium thiosulfate. Am J Kidney Dis 2009;53:133-137.

108. Kalb RE, Helm TN, Sperry H, et al. Gadolinium-induced nephrogenic systemic fibrosis in a patient with an acute and transient kidney injury. Br J Dermatol 2008;158:607-610.

109. Kane GC, Stanson AW, Kalnicka D, et al. Comparison between gadolinium and iodine contrast for percutaneous intervention in atherosclerotic renal artery stenosis: clinical outcomes. Nephrol Dial Transplant 2008;23:1233-1240.

110. Kelly B, Petitt M, Sanchez R. Nephrogenic systemic fibrosis is associated with transforming growth factor beta and Smad without evidence of renin-angiotensin system involvement. J Am Acad Dermatol 2008;58:1025-1030.

111. Khurana A, Nickel AE, Greene JF Jr, et al. Successful pregnancy in a hemodialysis patient and marked resolution of her nephrogenic systemic fibrosis. Am J Kidney Dis 2008;51:e29-e32.

112. Lu CF, Hsiao CH, Tjiu JW. Nephrogenic systemic fibrosis developed after recovery from acute renal failure: gadolinium as a possible aetiological factor. J Eur Acad Dermatol Venereol 2009;23:339-340.

113. Mathur K, Morris S, Deighan C, Green R, Douglas KW. Extracorporeal photopheresis improves nephrogenic fibrosing dermopathy/nephrogenic systemic fibrosis: three case reports and review of literature. J Clin Apher 2008;23:144-150.

114. Matthesen SK, Pedersen EB. [Nephrogen systemic fibrosis is reported in a dialysis patient after MR-angiography with a contrast medium]. Ugeskr Laeger 2008;170:655.

115. Naylor E, Hu S, Robinson-Bostom L. Nephrogenic systemic fibrosis with septal panniculitis mimicking erythema nodosum. J Am Acad Dermatol 2008;58:149-150.

116. O'Donnell PJ, Duke WH, Pantanowitz L. Absence of human herpes virus-8 (HHV8) in nephrogenic systemic fibrosis. BMC Res Notes 2008;1:82.

117. Pao VY, Chang S, Shoback DM, Bikle DD. Hypercalcemia and overexpression of CYP27B1 in a patient with nephrogenic systemic fibrosis: clinical vignette and literature review. J Bone Miner Res 2009;24:1135-1139.

118. Prince MR, Zhang H, Morris M, et al. Incidence of nephrogenic systemic fibrosis at two large medical centers. Radiology 2008;248:807-816.

119. Rydahl C, Thomsen HS, Marckmann P. High prevalence of nephrogenic systemic fibrosis in chronic renal failure patients exposed to gadodiamide, a gadolinium-containing magnetic resonance contrast agent. Invest Radiol 2008;43:141-144.

120. Schieren G, Tokmak F, Lefringhausen L, et al. C-reactive protein levels and clinical symptoms following gadolinium administration in hemodialysis patients. Am J Kidney Dis 2008;51:976-986.

121. Schietinger BJ, Brammer GM, Wang H, et al. Patterns of late gadolinium enhancement in chronic hemodialysis patients. JACC Cardiovasc Imaging 2008;1:450-456.

122. Schroeder JA, Weingart C, Coras B, et al. Ultrastructural evidence of dermal gadolinium deposits in a patient with nephrogenic systemic fibrosis and end-stage renal disease. Clin J Am Soc Nephrol 2008;3:968-975.

123. Shabana WM, Cohan RH, Ellis JH, et al. Nephrogenic systemic fibrosis: a report of 29 cases. AJR Am J Roentgenol 2008;190:736-741.

124. Shin K, Granter SR, Coblyn JS, Gupta S. Progressive arm and leg stiffness in a patient with chronic renal impairment. Nat Clin Pract Rheumatol 2008;4:557-562.

125. Weigle JP, Broome DR. Nephrogenic systemic fibrosis: chronic imaging findings and review of the medical literature. Skeletal Radiol 2008;37:457-464.

126. Wertman R, Altun E, Martin DR, et al. Risk of nephrogenic systemic fibrosis: evaluation of gadolinium chelate contrast agents at four American universities. Radiology 2008;248:799-806.

127. Wiginton CD, Kelly B, Oto A, et al. Gadolinium-based contrast exposure, nephrogenic systemic fibrosis, and gadolinium detection in tissue. AJR Am J Roentgenol 2008;190:1060-1068.

128. Zelasko S, Hollingshead M, Castillo M, Bouldin TW. CT and MR imaging of progressive dural involvement by nephrogenic systemic fibrosis. AJNR Am J Neuroradiol 2008;29:1880-1882.

129. Schieren G, Tokmak F, Lefringhausen L, et al. C-reactive protein levels and clinical symptoms following gadolinium administration in hemodialysis patients. Am J Kidney Dis 2008;51:976-986.

130. Schieren G, Wirtz N, Altmeyer P, et al. Nephrogenic systemic fibrosis—a rapidly progressive disabling disease with limited therapeutic options. J Am Acad Dermatol 2009;61:868-874.

131. Bainotti S, Rota E, Bertrero M, et al. Nephrogenic systemic fibrosis: the first Italian gadolinium-proven case. Clin Nephrol 2008;70:514-517.

132. Bertero M, Bainotti S, Comino A, et al. Nephrogenic fibrosing dermopathy/nephrogenic systemic fibrosis. Eur J Dermatol 2009;19:73-74.

133. Rota E, Nallino MG, Bainotti S, Formica M. Nephrogenic systemic fibrosis: an unusual scleroderma-like fibrosing disorder. Rheumatol Int 2010;30:1389-1391.

134. Deng AC, Bilu Martin D, Sina B, Gaspari A. Localized nephrogenic fibrosing dermopathy: Aberrant dermal repairing? J Am Acad Dermatol 2008;58:336-339.

135. Aluma MS, Restrepo R, Gaviria M. Nephrogenic fibrosing dermopathy: first Colombian case. Dermatol Online J 2007;13:24.

136. Anavekar NS, Chong AH, Norris R, et al. Nephrogenic systemic fibrosis in a gadolinium-naive renal transplant recipient. Australas J Dermatol 2008;49:44-47.

137. Digby S, Macduff E, Blessing K, Holmes S. Nephrogenic systemic fibrosis: a histopathological study of eight cases of a recently described entity. Histopathology 2008;52:531-534.

138. Edward M, Quinn JA, Mukherjee S, et al. Gadodiamide contrast agent 'activates' fibroblasts: a possible cause of nephrogenic systemic fibrosis. J Pathol 2008;214:584-593.

139. George DE, Lu R, George SJ, Hsu S. Nephrogenic fibrosing dermopathy: case report and review. Dermatol Online J 2006;12:7.

140. Kreuter A, Gambichler T, Weiner SM, Schieren G. Limited effects of UV-A1 phototherapy in 3 patients with nephrogenic systemic fibrosis. Arch Dermatol 2008;144:1527-1529.

141. Nagai Y, Hasegawa M, Shinmi K, et al. Nephrogenic systemic fibrosis with multiple calcification and osseous metaplasia. Acta Derm Venereol 2008;88:597-600.

142. Song J, Volkov S, Shea CR, et al. Nephrogenic systemic fibrosis associated with stromal and vascular calcification, report of two cases. J Cutan Pathol 2009;36(Suppl 1):31-34.

143. Abujudeh HH, Kaewlai R, Kagan A, et al. Nephrogenic systemic fibrosis after gadopentetate dimeglumine exposure: case series of 36 patients. Radiology 2009;253:81-89.

144. Al Habeeb A, Partington S, Rosenthal D, Salama S. Skin thickening in a hemodialysis patient: a case of nephrogenic fibrosing dermopathy. J Cutan Med Surg 2009;13:110-114.

145. Altun E, Martin DR, Wertman R, et al. Nephrogenic systemic fibrosis: change in incidence following a switch in gadolinium agents and adoption of a gadolinium policy—report from two U.S. universities. Radiology 2009;253:689-696.

146. Bahrami S, Raman SS, Sauk S, et al. Ten-year experience with nephrogenic systemic fibrosis: case-control analysis of risk factors. J Comput Assist Tomogr 2009;33:819-823.

147. Bhawan J, Swick BL, Koff AB, Stone MS. Sclerotic bodies in nephrogenic systemic fibrosis: a new histopathologic finding. J Cutan Pathol 2009;36:548-552.

148. Boyd AS, Sanyal S, Abraham JL. Tissue gadolinium deposition and fibrosis mimicking nephrogenic systemic fibrosis (NSF)-subclinical nephrogenic systemic fibrosis? J Am Acad Dermatol 2010;62:337-342.

149. Bridges MD, St Amant BS, McNeil RB, et al. High-dose gadodiamide for catheter angiography and CT in patients with varying degrees of renal insufficiency: Prevalence of subsequent nephrogenic systemic fibrosis and decline in renal function. AJR Am J Roentgenol 2009;192:1538-1543.

150. Christiansen RE, Sviland L, Sekse I, Svarstad E. Nephrogenic systemic fibrosis and use of MR contrast media. Tidsskr Nor Laegeforen 2009;129:180-182.

151. Chrysochou C, Buckley DL, Dark P, Cowie A, Kalra PA. Gadolinium-enhanced magnetic resonance imaging for renovascular disease and nephrogenic systemic fibrosis: critical review of the literature and UK experience. J Magn Reson Imaging 2009;29:887-894.

152. Deng A, Martin DB, Spillane A, et al. Nephrogenic systemic fibrosis with a spectrum of clinical and histopathological presentation: a disorder of aberrant dermal remodeling. J Cutan Pathol 2010;37:204-210.

153. Foss C, Smith JK, Ortiz L, Hanevold C, Davis L. Gadolinium-associated nephrogenic systemic fibrosis in a 9-year-old boy. Pediatr Dermatol 2009;26:579-582.

154. Heinz-Peer G, Neruda A, Watschinger B, et al. Prevalence of NSF following intravenous gadolinium-contrast media administration in dialysis patients with endstage renal disease. Eur J Radiol 2010;76:129-134.

155. Hope TA, Herfkens RJ, Denianke KS, et al. Nephrogenic systemic fibrosis in patients with chronic kidney disease who received gadopentetate dimeglumine. Invest Radiol 2009;44:135-139.

156. Hoppe H, Spagnuolo S, Froehlich JM, et al. Retrospective analysis of patients for development of nephrogenic systemic fibrosis following conventional angiography using gadolinium-based contrast agents. Eur Radiol 2010;20:595-603.

157. Kreuter A, Höxtermann S, Gambichler T, et al. Detection of clonal T cells in the circulation of patients with nephrogenic systemic fibrosis. Arch Dermatol 2009;145:1164-1169.

158. Lee CU, Wood CM, Hesley GK, et al. Large sample of nephrogenic systemic fibrosis cases from a single institution. Arch Dermatol 2009;145:1095-1102.

159. Mundim JS, Lorena Sde C, Elias RM, Romao Junior JE. Nephrogenic systemic fibrosis: mini-review. Clinics (Sao Paulo) 2009;64:482-484.

160. Nakai K, Takeda K, Kimura H, Miura S, Maeda A. Nephrogenic systemic fibrosis in a patient on long-term hemodialysis. Clin Nephrol 2009;71:217-220.

161. Perez-Rodriguez J, Lai S, Ehst BD, Fine DM, Bluemke DA. Nephrogenic systemic fibrosis: incidence, associations, and effect of risk factor assessment—report of 33 cases. Radiology 2009;250:371-377.

162. Ramaizel L, Sliwa JA. Rehabilitation in nephrogenic systemic fibrosis. PM R 2009;1:684-686.

163. Rodríguez Jornet A, Andreu Navarro FJ, et al. Gadolinium-induced systemic fibrosis in advanced kidney failure. Nefrologia 2009;29:358-363.

164. Schmiedl S, Wesselmann U, Lehmann P, Haage P, Grebe SO. Different time courses of nephrogenic systemic fibrosis: Is there a role for pharmacokinetic aspects in explaining a new clinical entity? Int J Clin Pharmacol Ther 2009;47:695-700.

165. So K, Macquillan GC, Adams LA, et al. Malignant fibrous histiocytoma complicating nephrogenic systemic fibrosis post liver transplantation. Intern Med J 2009;39:613-617.

166. Su HS, Nazarian RM, Scott JA. Case report. Appearance of nephrogenic fibrosing dermopathy on a bone scan. Br J Radiol 2009;82:e35-e36.

167. Tran KT, Prather HB, Cockerell CJ, Jacobe H. UV-A1 therapy for nephrogenic systemic fibrosis. Arch Dermatol 2009;145:1170-1174.

168. Wiedemeyer K, Kutzner H, Abraham JL, et al. The evolution of osseous metaplasia in localized cutaneous nephrogenic systemic fibrosis: a case report. Am J Dermatopathol 2009;31:674-681.

169. Wilford C, Fine JD, Boyd AS, et al. Nephrogenic systemic fibrosis: report of an additional case with granulomatous inflammation. Am J Dermatopathol 2010;32:71-75.

170. Wollanka H, Weidenmaier W, Giersig C. NSF after Gadovist exposure: a case report and hypothesis of NSF development. Nephrol Dial Transplant 2009;24:3882-3884.

171. Bangsgaard N, Marckmann P, Rossen K, Skov L. Nephrogenic systemic fibrosis: late skin manifestations. Arch Dermatol 2009;145:183-187.

172. Cuende E, Aldamiz M, Portu J, et al. Nephrogenic systemic fibrosis in a patient with a p-ANCA systemic vasculitis. Reumatol Clin 2009;5:264-267.

173. Davis RL, Abraham JL. Lanthanum deposition in a dialysis patient. Nephrol Dial Transplant 2009;24:3247-3250.

174. Ragunatha S, Palit A, Inamadar AC, et al. Nephrogenic fibrosing dermopathy. Indian J Dermatol Venereol Leprol 2009;75:63-67.

175. Becker S, Walter S, Witzke O, et al. The German registry for nephrogenic systemic fibrosis: findings from 23 patients. Clin Nephrol 2010;73:426-430.

176. Cuffy MC, Singh M, Formica R, et al. Renal transplantation for nephrogenic systemic fibrosis: a case report and review of the literature. Nephrol Dial Transplant 2011;26:1099-1101.

177. Edgar E, Woltjer R, Whitham R, et al. Nephrogenic systemic fibrosis presenting as myopathy: a case report with histopathologic correlation. Neuromuscul Disord 2010;20:411-413.

178. George SJ, Webb SM, Abraham JL, Cramer SP. Synchrotron X-ray analyses demonstrate phosphate-bound gadolinium in skin in nephrogenic systemic fibrosis. Br J Dermatol 2010;163:1077-1081.

179. Gist RS, Miller DW, Warren T. A difficult airway in a patient with nephrogenic sclerosing fibrosis. Anesth Analg 2010;110:555-557.

180. Kelly BC, Markle LS, Vickers JL, et al. The imbalanced expression of matrix metalloproteinases in nephrogenic systemic fibrosis. J Am Acad Dermatol 2010;63:483-489.

181. Kennedy C, Magee C, Eltayeb E, Gulmann C, Conlon PJ. Nephrogenic systemic fibrosis. Ir Med J 2010;103:208-210.

182. Knapp BA, Sepahpanah F. Nephrogenic systemic fibrosis in a patient with spinal cord injury: a unique case presentation. PM R 2010;2:1141-1144.

183. Lemy AA, del Marmol V, Kolivras A, et al. Revisiting nephrogenic systemic fibrosis in 6 kidney transplant recipients: a single-center experience. J Am Acad Dermatol 2010;63:389-399.

184. Quatresooz P, Paquet P, Hermanns-Le T, Pierard GE. Immunohistochemical aspects of the fibrogenic pathway in nephrogenic systemic fibrosis. Appl Immunohistochem Mol Morphol 2010;18:448-452.

185. Reddy IS, Somani VK, Swarnalata G, Maitra S. Nephrogenic systemic fibrosis following hair-dye ingestion induced acute renal failure. Indian J Dermatol Venereol Leprol 2010;76:400-403.

186. Swaminathan S, Arbiser JL, Hiatt KM, et al. Rapid improvement of nephrogenic systemic fibrosis with rapamycin therapy: possible role of phospho-70-ribosomal-S6 kinase. J Am Acad Dermatol 2010;62:343-345.

187. Kartono F, Basile A, Roshdieh B, et al. Findings of osseous sclerotic bodies: a unique sequence of cutaneous bone formation in nephrogenic systemic fibrosis. J Cutan Pathol 2011;38:286-289.

188. Charli-Joseph Y, Ruelas Villavicencio A, Garcia-Hidalgo L, Orozco-Topete R. Nephrogenic systemic fibrosis: Report of two cases. J Am Acad Dermatol 2010:AB91. Abstract P2603.

189. Davison R, Mead P. Nephrogenic systemic fibrosis (NSF): the role of tamoxifen. NDT Plus 2010;3:505.

190. Elmholdt TR, Jorgensen B, Ramsing M, et al. Two cases of nephrogenic systemic fibrosis after exposure to the macrocyclic compound gadobutrol. NDT Plus 2010;3:285-287.

191. Kitaura K, Harima K, Inami N, Kajiura T, Yamada K. Prolonged dural enhancement by iodine contrast agent mimicking subdural haematoma in a patient with nephrogenic systemic fibrosis. NDT Plus 2010;3:193-194.

192. Panos A, Milas F, Kalakonas S, Myers PO. Cardiac autotransplantation for aortic and mitral valve replacement in a patient with nephrogenic systemic fibrosis. Hellenic J Cardiol 2010;51:64-66.

193. Tsushima Y, Kanal E, Thomsen HS. Nephrogenic systemic fibrosis: risk factors suggested from Japanese published cases. Br J Radiol 2010;83:590-595.

194. Barker-Griffith A, Goldberg J, Abraham JL. Ocular pathologic features and gadolinium deposition in nephrogenic systemic fibrosis. Arch Ophthalmol 2011;129:661-663.

195. Elmholdt TR, Pedersen M, Jorgensen B, et al. Nephrogenic systemic fibrosis is found only among gadolinium-exposed patients with renal insufficiency: a case-control study from Denmark. Br J Dermatol 2011;165:828-836.

196. Kendrick-Jones JC, Voss DM, De Zoysa JR. Nephrogenic systemic fibrosis, in patients with end-stage kidney disease on dialysis, in the greater Auckland region, from 2000-2006. Nephrology 2011;16:243-248.

197. Robinson MR, Routhouska SB, Paspulati RM, Korman NJ. Alefacept therapy for nephrogenic systemic fibrosis: a case series. J Drugs Dermatol 2011;10:922-924.

198. Truong SV, Chen JK, Reinstadler A, Saedi N. Nephrogenic systemic fibrosis: a case report and review of the literature. J Drugs Dermatol 2011;10:622-624.

199. Matsumoto Y, Mitsuhashi Y, Monma F, et al. Nephrogenic systemic fibrosis: a case report and review on Japanese patients. J Dermatol 2012;39:449-453.

200. Aggarwal A, Froehlich AA, Essah P, et al. Complications of nephrogenic systemic fibrosis following repeated exposure to gadolinium in a man with hypothyroidism: a case report. J Med Case Rep 2011;5:566.

201. Hashemi P, Sina B, Rietkerk W, Safai B. The debate between gadolinium versus erythropoietin in a renal transplant patient with nephrogenic systemic fibrosis. J Nephrol 2013;26:48-54.

202. Becker S, Walter S, Witzke O, et al. Application of gadolinium-based contrast agents and prevalence of nephrogenic systemic fibrosis in a cohort of end-stage renal disease patients on hemodialysis. Nephron Clin Pract 2012;121:c91-c94.

203. Lima XT, Alora-Palli MB, Kimball AB, Kay J. Validation of a screening instrument for nephrogenic systemic fibrosis. Arthritis Care Res 2013;65:637-42.

204. Freed L, Hill J, Gooch D. Nephrogenic systemic fibrosis in the podiatric patient. J Am Podiatr Med Assoc 2012;102:419-421.

205. Galan A, Cowper SE, Bucala R. Nephrogenic systemic fibrosis (nephrogenic fibrosing dermopathy). Curr Opin Rheumatol 2006;18:614–617.

206. Cowper SE, Bucala R, Leboit PE. Nephrogenic fibrosing dermopathy/nephrogenic systemic fibrosis: setting the record straight. Semin Arthritis Rheum 2006;35:208–210.

207. Knopp EA, Cowper SE. Nephrogenic systemic fibrosis: early recognition and treatment. Semin Dial 2008;21:123–128.

208. Prince MR, Arnoldus C, Frisoli JK. Nephrotoxicity of high-dose gadolinium compared with iodinated contrast. J Magn Reson Imaging 1996;1:162–166.

209. Thomsen HS, Almen T, Morcos SK; Contrast Media Safety Committee of the European Society of Urogenital Radiology. Gadolinium-containing contrast media for radiographic examinations: a position paper. Eur Radiol 2002;12:2600–2605.

210. Agarwal R, Brunelli SM, Williams K, et al. Gadolinium-based contrast agents and nephrogenic systemic fibrosis: a systematic review and meta-analysis. Nephrol Dial Transplant 2009;24:856–863.

211. Kuo PH. Gadolinium-containing MRI contrast agents: important variations on a theme for NSF. J Am Coll Radiol 2008;5:29–35.

212. Cowper SE, Rabach M, Girardi M. Clinical and histological findings in nephrogenic systemic fibrosis. Eur J Radiol 2008;66:191–199.

213. Cowper SE. Nephrogenic fibrosing dermopathy: the first 6 years. Curr Opin Rheumatol 2003;15:785–790.

214. Bucala R. Circulating fibrocytes: cellular basis for NSF. J Am Coll Radiol 2008; 5:36–39.

215. Thomsen HS, Morcos SK, Almén T, et al. Nephrogenic systemic fibrosis and gadolinium-based contrast media: updated ESUR Contrast Medium Safety Committee guidelines. Eur Radiol 2013;23:307-318.

216. American College of Radiology. Nephrogenic Systemic Fibrosis. Manual of Contrast Media Version 8. Available from: http://www.acr.org/~/media/ACR/Documents/PDF/QualitySafety/Resources/Contrast%20Manual/Nephrogenic%20Systemic%20Fibrosis.pdf. Accessed February, 2013.

217. National Collaborating Centre for Chronic Conditions (UK). Chronic Kidney Disease: National Clinical Guideline for Early Identification and Management in Adults in Primary and Secondary Care. London: Royal College of Physicians (UK); 2008 Sep. (NICE Clinical Guidelines, No. 73.) Available from: http://www.ncbi.nlm.nih.gov/books/NBK51773/. Accessed February, 2013.

218. National Kidney Foundation. About Chronic Kidney Disease. Available from: http://www.kidney.org/kidneydisease/aboutckd.cfm. Accessed February, 2013.

219. Jaar BG, Khatib R, Plantinga L, Boulware LE, Powe NR. Principles of screening for chronic kidney disease. Clin J Am Soc Nephrol 2008;3:601–609.

220. Levey AS, Bosch JP, Lewis JB, et al. A more accurate method to estimate glomerular filtration rate from serum creatinine: a new prediction equation. Modification of Diet in Renal Disease Study Group. Ann Intern Med 1999;130:461–470.

221. Cockcroft DW, Gault MH. Prediction of creatinine clearance from serum creatinine. Nephron 1976;16:31–41.

222. Levey AS, Coresh J, Balk E, et al. National Kidney Foundation. National Kidney Foundation practice guidelines for chronic kidney disease: evaluation, classification, and stratification. Ann Intern Med 2003;139:137–147. Erratum in: Ann Intern Med 2003;139:605.

223. Stevens LA, Manzi J, Levey AS, et al. Impact of creatinine calibration on performance of GFR estimating equations in a pooled individual patient database. Am J Kidney Dis 2007;50:21–35.

224. Levey AS, Coresh J, Greene T, et al. Chronic kidney disease epidemiology collaboration. Expressing the modification of diet in renal disease study equation for estimating glomerular filtration rate with standardized serum creatinine values. Clin Chem 2007;53:766–772.

225. Levey AS, Coresh J, Greene T, et al. Chronic kdney disease epidemiology collaboration. Using standardized serum creatinine values in the modification of diet in renal disease study equation for estimating glomerular filtration rate. Ann Intern Med 2006;145:247–254.

226. Schwartz GJ, Munoz A, Schneider MF, et al. New equations to estimate GFR in children with CKD. J Am Soc Nephrol 2009;20:629-637.

227. FDA Drug Safety Communication: New warnings for using gadolinium-based contrast agents in patients with kidney dysfunction. Available at http://www.fda.gov/Drugs/DrugSafety/ucm223966.htm#. Accessed February, 2013.

228. European Medicines Agency. Assessment Report for Gadolinium Containing Contrast Agents. 1 July 2010. Available   at http://www.ema.europa.eu/docs/en_GB/document_library/Referrals_document/gadolinium_31/WC500099 538.pdf Accessed February, 2013.

229. Achenbach M, Figiel JH, Burbelko M, et al. Prospective comparison of image quality and diagnostic accuracy of 0.5 molar gadobenate dimeglumine and 1.0 molar gadobutrol in contrast-enhanced run-off magnetic resonance angiography of the lower extremities. J Magn Reson Imaging 2010;32:1166-1171.

230. Huang B, Liang CH, Liu HJ, et al. Low dose contrast-enhanced magnetic resonance imaging of brain metastases at 3.0T using high-relaxivity contrast agents. Acta Radiol 2012;51:78-84.

231. Noebauer-Huhmann IM, Pinker K, Barth M, et al. Contrast-enhanced, high-resolution, susceptibility-weighted magnetic resonance imaging of the brain. Dose-dependent optimization at 3 Tesla and 1.5 Tesla in healthy volunteers. Invest Radiol 2006;41:249–255.

232. Runge VM, Parker JR, Donovan M. Double-blind, efficacy evaluation of gadobenate dimeglumine, a gadolinium chelate with enhanced relaxivity, in malignant lesions of the brain. Invest Radiol 2002;37:269–280.

233. Baleriaux D, Colosimo C, Ruscalleda J, et al. Magnetic resonance imaging of metastatic disease to the brain with gadobenate dimeglumine. Neuroradiology 2002; 44:191-203.

234. Runge VM, Armstrong MR, Barr RG, et al. A clinical comparison of the safety and efficacy of MultiHance (gadobenate dimeglumine) and Omniscan (gadodiamide) in magnetic resonance imaging in patients with central nervous system pathology. Invest Radiol 2001;36:65–71.

235. Volk M, Strotzer M, Lenhart M, et al. Renal time-resolved MR angiography: Quantitative comparison of gadobenate dimeglumine and gadopentetate dimeglumine with different doses. Radiology 2001;220:484–488.

236. Schneider G, Ballarati C, Grazioli L, et al. Gadobenate dimeglumine – enhanced MR angiography: diagnostic performance of four doses for detection and grading of carotid, renal and aorto-iliac stenoses compared to digital subtraction angiography. J Magn Reson Imaging 2007;26:1020-1032.

237. Korperich H, Gieseke J, Esdorn H, et al. Ultrafast time-resolved contrast-enhanced 3D pulmonary venous cardiovascular magnetic resonance angiography using SENSE combined with CENTRA-keyhole. J Cardiovasc Magn Reson 2007;9:77–87.

238. Sandhu GS, Rezaee RP, Wright K, et al. Time-resolved and bolus-chase MR Angiography of the leg: branching pattern analysis and identification of septocutaneous perforators. Am J Roentgenol 2010;195:858-864.

239. Anzidei M, Cavallo Marincola B, Napoli A, et al. Low dose contrast-enhanced time-resolved MR angiography at 3 T: diagnostic accuracy for treatment planning and follow-up of vascular malformations. Clin Radiol 2011;66:1181-1192.

240. Knopp MV, Bourne MW, Sardanelli F, et al. Gadobenate dimeglumine-enhanced MRI of the breast: analysis of dose response and comparison with gadopentetate dimeglumine. AJR Am J Roentgenol 2003;181:663-676.

241. Sardanelli F, Iozzelli A, Fausto A, et al. Gadobenate dimeglumine–enhanced MR imaging breast vascular maps: Association between invasive cancer and ipsilateral increased vascularity. Radiology 2005;235:791-797.

242. Secchi F, Di Leo G, Papini GDE, et al. Optimizing dose and administration regimen of a high relaxivity contrast agent for myocardial MRI late gadolinium enhancement. Eur J Radiol 2011;80:96-102.

243. de Campos RO, Hredia V, Ramalho M, et al. Quarter dose (0.025 mmol/kg) gadobenate dimeglumine for abdominal MRI in patients at risk for nephrogenic systemic fibrosis: Preliminary observations. AJR Am J Roentgenol 2011;196:545-552.

244. Morcos SK, Thomsen HS, Webb JAW; Contrast Media Safety Committee of the European Society of Urogenital Radiology (ESUR). Dialysis and contrast media. Eur Radiol 2007;12:3026–3030.

245. Bennett CL, Qureshi ZP, Sartor AO, et al. Gadolinium-induced nephrogenic systemic fibrosis: the rise and fall of an iatrogenic disease. Clin Kidney J 2012;5:82-88.

Chapter 12   MRI Screening for Patients and Individuals

Ashok K. Saraswat, M.S., B.Ed., R.T. (R)(MR)

MRI Educational Program Director
Ohio State University
Wexner Medical Center
Clinical Instructor
Health & Rehabilitation Sciences
Columbus, OH

Mark A. Smith M.S., ABMP, R.T.(R)(MR)

MRI Physicist
Nationwide Children's Hospital
Clinical Instructor, Adjunct Faculty
Ohio State University
Wexner Medical Center
Columbus, OH

INTRODUCTION

The clinical applications of magnetic resonance imaging (MRI) have expanded rapidly in recent years, resulting in a greater percentage of the patient population undergoing diagnostic imaging using this modality. In addition, the number of patients and individuals possessing implantable devices continues to grow, as does the variation and complexity of these devices. Non-medical implants and materials such as body piercings, tattoos, and permanent cosmetics (e.g., eyeliner) have also increased in popularity. This progressive array of implanted patients and individuals, combined with the implementation of scanners with higher static magnetic fields (i.e., 3-Tesla) presents particular challenges for screening in the MRI environment. Indeed, accidents and injuries have increased over the years along with the increased use of MRI. Accordingly, this has captured the attention of various organizations and entities including the United States (U.S.) Food and Drug Administration (FDA), the Joint Commission, and the American College of Radiology (ACR). Public awareness of MRI-related hazards has heightened as well, particularly due to the fatality of a young boy in 2001. The majority of accidents and injuries that have occurred in the MRI setting have been the result of insufficient or no screening procedures. Unfortunately, considerable subjectivity remains among the policies and procedures implemented by MRI facilities, despite screening recommendations presented as far back as 1987 and periodically revised and updated to the present day (1-17).

This chapter presents the purpose of comprehensive MRI screening and discusses proper procedures. The recommended written screening forms to be used for individuals and patients are displayed and reviewed. Each section of these forms is explained, and justifications are given for the questions asked. Verbal MRI screening procedures are also reviewed, and the use of ferromagnetic detection systems as part of the screening process is discussed. Finally, secondary purposes and advantages of MRI screening are presented.

MRI SCREENING PROCEDURES

All patients undergoing MRI examinations must be screened prior to entering the MRI environment. Any other individual that needs to enter the MRI environment for any reason, even if just momentarily, must also be screened. This would include family members, friends, staff, visitors, field engineers, and emergency or security personnel such as firemen, police, and first responders. The screening process must include the completion of a written screening form by the patient or individual, followed by verbal MRI screening procedure conducted by the MRI technologist or other MRI safety-trained healthcare worker. All MRI facilities (clinical or research) should embrace a specific MRI screening process that is both consistent and thorough. This should be part of the MRI center's formal written policy, to be followed without exception. To stay current, MRI facilities need to revise and update the screening protocol, on an on-going and consistent basis.

SCREENING FORM AND PROCEDURES FOR PATIENTS

A standard, two page MRI screening form for patients developed by the Institute for Magnetic Resonance Safety Education and Research (www.IMRSER.org) is presented in **Figure 1** and **Figure 2** (the Spanish language version is displayed in **Figure 3** and **Figure 4**). The ACR (American College of Radiology, www.ACR.org) also offers a similar MRI screening form (14). Before each MRI examination, proper MRI screening must be conducted for each patient. To avoid confusion, this chapter will focus on the written screening form developed by the Institute for Magnetic Resonance Safety Education and Research.

SAFETY QUESTIONS AND INFORMATION

The upper section on the first page of the screening form (**Figure 1**) asks for patient identification (ID) and demographics. This section must be completed and double checked against the patient ID band and MRI order or request. An incorrect patient or examination problem can easily occur during the fervor of a booked clinical schedule. The referring physician's name and telephone number should also be filled out, but this information may be different than the "ordering" physician or resident. The rest of the first page of the screening form lists various medical and surgical history questions for the patient (note: certain

Figure 1. The MRI Screening Form used to screen patients, page one.

MAGNETIC RESONANCE (MR) PROCEDURE SCREENING FORM FOR PATIENTS

Date _____/_____/_____   Patient Number _____

Name _____ Age _____ Height _____ Weight _____
       Last name   First name   Middle Initial

Date of Birth _____/_____/_____   Male ☐ Female ☐   Body Part to be Examined _____
       month day year
Address _____   Telephone (home) (____) ____-_____

City _____   Telephone (work) (____) ____-_____

State _____ Zip Code _____

Reason for MRI and/or Symptoms _____

Referring Physician _____   Telephone (____) ____-_____

---

1. Have you had prior surgery or an operation (e.g., arthroscopy, endoscopy, etc.) of any kind?   ☐ No   ☐ Yes
   If yes, please indicate the date and type of surgery:
   Date _____/_____/_____   Type of surgery _____
   Date _____/_____/_____   Type of surgery _____
2. Have you had a prior diagnostic imaging study or examination (MRI, CT, Ultrasound, X-ray, etc.)?   ☐No   ☐ Yes
   If yes, please list: Body part   Date   Facility
MRI   _____ ___/___/___ _____
CT/CAT Scan   _____ ___/___/___ _____
X-Ray   _____ ___/___/___ _____
Ultrasound   _____ ___/___/___ _____
Nuclear Medicine _____ ___/___/___ _____
Other_____   _____ ___/___/___ _____

3. Have you experienced any problem related to a previous MRI examination or MR procedure?   ☐ No   ☐ Yes
   If yes, please describe: _____
4. Have you had an injury to the eye involving a metallic object or fragment (e.g., metallic slivers,
   shavings, foreign body, etc.)?   ☐ No   ☐ Yes
   If yes, please describe: _____
5. Have you ever been injured by a metallic object or foreign body (e.g., BB, bullet, shrapnel, etc.)?   ☐ No   ☐ Yes
   If yes, please describe: _____
6. Are you currently taking or have you recently taken any medication or drug?   ☐ No   ☐ Yes
   If yes, please list: _____
7. Are you allergic to any medication?   ☐ No   ☐ Yes
   If yes, please list: _____
8. Do you have a history of asthma, allergic reaction, respiratory disease, or reaction to a contrast
   medium or dye used for an MRI, CT, or X-ray examination?   ☐ No   ☐ Yes
9. Do you have anemia or any disease(s) that affects your blood, a history of renal (kidney)
   disease, renal (kidney) failure, renal (kidney) transplant, high blood pressure (hypertension),
   liver (hepatic) disease, a history of diabetes, or seizures?   ☐ No   ☐ Yes
   If yes, please describe: _____

For female patients:
10. Date of last menstrual period:_____/_____/_____   Post menopausal?   ☐ No   ☐ Yes
11. Are you pregnant or experiencing a late menstrual period?   ☐ No   ☐ Yes
12. Are you taking oral contraceptives or receiving hormonal treatment?   ☐ No   ☐ Yes
13. Are you taking any type of fertility medication or having fertility treatments?   ☐ No   ☐ Yes
    If yes, please describe: _____
14. Are you currently breastfeeding?   ☐ No   ☐ Yes

Figure 2. The MRI Screening Form used to screen patients, page two.

 WARNING: Certain implants, devices, or objects may be hazardous to you and/or may interfere with the MR procedure (i.e., MRI, MR angiography, functional MRI, MR spectroscopy). Do not enter the MR system room or MR environment if you have any question or concern regarding an implant, device, or object. Consult the MRI Technologist or Radiologist BEFORE entering the MR system room. The MR system magnet is ALWAYS on.

Please indicate if you have any of the following:

- ☐ Yes ☐ No Aneurysm clip(s)
- ☐ Yes ☐ No Cardiac pacemaker
- ☐ Yes ☐ No Implanted cardioverter defibrillator (ICD)
- ☐ Yes ☐ No Electronic implant or device
- ☐ Yes ☐ No Magnetically-activated implant or device
- ☐ Yes ☐ No Neurostimulation system
- ☐ Yes ☐ No Spinal cord stimulator
- ☐ Yes ☐ No Internal electrodes or wires
- ☐ Yes ☐ No Bone growth/bone fusion stimulator
- ☐ Yes ☐ No Cochlear, otologic, or other ear implant
- ☐ Yes ☐ No Insulin or other infusion pump
- ☐ Yes ☐ No Implanted drug infusion device
- ☐ Yes ☐ No Any type of prosthesis (eye, penile, etc.)
- ☐ Yes ☐ No Heart valve prosthesis
- ☐ Yes ☐ No Eyelid spring or wire
- ☐ Yes ☐ No Artificial or prosthetic limb
- ☐ Yes ☐ No Metallic stent, filter, or coil
- ☐ Yes ☐ No Shunt (spinal or intraventricular)
- ☐ Yes ☐ No Vascular access port and/or catheter
- ☐ Yes ☐ No Radiation seeds or implants
- ☐ Yes ☐ No Swan-Ganz or thermodilution catheter
- ☐ Yes ☐ No Medication patch (Nicotine, Nitroglycerine)
- ☐ Yes ☐ No Any metallic fragment or foreign body
- ☐ Yes ☐ No Wire mesh implant
- ☐ Yes ☐ No Tissue expander (e.g., breast)
- ☐ Yes ☐ No Surgical staples, clips, or metallic sutures
- ☐ Yes ☐ No Joint replacement (hip, knee, etc.)
- ☐ Yes ☐ No Bone/joint pin, screw, nail, wire, plate, etc.
- ☐ Yes ☐ No IUD, diaphragm, or pessary
- ☐ Yes ☐ No Dentures or partial plates
- ☐ Yes ☐ No Tattoo or permanent makeup
- ☐ Yes ☐ No Body piercing jewelry
- ☐ Yes ☐ No Hearing aid
  (Remove before entering MR system room)
- ☐ Yes ☐ No Other implant _____
- ☐ Yes ☐ No Breathing problem or motion disorder
- ☐ Yes ☐ No Claustrophobia

Please mark on the figure(s) below the location of any implant or metal inside of or on your body.

RIGHT   LEFT   LEFT   RIGHT

⚠ **IMPORTANT INSTRUCTIONS**

Before entering the MR environment or MR system room, you must remove **all** metallic objects including hearing aids, dentures, partial plates, keys, beeper, cell phone, eyeglasses, hair pins, barrettes, jewelry, body piercing jewelry, watch, safety pins, paperclips, money clip, credit cards, bank cards, magnetic strip cards, coins, pens, pocket knife, nail clipper, tools, clothing with metal fasteners, & clothing with metallic threads.

Please consult the MRI Technologist or Radiologist if you have any question or concern BEFORE you enter the MR system room.

NOTE: You may be advised or required to wear earplugs or other hearing protection during the MR procedure to prevent possible problems or hazards related to acoustic noise.

I attest that the above information is correct to the best of my knowledge. I read and understand the contents of this form and had the opportunity to ask questions regarding the information on this form and regarding the MR procedure that I am about to undergo.

Signature of Person Completing Form: _____   Date ____/____/____
                                        Signature

Form Completed By: ☐ Patient ☐ Relative ☐ Nurse _____   _____
                                                      Print name   Relationship to patient

Form Information Reviewed By: _____   _____
                                        Print name   Signature

☐ MRI Technologist   ☐ Nurse   ☐ Radiologist   ☐ Other_____

Figure 3. The MRI Screening Form used to screen patients, Spanish language version, page one.

**CUESTIONARIO PREVIO A ESTUDIO CON RESONANCIA MAGNÉTICA (MR)
PARA PACIENTES**

Fecha ____/____/____   Número de paciente_____

Nombre_____   Edad _____ Altura_____ Peso_____
     Apellido   Primer Nombre   Segundo Nombre

Fecha de nacimiento____/____/____   Varón☐ Hembra☐   Parte del cuerpo a ser examinada_____
          Mes Día Año
Dirección_____   Teléfono (domicilio) (____) _____-_____

Ciudad_____   Teléfono (trabajo)   (____) _____-_____

Provincia _____   Código Postal _____

Motivo para el estudio de MRI y/o síntomas_____

Médico que le refirió _____   Teléfono (____) - _____

1. Anteriormente, ¿le han hecho alguna cirugía u operación (e.g., artroscopía, endoscopía, etc.) de cualquier tipo?   ☐ No ☐ Sí
Si respondió afirmativamente, indique la fecha y que tipo de cirugía:
Fecha ____/____/____ Tipo de cirugía _____
Fecha ____/____/____ Tipo de cirugía _____
2. Anteriormente, ¿le han hecho algún estudio o exámen de diagnóstico (MRI, CT, Ultrasonido, Rayos-X, etc.)?   ☐ No ☐ Sí
Si respondió afirmativamente, descríbalos a continuación:

Parte del Cuerpo	Fecha	Lugar/Institución
MRI _____	___/___/___	_____
CT/CAT _____	___/___/___	_____
Rayos-X _____	___/___/___	_____
Ultrasonido _____	___/___/___	_____
Medicina Nuclear _____	___/___/___	_____
Otro_____	___/___/___	_____

3. ¿Ha tenido algún problema relacionado con estudios ó procedimientos anteriores con MR?   ☐ No ☐ Sí
  Si respondió afirmativamente, descríbalos: _____
4. ¿Se ha golpeado el ojo con un objeto ó fragmento metálico (e.g., astillas metálicas, virutas, objeto extraño, etc.)?   ☐ No ☐ Sí
  Si respondió afirmativamente, describa el incidente: _____
5. ¿Ha sido alcanzado alguna vez por un objeto metálico u objeto extraño (e.g. perdigones, bala, metralla, etc.)?   ☐ No ☐ Sí
  Si respondió afirmativamente, describa el incidente: _____
6. ¿Esta actualmente tomando ó ha recientemente tomado algún medicamento o droga?   ☐ No ☐ Sí
  Si respondió afirmativamente, indique el nombre del medicamento:_____
7. ¿Es Ud. alérgico/a á algún medicamento?   ☐ No ☐ Sí
  Si respondió afirmativamente, indique el nombre del medicamento:_____
8. ¿Tiene historia de asma, reacción alérgica, enfermedad respiratoria, ó reacción a contrastes ó tinturas usados en MRI, CT, ó
  Rayos-X?   ☐ No ☐ Sí
9. ¿Tiene anemia u otra enfermedad que afecte su sangre, algún episodio de enfermedad de riñón, fracaso de riñón,
un transplante de riñón, hipertensión, la historia de la diabetes, relativo al hígado ó de ataques epilépticos?
Si respondió afirmativamente, descríbalos: _____   ☐ No ☐ Sí

Para los pacientes femeninos:
10. Fecha de su último periodo menstrual: ____/____/____   En la menopausia?   ☐ No ☐ Sí
11. ¿Está embarazada ó tiene retraso con su periodo menstrual?   ☐ No ☐ Sí
12. ¿Está tomando contraceptivos orales ó recibiendo tratamiento hormonal?   ☐ No ☐ Sí
13. ¿Está tomando algún tipo de medicamento para la fertilidad ó recibiendo tratamientos de fertilidad?   ☐ No ☐ Sí
  Si responde afirmativamente, descríbalos a continuación: _____
14. ¿Está amamantado a su bebé?   ☐ No ☐ Sí

Translated with permission 5/05 Olga Fernandez-Flygare, M.S., Brain
Mapping Center, UCLA School of Medicine, Los Angeles, CA

Figure 4. The MRI Screening Form used to screen patients, Spanish language version, page two.

ADVERTENCIA: Ciertos implantes, dispositivos, u objetos pueden ser peligrosos y/o pueden interferir con el procedimiento de resonancia magnética (es decir, MRI, MR angiografía, MRI funcional, MR espectroscopía). **No entre** a la sala del escáner de MR o a la zona del laboratorio de MR si tiene alguna pregunta o duda relacionadas con un implante, dispositivo, u objeto. Consulte con el técnico o radiólogo de MRI ANTES de entrar a la sala del escáner de MR. **Recuerde que el imán del sistema MR está SIEMPRE encendido.**

Por favor indique si tiene alguno de los siguientes:

- ☐ Sí ☐ No   Pinza(s) de aneurisma
- ☐ Sí ☐ No   Marcapasos cardíaco
- ☐ Sí ☐ No   Implante con desfibrilador para conversión cardíaca (ICD)
- ☐ Sí ☐ No   Implante electrónico ó dispositivo electrónico
- ☐ Sí ☐ No   Implante ó dispositivo activado magnéticamente
- ☐ Sí ☐ No   Sistema de neuroestimulación
- ☐ Sí ☐ No   Estimulador de la médula espinal
- ☐ Sí ☐ No   Electrodos ó alambres internos
- ☐ Sí ☐ No   Estimulador de crecimiento/fusión del hueso
- ☐ Sí ☐ No   Implante coclear, otológico, u otro implante del oído
- ☐ Sí ☐ No   Bomba de infusión de insulina ó similar
- ☐ Sí ☐ No   Dispositivo implantado para infusión de medicamento
- ☐ Sí ☐ No   Cualquier tipo de prótesis (ojo, peneal, etc.)
- ☐ Sí ☐ No   Prótesis de válvula cardiaca
- ☐ Sí ☐ No   Muelle ó alambre del párpado
- ☐ Sí ☐ No   Extremidad artificial ó prostética
- ☐ Sí ☐ No   Malla metálica (stent), filtro, ó anillo metálico
- ☐ Sí ☐ No   Shunt (espinal ó intraventricular)
- ☐ Sí ☐ No   Catéter y/u orificio de acceso vascular
- ☐ Sí ☐ No   Semillas ó implantes de radiación
- ☐ Sí ☐ No   Catéter de Swan-Ganz ó de termodilución

- ☐ Sí ☐ No   Parche de medicamentos (Nicotina, Nitroglicerina)
- ☐ Sí ☐ No   Cualquier fragmento metálico ó cuerpo extraño
- ☐ Sí ☐ No   Implante tipo malla
- ☐ Sí ☐ No   Aumentador de tejidos (e.g. pecho)
- ☐ Sí ☐ No   Grapas quirúrgicas, clips, ó suturas metálicas
- ☐ Sí ☐ No   Articulaciones artificiales (cadera, rodilla, etc.)
- ☐ Sí ☐ No   Varilla de hueso/coyuntura, tornillo, clavo, alambre, chapas, etc.
- ☐ Sí ☐ No   Dispositivo intrauterino (IUD), diafragma, ó pesario
- ☐ Sí ☐ No   Dentaduras ó placas parciales
- ☐ Sí ☐ No   Tatuaje ó maquillaje permanente
- ☐ Sí ☐ No   Perforación (piercing) del cuerpo
- ☐ Sí ☐ No   Audífono *(Quíteselo antes de entrar a la sala del escáner de MR)*
- ☐ Sí ☐ No   Otro implante_____
- ☐ Sí ☐ No   Problema respiratorio ó desorden del movimiento
- ☐ Sí ☐ No   Claustrofobia

Por favor marque en la imagen de abajo la localización de cualquier implante o metal en su cuerpo.

DERECHA   IZQUIERDA   DERECHA

⚠ **¡AVISO IMPORTANTE!**

Antes de entrar a la zona de MR ó a la sala del escáner de MR, tendrá que quitarse todo objeto metálico incluyendo audífono, dentaduras, placas parciales, llaves, beeper, teléfono celular, lentes, horquillas de pelo, pasadores, todas las joyas (incluyendo "body piercing"), reloj, alfileres, sujetapapeles, clip de billetes, tarjetas de crédito ó de banco, toda tarjeta con banda magnética, monedas, plumas, cuchillos, corta uñas, herramientas, ropa con enganches de metal, y ropa con hilos metálicos.

Por favor consulte con el Técnico de MRI ó Radiólogo si tiene alguna pregunta o duda ANTES de entrar a la sala de escáner de MR.

NOTA: Es posible se le pida usar auriculares u otra protección de sus oídos durante el procedimiento de MR para prevenir problemas ó riesgos asociados al nivel de ruido en la sala del escáner de MR.

Atestiguo que la información anterior es correcta según mi mejor entender. Leo y entiendo el contenido de este cuestionario y he tenido la oportunidad de hacer preguntas en relación a la información en el cuestionario y en relación al estudio de MR al que me voy a someter a continuación.

Firma de la persona llenando este cuestionario: _____   Fecha____/____/____

Firma

Cuestionario lleno por: ☐Paciente ☐Pariente ☐Enfermera _____   _____

Nombre en letra de texto   Relación con el paciente

Información revisada por: _____

Nombre en letra de texto   Firma

☐ Técnico de MRI   ☐Enfermera   ☐ Radiólogo   ☐ Otro _____

Translated with permission Olga Fernandez-Flygare, M.S., Brain Mapping Center, UCLA School of Medicine, Los Angeles, CA

questions pertain to female patients, only). Explanations of the questions and their importance to MRI screening are provided below.

Question #1 asks about previous surgeries or procedures. Many patient safety concerns in MRI are impacted by the response to this question, so it cannot be left unanswered. If the answer to Question #1 is "yes", additional information must be given on types and dates of all surgeries and/or related procedures. Accuracy is paramount here, since information on potential implants, devices, and materials can be discovered. If the patient is a minor or is not fully aware of this information, a parent, guardian or other knowledgeable caregiver must assist in providing and verifying this information. Further review of the patient's chart or medical records may be necessary. If previous surgery or other procedural information is not available at the time of the MRI examination, as with an outpatient who has arrived with a limited history, MRI must be postponed or rescheduled until this information can be captured and verified.

Question #2 asks about previous diagnostic imaging studies (MRI, computed tomography or CT, X-ray, ultrasound, nuclear medicine, etc.). The results of these examinations can help verify the patient's surgical or other procedural history and assist in identifying the presence of an implant, device, or foreign body that may be of concern.

Question #3 asks the patient about problems related to a prior MRI examination. If the answer to this question is "yes", the patient is asked to describe the problem, prompting the MRI technologist to investigate and otherwise consider this matter further. Notably, if the answer to this question is "no", the patient cannot simply bypass the MRI screening process. A written screening form must still be completed, in case the patient that had a previous MRI exam performed had the placement of an implant, device, material, or encountered a foreign body. Assumptions should not be made that non-incidental, previous MRI examinations permit subsequent incident-free MRI procedures. Factors related to the MRI examination such as the strength of the static magnetic field, maximum spatial gradient magnetic field of the magnet, patient orientation in the MR system, time-varying or gradient magnetic fields, type of RF coil used, and pulse sequence parameters can vary significantly among different MR systems. Careful investigation is indicated for implants or devices assumed to be "MR safe" for a previous MR system, as this can change to "MR conditional" or even "MR unsafe" based on the MR system factors indicated above (15). The MRI technologist or radiologist can refer to the latest version of the *Reference Manual for Magnetic Resonance Safety, Implants, and Devices* (16), or visit the website, www.MRIsafety.com, for specific information pertaining to information for implants and devices. Notably, it may be necessary to consult the manufacturer of the implant or device for more information, especially if an electronically-activated implant is encountered (16).

Questions #4 and #5 ask the patient about personal injury involving a metallic object or foreign body. If the answer to either question is "yes", further questioning must be conducted as to whether the object was removed entirely, and if not, the location and composition of the object must be investigated further. In the case of injuries involving the eyes, it is important to negate the presence of any remaining metal. If the patient answers that an orbital metal foreign body (e.g., fragment, sliver, bullet, BB, shrapnel, welding slag, etc.) does remain or is unsure, the MRI exam must be postponed or rescheduled, and the patient is not allowed to enter the MRI environment. If the patient cannot recount with confidence that all metallic foreign bodies within the orbit(s) have been removed, an X-ray is indicated to determine the presence of metal. If the X-ray is unremarkable, and MRI screening is otherwise complete, the examination can be performed. If the X-ray identifies the presence of any non-surgical orbital metal, the MRI examination must be cancelled. Under certain circumstances, the radiologist may allow the MRI procedure to proceed if the X-rays show the metal is of relatively low mass, located in an extra-orbital, non-threatening position, or it has been determined that the metal is non-ferrous.

Questions #6 and #7 ask the patient about current medications and allergies to medications. These questions may not be directly related to MRI safety, but if the patient needs to receive emergency medical attention, such information could be vital. Some patients may complain of problems such as vertigo, headache, or memory loss immediately following MRI, or days after the exam. In such cases, it can be helpful to the radiologist or clinician to check the written screening form for medications the patient listed, as these may help explain the patient's symptoms. Many radiologists can attest to incidents where patients mistakenly associated medical problems with an MRI procedure or other imaging modality.

Question #8 asks about asthma, allergic reaction, or respiratory disease, but also specifically asks about prior reaction to contrast medium used in MRI, CT, or X-ray. It is not uncommon for patients to cite previous episodes of transient flushing, metallic taste, or nausea immediately following an injection. Unpleasant as it is for the patients, such transient symptoms are usually harmless. Notably, adverse reactions to MRI contrast agents can occur, although serious reactions such as anaphylactic responses to a gadolinium-based contrast agent (GBCA) are extremely rare. If the patient indicates a previous reaction to what they perceive as "dye", further questioning will be needed to clarify this matter. The patient may not make the distinction between CT and MRI, nor between GBCAs and iodinated contrast agents used in X-ray and CT. A polite but thorough interview with the patient should be able to determine the severity of a previous adverse event and which contrast agent was administered. If available, a review of the patient's chart or medical records should be done for clarification.

Question #9 asks about anemia or other blood diseases, renal or hepatic disease, diabetes, and seizures. Importantly, MRI contrast agents may be contraindicated for some of these conditions. For example, the use of GBCAs has recently emerged as an MRI safety concern in patients with renal insufficiency, as certain GBCAs are implicated in causing nephrogenic systemic fibrosis (NSF). Hence, the results of a glomerular filtration rate (GFR) test must be obtained prior to a GBCA administration in patients with suspected renal insufficiency. This important topic is discussed in considerable detail in another chapter of this textbook.

Questions #10 through #14 pertain to female patients, asking about possible pregnancy, menstrual cycle, and breastfeeding. Prior to entering the MRI environment, any patient who is possibly pregnant must undergo a pregnancy test. If the patient is pregnant, a consultation between the patient, radiologist and referring clinician is required in assessing the risk versus benefit of performing the MRI examination. The ACR recommends MRI examinations in pregnant patients if other non-ionizing imaging modalities are diagnostically inadequate, or ionizing procedures would otherwise have to be performed to answer critical clinical questions about the patient or fetus (15). Furthermore, MRI may be performed without written or verbal informed consent in pregnant patients (15).

Non-pregnant patients should still answer questions #10 through #14 to the best of their ability, especially if they are scheduled for a breast or pelvic MRI. This information can aid the radiologist to interpret the results of the MRI procedure since hormonal changes induced by menstrual cycle, fertility treatments, and breastfeeding can alter tissue contrast on MR images. In particular, hormonal changes directly impact the timing and rate of breast tissue enhancement following the administration of a GBCA. Also, breastfeeding patients (question #14) will be instructed to refrain from breastfeeding for 24-hours following administration of a GBCA (while continuing to express and discard the breast milk). This will help ensure that suckling infants ingest negligible amounts of gadolinium chelates.

The top of the second page of the written screening form for patients is intended to capture the attention of the patient or individual filling out the form (**Figure 2**). A "bold" warning statement is issued that certain implants, devices, or objects may be hazardous, and/or interfere with the MRI procedure. Thus, the patient is instructed not to enter the MRI environment if he or she has any question concerning an implant, device or object, and to consult the radiologist or MRI technologist before entering the MR system room. The patient or individual is also reminded that the "MR system magnet is ALWAYS on!" This warning statement is not intended to frighten patients or individuals who may already be anxious about their ensuing exam, but rather to discourage those who otherwise might wander into restricted areas in the MRI environment.

The middle section of page 2 of the screening form lists thirty-three implant or device categories of potential concern. The patient or individual filling out the form is asked to indicate whether he or she possesses any implant or device by checking a "Yes" or "No" box. By doing so, the patient or individual may recall previous forgotten surgeries or procedures that involved the implants or devices listed. If the patient has an implant or device not listed, the patient is asked to write it down at the bottom of the list. If the patient or individual does possess an implant, device, object, or metal on or in the body, he or she is instructed to indicate the location(s) on the diagrams of the human body (anterior and posterior views) provided on the form.

Below the diagrams, the patient or individual is reminded to remove all metal objects such as hearing aides, dentures, jewelry, eyeglasses, keys, cell phones, belts, and other objects before entering the MR system room. Articles of clothing containing metal such as buttons, zippers and wires should also be removed. The metal in the clothing may be nonferrous but can degrade image quality if located proximal to the region being scanned. More importantly, the metal may excessively heat during certain MRI conditions, causing a burn injury. As a critical policy, many MRI facilities require patients to remove clothing and change into a gown or scrubs that have no pockets as part of the screening process. Lockers must be provided to secure the belongings of patients and other individuals. Without harsh interrogation or inappropriate searching, the MRI technologist must always check the patient or individual to verify that all metal of concern has been removed prior to entering the MR system room. Some facilities refer to this second check as the "final screening".

Questions are also asked about breathing problems, motion disorders, or claustrophobia. These questions are used to assess the patient's general ability to hold still and tolerate the MRI procedure. These issues are not too critical for safety, but may determine whether the patient needs sedation, which will dictate scheduling times and different MRI facility staffing needs.

Hearing protection for the patient or individual is also recommended on the written MRI screening form, which reflects many early guidelines pertaining to this matter as well as current ACR recommendations (15). In the distribution of hearing protection such as disposable earplugs, the MRI technologist or trained healthcare worker should assist the patient or individual in placement of the disposable earplugs. Some individuals will have difficulty in properly positioning the earplugs, especially if the ear canal is curved. At times, it may be necessary to immobilize the earplugs in place by using hypoallergenic tape to prevent them from loosening during the exam. The ear canals of small infants often will not accommodate conventional foam earplugs, but the earplugs can easily be cut to fit (any cutting with tools such as scissors or knives must of course be done outside the MRI environment) or alternative hearing protection devices can be used in these cases.

The last section on page 2 of the MRI screening form provides a place for the person completing the form to sign, print his or her name, and date the form. When signing, the patient attests that the information provided on the form is correct. For a minor, a parent or legal guardian should sign the form. If the patient is unable to sign the form, an authorized relative or knowledgeable healthcare professional may need to sign. The MRI technologist, or other trained staff who reviewed the form and conducted the verbal interview must also print and sign this document. If the completed form is handed off to another MRI technologist to perform the MRI examination, care must be taken that the scanning MRI technologist checks the form to be sure that it was reviewed and signed. This final step must be done prior to escorting the patient or individual into the MR system room (**Figure 6**).

In the event that the patient is comatose or for whatever reason unable to verbally communicate, the written screening form should be completed by the most qualified individual (e.g., physician, family member, etc.) that has knowledge about the patient's medical history and present condition. If the screening information is inadequate, it is advisable to look for surgical scars on the patient and/or to obtain plain films of the skull and/or chest to search for implants that may be particularly hazardous in the MRI environment (e.g., aneurysm clips, cardiac pacemakers, neuromodulation systems, etc.)(16).

WRITTEN SCREENING FORM AND PROCEDURES FOR INDIVIDUALS

As stated previously, any individual other than the patient that needs to enter the MRI environment for any reason must also complete a written screening form (**Figure 5**). This form is basically an abbreviated version of the patient MRI screening form. Whether the MRI facility is in a hospital, clinic, or free standing imaging center, a certain amount of employee turnover is inevitable. New physicians, MRI technologists, nurses, assistants, students, and other staff members will rotate through the MRI center, some of which will need to enter the MRI environment. No one is exempt from completing the screening form and process prior to entering the MRI environment. For individuals that must frequently

Figure 5. The MRI Screening Form used to screen individuals.

MAGNETIC RESONANCE (MR) ENVIRONMENT SCREENING FORM FOR INDIVIDUALS*

The MR system has a very strong magnetic field that may be hazardous to individuals entering the MR environment or MR system room if they have certain metallic, electronic, magnetic, or mechanical implants, devices, or objects. Therefore, all individuals are required to fill out this form BEFORE entering the MR environment or MR system room. Be advised, the MR system magnet is ALWAYS on.

*NOTE: If you are a patient preparing to undergo an MR examination, you are required to fill out a different form.

Date ____/____/____   Name _____   Age _____
      month day year   Last Name   First Name   Middle Initial

Address _____   Telephone (home) (____) ____-_____

City _____   Telephone (work) (____) ____-_____

State _____   Zip Code _____

1. Have you had prior surgery or an operation (e.g., arthroscopy, endoscopy, etc.) of any kind?   ❑ No ❑ Yes
   If yes, please indicate date and type of surgery: Date ___/___/___ Type of surgery_____
2. Have you had an injury to the eye involving a metallic object (e.g., metallic slivers, foreign body)?   ❑ No ❑ Yes
   If yes, please describe: _____
3. Have you ever been injured by a metallic object or foreign body (e.g., BB, bullet, shrapnel, etc.)?   ❑ No ❑ Yes
   If yes, please describe: _____
4. Are you pregnant or suspect that you are pregnant?   ❑ No ❑ Yes

WARNING: Certain implants, devices, or objects may be hazardous to you in the MR environment or MR system room. Do not enter the MR environment or MR system room if you have any question or concern regarding an implant, device, or object.

Please indicate if you have any of the following:
❑ Yes ❑ No Aneurysm clip(s)
❑ Yes ❑ No Cardiac pacemaker
❑ Yes ❑ No Implanted cardioverter defibrillator (ICD)
❑ Yes ❑ No Electronic implant or device
❑ Yes ❑ No Magnetically-activated implant or device
❑ Yes ❑ No Neurostimulation system
❑ Yes ❑ No Spinal cord stimulator
❑ Yes ❑ No Cochlear implant or implanted hearing aid
❑ Yes ❑ No Insulin or infusion pump
❑ Yes ❑ No Implanted drug infusion device
❑ Yes ❑ No Any type of prosthesis or implant
❑ Yes ❑ No Artificial or prosthetic limb
❑ Yes ❑ No Any metallic fragment or foreign body
❑ Yes ❑ No Any external or internal metallic object
❑ Yes ❑ No Hearing aid
❑ Yes ❑ No Other implant_____
❑ Yes ❑ No Other device_____

⚠ IMPORTANT INSTRUCTIONS

Remove all metallic objects before entering the MR environment or MR system room including hearing aids, beeper, cell phone, keys, eyeglasses, hair pins, barrettes, jewelry (including body piercing jewelry), watch, safety pins, paperclips, money clip, credit cards, bank cards, magnetic strip cards, coins, pens, pocket knife, nail clipper, steel-toed boots/shoes, and tools. Loose metallic objects are especially prohibited in the MR system room and MR environment.

Please consult the MRI Technologist or Radiologist if you have any question or concern BEFORE you enter the MR system room.

I attest that the above information is correct to the best of my knowledge. I have read and understand the entire contents of this form and have had the opportunity to ask questions regarding the information on this form.

Signature of Person Completing Form: _____   Date ____/____/____
                                        Signature

Form Information Reviewed By: _____   _____
                              Print name   Signature

❑ MRI Technologist   ❑ Radiologist   ❑ Other _____

Figure 6. MRI technologist shown conducting a verbal interview and a review of the written screening form with the patient.

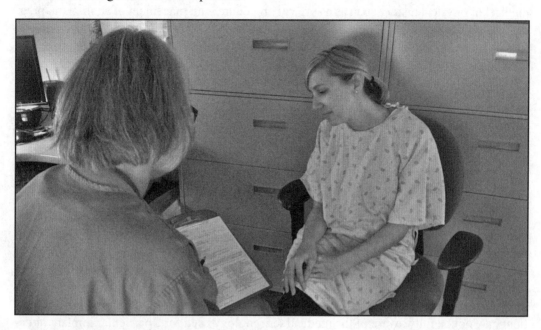

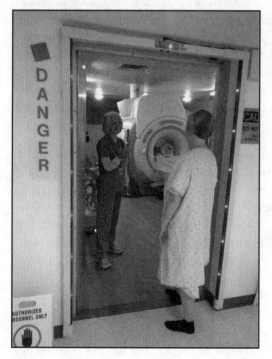

Figure 7. Following the completion of MRI screening, the MRI technologist escorts the patient through a ferromagnetic detection system and into the MR system room.

enter the MRI environment as part of their duty, such as an MRI technologist, the screening form can be completed initially and kept on file. Any subsequent changes to an individual's medical or physical history such as a surgical procedure with placement of an implant, pregnancy, exposure to shrapnel or other similar matter will void the prior MRI clearance on file. It is the individual's responsibility to make this known so that the re-screening and/or updating of screening history can take place.

Importantly, if for any reason the individual undergoing screening may need to enter the MR system itself (e.g., moving partially into the bore of the scanner to help manage the patient) and, thus, become exposed to the electromagnetic fields used for the MRI procedure, this person must be screened using the detailed form for patient screening.

VERBAL SCREENING PROCEDURES

Equally important to the completion of the written MRI screening forms for both patients and other individuals is the verbal screening procedure or interview (**Figure 6**). Additional information or clarification of information about prior surgeries, procedures, or incidents is often obtained during this time. The interview provides a mechanism for clarification or confirmation of the answers to the questions posed to the patient so that there is no miscommunication regarding important MRI safety issues. In addition, because the patient may not be fully aware of the medical terminology used for a particular implant or device, it is imperative that this particular information on the form be discussed during the verbal interview. Additionally, a patient might be reluctant to indicate a pregnancy or foreign body on the written form in the presence of family or friends, but honesty might prevail in a private interview with the MRI technologist or MRI safety-trained healthcare worker. Due to cultural or religious reasons, some patients may ask for a male or female MRI technologist to conduct the interview. Questions, misconceptions, and fears that the patient might harbor can also be discussed and answered. Both the stress of the patient and the difficulty of the MRI examination can be reduced as a result of a satisfactorily performed, verbal screening procedure.

With the use of any type of written questionnaire, limitations exist related to incomplete or incorrect answers provided by the patient or individual. For example, there may be difficulties associated with patients that are impaired with respect to their vision, language fluency, or level of literacy. Therefore, an appropriate accompanying family member or other individual (e.g., referring physician) should be involved in the screening process to verify information that may impact patient safety. Versions of the screening form should be available in other languages, as needed (i.e., specific to the demographics of the MRI facility).

THE USE OF FERROMAGNETIC DETECTION SYSTEMS IN MRI SCREENING

The use of conventional metal detectors as a MRI screening tool has not been recommended in the past mainly as a result of false positive and false negative alarms, resulting in "alarm fatigue". Such detectors have exhibited inconsistent sensitivities, operator error, and the inability to distinguish between ferrous and non-ferrous metals. In recent years, however, new ferromagnetic detection systems have emerged that have proven helpful in the screening process. These ferromagnetic detection systems are typically installed at the threshold of the entrance into the MR system room (**Figure 7**). Additionally, one hand-held and "pillar" versions of ferromagnetic detection systems exist. These devices are consistently sensitive to small ferromagnetic objects external to the patient or individual, giving visual and audible alarms, as the offending object is detected. The ACR recommends the use of ferromagnetic detection systems, but only as an adjunct to a thorough and competent MRI screening process (15). Interestingly, recent research has suggested that ferromagnetic detection systems may also be used to identify implanted ferromagnetic implants or embedded foreign bodies (e.g., armor-piercing bullets)(18-20).

SECONDARY PURPOSES AND ADVANTAGES OF MRI SCREENING

Obviously, the primary purpose of MRI screening is safety, but screening serves secondary purposes and advantages, as presented below.

Optimizing the Diagnostic Value of the MRI Examination

Many implants and devices do not pose safety issues, but some can significantly degrade image quality, especially when in or near to the anatomical region of interest. Information gathered during MRI screening regarding the type and location of a metallic implant or foreign body can allow for strategies and/or adjustments in the MRI protocol to minimize signal loss and/or distortion. For example, an adolescent with extensive orthodontic work who is scheduled for a pituitary study might be scanned on a 1.5-Tesla MR system rather than a 3-Tesla scanner in an effort to reduce susceptibility artifacts. Alternatively, the optimization of imaging parameters that are known to reduce artifacts related to metallic objects may be necessary in order to maintain the diagnostic aspects of the MRI examination.

Appropriate Patient Management Aided by MRI Screening

A physician ordering a clinical MRI examination must state a "reason for exam". Based on this information, the attending MRI-trained physician will then select an appropriate protocol (i.e., with consideration given to the type of transmit/receive RF coil to be used, pulse sequences, etc.), which is unique for the desired outcome for that specific patient. Additional communication between the ordering/referring physician and the radiologist may be necessary if this information and justification for the MRI procedure is vague.

If the patient arrives for the MRI appointment with a limited history, and the ordering physician is not available for consultation, the screening information that is obtained may be helpful to the radiologist. For instance, if the reason for the examination simply indicates "headache", and the screening procedure reveals that the patient has not had a prior MRI procedure, the radiologist may optimize the scan protocol with more diagnostic emphasis. Conversely, if MRI screening reveals previous MRI studies, and the present MRI exam is for surgical planning, the radiologist may optimize the scan protocol with this in mind. Otherwise, the radiologist may simply protocol "repeat prior study" or the MRI protocol may involve performing additional sequences, possibly with an injection of an MRI contrast agent.

INITIAL MRI SCREENING

In the current age of faxing, email, and the use of other electronic media, MRI facilities can readily distribute electronic versions of the written MRI screening forms to referring physician's offices, clinics, or any service that may order an MRI. Once the physician has seen the patient and has decided that an MRI procedure is indicated, the patient can be given the MRI screening form to fill out, or at a minimum, answer key MRI screening questions. This information can then be returned to the MRI facility prior to the appointment date. Such a practice has multiple purposes and advantages, including:

Early Discovery of Implants, Devices, or Other Objects

Initial MRI screening of a patient can reveal MR conditional or MR unsafe implants, devices, or other objects. The MRI facility can then investigate the item ahead of time and decide, under what conditions, the patient can be scanned, if at all. Patients with non-medical objects such as piercings or excessive jewelry can be instructed to remove these items prior to their MRI appointments.

Management of Severe Anxiety or Claustrophobia

If the MRI facility receives early notification that a patient suffers from severe anxiety or claustrophobia, then the patient may be scheduled on an "open" or wide-bore MR system, or the facility staff can prepare to coach or sedate the patient for the procedure.

Patient Body Habitus Management

MR systems typically have weight and/or dimensional limits for patients. If an MRI examination has been ordered on an excessively large patient, the weight and dimensions of the patient should be recorded and relayed to the MRI facility during the initial MRI screening procedure to ensure that the scanner can accommodate the patient. This can save time and embarrassment for all involved.

Anticipation and Preparation of the MRI Facility's Staffing Needs

Patients who need special assistance, sedation, or high-risk patients who may need general anesthesia require specific and additional staff at the time of the MRI examinations. Furthermore, additional time will likely be needed to complete the MRI procedure and, possibly, to manage the patient after the exam (e.g., in the case of needing to recover a patient after general anesthesia). Initial MRI screening information is particularly beneficial for managing the afore-mentioned patients, because the MRI facility will need to prepare and schedule these patients, accordingly.

"No Show" Rate Reduction

Initial MRI screening (i.e., using verbal or written methods) can help reduce the "no show" rate of an MRI facility. During the initial screening process, certain patients may refuse the MRI examination, despite the physician's recommendation. Common MRI contraindications are limitations are also exposed during this time. Thus, it may not be possible to schedule such patients right away. Frequently, MRI facilities dedicate a staff member to review the MRI screening information while placing "reminder" telephone calls to patients a few days before their appointments. At the time of the call, the patient may indicate that he or she is unable to honor the appointment, and the appointment will need to be re-scheduled or canceled. In either case, a likely "no show" can be averted by following simple tasks involved in initial MRI screening.

SUMMARY AND CONCLUSIONS

The process of MRI screening is absolutely critical to avoid MRI-related accidents and injuries, as well as to ensure safety for staff members and others. MRI screening must never be performed in haste, but rather, in a consistent and thorough manner. If a reduction in MRI incidents is to be realized, adhering to comprehensive MRI screening protocols and revising screening criteria must be an integral part of MRI policies and procedures. As emphasized throughout this chapter, MRI screening of patients and individuals must, at a minimum, include completion of a written screening form and a subsequent verbal interview, and have the form signed-off by the MRI technologist or other MRI safety-trained healthcare worker. Beyond MRI safety, screening proves efficacious by providing information that allows proper scheduling of the patient and preparation of the MRI facility to accommodate the patient's needs for effective customer service standards, improved business, and optimal patient-care outcomes.

REFERENCES

1. Gangarosa RE, Minnis JE, Nobbe J, Praschan D, Genberg RW. Operational safety issues in MRI. Magn Reson Imaging 1987;5:287-92.

2. Shellock FG, Kanal E. Policies, guidelines, and recommendations for MR imaging safety and patient management. J Magn Reson Imaging 1991;1:97-101.

3. Shellock FG, Kanal E. SMRI Report. Policies, guidelines and recommendations for MR imaging safety and patient management. Questionnaire for screening patients before MR procedures. J Magn Reson Imaging 1992;2:247-8.

4. Shellock FG, Kanal E. Guidelines and recommendations for MR imaging safety and patient management. III. Questionnaire for screening patients before MR procedures. The SMRI Safety Committee. J Magn Reson Imaging. 1994;4:749-51.

5. Elster AD, Link KM, Carr JJ. Patient screening prior to MR imaging: a practical approach synthesized from protocols at 15 U.S. medical centers. AJR Am J Roentgenol 1994;162:195-9.

6. Shellock FG, Kanal E. Magnetic Resonance: Bioeffects, Safety, and Patient Management. New York: Lippincott-Raven Press: 1996.

7. Sawyer-Glover AM, Shellock FG. Pre-MRI procedure screening: recommendations and safety considerations for biomedical implants and devices. J Magn Reson Imaging 2000;12:510-515.

8. Shellock FG. New recommendations for screening patients for suspected orbital foreign bodies. Signals 2001;36:8-9.

9. Sawyer-Glover A, Shellock FG. Pre-Magnetic Resonance Procedure Screening. In: Magnetic Resonance Procedures: Health Effects and Safety. Shellock FG, Editor. Boca Raton: CRC Press, LLC; 2001.

10. Kanal E, Borgstede JP, Barkovich AJ, et al. American College of Radiology. American College of Radiology white paper on MR safety. AJR Am J Roentgenol 2002;178:1335-47.

11. Shellock FG, Crues JV. Commentary. MR safety and the American College of Radiology white paper. American Journal of Roentgenology 2002;178:1349-1352.

12. Shellock FG, Crues JV. MR procedures: biologic effects, safety, and patient care. Radiology 2004;232:635-652.

13. Kanal E, Barkovich AJ, Bell C, et al. ACR Blue Ribbon Panel on MR Safety. ACR guidance document for safe MR practices: 2007. AJR Am J Roentgenol. 2007;188:1447-74.

14. Shellock FG, Spinazzi A. MRI Safety Update: 2008, Part 2, Screening patients for MRI. American Journal of Roentgenology 2008;191:12-21.

15. Expert Panel on MR Safety, Kanal E, Barkovich AJ, Bell C, et al. ACR guidance document on MR safe practices: 2013. J Magn Reson Imaging 2013;37:501-30.

16. Shellock FG. Reference Manual for Magnetic Resonance Safety, Implants, and Devices: 2013 Edition. Biomedical Research Publishing Group, Los Angeles, CA, 2013.

17. Boutin RD, Briggs JE, Williamson MR. Injuries associated with MR imaging: survey of safety records and methods used to screen patients for metallic foreign bodies before imaging. AJR Am J Roentgenol 1994;162:189-94.

18. James CA, Karacozoff AM, Shellock FG. Undisclosed and undetected foreign bodies during MRI screening resulting in a potentially serious outcome. Magn Reson Imaging 2013; 31:630-3.

19. Karacozoff AM, Shellock FG. Armor-piercing bullet: 3-Tesla MRI findings and identification by a ferromagnetic detection system. Military Medicine 2013; 178(3):e380-5.

20. Shellock FG, Karacozoff AM. Detection of implants and other objects using a ferromagnetic detection system: implications for patient screening prior to MRI. AJR Am J Roentgenol (In Press)

Chapter 13 Using Ferromagnetic Detection Systems in the MRI Environment

MARK N. KEENE, PH.D.

Chief Technology Officer
Metrasens, Ltd.
Worcestershire
United Kingdom

INTRODUCTION

Magnetic resonance imaging (MRI) is an important diagnostic modality that utilizes a powerful static magnetic field that may pose serious hazards. The potentially violent attraction of ferromagnetic objects into the bore of a magnetic resonance (MR) system is referred to as the missile (or projectile) effect. Magnetic field interactions acting on a highly ferromagnetic object brought too close to the magnet of the scanner can become so substantial as to be unstoppable by human effort. Items such as steel gas cylinders and fire extinguishers can enter a magnet at 30- to 40-mph, the same speed they would reach if dropped from a 40-foot building to the ground. The kinetic energy gained by a steel cylinder that becomes a missile as it rapidly moves towards a magnet is dissipated on impact. A 15-lb cylinder acting as a projectile can critically injure an individual and/or or severely damage the MR system.

Recently, a new device, referred to as a ferromagnetic detection system (FMDS), has become available for use in the MRI environment. Various versions of the FMDS currently exist. These devices are specially designed to only detect ferromagnetic objects. Other materials, such as aluminum and copper, are non-ferromagnetic and, therefore, are not detected by an FMDS. There are many ferromagnetic metals but, by far, the most common is steel. An FMDS will detect a steel gas cylinder and indicate a positive alarm, but it will not detect or alarm on an aluminum one. Thus, the FMDS will only alarm on potentially dangerous objects relative to issues related to magnetic field interactions. Utilizing an FMDS in the MRI environment is recommended by several influential organizations concerned with MRI safety, including the American College of Radiology (ACR) and the Joint Commission (1-5).

This chapter discusses the missile effect and its causes and consequences. The unique detection technology utilized by a ferromagnetic detection system is then presented. Included in this chapter is a practical guide to working with an FMDS in the MRI environment. The relatively new area of patient screening involving identifying implanted ferromagnetic devices and foreign bodies using an FMDS is also discussed, followed by a view on the future of these devices.

THE MISSILE EFFECT AND ITS CONSEQUENCES

The Fringe Field Associated with an MR System

A properly functioning clinical MR system has a powerful and highly uniform static magnetic field (6). The vast majority of scanners use superconducting electromagnets because these provide substantially higher static magnetic fields and considerably lower power consumption than electromagnets. Superconducting electromagnets have the fascinating property that the massive electrical currents in their coils will flow perpetually without the need for a power supply as long as they are kept cold enough to remain superconducting. A superconducting magnet does need high power to establish the field while the magnet is being "ramped up". The energy that is used during this time is stored in the magnetic field. This stored energy will only be released when the magnet is "ramped-down" or quenched.

From a safety consideration, it is important to understand that a magnetic field is an "energy store". An analogy might be a gas cylinder insofar as it requires energy to compress a gas into the cylinder. Once there (and with the valve closed), no power or energy is required to maintain it. The stored energy is only released when the gas is let out. With the gas cylinder, the energy is stored safely within the walls of the cylinder. However, with a magnet used by an MR system, the energy is stored in the magnetic field on the *outside*, through which staff members, patients, and other individuals walk through and work in every day. It is a common misconception that the energy in an MR system's magnet is stored in the electrical current in the windings, safely within the scanner. However, that is not the case. Inside the bore of the magnet and in the area surrounding the magnet there is an energy field that cannot be felt, seen, heard, tasted, or smelled. The only sense of the presence and power of this energy field is when a ferromagnetic object is taken into the area and the forces are felt that are exerted on the object.

During the planning of an MRI facility, a plot showing the magnetic contours surrounding the MR system is typically provided, an example of which is shown in **Figure 1**. Normally, MR system rooms are designed such that where there are walls adjoining areas occupied by people, the fringe field is less than 5-gauss (7). This is considered to be the generally permissible magnetic field level that ensures safety for individuals with electronically activated devices, such as cardiac pacemakers. Frequently, the 5-gauss line is contained well within the MRI environment, usually at or within a controlled area.

The fringe field associated with the magnet of the MR system falls away in all directions, getting weaker as the distance increases. The rate of change of the magnetic field with distance is called the spatial gradient magnetic field. If field is B, then the gradient is

Figure 1. Example of a magnetic field contour plot for the fringe field of a 1.5-T magnet. The contours are of constant field magnitude (i.e., irrespective of the field orientation). The field value for each contour is as marked.

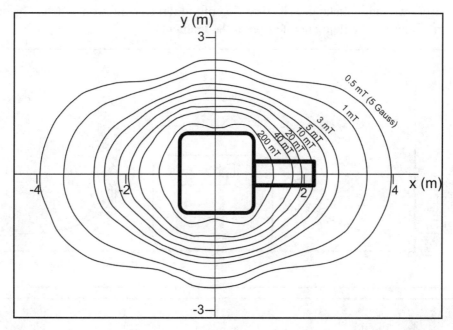

$\partial B/\partial x$, where x is the distance in the x-direction. An illustration of the fringe field and gradient profiles are shown in **Figure 2(a)** and **Figure 2(b)**.

How Magnetic Fields Interact With Metals

There are four primary mechanical effects that a magnetic field could impart on a metallic object: (1) motion damping, (2) magnetization effects, (3) torque (rotational force), and (4) linear force. These mechanical effects are described below.

Motion Damping

This is the only main effect that all metals experience whether or not they are ferromagnetic. It is a mechanism that is a function of the electrical conductivity of the metal and its shape. If a metal object moves through a field gradient so that the field it experiences changes with time, then eddy currents are generated within the metal, obeying Faraday's Law of Induction, also known as the dynamo effect. The eddy currents circulate, according to Lenz's Law (8) in a manner that generates their own magnetic field that opposes the movement (i.e., the objects resist motion).

Instead, if the object is rotated in a magnetic field such that its cross-section changes with respect to the direction of the field (e.g., like spinning a coin), then eddy currents will flow to oppose the rotation. The better the conductor, the stronger these effects are, so that the effect is greater in objects made from aluminum and copper than in those made from steel or titanium. The reason this is discussed here is because a ferromagnetic missile ac-

Figure 2. Illustrations showing examples of the fringe field and spatial gradient. **(a)** The magnetic field amplitude in the x direction is nearly constant within the bore of the magnet and decays rapidly with distance away from the bore. **(b)** The magnetic field gradient, $\partial B_x/\partial x$, as a function of distance. The direction of the force on a ferromagnetic object is shown in relation to the field and the sign of the gradient.

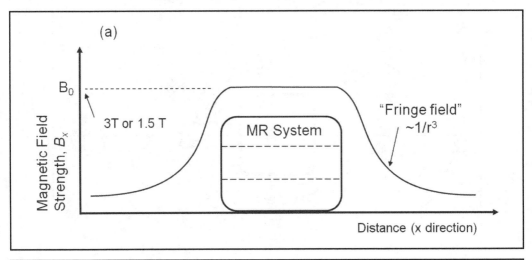

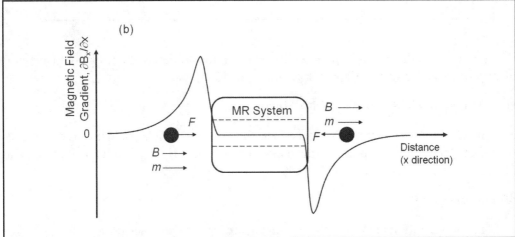

celerating toward the bore of the magnet is slowed down by this effect. Without this effect, missile incidents would be even more damaging.

Magnetization Effects

This only occurs in ferromagnetic objects. The magnetization of a ferromagnetic object increases with the applied magnetic field. This means that the closer a ferromagnetic object approaches to the magnet of the MR system, the more magnetized it becomes.

Torque

This is when a ferromagnetic object, in the presence of a magnetic field, experiences a torque to rotate or align it with respect to the direction of the magnetic field. Once in the preferred direction, there is no further rotation, however, torque will oppose any attempt to orient the object in another direction. This is the principle that magnetic compasses use to indicate the direction of the Earth's magnetic poles. A long ferromagnetic object (e.g., a steel oxygen cylinder, pen, etc.) becomes magnetized along its long axis in preference to another direction. Unless the object is spherical, it will usually experience torque.

Linear Force

This is the mechanism that causes the missile or projectile effect. It occurs because an object, having been magnetized by the magnetization effect, or by its previous magnetization state (or both) becomes attracted to the magnet of the MR system. The spatial gradient of the magnetic field is responsible for linear force. The position at which the magnetic field is highly uniform, such as in the middle of the bore of the MR system, the linear force is close to zero. This is discussed in more detail later in this chapter.

When an individual approaches the magnetic field of the MR system with a ferromagnetic object, the object will typically first encounter torque as the first effect to be noticed. The linear force acting on the object is often felt closer to the scanner.

The motion damping effect is not that noticeable but can be experienced if an aluminum sheet is taken into the magnetic field and moved around. A favorite trick MRI physicists like to display is to take a half-inch thick slab of aluminum or similar object (like a pizza pan), stand it edgeways on the patient table near the bore of the MR system, and then tip it over. This object falls in a surprisingly slow manner.

The Missile Effect

Although the missile effect is predominantly caused by the linear force acting on a ferromagnetic object, each of the four interactions described above plays a part. Let's begin by considering the linear force in more detail. As a ferromagnetic object approaches the magnet, the force it experiences increases dramatically. Thus, every time the range to the magnet is reduced by 10%, the force doubles, so small changes in range equate to large changes in the force acting on the object. Decreasing the distance to the magnet of half increases the force by approximately 130 times.

This highly non-linear range dependence on the force causes problems for individuals carrying ferromagnetic objects close to the MR system. When the forces begin to get strong, muscle control typically cannot cope with the non-linearity. Thus, there is a point at which the ferromagnetic object can no longer be restrained. The force is so highly non-linear that it is rare for individuals to experience or encounter similar forces under other circumstances because we are naturally more accustomed to sensations involving constant or linear forces. It is often an unconscious assumption by people who deliberately take ferromagnetic objects into the MR system room that the force will increase more smoothly than it actually does, as the ferromagnetic object gets close to the scanner. This incorrect assumption has led to many missile accidents. In various videos posted on the Internet of individuals deliberately demonstrating the missile effect, one can see the sudden attraction of a ferromagnetic object into the bore of the MR system. Additional information on this topic directed towards the interests of the MRI physicist may be obtained from the comprehensive publication by Bleaney and Bleaney (9).

TERMINOLOGY USED FOR IMPLANTS AND DEVICES

Descriptions of the current terminology and classifications used for implants and devices, including patient support equipment, have been presented by Shellock, et al. (10). One important aspect of the classifications is the item's susceptibility to becoming a missile hazard. For example, MR Safe items are those defined as, amongst other things, "nonmetallic, nonmagnetic" objects (10). MR Unsafe items are "known to pose hazards in all MR environments" (10). Objects made from steel or iron are, obviously, MR Unsafe. MR Conditional items have, "been demonstrated to pose no known hazards in a specified MR environment with specified conditions of use. Field conditions that define the MR environment include static magnetic field strength...."(10). As far as missile hazards are concerned, this classification refers to items that are either very weakly magnetic or composite items that have small amounts of ferromagnetic materials. For implants, the counterforces present for certain MR Conditional items may be taken into consideration because these can prevent risks related to movement or displacement relative to the use of MRI.

An important area to consider is composite equipment that is classified as MR Conditional, where the majority of the materials that are used are non-magnetic but there may be ferromagnetic components, as well. Most MR Conditional gurneys, wheelchairs, and removable patient tables are in this category. The ferromagnetic materials found in composite equipment always experiences forces of attraction in association with an MR system, so an interesting question is, when does an object become too magnetic and in danger of becoming a missile? On one level the answer is simple. It is when the attractive force of the magnet overcomes the restraining or counterforce holding the object back. For a piece of patient support equipment, such as a wheelchair, there are two primary forces that can prevent it from becoming a missile: the weight which acts in a downward direction and the friction due to contact with the ground, which acts along the floor in the opposite direction of the force, as illustrated in **Figure 3**. The force of attraction is generally towards the nearest edge of the bore of the magnet. In **Figure 3**, the magnetic force is shown resolved into its horizontal and vertical components. The forces of gravity and friction are in opposition to these components.

First, consider the friction. This has the property that frictional force increases to exactly match any horizontal force on the object up to a point called F_{max}, beyond which it will begin to slide toward the magnet. A full analysis is complicated because F_{max} is proportional to the object's weight and it also depends on the properties of the two surfaces in contact. For a given object, there will be an area surrounding the MR system's magnet, outside of which the object will remain stationary on the floor, and inside of which it will become a missile, due to horizontal forces. Objects with wheels have intrinsically low F_{max} because that is the point of having wheels in the first place, that is, to allow devices such as wheelchairs, gurneys, and trolleys to move horizontally with very low friction. This means special care should be taken with wheeled items when present in the MRI environment so that these

Figure 3. An illustration of the forces acting on an object in the fringe field of an MR system's magnet. The magnetic attraction force is shown resolved into vertical and horizontal components that oppose gravity and friction.

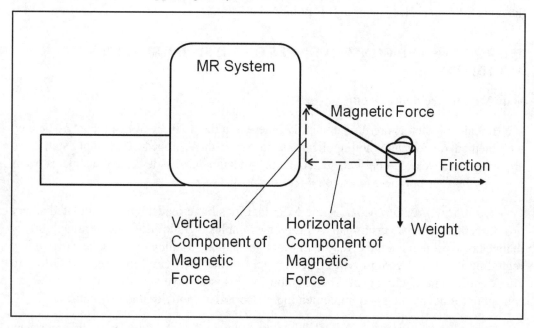

devices are not moved closer than allowed based on the approved MR Conditional labeling. For example, certain patient support devices are labeled as MR Conditional and the conditions specify use at 500-gauss or less. Moving the device closer than 500-gauss may pose a missile-related hazard.

The vertical forces are different in nature. An object of a given weight will remain on the floor until the vertical component of the magnetic force exceeds it. Then, it may become a missile, as it rises off the floor and moves towards the magnet. This cannot be disentangled from the horizontal forces because F_{max} depends on the force pressing the object to the floor, which is the difference between its weight and the opposing vertical magnetic force component. Because of this, objects positioned on the floor will tend to first travel along the floor, move near the magnet, and then leap up off the floor into the MR system.

Again, it should be noted that the magnetic force is related to the spatial gradient of the magnetic field and not to the strength of the static magnetic field. While it is generally true that a ferromagnetic object in the presence of a 3-Tesla MR system will tend to be more strongly attracted than in association with a 1.5-Tesla MR system, with the emergence of new "open", vertical field MR systems it is conceivable that a lower strength magnet can have larger spatial gradients than a higher field strength one. The take home message is that it is always prudent to be cautious when introducing an MR Conditional item into an MR system room for the first time, even if the condition relative to the static magnetic field is met. What is important is the allowable fringe field (e.g., 500-gauss or less) for which the device is labeled and where that value exists in the specific room where the device is intended for use.

For handheld items, the restraining force is muscular. Like the frictional force, muscles can also restrain a ferromagnetic object up to a point. Beyond this, the object may be snatched away from the person's grasp and become a missile. Normally, torque acting on the object is experienced prior to this point.

THE CAUSES AND CONSEQUENCES OF MISSILE-RELATED ACCIDENTS

Why Missile Accidents Occur

Human risk factors are fundamentally inherent in the delivery of healthcare associated with medical devices and their applications during medical procedures. Simply stated, we are human and we are imperfect, so accidents will happen. Missile-related accidents occur for many reasons but there tends to be five main causes.

(1) Faulty safety protocols. Some MRI facilities have inadequate or outdated safety protocols that have dangerous gaps. Common examples include allowing untrained staff or maintenance people into the MR system room, inadequate training regimes, lack of a policy regarding the use of certain types of equipment in the MRI environment, and failure to check equipment labeling (11). The solution for this is to have an MRI Safety Officer responsible for developing and implementing proper safety policies and procedures.

(2) Ignorance of safety protocols by staff members. This occurs when staff members have not been properly educated and trained to follow the MRI facility's safety protocols and, thus, they are ignorant or unaware of them. Common accidents where this is the cause involve cleaning and maintenance staff as well as non-MRI medical staff. The prevention of this problem involves a concerted effort to educate and train all of those involved in the MRI environment.

(3) Unintentional disregard for safety protocols. Staff members may unintentionally disregard safety protocols due to lapses in concentration, or making wrong decisions under high pressure or in emergency situations (12). This can, and often does, occur with highly experienced staff members. Long experience and a good previous record will not ensure safety due to this cause. There is no practical mitigation against this, although regular practice of emergency situations may help.

(4) Deliberate disregard of safety protocols. This is the "I know better than the MRI Safety Officer" or "It will never happen to me" attitude. Some staff members guilty of such attitudes may decide that some aspects of their safety protocols are unnecessary or incorrect, and have decided to ignore them. Fundamentally, this is about the personality of the staff member. Strong character traits of arrogance, pride, or an attraction to risk may lead to this. Prevention of this problem is difficult, but training and safety inspections help. Disciplinary action should be considered for staff members caught disregarding safety protocols.

(5) Incorrect or absent information on MR Safe or MR Conditional equipment. Proper MRI labeling was instituted in 2005. Equipment labeling prior to 2005 may not have updated labeling applied. Even now, some equipment labeled MR Safe is not. Thus, the regular review of equipment and application of proper labeling are important procedures for MRI

facilities. Additionally, MR Conditional equipment does not always have the conditions for use marked on the devices (13). Also, an MRI facility may have recently upgraded from a 1.5-T magnet to a 3-T MR system. Prevention of this issue involves regular equipment inspections and review, particularly with regard to MRI labeling.

Frequency of Occurrence

It is well known that the majority of missile-related incidents are not reported. This is because, in many instances, missile-related incidents that do not hurt individuals don't tend to be reported. Also, at least in the United States (U.S.), only a small minority of medical incidents of all kinds that result in patient harm are reported (14). For accidents involving the missile effect, estimates vary between 5% and 20% for the proportion of potentially harmful incidents that are actually reported. Despite the unknown scale of the problem, the missile effect is often quoted as one of the most serious hazards in the U.S. healthcare system (5).

Fatalities are very rare, but it is estimated that major injuries occur approximately once a year across 20,000 MR systems. For minor injuries, there are no reliable statistics, but these are believed to be far more common. Expensive accidents resulting in damage to the MR system and downtime are thought to be relatively common. However, again, there are no reliable statistics in the public domain pertaining to this matter. Small accidents involving scissors, pens, paper clips, and other similar items that can be removed from MR systems without the need to quench the scanner are very common. Most MRI facilities have several stories of such incidents but there are no known statistics that document how often these problems occur.

Consequences of Missile-Related Accidents

An Internet search for MRI accidents will reveal many photographs and reports of some of the more serious cases. Floor buffers, gas cylinders, and office chairs are amongst the most common missiles, although monitoring equipment, ventilators, tools and even handguns and knives may be seen. There are also many links to news reports describing accidents involving victims and near misses.

If a patient or staff member is injured or killed, then there is a high risk of expensive litigation, and a significant loss of reputation for the hospital or the MRI facility. Larger ferromagnetic objects cannot be manually removed from the MR system while it is at field. Therefore, it is usual for the manufacturer of the MR system to provide technical support to ramp the magnet down, remove the item, and repair any damage. After that, the magnetic field of the MR system needs to be ramped-up and shimmed. The process can take several days, resulting in a significant loss of imaging time. Estimates for the average cost of a missile-related accident not involving human injury vary between $20,000 to more than $200,000. Where injuries are involved, the monetary costs can be excessive, not including any commercial damage due to loss of reputation.

FERROMAGNETIC DETECTION SYSTEMS

Introduction To Ferromagnetic Detection Systems

Ferromagnetic Detection Systems (FMDS) designed for the MRI environment appeared in 2002, shortly after the tragic death of Michael Colombini in 2001, who was struck by a steel oxygen that was brought into the MR system room while he was in the scanner (15). Prior to this, conventional archway metal detectors and some forms of magnetometers were tried at MR system room doorways, but these were not found to be useful. Conventional metal detectors "alarm" on all metals, ferromagnetic and non-ferromagnetic and, therefore, may detect many objects that can be legitimately taken into the MR system room which do not pose a missile-related hazard.

The first example of a modern FMDS was installed in the Royal Hospital Haslar in the United Kingdom in November 2002. Since then, three primary companies specializing in FMDS have supplied these devices commercially (16-18).

As the name suggests, ferromagnetic detection systems selectively detect ferromagnetic objects, ignoring non-ferromagnetic objects. Because only ferromagnetic objects pose a missile-related hazard, an FMDS selectively detects threats and work by monitoring the ambient magnetic field using magnetic sensors. The ambient field is a combination of the fringe field of the magnet and the Earth's magnetic field plus the contribution from architectural steel and any other stationary steel objects in the vicinity. A ferromagnetic object distorts the ambient field in its vicinity. If it is brought close to an FMDS, the distortion is detected as a changing magnetic field and an alert is triggered. This is illustrated in **Figure 4**, where the ambient field is illustrated as parallel horizontal lines. A person who is not carrying any ferromagnetic material does not modify this field in any way and can walk past the FMDS undetected, as seen in **Figure 4(a)**. **Figure 4(b)** shows how a ferromagnetic object carried by a person perturbs the ambient magnetic field. Note that the perturbation in the field is local to the object. Because the person is far from the FMDS, the ambient field is unchanged, so the FMDS has not detected the object, as of yet. In **Figure 4(c)**, the person carrying the ferromagnetic object is now close enough to the FMDS such that the perturbation in the field surrounding the object has caused a change of the ambient field at the FMDS. This change triggers an alarm.

Importantly, an FMDS ignores static magnetic fields (i.e., magnetic fields that do not change with time). In practice, this means that the FMDS is only sensitive to changing magnetic fields, or moving ferromagnetic objects. They are insensitive to a stationary ferromagnetic object, so if an object is placed near to an FMDS it will be detected as it is put in place but thereafter ignored, until it is moved again. The reason for this is that the ambient magnetic fields are very large compared with the magnetic perturbations caused by a ferromagnetic object, and it is difficult to measure tiny changes on a large background field. The large static background is therefore removed by the FMDS by filtering it out, irrespective of whichever components make up that static magnetic field including the magnet of the MR system, the Earth's magnetic field, or a metal cabinet next to the FMDS.

Figure 4. An example of the operation of an FMDS. **(a)** With no ferromagnetic object present, the ambient field lines are not affected, and as the person passes the FMDS, there is no alarm. **(b)** With a ferromagnetic object present, the ambient field becomes perturbed in the vicinity of the object. **(c)** The changing field caused by the ferromagnetic object is detected by the FMDS, causing an alarm.

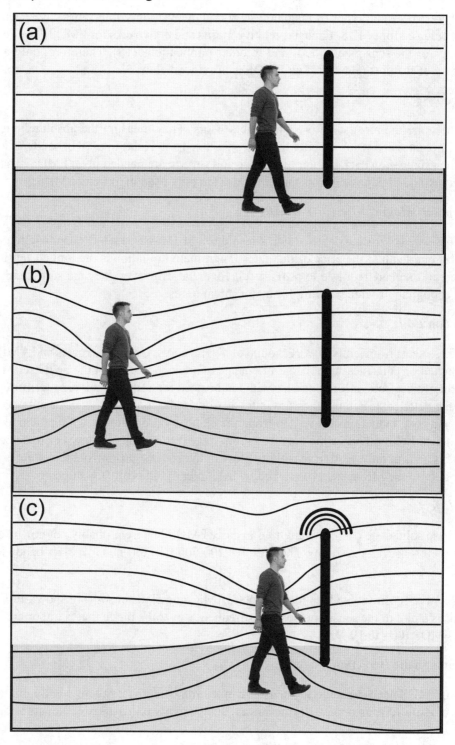

For a handheld FMDS, the object may be stationary but the FMDS is moved, so it is the relative motion that is important when using this type of device. A stationary FMDS detects moving ferromagnetic objects only.

Magnetic Sensors

There are several types of magnetic sensors, however, only four types have been used in devices used for FMDS. Each has relative merits and drawbacks for FMDS. The detailed workings of the sensors can be found in other publications (19). Therefore, only a brief summary of features relevant to an FMDS is provided below.

Fluxgates

These are the most sensitive magnetic sensors. They measure the absolute magnetic field. Fluxgates can resolve better than 20-pT (20×10^{-12}-Tesla) in a 1-Hz bandwidth at 1-Hz. Their main drawback is their high price and several are needed in an FMDS. The high sensitivity and high price means that fluxgates are only used in top-end FMDS.

Amorphous Magneto-Resistive (AMR)

These are solid-state devices with a resolution of 350-pT in a 1-Hz bandwidth at 1-Hz and cost one-tenth of the price of fluxgates. Their main limitation is the limited sensitivity, so more of them are required to provide full coverage. However, they are sufficiently sensitive enough to provide warning for major threat items.

Induction Coils

These sensors are coils of wire wound on ferrite cores. Unlike fluxgates and AMR sensors, induction coils measure the rate-of-change of magnetic field, not the field itself. Therefore, they reject static magnetic fields without the need for a filter. Their sensitivity depends upon the detailed design but they are intrinsically similar to an AMR sensor in both sensitivity and cost. Induction coil FMDS from one company use magnets within them to boost the ambient field and hence the magnetization of the ferrous objects they seek to detect (18, 20). This adds to the effective sensitivity close to the FMDS sensors, but the effect is small at the door to the MR system room where the ambient field is already large.

Hall Effect

These solid-state devices were tried in early FMDS but are probably not now used because their sensitivity is so low. They resolve 200,000-pT (200-nT) in a 1-Hz bandwidth at 1-Hz.

Relative sensitivity values for fluxgates, AMR, and Hall sensors are shown in **Figure 5**. This is a plot of the sensor noise verses frequency over the range that is important to use in an FMDS (0.1- to 10-Hz).

Ferromagnetic Detection Systems

An FMDS needs to be highly sensitive in its immediate vicinity but highly immune to large moving ferrous objects further away, such as cars on roads and elevator counter-

Figure 5. The spectral noise density for typical fluxgate AMR and Hall effect sensors used in FMD devices showing relative sensitivity differences. Lower noise equates to higher resolution. Induction coil sensors (not shown) are similar or slightly better than AMR sensors.

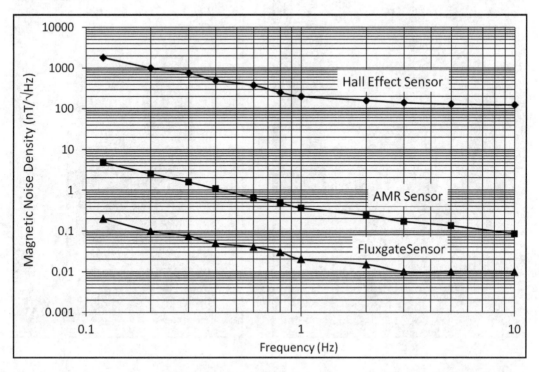

weights. To achieve this, the magnetic sensors are usually configured into pairs such that each pair produces a signal that is the difference in the magnetic field between the two sensors. If the two sensors in a pair were co-located (i.e., they share the same position), then they would not measure anything because both sensors "see" the same field and cancel each other out. However, if they are separated by a distance called the "baseline", then they can detect field differences caused by a nearby ferromagnetic object, particularly if it is within a distance comparable to the baseline of the sensor pairs. For magnetic sources that are distant compared to the baseline, the sensors appear to be more co-located and will, therefore, provide a smaller signal than an individual sensor would.

Physicists will be familiar with this as a magnetic gradiometer system. At long ranges, the field from a magnetic dipole source falls as $B \propto 1 / r^3$ and its gradient as $\partial B / \partial r \propto -3/r^4$. Therefore, a gradiometer measures less signal than a magnetometer for distant targets. At ranges smaller than the baseline, the FMDS does not behave as a gradiometer. Its sensitivity is generally similar to that of a single magnetometer but the situation is more complicated due to geometrical effects beyond the scope of this chapter.

An FMDS will consist of one or more magnetic gradiometers along with the necessary amplifiers and filters. Following this is the detection stage. Detection can be done in several ways but the simplest is to rectify the signals so that they are always positive and compare them with a threshold level. If the threshold is exceeded by the magnetic signal, an audible

Figure 6. Examples of entryway or portal-type ferromagnetic detection systems. (a) Photograph courtesy of Metrasens, Ltd. (b) Photograph courtesy of Kopp Development, Inc.

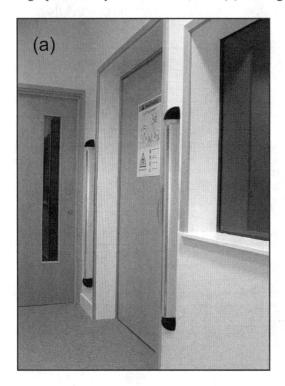 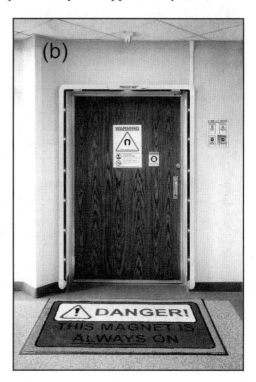

and visual alarm will result. Adjusting the threshold adjusts the sensitivity of the system. That is, a higher threshold means the magnetic signal has to be larger to exceed it and vice versa.

Because there may be ferromagnetic objects that are moving close to the FMDS that are not intended to go into the MR system room, most manufacturers have techniques for suppressing the alarm unless the object is actually passing into the scanner room itself. This cuts down on unwanted or nuisance alarms (21). Because doors leading into the MR system room tend to be relatively wide, to get good coverage across the width, the FMDS will have sensors on both sides of the door. This may be in the form of two wall-mounted units as illustrated in **Figure 6(a)**, a frame surrounding the door as shown in **Figure 6(b)**, or two free-standing units which are upright poles with bases, although these are less common. Freestanding units consist of upright poles with sensors and a base that can be moved around.

It is important to note that the sensors are housed in the upright sections of the FMDS, and the closer these are together the more sensitive the system will be in its least sensitive position, that is, at the midpoint of the uprights. **Figure 7** shows illustratively how the field perturbation from a ferromagnetic object decays with distance as $B \propto 1 / r^3$. An object at position A has a larger field, B_A at the FMDS sensors than it would if it were at the midpoint, position B. This can more usefully be looked at from the viewpoint of what the signal is

Figure 7. Illustration of the relationship between the position of a ferromagnetic object across the door to the MR system room and the FMDS signal. **(a)** This shows how the decaying field from a ferrous object impacts an FMDS when it is to one side, position A, and in the center, position B. The magnetic fields at the FMDS are B_A and B_B respectively. **(b)** The resulting FMDS signal (proportional to the measured magnetic field) as a function of the ferromagnetic object's position across the door.

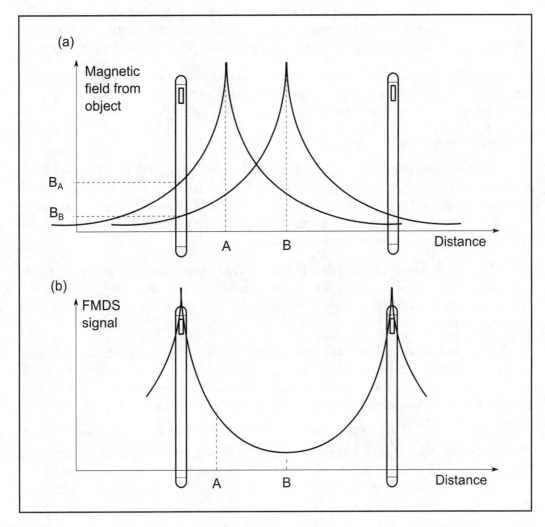

measured by the FMDS as a function of the ferrous object's position across the door to the MR system.

Note that the FMDS response is highly non-uniform and has a minimum for objects at the midpoint, point B (**Figure 7**). If the FMDS uprights were further apart, the minimum would be lower. At some separation, the minimum will dip to below the sensitivity threshold of the FMDS. Then there will be a gap through which a ferromagnetic object could pass undetected.

Although originally devised as a system to be sited at the entrance to the MR system room, an FMDS used in the patient preparation area has recently been developed. This type of FMDS is primarily aimed at ensuring that patients are free from even small ferromagnetic objects. The patient screening FMDS comes in two forms, wall-mounted in a single upright unit or as a handheld unit. These will be discussed in more detail later in this chapter.

To distinguish the different types of FMDS that exist, the following nomenclature is used in this chapter:

Entryway FMDS. The purpose of this FMDS is to protect the MR system room. The entryway FMDS is a system that is normally mounted at or near to the entrance of the scanner room, ideally with the purpose of providing a warning prior to entry into the room.

Patient Screening FMDS. This is a system mounted in or near to a patient preparation area with the purpose of warning if a patient who is about to be scanned is carrying a ferromagnetic object. This type of FMDS may be a wall-mounted or handheld device.

Installation Issues

The effectiveness of an FMDS depends not only upon the quality of the system itself, but where it is sited and what its environment is. We first consider the entryway FMDS. It is important that an FMDS is sited such that anyone entering the MR system room must pass through it. There are many different architectural layouts for MR system rooms, but there are five main MRI entrance types, as follows:

Off an atrium. In this case, the door is in the wall of a room that may have an open control room (or several) or a waiting area. In some facilities, these are highly compact with control room desks and patient transfer equipment in a confined space. Others have large uncluttered areas.

With an anti-chamber. Here, stub walls are built out from both sides of the MR system doorway, usually to a distance of 1.5-m to 2-m. These may be built for a variety of reasons, but most commonly for allowing extra control desk area, or dedicated space for outward opening MR system room doors to swing into. Sometimes these are built especially to accommodate an FMDS.

End of a corridor. Due to being at the end, the last section of the corridor is dedicated to the MR scanner. In this respect it is similar to the anti-chamber setting. The system control room will often have a door to the side of the corridor shortly before the MR system door itself.

Side of a corridor. This is a common layout but the least safe. This layout is poor practice from a safety consideration unless the corridor can be a controlled area.

Mobile MRI trailer. This a highly compact setting and a smaller than standard MR system door is usually installed. The control room is in very close proximity to the door.

For each of these entrance types, the door may be swing-in or swing-out (although swing-out is rare for a side of a corridor entrance). Usually the FMDS will be installed on the immediate surrounding area of the door itself because there is normally available wall space. However, there is a disadvantage with this. The door may be magnetic and, thus, strongly detected by the FMDS when it is in motion, causing unwanted alarms. Therefore, it is preferable to have the FMDS offset in front of the door so the person entering has been screened by the FMDS before the door is opened. This can only be practically achieved with anti-chamber or end of corridor layouts.

When the FMDS is mounted at the doorway, it is incumbent upon the MRI technologists to wait until the door has stopped moving until passing through the FMDS otherwise an alarm will occur. This is discussed in more detail in the following section. Where possible, mounting an FMDS at a distance of 1.5-m to 2-m before the door overcomes this problem. Recently, an FMDS has become available that has immunity to the door that alleviates the need for this (16).

Swing-out doors open through an FMDS mounted on the outside of the door. This presents an issue because the FMDS needs to distinguish between the door opening and a person carrying a ferrous object. In both cases, a moving ferromagnetic object is passing through the FMDS, the door is safe and the person is unsafe. Different FMDS manufacturers have developed different solutions. One manufacturer has developed a solution that allows the FMDS to be mounted on the outside of a swing-out door and operate normally (22). Another has elected to install the FMDS on the inside of the MR system room, so that the door swings outwards away from the system, not through it (17). Some MRI facilities regard this as providing a warning too late, but others accept it.

Wall-mounted and handheld patient screening devices have two requirements on their installation location. First, this type of FMDS needs to be located in a convenient position from the point of view of efficient workflow. This will normally be in the patient changing or preparation area, or sometimes in the close proximity to the MR system room. The second requirement is that it is located sufficiently far away from interfering magnetic sources to that it can be set to maximum sensitivity. Interfering sources may include public corridors, roads, and elevators.

WHAT THE FMDS WILL AND WILL NOT DETECT: ADVANTAGES AND LIMITATIONS

Magnetic Qualities of Potentially Dangerous Objects

The physics involved with magnetics is not intuitive. There are two common misconceptions that individuals have when they consider using an FMDS in the MRI environment. It is often expected that identical objects will have identical magnetic qualities but, in fact, they can magnetically vary by several orders of magnitude. Another is that larger ferrous objects will be magnetically stronger (and pose a greater risk) than smaller ones. This premise can be true but so can the converse. Probably the most common question asked of the FMDS manufacturer is, *what is the smallest object that can be detected?* It is one of the most difficult questions to answer because a ferromagnetic object's size is not strongly related to its magnetic properties. Furthermore, because of the strong dependence on range, very small ferromagnetic objects may be detected close to an FMDS sensor, whereas at longer distances to the FMDS, the same or larger objects may not be detected.

In general, the magnetic properties of a ferromagnetic object depend primarily on the material and shape of the object (23). For objects with different sizes but made of the iden-

Figure 8. The magnetic signal strength of control room objects measured at the mid-point of an FMDS in a 1-gauss fringe field.

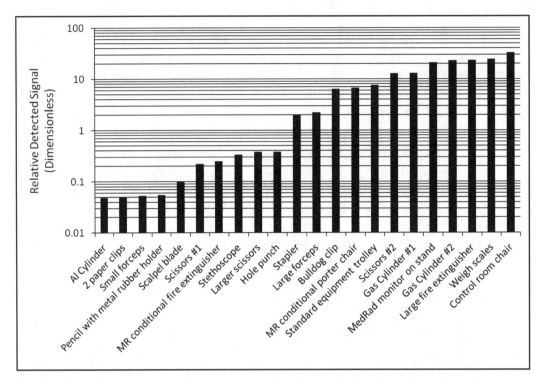

tical material, there is potential for the larger objects to be more heavily magnetized than the smaller ones. Also, for objects of identical size but made from different materials, there is potential for the objects with higher magnetic permeability to be more heavily magnetic than those with lower magnetic permeability. For example, a "weakly magnetic" pair of scissors made from steel can be magnetized more than a stainless steel pair of the same size and shape.

Very small objects have only a limited potential to achieve high magnetic moments. Most magnets associated with MR systems will have very minor missile-related occurrences by paper clips, pens, or other small objects. The limited magnetic qualities along with the very light weight of certain objects means that they cannot accumulate enough kinetic energy to do damage or cause much inconvenience (unless the object impacts a particularly delicate area, such as the human eye). There is clearly a grey-scale between this and a missile-related accident with larger objects that will be inevitably serious. Using an FMDS at the MR system door should, at the mid-point of the door, at least detect the latter.

The relative signal strength related to the magnetic qualities of different objects that may be commonly found in the MRI setting has been measured (M.N. Keene, unpublished data) (**Figure 8** and **Figure 9**). These measurements were made in the fringe field, just outside of an MR system room at 1-gauss and at the mid-point, 75-cm from the uprights of the FMDS. The average of several movements past the FMDS for each object are shown. **Figure 8** shows data for objects commonly found in control rooms and **Figure 9** shows data

Figure 9. The magnetic signal strength of personal items measured at the mid-point of an FMDS in a 1-gauss fringe field.

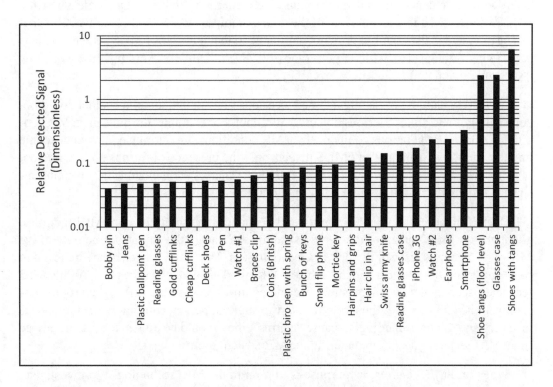

for personal items. The vertical scale is consistent for **Figure 8** and **Figure 9**. Depending upon the type of sensor used (or brand of FMDS), the maximum sensitivity that is available is between 0.06 and 0.3 on this scale. Notably, the signals are much higher if the objects are near to the FMDS uprights.

PRACTICAL ASPECTS OF MRI ENTRYWAY PROTECTION

Working With an FMDS

The ideal FMDS (which does not yet exist, by the way) would have the following two qualities: (1) no adaptations to workflow would be needed to accommodate the FMDS and (2) the FMDS would never alarm unless there was a ferromagnetic object entering the MR system room. It is not ideal for MRI technologists to have to modify their behavior to accommodate an FMDS. The door to the MR system room being magnetic is a common issue when the MRI technologist opens the door and passes through while it is still moving. Waiting for the door to stop before moving into the room is a minor workflow interruption. This is particularly important for swing-in doors where, to open them fully, there is a tendency to follow the door into the MR system room. There are two common responses. In one case, the MRI technologists may accept the short delay. It provides a momentary pause and an opportunity to take a brief "time-out" to think before entering the room. In the other case, many MRI technologists allow the alarm to occur as they operate the door, on the assumption that they are not carrying anything dangerous into the area. Although the FMDS is not effectively screening them in this case, the MRI technologists will often watch the patients move through the FMDS with a stationary door. These approaches are not ideal because safety and convenience are traded off against each other. The door is not an issue where the FMDS is mounted a few feet in front of the door. An improved FMDS is now available that can be mounted at the door but does not alarm due to the door. This FMDS screens the person moving through (16). Utilizing this type of FMDS effectively overcomes the workflow issue while maintaining the safety level.

An FMDS cannot yet distinguish between loose ferromagnetic objects that could become missiles and "fixed" ferrous objects that cannot. For example, the bolts in an MR conditional gurney or the ferrous components in MR conditional monitoring equipment become problematic for screening. The FMDS detects only the presence of ferrous objects and not whether they are free to move. Therefore, extraneous alarms are inevitable in some circumstances and are discussed in more detail in the following section.

Overall, the use of an FMDS significantly enhances the safety level of MRI facilities, although non-ideal aspects of the current systems can impact the day-to-day activity of the MRI staff members, especially the MRI technologists. The individuals who are believed to cause most missile-related accidents are non-MRI workers who enter the room. While MRI technologists may not be able to supervise and control access to the MR system room constantly an FMDS can and, thus, provides a warning to a person entering when the door is unsupervised. If non-technologists cause "alarms", they should be trained to seek the advice of an MRI technologist before entering the MR system room.

When an FMDS alarms, its purpose is to prompt the MRI technologist to investigate. As an example, an MRI technologist pushes an MR Conditional gurney into the room and the alarm sounds, as always, because the gurney has ferromagnetic components. The correct response of the MRI technologist is to stop and to perform a final check of the gurney. Is the gurney acceptable to use with this particular MR system? Is there an oxygen cylinder or IV pole present that is MR Unsafe? Is there a ferromagnetic object under the sheets? The incorrect response is to ignore the alarm because an MR conditional gurney will always trigger an alarm. Many accidents have occurred because of ferromagnetic items being placed on top of gurneys or underneath sheets. In this case, the alarm from the FMDS acts as a reminder to do a final check.

Extraneous Alarms and False Alarms: Causes and Prevention

There is an important distinction between false alarms and extraneous alarms. A false alarm occurs when there is no ferrous material passing through the FMDS but the alarm is activated. This may be due to some external factor causing a magnetic disturbance at the same time as a magnetically "clean" person passes through or by the FMDS. False alarms are rare when the FMDS has been installed and set up properly. The most common cause of false alarms are control room chairs when they get close to the FMDS.

An extraneous alarm occurs when ferromagnetic material is deliberately passed through the FMDS because it is known to not present a missile-related hazard. The most common causes of extraneous alarms are, the following: the door to the MR system room moving as individuals pass through; MR Conditional equipment (e.g., gurneys, wheelchairs, monitoring equipment, patient tables, etc.) passing by the FMDS, staff clothing and accessories (e.g., underwire bras, watches, shoes with metal, etc.); and patient clothing and accessories. Notably, with extraneous alarms, the FMDS is functioning normally and doing its job.

If the frequency of extraneous alarms is too high, alarm fatigue sets in and staff members soon begin to ignore the FMDS. When this occurs, the FMDS is reduced in effectiveness during the working hours of the MRI facility, although it still remains effective for non-MRI staff members. However, most of the causes of extraneous alarms are preventable and within the power of the MRI technologists to remediate them. Certain solutions exist to prevent extraneous alarms including, the following:

The door to the MR system room. There are several alternatives for this problem. For example site the FMDS a suitable distance in front of the door, if possible; select an FMDS that can ignore the door; or always ensure that the door is stationary before passing through the FMDS.

MR Conditional equipment. For patient transfer equipment, there are products that are commercially available that are entirely non-ferromagnetic and, thus, will not cause extraneous alarms. The use of ferrous-free transfer equipment means an FMDS will alarm only on ferrous materials. For docking tables, patient monitors, and other equipment there is currently no solution. It is recommended that the extraneous alarm should be used for the purpose of taking the time to check the equipment for objects placed upon them before proceeding into the MR system room.

Staff clothing and accessories. This can be one of the biggest causes of extraneous alarms. One of the most common items is the underwire bra. Considering the activities of female MRI technologists, these may come into close proximity with the MR system's magnet and, thus, become highly magnetized. Other objects such as watches, bracelets, and shoes with tangs or metallic supports can also trigger the FMDS. Alternatives for all such clothing and accessories are readily available. Watches and ferromagnetic jewelry can easily be removed.

Patient clothing and accessories. It is always best practice to place patients in gowns or scrubs that have no pockets in preparation for MRI examinations. Accordingly, any FMDS alarm will be real and not extraneous. Underwire bras, shoes with metal and jewelry issues are the same as for staff members.

Safety Level for Avoidance of Missile-Related Accidents

The effectiveness of an entryway FMDS for improving safety depends predominantly on the attitude of the MRI facility's MRI technologists and managers. The introduction of an FMDS significantly increases the potential for safety improvements, but this may not be realized due to various factors. To illustrate this, two examples are given.

MRI Facility A purchased several entryway FMDS to protect their MR system rooms. The patient transfer equipment was replaced with entirely non-ferromagnetic equivalents. A policy of "zero tolerance" to ferrous materials was introduced with the exception of patient monitors. Staff members are required to be ferrous-free, adopting the same standard of "magnetic cleanliness" as the patients. Each patient is gowned and checked with a screening

FMDS prior to entry into the MR system room. The doors to the MR system rooms are always stationary when individuals pass through. The low extraneous alarm rate that resulted from these measures allowed each FMDS to be set at a very high sensitivity, such that it could detect very small ferromagnetic objects. The staff members have regular safety training and are able to contribute to the evolving safety protocols for the facility.

MRI Facility B also purchased several entryway FMDS to protect their MR system rooms. The ferromagnetic detection systems were purchased by an inexperienced manager without consultation with the MRI technologists. The staff members were unwilling to change the way they clothed, and the managers were unwilling to enforce a clothing policy. They kept their regular MR Conditional transfer equipment. Staff members resisted making any workflow concessions with regard to the doors to the MR system rooms. Patients were not gowned and their family members were allowed into the MR system rooms. There was no patient screening FMDS. Despite being set to a low sensitivity to reduce extraneous alarms, each FMDS alarmed on almost all entrance and exit occurrences. When this became intolerable each FMDS was switched off.

For any MRI facility, improving safety with regard to missile-related accidents using an FMDS is a journey. Some facilities choose to make that journey in one leap with a radical culture change to become like *MRI Facility A*. For most facilities, it is a more of a gradual change. An FMDS may be set to modest sensitivity initially and as the MRI technologists improve their protocols and the surrounding environmental factors, the sensitivity of the FMDS may be increased, accordingly, as time goes by.

The examples of *MRI Facility A* and *MRI Facility B* may be regarded as being at opposite ends of a safety level where one facility has maximized its safety standard and represents best practice, while the other facility is unchanged from its initial poor practice. Every MRI facility ought to be aware of where it is on this scale and where it should ultimately be. **Table 1** shows a form that provides an approximate means of assessing the safety level for an MRI facility with regard to missile-related hazards.

Workflow Aspects of Using an FMDS

The FMDS should be sited where workflow is least affected. For an MRI facility that is high on the safety scale where extraneous alarms are low, there is very little impact on workflow. Where there are a substantial number of extraneous alarms and each one is investigated, the impact increases. In many facilities the workflow is a key priority that will not be compromised. There are two common responses to this. One is to ignore the FMDS, which reduces safety levels. The other is to move up the safety scale to reduce the extraneous alarms. Both responses retain the workflow, but one increases safety while the other reduces it. For example, implementing a ferrous-free clothing policy tends to make the biggest impact on maintaining workflow in a positive safety direction followed by changing to ferrous-free patient transfer equipment.

FERROMAGNETIC DETECTION SYSTEMS FOR PATIENT SCREENING

Using an FMDS for patient screening is becoming more common (24-28). The main purpose of this device is to check patients for ferromagnetic objects just prior to the MRI

Table 1. Form that may be used to assess the safety level for an MRI facility with regard to missile-related hazards. Provided by Metrasens, Ltd. with permission.

No.	MRI Facility & Staff	Score	Max Pts.
\multicolumn{4}{l}{**MRI FACILITY MISSILE-RELATED HAZARD FORM**}			
\multicolumn{4}{l}{**Instructions:** For each question, score your facility's response up to the maximum points for that question. On completion sum the score.}			
1	Do staff members have formal training and regular refreshers in MRI safety?		4
2	Are there danger signs on the MR system room door?		4
3	Are all of the MR Safe and MR Conditional equipment clearly marked?		2
4	Are all fire extinguishers and hand tools in the immediate vicinity MR Safe or MR Conditional and marked as such?		2
5	Is there a zero tolerance policy for un-marked metallic objects being taken into the MR system room? (e.g. stethoscopes, pens, etc.)		3
6	Is the MR system room locked when no staff member is present?		3
7	Does the MRI have an entryway ferromagnetic detection system? High quality Modest Quality		5 3
8	Are MRI staff members required to wear clothing with no ferrous metals?		2
9	Are MRI staff members required to screen themselves using an FMD at the start of their shift?		1
10	Is the patient gurney/wheelchair ferrous-free?		3
11	Are all untrained staff or visitors into the MR system room pre-screened?		2
12	Do cleaners, janitors, & maintenance staff with access to the MR system room have MRI safety training?		3
13	Are safety protocols regularly reviewed and updated?		3
\multicolumn{2}{l}{**Patient Pre-screen and scanning**}	**Score**	**Max Pts.**
14	Are non-trained or non-screened people forbidden to accompany patients during scans?		2
15	Are all patients changed into ferrous-free clothing prior to exam?		2
16	Are removed clothes/metal items kept outside of the MR system room?		3
17	Does the MRI safety trained staff member perform a final screening and visual inspection of patients prior to entry into the MR system room?		1
18	Are patients pre-screened with a ferromagnetic detection system prior to entry into the MR system room? High quality Modest Quality		5 3
	SCORE		/50

examination. The utilization of an FMDS will help to prevent potential missile-related in-cidents from devices a patient may bring into the MR system room and to reduce scanning artifacts due to small and well-hidden ferromagnetic objects such as bobby pins.

There are two types available, wall-mounted as shown in **Figures 10(a)** and **10(b)** and a handheld device, **Figure 10(c)**. For the wall-mounted FMDS, the patient approaches the unit and rotates in front of it. This brings all parts of the surface of the patient within a few inches of the FMDS, which has a twofold purpose: (1) the small range between a ferrous object and the magnetic sensors means that far smaller (i.e., lower magnetic susceptibility) objects can be detected and (2) it provides the necessary motion of the ferrous object relative to the FMDS. A handheld device is used to scan over the surface of the patient.

Performing patient screening using an FMDS does not tend to have extraneous alarms because only the patient is screened and should essentially be clean of ferrous objects. Staff members and equipment are not screened this way unless there is a policy for this procedure. However, patient screening using an FMDS is subject to false alarms if there is a moving ferromagnetic object nearby when the patient undergoes screening. Normally, the MRI tech-nologist can identify this situation by observation, and repeat the screening, as needed.

Figure 10. (a) and **(b)** Examples of wall-mounted ferromagnetic detection systems where patients are screened by rotating in front of these devices. **(c)** Handheld FMDS that is swept over the patient's body. (Photographs provided courtesy of Metrasens Ltd., Kopp Development Inc., and Mednovus, Inc.)

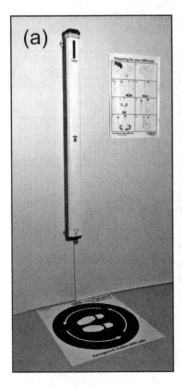
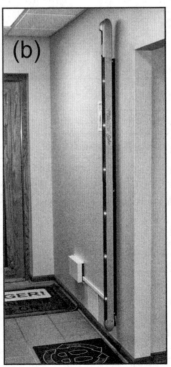
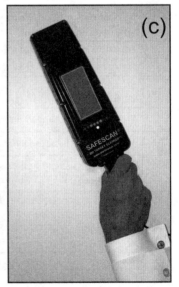

The Patient Screening Process Using an FMDS

Screening the patient using an FMDS is an additional step in the screening process and is the last step before the MRI examination. It is important to note that it is not a replacement for any aspect of the screening procedure but rather it is an addendum that adds a final objective check prior to performing MRI (28). This type of screening normally takes less than one minute to complete provided that there is no positive alarm. It takes somewhat longer to use a handheld FMDS because it has to be manually scanned over the entire area of the patient's body. Ideally, there will be a line at the bottom of the screening questionnaire that records the result of FMDS screening and any observations or actions as a result.

If a patient passes the FMDS screening without a detection occurring (i.e., no positive alarm), this should be documented on the screening form and the patient may then proceed with the MRI examination. If an alarm occurs, then the patient must be investigated for the presence of a ferromagnetic object and it should be removed (if possible). Once this has been done, the patient should be re-screened using the FMDS. If a ferrous object cannot be found, the FMDS screening should be repeated in case the original result was a false alarm. For genuine alarms that cannot be resolved, the MRI technologist must then suspect the possibility that the ferromagnetic object is internal, being either an implant or a foreign body (25-28). The patient's history should then be thoroughly checked before proceeding to MRI.

Detection Performance

The earlier discussion concerning the size of ferromagnetic objects that can be detected using an entryway FMDS applies to patient screening utilizing an FMDS, as well. However, due to the shorter range when using a patient screening FMDS, magnetically weaker objects can be more reliably detected. In general, bobby pins, hair barrettes, and some jewelry can be reliable detected with the best performing patient screening FMDS. Obviously, this feature is good for artifact reduction and will save time re-scanning individuals in the MRI setting. However, very small ferrous objects are not likely to be detected, such as small metallic fragments in the eye.

Some investigations have been performed on the performance of using a patient screening FMDS but most are unpublished. A summary of this information is provided in **Table 2**. It is interesting to note that although the patients in each of these studies were gowned, there were a surprising number of positive alarms. These alarms were mainly associated with removable dental implants, eyeglasses, bras, jewelry, and other objects.

Using a Wall-Mounted Versus Handheld FMDS

The use of a wall-mounted FMDS provides head-to-toe, whole-body screening that is easy to accomplish and fast to perform for cooperative ambulatory patients. For non-ambulatory patients the only means of screening with a wall-mounted FMDS is to use a ferrous-free gurney or wheelchair and perform a "drive-by" in two directions parallel to the wall, pushed by a ferrous-free MRI technologist. However, this process will not provide the close range required to detect the smallest objects, but is nonetheless useful for the detection of larger personal items.

Table 2. Summary of five patient screening studies using FMDS technology. All studies involved patients who were in gowns.

	Hospital 1	Hospital 2	Hospital 3	Hospital 4	Hospital 5
No. of patients presenting to MRI	75	20	38	91	340
No. of screens performed	95	20	26	55	340
No. of alerts raised	27	3	8	5	16
% of alerts / screening	28.4%	15%	30.8%	9.1%	4.7%

1- U.S. Out-Patient Facility, Unpublished
2- English NHS Trust, Unpublished
3- Scottish Health Board Twin Site, Unpublished
4- Scottish General Hospital, Unpublished
5- University Hospital, Jena, Germany

The use of a handheld FMDS (18) is somewhat similar to using a handheld metal detector (e.g., the type used at airports), insofar as it must be swept or scanned over the surface of the body at close range, usually within 5-cm of the surface. The sensing area is quite small (approximately 5-cm x 9-cm) so care must be taken to ensure that screening occurs with no gaps while maintaining a relatively short, stand-off distance. Due to this being a manual process, the quality and reliability of the screening depends on the person performing the scan using the handheld FMDS. Staff members may be reluctant to screen an intimate patient area, such as the groin (25). Notably, the only available handheld FMDS at this time has a strong permanent magnet within it to boost the magnetization of ferrous objects. Because of this, this type of handheld FMDS should not be used close the eyes or near cardiac pacemakers or other similar implanted devices in case the magnetic field poses possible problems. A handheld FMDS can be used for a non-ambulatory patient on an MR Conditional gurney or wheelchair, as opposed to ferrous-free ones. With a gurney, the patient needs to turn over from one side to the other to get full coverage. With a wheelchair, it is more difficult to get full coverage unless the patient can stand for a short while.

Screening for Metallic Implants, Devices, and Foreign Bodies

The question surrounding the detection of ferromagnetic implants, devices, and foreign bodies is a current research topic with growing international interest (24-28). Currently the use of a patient screening FMDS is not approved by a governmental entity or organization and, thus, is not intended to be used for the specific purpose of detecting implanted objects. However, because human flesh is effectively transparent to ferromagnetic detection, the distinction between *ex vivo* and *in vivo* ferrous objects is merely one of range. Some initial studies on implant detection have been conducted as well as on foreign bodies (24-28). Although research is at an early stage, the initial results seem to indicate that the use of a patient screening FMDS is capable of detecting many *in vivo* ferrous objects and this has important implications for patient safety in the MRI environment.

CONCLUSIONS

The safety of patients, staff, equipment, and reputation of an MRI facility should be recognized as a holistic issue, not just about the use of an FMDS, but the whole culture. This culture should be characterized by an adoption of best practice in safety procedures, staff training and education, vigilance and safety technology, together with a striving for continuous further improvement at all levels. Unfortunately, there is a notion that adopting a culture of high safety standards often works against high throughput or efficiency within the MRI facility. This is a dangerous and incorrect perspective.

The availability of ferromagnetic detection as a safety technology has substantially increased the potential safety levels that a facility may attain. If these devices are adopted with the view that they are one key element of an overall safety improvement program, they will be most effective. If they are adopted as an excuse to do nothing more on training or safety procedures, they will have a much more limited positive benefit.

Earlier in this chapter, the ideal FMDS was defined. As the technology continues to develop, systems will move toward this ideal. The main non-ideal issue present with an FMDS relates to extraneous alarms, which are partly a result of the introduction of the FMDS into a setting where unnecessary ferrous objects may be routinely carried into the MR system room and partly due to problematic siting (i.e., with regard to the position of the door to the MR system). Hopefully, FMDS technology will evolve to eventually overcome these matters.

An FMDS is not currently subject to regulatory standards so there is no minimum performance standard defined for this device. When selecting an FMDS, an MRI facility currently has to rely on the manufacturer's claims, recommendations from other MRI centers, or whether or not a satisfactory experience occurred during the demonstration of the product.

At some point, the use of an FMDS may become an essential screening tool for MRI facilities. To date, the statistical impact these devices have on safety has yet to be investigated and, therefore, it is difficult to know how many accidents have been avoided. There have been many anecdotal reports of successful prevention of dangerous objects entering MR system rooms. As the recognition of the need to improve MRI safety spreads, and as the use of FMDS technology correspondingly widens, the global MRI community will hopefully become substantially safer.

REFERENCES

1. Kanal E, Barkovich J, Bell C, et al. ACR guidance document for safe MR practices: 2007. American Journal of Roentgenology 2007;188:1447.

2. Kanal E, Barkovich AJ, Bell C, et al. ACR guidance document on MR safe practices: 2013. J Magn Reson Imaging 2013;37:501-530.

3. Joint Commission. Preventing accidents and injuries in the MRI suite. Sentinel Event Alert, Issue 38, February 14, 2008.

4. United States Department of Veterans Affairs. MRI Design Guide April 2008:2-25 – 2-28.

5. ECRI Institute, Health Devices. 2010 Top 10 Technology Hazards; November 2009;38:No. 11:1-10.

6. Schwartz GM, Huang Y. Chapter 2. MRI for Technologists. Magnetic Resonance: A Technical Overview. In: Woodward P, Editor. MRI for Technologists, Second edition. New York: McGraw-Hill Medical Publishing Division; 2001, pp.13-26.

7. Karpowicz J, Gryz K. Health risk assessment of occupational exposure to a magnetic field from magnetic resonance imaging devices. International Journal of Occupational Safety and Ergonomics (JOSE) 2006;12:155–167.

8. Duffin WJ. Electricity and Magnetism, Third Edition. London: McGraw-Hill; 1980. pp. 230-232.

9. Bleaney BI, Bleaney B. Electricity and Magnetism. Third Edition. Oxford: Oxford University Press; 1978. pp. 101-107.

10. Shellock FG, Woods TO, Crues JV. MRI labeling information for implants and devices: Explanation of terminology. Radiology 2009;253:26-30.

11. Kanal E, Borgstede JP, Barkovich AJ. American College of Radiology white paper on MR safety. American Journal of Roentgenology 2002;178:1335-1347.

12. Kohn LT, Corrigan JM, Donaldson MS, Editors. To Err is Human: Building a Safer Health System. Washington, DC: National Academy Press, Institute of Medicine; 1999.

13. Riva D. Magnetic Resonance Imaging (MRI) Safety. Introduction to Public Workshop. Public Workshop, Magnetic Resonance Imaging Safety, U.S. Food and Drug Administration, White Oak Campus, Silver Spring, MD, 2011.

14. Levinson DR. Hospital incident reporting systems do not capture most patient harm. Department of Health and Human Services, Office of Inspector General, OEI-06-09-0009, 2012.

15. Chen DW. Boy, 6, dies of skull injury during MRI. New York Times. July 31, 2001:B1-B5.

16. Metrasens Ltd., www.metrasens.com.

17. Kopp Development, Inc., www.koppdevelopment.com.

18. Mednovus Inc., www.mednovus.com.

19. Ripka P, Editor. Magnetic Sensors and Magnetometers. Boston: Artech House; 2001.

20. Czipott PV, Kumar S, Wolff S, et al. Magnetic Resonance Imaging Screening Method and Apparatus. 2008; United States Patent. No. US 7,315,166 B2.

21. Keene MN. Ferromagnetic Object Detector. 2006; United States Patent. No. US 7,113,092 B2.

22. Wooliscroft MJ. Apparatus For Detecting Ferromagnetic Objects and a Protected Doorway Assembly. 2012; World Intellectual Property Organization, International Publication Number WO 2012/022971 A2.

23. Jiles DC. Introduction to Magnetism and Magnetic Materials, Second Edition. Florida: Chapman & Hall/CRC Press; 1998.

24. Heinrich A, Guttler F, Jager U, Teichgraber U. Can ferromagnetic metal detectors improve MRI safety? Proc Biomed Tech 2012;57(Suppl. 1):709.

25. James CA, Karacozoff AM, Shellock FG. Undisclosed and undetected foreign bodies during MRI screening resulting in a potentially serious outcome. Magnetic Resonance Imaging 2013;31:630-633.

26. Keene MN, Shellock FG, Karacozoff AM. Detection of ferromagnetic implants using a ferromagnetic detection system: Implications for patient screening prior to MRI. MR Safety in Practice: Now and In the Future. International Society for Magnetic Resonance in Medicine, Scientific Workshop, 2012; Lund, Sweden, 2012.

27. Karacozoff AM, Shellock FG. Armor-piercing bullet: 3-Tesla MRI findings and identification by a ferromagnetic detection system. Military Medicine 2013;178:e380- e385.

28. Shellock FG, Karacozoff AM. Detection of implants and other objects using a ferromagnetic detection system: implications for patient screening prior to MRI. American Journal of Roentgenology 2013;201:720-725.

Chapter 14   Patient Monitoring in the MRI Environment

NANDA DEEPA THIMMAPPA, M.D.

Fellow, Body MRI
Department of Radiology
Weill Cornell Medical College
New York, NY

FRANK G. SHELLOCK, PH.D.

Adjunct Clinical Professor of Radiology and Medicine
Keck School of Medicine, University of Southern California

Adjunct Professor of Clinical Physical Therapy
Division of Biokinesiology and Physical Therapy
School of Dentistry, University of Southern California

Director for MRI Studies of Biomimetic MicroElectronic Systems
National Science Foundation, Engineering Research Center
University of Southern California

Institute for Magnetic Resonance Safety, Education, and Research
President, Shellock R & D Services, Inc.
Los Angeles, CA

INTRODUCTION

Conventional physiological monitoring equipment and accessories were not designed to operate in the harsh magnetic resonance imaging (MRI) environment where static, gradient, and radiofrequency (RF) electromagnetic fields can adversely affect or alter the operation of these devices (1). Fortunately, various monitors and other patient support devices have been developed or specially modified to perform properly during MRI procedures (1-32). Thus, commercially available MR Conditional monitors and other devices (some of which are MR Safe) are readily available and can be used routinely for patients in the MRI environment (1-32).

MRI healthcare professionals must carefully consider the ethical and medicolegal ramifications of providing proper patient care that includes identifying patients who require monitoring in the MRI setting and following a proper protocol to ensure their safety by using appropriate equipment, devices, and accessories (1, 33-43). The early detection and treatment of complications that may occur in high-risk, critically ill, or sedated patients undergoing MRI can prevent relatively minor problems from becoming life-threatening situations.

This chapter provides information, recommendations, and guidelines for patient monitoring in the MRI environment. In addition, techniques, equipment, and devices that may be used to monitor and support patients undergoing MRI examinations are described herein.

RECOMMENDATIONS AND GUIDELINES FOR PATIENT MONITORING

General Policies and Procedures

In general, monitoring during an MRI examination is indicated whenever a patient requires observations of vital physiologic parameters due to an underlying health problem or whenever a patient is unable to respond or alert the MRI technologist or another healthcare worker regarding pain, respiratory problem, cardiac distress, or other difficulty that might arise during the examination (1-3). In addition, a patient should be monitored if there is a greater potential for a change in physiologic status during the MRI procedure (1-3). Besides patient monitoring, various support devices and accessories may be needed for use in the high-risk patient to ensure safety (1-32).

With the advent of advanced MRI applications such as MRI-guided interventional or intraoperative procedures, there is an increased need to monitor patients, especially since these patients are typically anesthetized for the procedures. Additionally, patients (or volunteer subjects) undergoing MRI examinations using experimental MR systems, experimental MRI accessories (e.g., transmit radiofrequency coils), or experimental pulse sequences should be monitored continuously to ensure their safety due to potential risks that may be encountered.

Because of the widespread use of MRI contrast agents and the potential for adverse effects or idiosyncratic reactions to occur, it is prudent to have appropriate monitoring equipment and accessories readily available for the proper management and support of patients who may experience deleterious side-effects (1-3). This is emphasized because adverse events, while extremely rare, may be serious or fatal.

In 1992, the Safety Committee of the Society for Magnetic Resonance Imaging published guidelines and recommendations concerning the monitoring of patients during MRI procedures (2). The information indicated that all patients undergoing MRI should, at the very least, be visually (e.g., using a camera system) and/or verbally (e.g., intercom system) monitored, and that patients who are sedated, anesthetized, or are unable to communicate should be physiologically monitored and supported by the appropriate means (2).

Severe injuries and fatalities have occurred in association with MRI that could have been prevented with the proper use of monitoring equipment and devices (1, 3). Notably,

Table 1. Patients who may require physiological monitoring and support during MRI procedures.

• Patients that are physically or mentally unstable.
• Patients that have compromised physiologic functions.
• Patients that are unable to communicate.
• Neonatal and pediatric patients.
• Sedated or anesthetized patients.
• Patients undergoing MRI-guided interventional/intraoperative procedures.
• Patients undergoing MRI procedures using experimental MR systems.
• Patients undergoing MRI procedures using experimental techniques.
• Patients that may have a reaction to an MRI contrast agent.
• Critically ill or high-risk patients.

recommendations issued by the Joint Commission state that MRI facilities should proactively plan for managing critically ill patients who require physiologic monitoring and continuous use of life-sustaining drugs while in the MRI suite (33).

The American Society of Anesthesiology (ASA) issued a Practice Advisory on anesthetic care for MRI, which considers several aspects of patient monitoring important for safe patient management (34). These include routine monitoring, anesthetic care, airway management, and management of emergencies. In order to achieve safe monitoring conditions, the Practice Advisory suggests the use of appropriate equipment (e.g., MR Conditional monitors and other devices) and compliance with ASA standards (34). The American College of Radiology's (ACR) guidance document on MRI safe practices also provides guidelines that are applicable to physiological monitoring (35).

Other organizations similarly recommend the need to monitor certain patients using proper equipment and techniques in the MRI setting (36-38). **Table 1** summarizes the types of patients who may require physiological monitoring and support during MRI procedures (1).

Selection of Parameters to Monitor

The proper selection of the specific physiologic parameter(s) that should be monitored during MRI is crucial for patient safety. Various factors must be considered including the patient's medical history, present condition, the use of medication and possible side-effects, as well as the aspects of the MRI procedure to be performed (1-3, 34-38). For example, if the patient is to receive a sedative, it is generally necessary to monitor respiratory rate, apnea, and/or oxygen saturation (34-38). If the patient requires general anesthesia during MRI, monitoring multiple physiologic parameters is required (1, 3, 34-38).

Policies and procedures for the management of the patient in the MRI environment with respect to monitoring should be comparable to those used in the operating room or critical care setting, especially with respect to monitoring and support requirements. Specific recommendations for physiologic monitoring of patients during MRI procedures should be developed in consideration of "standard of care" issues as well as in consultation with anesthesiologists, critical care specialists, and other similar healthcare professionals (1, 3, 11, 28, 29, 34-40).

Personnel Involved in Patient Monitoring

Only healthcare professionals with appropriate training and experience should be permitted to be responsible for monitoring patients during MRI (1, 3, 28, 29, 34-40). This includes several facets of training and experience. The healthcare professional must be well acquainted with the operation of the monitoring equipment and accessories used in the MRI environment and should be able to recognize equipment malfunctions, device problems, and recording artifacts. Furthermore, the person responsible for monitoring the patient should be well versed in screening patients for conditions that may complicate the procedure. For example, patients with asthma, congestive heart failure, obesity, obstructive sleep apnea, and other underlying health conditions are at increased risk for having problems during sedation (29). Also, this healthcare professional must be able to identify and manage adverse events using appropriate equipment and procedures in the MRI environment (1, 3, 11, 28, 29, 34-40).

If a sedated patient suddenly exhibits a rapid decline in oxygen saturation during MRI, the healthcare professional should be able to recognize this problem, assess the patient for potential causes, and rapidly determine if intervention is necessary. At the very minimum, the individual should be capable of recognizing and responding quickly to contact an emergency team in the event that an adverse event is experienced by the patient.

Additionally, there must be policies and procedures implemented to continue appropriate physiologic monitoring of the patient by trained personnel after the MRI procedure is performed. This is especially needed for a patient recovering from the effects of a sedative or general anesthesia.

The monitoring of physiologic parameters and management of the patient during MRI may be the responsibility of one or more individuals depending on the level of training for the healthcare worker and in consideration of the condition, medical history, and procedure that is to be performed on the patient. These individuals include anesthesiologists, nurse anesthetists, and registered nurses (34-40).

Emergency Plan

The development, implementation, and regular practice of an emergency plan that addresses and defines the activities, use of equipment, and other pertinent issues pertaining to a medical emergency are important for patient safety in the MRI environment (1, 3, 29, 35-38). For example, a plan needs to be developed for removing the patient from the MR system room to perform cardiopulmonary resuscitation in the event of a cardiac or respiratory arrest. Obviously, taking vital equipment such as a cardiac defibrillator, intubation instruments, or other similar devices near the MR system could pose a substantial hazard to patients and healthcare professionals since these items tend to be unsafe for use in the MRI environment. Appropriately-trained healthcare professionals that are in charge of the emergency or code blue team, maintaining the patient's airway, administering drugs, recording events, and conducting other emergency-related duties must be identified, trained, and continuously practiced in the performance of these critical activities in the MRI setting.

Attempting to manage an emergency in the MR system room is considered unsafe (1, 3, 28, 29, 34-38). This is primarily because unacceptable equipment may be brought into the room by first responders unaware of the dangers associated with the MRI environment. Therefore, for emergencies, it is important that there is a policy to immediately remove the patient from the MR system room and to transfer the patient to a suitable location where patient management may be safely conducted with appropriate equipment and devices readily available (1, 3, 28, 29, 34-38).

For out-patient or mobile MRI facilities, it is usually necessary to have an advanced agreement with outside emergency personnel and an acute care hospital willing to take care of their patients. Typically, MRI facilities not affiliated with or in close proximity to a hospital must contact paramedics to handle medical emergencies and to transport patients to the hospital for additional care. Therefore, personnel responsible for summoning the paramedics, notifying the hospital, and performing other integral activities must be designated beforehand to avoid problems and confusion during an actual emergency event.

TECHNIQUES AND EQUIPMENT FOR PATIENT MONITORING AND SUPPORT

Physiologic monitoring and support of patients is not a trivial task in the MRI environment. A variety of potential problems and hazards exist. Furthermore, the types of equipment used for patient monitoring and support must be considered carefully and implemented properly to ensure the safety of both patients and MRI healthcare professionals.

During the early days of MRI, MR Conditional monitoring equipment did not exist. Therefore, it was a common practice to modify conventional physiologic monitoring equipment in order for it to be used on patients undergoing MRI (2-21, 28). Over the years, monitoring equipment was specially designed to be acceptable for use in the MRI setting (i.e., labeled MR Conditional) and there are now many commercially available devices that may be used to monitor patients during MRI which include stand-alone individual monitors (e.g.,

Table 2. List of manufacturers and suppliers of physiological monitors and support devices for use in the MRI environment.

Company	Products
Draeger Medical, Inc. (www.draeger.com)	ventilators
Invivo Corporation (www.invivocorp.com)	monitors, patient support equipment
Magmedix, Inc. (www.magmedix.com)	monitors, patient support equipment
Maquet, Inc. (www.maquet.com)	ventilators
Medrad, Inc. (www.Medrad.com)	monitors, patient support equipment
MRIEquip (www.mriequip.com)	monitors, patient support equipment
MRI Med (www.mrimed.com)	patient support equipment
Nonin Medical, Inc. (www.nonin.com)	pulse oximeter
Schiller (www.schillerservice.com)	monitors, patient support equipment
Smiths Medical (www.smiths-medical.com)	ventilators

used to record heart rate, blood pressure, oxygen saturation, temperature, etc.) as well as more sophisticated, multi-parameter systems that are similar to those found in the operating room or critical care setting (**Table 2**).

Potential Problems and Hazards

Several potential problems and hazards are associated with the performance of patient monitoring and support in the MRI environment. Conventional or even MR Conditional physiologic monitors and other accessories that contain ferromagnetic components (e.g., transformers, power supplies, batteries, etc.) may be strongly attracted by the static magnetic field of the MR system, posing a serious missile or projectile hazard to patients and MRI healthcare professionals. Notably, several incidents and one fatality occurred as a result of bringing MR Unsafe gas cylinders into the MR system room (1, 3, 41-44). The MR system may sustain substantial damage as a result of being struck by a large ferromagnetic object and further expense is incurred if it is necessary to quench a superconducting magnet associated with a scanner in order to remove the object (43).

If possible, MR Conditional devices that have specific gauss-level ratings as part of the specified conditions of use (e.g., a device that is labeled to state that it must not be used in a gauss level above 300-gauss) such as monitoring equipment, gas anesthesia machines, and ventilators because of the presence of ferromagnetic materials or operational components that may be damaged by exposure to higher magnetic fields should be permanently fixed to the floor or otherwise "tethered" to prevent them from becoming projectiles. Furthermore, these devices must have prominent warning labels to inform MRI healthcare professionals that they should not move this equipment too close to the MR system. Importantly, all personnel involved with the MRI procedures should be trained and made aware of the importance of the placement and use of the equipment in the MR system room, especially with regard to the hazards of moving portable devices too close to the scanner.

Radiofrequency (RF) fields from the MR system can significantly effect the operation of conventional monitoring equipment, especially those with displays that involve electron beams (i.e., cathode ray tube, CRT) or video display screens (with the exception of those that use a liquid crystal display, LCD). In addition, the monitoring equipment itself may emit spurious noise that, in turn, produces distortion or artifacts on the MR images (**Figure 1**).

Physiologic monitors that contain microprocessors or other similar components may "leak" RF, producing electromagnetic interference that can substantially alter MR images (1, 3). To prevent adverse radiofrequency-related interactions with physiologic monitors, RF-shielded cables, RF filters, special outer RF-shielded enclosures, or fiber-optic techniques can be utilized to prevent image-related or other problems in the MRI environment (1, 3, 28).

During the operation of the MR system, electrical currents may be generated in the conductive materials of monitoring equipment that are used as the interface to the patient (e.g., cables, leads, probes, etc.). These currents may be of sufficient magnitude to cause excessive heating and thermal injury to the patient (1-3, 41, 46-60). The primary bioeffect associated with the RF radiation used during MRI is related to the thermogenic qualities of this elec-

Figure 1. T1-weighted, MR image of a fluid-filled phantom showing substantial artifacts related to electromagnetic interference associated with the operation of a monitor in the MR system room.

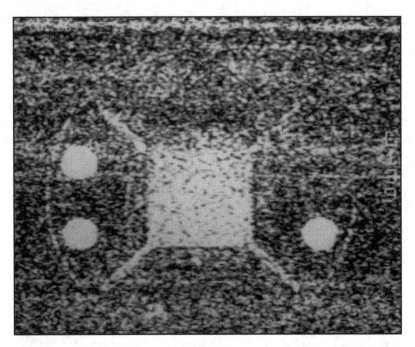

tromagnetic field (1). Numerous burns have occurred in association with MRI procedures that were directly attributed to the use of monitoring devices (1, 3, 46-60). These thermal injuries have been related to the use of electrocardiographic (ECG) leads, ECG electrodes, plethysmographic gating systems, pulse oximeters, intracranial pressure monitoring catheters, and other types of monitoring equipment comprised of wires, cables, and catheters with thermistors or similar components made from conductive materials (1, 3, 46-60). Patient burns related to the use of monitoring equipment and other devices in the MRI environment are a frequent problem that may be avoided by following recommendations indicated in **Table 3**.

Monitoring Equipment and Support Devices

This section describes the physiologic parameters that may be assessed in patients during MRI procedures using MR Conditional monitoring equipment. In addition, various devices and accessories that are useful for the support and management of patients in the MRI setting are presented.

Electrocardiogram and Heart Rate

Monitoring the patient's electrocardiogram (ECG) in the MR system room is particularly challenging because of the inherent distortion of the ECG waveform that occurs (1, 3, 11, 18, 19, 22, 27, 28). This effect is observed as blood, a conductive fluid, flows through the large vascular structures in the presence of the static magnetic field of the MR system

Table 3. Recommendations to prevent excessive heating and possible burns in association with MRI procedures.

- Prepare the patient for the MRI procedure by ensuring that there are no unnecessary metallic objects contacting the patient's skin (e.g., metallic drug delivery patches, jewelry, necklaces, bracelets, key chains, etc.).

- Prepare the patient for the MRI procedure by using insulation material (i.e., appropriate padding) to prevent skin-to-skin contact points and the formation of "closed-loops" from touching body parts.

- Insulating material (minimum recommended thickness, 1-cm) should be placed between the patient's skin and transmit RF coil that is used for the MRI procedure (alternatively, the RF coil itself should be padded). For example, position the patient so that there is no direct contact between the patient's skin and the transmit RF body coil of the MR system. This may be accomplished by having the patient place his/her arms over his/her head or by using elbow pads or foam padding between the patient's tissue and the body RF coil of the MR system. This is especially important for those MRI examinations that use the body coil or other large RF coils for transmission of RF energy.

- Use only electrically conductive devices, equipment, accessories (e.g., ECG leads, electrodes, etc.), and materials that have been thoroughly tested and determined to be MR Safe and/or MR Conditional for MRI procedures.

- Carefully follow specific MRI safety criteria and recommendations for implants made from electrically conductive materials (e.g., bone fusion stimulators, neurostimulation systems, etc.).

- Before using electrical equipment, check the integrity of the insulation and/or housing of all components including surface RF coils, monitoring leads, cables, and wires. Preventive maintenance should be practiced routinely for such equipment.

- Remove all non-essential electrically conductive materials from the MR system (i.e., unused surface RF coils, ECG leads, cables, wires, etc.).

- Keep electrically conductive materials that must remain in the MR system from directly contacting the patient by placing thermal and/or electrical insulation between the conductive material and the patient.

- Keep electrically conductive materials that must remain within the transmit RF body coil or other transmit RF coil of the MR system from forming conductive loops. Note: The patient's tissue is conductive and, therefore, may be involved in the formation of a conductive loop, which can be circular, U-shaped, or S-shaped.

- Position electrically conductive materials to prevent "cross points". For example, a cross point is the point where a cable crosses another cable, where a cable loops across itself, or where a cable touches either the patient or sides of the transmit RF coil more than once. Notably, even the close proximity of conductive materials with each other should be avoided because some cables and RF coils can capacitively couple (without any contact or crossover) when placed close together.

- Position electrically conductive materials to exit down the center of the MR system (i.e., not along the side of the MR system or close to the body RF coil or other transmit RF coil).

Table 3. (Continued)

- Do not position electrically conductive materials across an external metallic prosthesis (e.g., external fixation device, cervical fixation device, etc.) or similar device that is in direct contact with the patient.

- Allow only properly trained individuals to operate devices (e.g., monitoring equipment) in the MRI environment.

- Follow all manufacturer instructions for the proper operation and maintenance of physiologic monitoring or other similar electronic equipment intended for use during MRI procedures.

- Electrical devices that do not appear to be operating properly during the MRI procedure should be removed from the patient immediately.

- Closely monitor the patient during the MRI procedure. If the patient reports sensations of heating or other unusual sensation, discontinue the MRI procedure immediately and perform a thorough assessment of the situation.

- RF surface coil decoupling failures can cause localized RF power deposition levels to reach excessive levels. The MR system operator will recognize such a failure as a set of concentric semicircles in the tissue on the associated MR image or as an unusual amount of image non-uniformity related to the position of the RF coil.

(38). The resulting induced biopotential is seen primarily as an augmented T-wave amplitude, although other non-specific waveform-changes are also apparent on the ECG (1, 3, 61-63). Since altered T-waves or ST segments may be associated with cardiac disorders, static magnetic field-induced ECG-distortions can be problematic. For this reason, it may be necessary to obtain a baseline recording of the ECG prior to placing the patient inside of the MR system and compare it to a recording obtained immediately after the MRI procedure in order to determine the cardiac status of the patient (1, 3).

Additional artifacts caused by the static, gradient, and RF electromagnetic fields can severely distort the ECG, making observation of morphologic changes and detection of arrhythmias quite difficult (**Figure 2**). To minimize some of these artifacts, a variety of filtering techniques, including active and passive techniques, may be used.

Active techniques involve the use of low pass filters or the electronic suppression of noise that decrease the artifacts from the gradient and RF electromagnetic fields, while maintaining the intrinsic qualities of the ECG. Passive techniques include the use of special cable and lead preparation methods along with the proper placement of leads that will minimize the artifacts seen on the ECG in the MRI environment (1, 3).

ECG artifacts that occur in the MRI environment may also be decreased substantially by implementing several simple techniques that include, the following (1-3): (a) using ECG electrodes that have minimal metal; (b) selecting electrodes and cables that contain no ferromagnetic metals; (c) placing the limb electrodes in close proximity to one another; (d) positioning the line between the limb electrodes and leg electrodes parallel to the magnetic field flux lines; (e) maintaining a small area between the limb and leg electrodes; (f) placing

Figure 2. Electrocardiogram recorded in a patient in the MR system room: (Top panel) Five-feet from a 1.5-Tesla magnet (MR system); (Middle panel) At isocenter; and (Bottom panel) Inside the MR system during MRI. Note the augmented T-wave resulting from the induced flow potential as well as the other nonspecific changes caused by the static magnetic field of the MR system. During MRI, Onset of Gating, there is severe distortion of the electrocardiographic waveform.

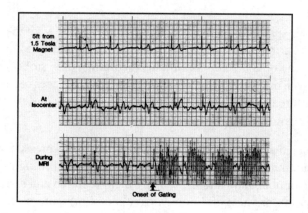

the anatomic area of the electrodes near or in the center of the MR system; and (g) twisting or braiding the ECG cables.

The use of proper ECG electrodes is strongly recommended to ensure patient safety and proper recording of the electrocardiogram in the MRI environment (22). Accordingly, this means that only the ECG electrodes recommended or otherwise approved by the manufacturer of the ECG recording equipment should be used in order to protect the patient from potentially hazardous conditions. Similarly, the ECG leads and cables should also be those recommended by the manufacturer and deemed acceptable for use in the MR system room.

As previously indicated, it is well known that the use of standard ECG electrodes, leads, and cables may cause heating that results in patient burns at the electrode sites or where the leads and cables are in contact with the patient's tissues. Additionally, MR Conditional, ECG monitoring equipment has been responsible for patient burns in association with MRI as the result of improper uses of the devices.

Various techniques have been developed to prevent excessive heating related to the use of ECG recording equipment in the MRI environment, including using fiber-optic technology and/or wireless methods to record the ECG. For example, the use of the fiber-optic technique combined with a wireless method to monitor the ECG during MRI eliminates the potential for burns associated with hard-wired ECG systems by removing the conductive patient leads and cable and the "antenna effects" that are typically responsible for excessive heating during MRI. Accordingly, most modern-day, MR Conditional ECG monitors employ these technological solutions to ensure patient safety.

Heart rate may be monitored in the MR system room using a few different methods. Besides using the ECG monitor to record heart rate in patients undergoing MRI, this physiologic parameter may be determined continuously using MR Conditional devices such as the photoplethysmograph found with a pulse oximeter or a noninvasive, heart rate/blood pressure monitor (see section below) that can also be utilized to obtain intermittent or semicontinuous recordings of heart rate during MRI procedures (see section below) (1, 3, 11).

Blood Pressure

MR Conditional, sphygmomanometers are commercially available to measure blood pressure in patients during MRI. MR Conditional blood pressure monitors that use the oscillometric method can obtain semi-continuous recordings of systolic, diastolic, and mean blood pressures as well as pulse rate in patients. Thus, these devices can be utilized to record systemic blood pressure in adult, pediatric, and neonatal patients by selecting the appropriate size for the blood pressure cuff.

It should be noted that the intermittent inflation of the blood pressure cuff from a manual or an automated, noninvasive blood pressure device may disturb lightly-sedated patients, especially pediatric or neonatal patients, causing them to move and disrupt the MRI examination. For this reason, the use of a noninvasive blood pressure monitor may not be the best instrument to perform physiologic monitoring in every type of patient.

Intravascular, Intracardiac, and Intracranial Pressures

Direct monitoring of intravascular, intracardiac, or intracranial pressures may be performed in patients during MRI using specially designed, fiber-optic pressure transducers or nonferromagnetic, micromanometer-tipped catheters. However, this type of monitoring is not commonly performed in this setting (1, 6, 9). These monitoring devices are unaffected by the electromagnetic fields used for MRI and are capable of invasively recording pressures that are comparable to those obtained using conventional recording equipment (6, 9, 11, 46, 47).

Monitoring intracranial pressure (ICP) is essential in the management of severe head injuries. Unfortunately, most ICP monitoring devices are unacceptable for use during MRI and may cause patient injuries, as reported by Tanaka, et al. (1, 45).

Respiratory Rate and Apnea

Because respiratory depression and upper airway obstruction are frequent complications associated with the use of sedatives and anesthetics, monitoring techniques that detect a decrease in respiratory rate, hypoxemia, or airway obstruction should be used during the administration of these drugs (1, 3, 29, 34, 36-38). This is particularly important in the MRI environment because visual observation of the patient's respiratory efforts is often difficult, especially when the patient is entirely inside the bore of an MR system.

Respiratory rate monitoring can be performed during MRI procedures by various techniques. The impedance method that utilizes chest leads and electrodes (similar to those used to record the ECG) can be used to record respiratory rate. This method of recording respiratory rate measures a difference in electrical impedance induced between the leads that correspond to changes in respiratory movements. Unfortunately, the electrical impedance method of assessing respiratory rate may be inaccurate in pediatric patients because of the small volumes and associated motions of the relatively small thorax area.

Respiratory rate may also be monitored during MRI procedures using a rubber bellows placed around the patient's thorax or abdomen (i.e., for "chest" or "belly" breathers) (1, 3, 11). The bellows device is attached to a remote pressure transducer that records changes in body movements associated with inspiration and expiration. However, the bellows monitoring technique, like the electrical impedance method, is only capable of recording body movements associated with respiratory efforts. Therefore, these techniques of monitoring respiratory rate do not detect apneic episodes related to upper airway obstruction (i.e., absent airflow despite respiratory effort) and, thus, may not provide sufficient sensitivity for assessing patients during MRI examinations. For this reason, assessment of respiratory rate and detection of apnea should be accomplished using other, more appropriate monitoring methods.

Respiratory rate and apnea may be monitored during MRI using an MR Conditional, end-tidal carbon dioxide monitor or a capnometer. These devices measure the level of carbon dioxide during the end of the respiratory cycle (i.e., end-tidal carbon dioxide), when carbon dioxide is at its maximum level. Additionally, capnometers can provide quantitative data with respect to end-tidal carbon dioxide that is important for determining certain aspects of gas exchange in patients. The waveform provided on end-tidal carbon dioxide monitors is also useful for assessing whether the patient is having difficulties breathing. Importantly, the interface between the patient for the end-tidal carbon dioxide monitor and capnometer is a nasal or oro-nasal cannula that is made out of plastic and, thus, it is MR Safe. Obviously, this type of interface prevents any potential adverse interaction between the monitor and the patient during an MRI procedure.

Oxygen Saturation

Oxygen saturation is a critical variable to measure in high-risk, sedated or anesthetized patients, especially in the MRI setting (1, 3, 11, 14, 24, 29, 34-40). This physiologic parameter is measured using pulse oximetry, a technique that assesses the oxygenation of tissue, which may be accomplished using an MR Conditional pulse oximeter. Because oxygen-saturated blood absorbs differing quantities of light compared with unsaturated blood, the amount of light that is absorbed by the blood can be readily used to calculate the ratio of oxygenated hemoglobin to total hemoglobin and displayed as the oxygen saturation. Additionally, the patient's heart rate may be calculated using a pulse oximeter by measuring the frequency that pulsations occur as the blood moves through the vascular bed. Thus, the pulse oximeter determines oxygen saturation and pulse rate on a continuous basis by measuring the transmission of light through a vascular measuring site such as the ear lobe, fingertip, or toe. Importantly, the use of pulse oximetry is considered by anesthesiologists as the standard practice for monitoring sedated or anesthetized patients (34, 36, 37).

Conventional pulse oximeters typically have hard-wire cables which are of great concern and have been responsible for causing burns in patients in the MRI setting (1, 3, 24, 48, 53). Fortunately, pulse oximeters have been developed that use fiber-optic technology to obtain and transmit the physiologic signals from the patient (1, 3, 24). It is physically

Figure 3. Example of MR Conditional pulse oximeter used to record oxygen saturation and heart rate (Nonin Medical, Inc.).

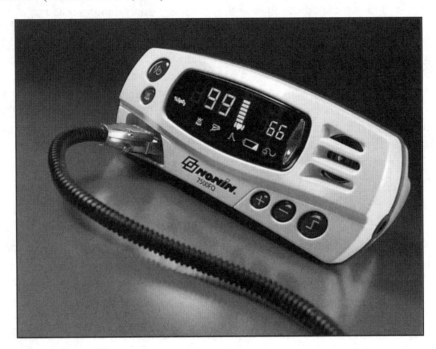

Figure 4. Example of MR Conditional pulse oximeter used to record oxygen saturation and heart rate (Invivo Corporation).

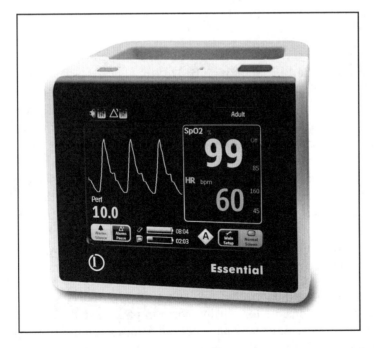

impossible for a patient to be burned by a fiber-optic pulse oximeter during an MRI procedure because there are no conductive pathways formed by metallic materials connecting to the patient. These commercially available, MR Conditional devices operate without interference from the electromagnetic fields used during MRI. **Figure 3** and **Figure 4** show examples of MR Conditional pulse oximeters that can be used to record oxygen saturation and heart rate.

Temperature

In human subjects, "deep" body or core temperature is regulated between 36°C and 38°C by the hypothalamus and continuously fluctuates due to diurnal, internal, and external factors (64). Importantly, the regulation of body temperature is suppressed by anesthesia and generally results in the patients becoming hypothermic (65, 66). Health conditions related to a decrease in body temperature can range from hypovolemia, myocardial ischemia, cardiac arrhythmia, pulmonary edema, and decreased cerebral blood flow in cases of mild hypothermia, to mortality related to extreme hypothermia (67). In the MRI setting, besides monitoring body temperature in anesthetized patients it is also important to record temperatures in neonates because they have inherent problems retaining body heat, a tendency that is augmented during sedation and anesthesia. Accordingly, body temperature is an important parameter to record in various patients undergoing MRI.

With further regard to patients who are anesthetized during MRI, some patients may experience malignant hyperthermia, which is a rare life-threatening condition that may be triggered by exposure to certain drugs used for general anesthesia. In susceptible individuals, these drugs can induce a drastic and uncontrolled increase in skeletal muscle oxidative metabolism, which overwhelms the body's capacity to supply oxygen, remove carbon dioxide, and regulate body temperature. Malignant hyperthermia can eventually lead to circulatory collapse and death if not quickly identified and treated.

As previously indicated, the anesthesiologist or nurse anesthetist may not be able to clearly visualize or have close access to the patient during the MRI procedure due to the design of the MR system. Therefore, it is imperative to continuously monitor body temperature in certain patients, obtaining real-time information for the anesthesia provider. Notably, it is also important that the measurement site has clinical relevance and a relatively "fast" response time to any fluctuation in body temperature because the anesthesiologist or nurse anesthetist is unable to visualize the discoloration of the patient's skin in cases of sudden temperature changes.

The accuracy and efficacy of the measurement of body temperature has been a topic of discussion for many years (64, 68-70). Temperature measurements in human subjects are affected by many factors, including (64, 70, 71): (a) the site of measurement (e.g., skin, oral, esophagus, rectal, pulmonary artery, hypothalamus, bladder, tympanic membrane, axillary area); (b) environmental conditions (i.e., temperature and humidity); and (c) the measurement technique (e.g., mercury thermometer, electronic thermometer, thermistor probe or catheter, thermocouple-based probe, infrared radiation readers, fiber optic method).

The most accurate deep body temperature is measured at the hypothalamus, but this site is not accessible by any practical means. Therefore, a "deep" body site that directly reflects the temperature "sensed" by the hypothalamus will provide clinically relevant information (14). For example, sites that provide high levels of accuracy and correlation to deep body temperature are pulmonary artery blood, urinary bladder, the esophagus, and rectum (18, 19, 22). However, the temporal resolution for each site varies, which can dramatically impact the ability to recognize clinically important changes that may require prompt patient management (64, 68).

When monitoring temperature during MRI, the decision on which body site to use should be based on accuracy as well as accessibility. There may be limitations on the type of equipment available for temperature measurements in the MR system room. For example, hard wire thermistor or thermocouple-based sensors are prone to measurement errors due to electromagnetic interference (EMI) and can introduce artifacts in the MR images (1-3). Fiber-optic sensors (i.e., fluoroptic thermometry) are optimally used to record temperatures in the MRI environment because they are safe and unaffected by EMI (3).

In the MRI setting, anesthesiologists, nurse anesthetists, and clinicians may feel that they are limited to measure "surface" temperatures, such as the temperatures of the skin, axilla, or groin. However, these temperature measurement sites are very problematic insofar as they do not properly reflect "deep" body temperature. Another option is to use minimally invasive measurement techniques to record the temperature in the rectum or esophagus.

While a so-called "surface" temperature site (i.e., skin, axilla, and groin) tends to be used for temperature recordings during MRI mainly because of the ease of obtaining the measurement with currently available equipment, this method does not provide an accurate representation of body temperature and is susceptible to substantial variations and erroneous information relative to the core or "deep" body temperature due to the specific site selected for temperature probe placement, patient movement, and environmental conditions (64, 69, 70).

Notably, the level of the patient's perspiration due to RF-induced heating and the use of blankets or air circulation from the fan in the bore of the MR system can influence the recording of skin or surface temperature during MRI. Additionally, investigations have demonstrated that peripheral vasoconstriction resulting from skin surface cooling decreases the surface temperature measurement without influencing the deep body temperature (64). By comparison, deep body temperature measurements require additional set up time and somewhat invasive, but provide a more accurate representation of the body temperature (64).

Two of the most prevalent core temperature measurement sites used during MRI procedures are the rectum and esophagus. Rectal temperature measurements are highly accurate and within 0.6°C of deep body temperature (64). The main drawback to this temperature measurement site is associated with a lag or delay in the temporal response to a changing body temperature due to the presence of thermal inertia from the intervening tissues (i.e., between the rectum and hypothalamus). This temporal delay may also be caused by the presence of feces and poor blood supply in the rectum (64, 65). A clinical investigation reported that the rectal temperature substantially lagged in response to changes in body temperature (74). This lack of proper temporal resolution can expose the patient to a hypothermic or hyperthermic condition for an extended period without being recognized

Figure 5. Examples of MR Conditional, multi-parameter physiologic monitoring systems. **(A)** Multi-parameter monitor set up in a 3-Tesla MR system room.

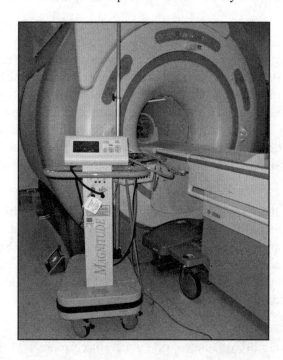

Figure 5. (B) Multi-parameter monitor set up in a 1.5-Tesla MR system room. Note the additional monitor placed in the control room that communicates directly with the monitoring equipment in the scanner room.

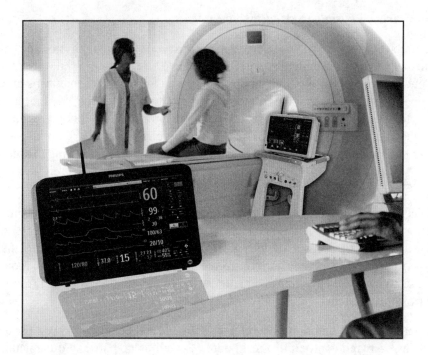

by the clinician. Also, special care must be taken when placing a rectal temperature probe in a neonatal or pediatric patient in order to prevent perforation or infection (64, 65).

Measurement of esophageal temperature provides a high level of accuracy and good temporal correlation to core body temperature due to the close proximity to the aorta, a deep body site (64, 70). In addition to this accuracy, the temperature recorded in the esophagus is responsive to fluctuations in body temperature and readily tracks changes compared to rectal or surface temperature measurement sites (64, 65). The only caveat is that the accuracy of measuring temperature in the esophagus is directly linked to the proper positioning of the probe (64, 69). Airflow in the trachea can impact the measured temperature if the probe is not inserted deep enough into the esophagus. The recommended placement of the sensor is in the lower one-third of the esophagus for an accurate core temperature measurement (64).

In consideration of the available temperature measurement sites that may be monitored during MRI, especially with regard to which site provides the most accurate information along with the best temporal resolution, the temperature of the esophagus is considered to be site of the most acceptable and clinically relevant information. Furthermore, esophageal temperature is insensitive to ambient air circulation and has the added benefit of fast response time to temperature fluctuations in the body compared to the measurement of temperature in the rectum.

The current availability of fiber-optic temperature probes and recording equipment properly designed for use in the MRI setting permits the monitoring of body temperature in the esophagus, which provides physiologic information that is vital to patient care. Temperature monitoring capabilities are typically found in association with multi-parameter physiologic monitoring equipment.

Multi-Parameter, Physiologic Monitoring Systems

In certain cases, it may be necessary to monitor several different physiologic parameters simultaneously in patients undergoing MRI (1, 3, 11, 29, 32, 36-40). While several different stand-alone units may be used to accomplish this task, the most efficient means of recording multiple parameters is by utilizing a monitoring system that permits the measurement of different physiologic functions such as heart rate, respiratory rate, blood pressure, oxygen saturation, and temperature (**Figure 5**). Currently, there are several MR Conditional, multi-parameter patient monitoring systems available for use in the MRI setting (**Table 2**).

Ventilators

Devices used for mechanical ventilation of patients typically contain mechanical switches, microprocessors, and ferromagnetic components that may be adversely affected by the electromagnetic fields used during MRI (1, 3, 8, 11, 15, 75). Ventilators that are activated by high-pressure oxygen and controlled by the use of fluidics (i.e., no requirements for electricity) may still have ferromagnetic parts that can malfunction as a result of interference from MR systems.

Fortunately, MR Conditional ventilators have been specially designed for use in the MR system room and can be utilized in adult as well as pediatric and neonatal patients

Figure 6. Example of MR Conditional ventilator system (SERVO-i, Maquet Inc., Wayne, NJ). This system includes the ventilator, mobile cart, and battery packs.

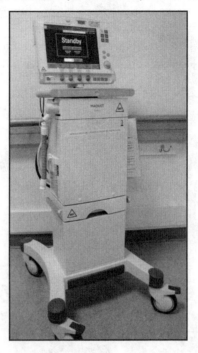

Figure 7. Example of MR Conditional ventilator system. This equipment includes a magnetic field strength alarm system (arrow) (GaussAlert, Kopp Development Inc., Jensen Beach, FL) that is designed to help keep MR Conditional equipment outside of a particular MRI exclusion zone (e.g., 300-gauss).

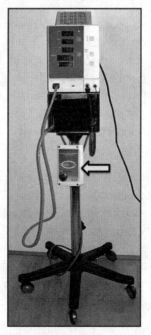

Figure 8. Example of MR Conditional gas anesthesia machine and related accessories.

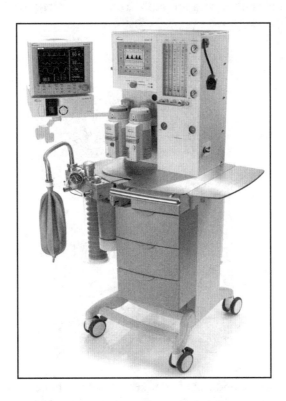

(**Table 2**). These devices are constructed from nonferromagnetic materials and have undergone pre-clinical evaluations to ensure that they operate properly in the MRI environment, without producing artifacts on MR images (**Figure 6** and **Figure 7**).

Importantly, many MR Conditional ventilators classified as MR Conditional have specific fringe field requirements (e.g., the device may not be used in a field greater than 300-gauss) due to the presence of ferromagnetic parts or functional aspects that may be compromised in association with static magnetic fields. Therefore, as always, to prevent accidents and incidents, it is vital for all healthcare professionals working in the MRI environment to have an understanding of the issues related to the use of all potentially dangerous equipment, particularly if ferromagnetic objects, such as ventilators, are unknowingly brought into the MR system room.

If the ventilator must be maintained at a designated gauss level relative to the MR system, this area should be clearly demarcated on the floor of the scanner room and all healthcare personnel must be educated regarding the importance of maintaining the device at or behind this marked area. One way to ensure this would be to attach a tether or restraint strap to the ventilator that provides a mechanism that could "catch" in order to prevent encroachment of the device to an unsafe area. The tether system should only be used to prevent disaster and not relied on as the primary restraint mechanism.

Alternatively, the device called the GaussAlert (Kopp Development Inc., Jensen Beach, FL) can be utilized to maintain an MR Conditional ventilator (or other similar equipment such as infusion pumps, contrast injectors, patient monitors, gas anesthesia machines, etc.) outside of a particular MRI exclusion zone (**Figure 7**). This magnetic field strength alarm system was specifically designed for this task and produces an audio alert when a preset magnetic field strength is exceeded.

Additional Devices and Accessories

A variety of devices and accessories are often necessary for support and management of patients in the MRI environment. MR Safe or MR Conditional gurneys, oxygen tanks, stethoscopes, suction devices, infusion pumps, power injectors, gas anesthesia systems, and other similar devices and accessories are commercially available and may be obtained from various manufacturers and distributors (**Figure 8**) (**Table 2**).

CONCLUSIONS

The care and management of high-risk, critically ill, or sedated/anesthetized patients undergoing MRI procedures presents special challenges. These challenges are related to requirements for MR Safe and MR Conditional equipment and devices as well as the need for MRI facilities to implement proper policies and procedures. Policies, procedures, recommendations, and guidelines have been developed and are available from well-established professional organizations and other resources.

REFERENCES

1.   Shellock FG. Reference Manual for Magnetic Resonance Safety: 2013 Edition. Los Angeles: Biomedical Research Publishing Group; 2013.

2.   Kanal E, Shellock FG. Policies, guidelines, and recommendations for MR imaging safety and patient management. Patient monitoring during MR examinations, J Magn Reson Imaging 1992;2:247-8.

3.   Shellock FG. Chapter 4. Magnetic Resonance Imaging: Safety and Bioeffects. In: Open MRI. Philadelphia: Lippincott Williams and Wilkins;1998. pp. 23-38.

4.   Barnett GH, Roper AHD, Johnson AK. Physiological support and monitoring of critically ill patients during magnetic resonance imaging. J Neurosurg 1988;68:246.

5.   Boutros A, Pavlicek W. Anesthesia for magnetic resonance imaging. Anesth Analg 1987;66:367.

6.   Dell'Italia LJ, Carter B, Millar H, Pohost GM. Development of a micromanometer-tip catheter to record high-fidelity pressures during cine-gated NMR without significant image distortion. Magn Reson Med 1991;17:119-25.

7.   Fisher DM, Litt W, Cote CJ. Use of oximetry during MR imaging of pediatric patients. Radiology 1991;178:891-892.

8.   Dunn V, Coffman CE, McGowan JE, Ehrardt JC. Mechanical ventilation during magnetic resonance imaging. Magn Reson Imaging 1985;3:169-72.

9.   Roos CF, Carrol FE. Fiber-optic pressure transducer for use near MR magnetic fields. Radiology 1985;156:548.

10. Geiger RS, Cascorbi HF. Anesthesia in an NMR scanner. Anesth Analg 1984;63:622-3.

11. Holshouser B, Hinshaw DB, Shellock FG. Sedation, anesthesia, and physiologic monitoring during MRI. J Magn Reson Imaging 1993;3:553-558.

12. Hubbard A, Markowitz R, Kimmel B, Kroger M, Bartko M. Sedation for pediatric patients undergoing CT and MRI. Journal of Computer Assisted Tomography 1992;16:3-6.

13. Karlik S, Heatherley T, Pavan F, et al. Patient anesthesia and monitoring at a 1.5 T MRI installation. Magn Reson Med 1988;7:210-21.

14. McArdle C, Nicholas D, Richardson C, Amparo E. Monitoring of the neonate undergoing MR imaging: Technical considerations. Radiology 1986;159:223-6.

15. McGowan JE, Erenberg A. Mechanical ventilation of the neonate during magnetic resonance imaging. Magn Reson Imaging 1989;7:145-8.

16. Mirvis SE, Borg U, Belzberg H. MR imaging of ventilator-dependent patients: preliminary experience. Am J Roentgenol 1987;149:845-6.

17. Rejger VS, Cohn BF, Vielvoye GJ, De-Raadt FB. A simple anesthetic and monitoring system for magnetic resonance imaging. European Journal of Anesthesiology 1989;6:373-8.

18. Rokey RR, Wendt RE, Johnston DL. Monitoring of acutely ill patients during nuclear magnetic resonance imaging: use of a time-varying filter electrocardiographic gating device to reduce gradient artifacts. Magn Reson Med 1988;6:240-5.

19. Roth JL, Nugent M, Gray JE, et al. Patient monitoring during magnetic resonance imaging. Anesthesiology 1985;62:80-3.

20. Selden H, De Chateau P, Ekman G, et al. Circulatory monitoring of children during anesthesia in low-field magnetic resonance imaging. Acta Anesthesiol 1990;34:41-3.

21. Shellock FG. Monitoring during MRI. An evaluation of the effect of high-field MRI on various patient monitors. Med Electron 1986;17:93-7.

22. Shellock FG. MRI and ECG electrodes. Signals 1999;29:10-14.

23. Shellock FG. Monitoring sedated patients during MRI (letter). Radiology 1990;177:586.

24. Shellock FG, Myers SM, Kimble K. Monitoring heart rate and oxygen saturation during MRI with a fiber-optic pulse oximeter. Am J Roentgenology 1991;158:663-4.

25. Smith DS, Askey P, Young ML, Kressel HY. Anesthetic management of acutely ill patients during magnetic resonance imaging. Anesthesiology 1986;65:710-1.

26. Taber K, Layman H. Temperature monitoring during MR imaging: Comparison of fluoroptic and standard thermistors. J Magn Reson Imaging 1992;2:99.

27. Wendt RE, Rokey R, Vick GW, Johnston DL. Electrocardiographic gating and monitoring in NMR imaging. Magn Reson Imaging 1988;6:89.

28. Kanal E, Shellock FG. Patient monitoring during clinical MR imaging. Radiology 1992;185:623-9.

29. Reinking Rothschild, D. Chapter 5. Sedation for Open Magnetic Resonance Imaging. In: Rothschild PA, Rothschild DR, Editors. Open MRI. Philadelphia: Lippincott, Williams and Wilkins; 2000. pp. 39-53.

30. Tobin JR, Spurrier EA, Wetzel RC. Anaesthesia for critically ill children during magnetic resonance imaging. Br J Anaesth 1992;69:482-6.

31. Szelenyi A, Gasser T, Seifert V. Intraoperative neurophysiological monitoring in an open low-field magnetic resonance imaging system: clinical experience and technical considerations. Neurosurgery 2008;63(4 Suppl 2):268-75.

32. Menon DK, Peden CJ, Hall AS, Sargentoni J, et al. Magnetic resonance for the anesthetist, Part II: anesthesia and monitoring in MR units. Anesthesia 1992;47:508-17.

33. The Joint Commission. Sentinel Event Alert. Preventing accidents and injuries in the MRI suite. Issue 38, 2008.

34. Practice advisory on anesthetic care for magnetic resonance imaging: a report by the Society of Anesthesiologists Task Force on Anesthetic Care for Magnetic Resonance Imaging. Anesthesiology 2009;110:459-79.

35. Kanal E, Barkovich AJ, Bell C, et al. ACR guidance document on MR safe practices: 2013. J Magn Reson Imaging 2013;37:501-30.

36. Guidelines for monitoring and management of pediatric patients during and after sedation for diagnostic and therapeutic procedures: An update. Pediatrics 2006;118:2587-2602.

37. Special article. practice guidelines for sedation and analgesia by non-anesthesiologists. An updated report by the American Society of Anesthesiologists Task Force on Sedation and Analgesia by Non-Anesthesiologists. Anesthesiology 2002;96:1004–17.

38. American College of Radiology (ACR), Society of Interventional Radiology (SIR) Practice Guideline for Sedation/Analgesia. [online publication]. American College of Radiology (ACR), 2010.

39. Menon DK, Peden CJ, Hall AS, et al. Magnetic resonance for the anesthetist, Part II: anesthesia and monitoring in MR units. Anesthesia 1992;47:508-17.

40. Rotello LC, Radin EJ, Jastremski MS, Craner D, Milewski A. MRI protocol for critically ill patients. Am J Crit Care 1994;3:187-90.

41. Shellock FG, Crues, JV. MR procedures: biologic effects, safety, and patient care. Radiology 2004;232:635-52.

42. Chaljub G, Kramer LA, Johnson RF III, Singh H, Crow WN. Projectile cylinder accidents resulting from the presence of ferromagnetic nitrous oxide or oxygen tanks in the MR suite. AJR Am J Roentgenol 2001;177:27–30.

43. Colletti PM: Size "H" oxygen cylinder: Accidental MR projectile at 1.5 Tesla. J Magn Reson Imaging 2004;19:141–3.

44. ECRI hazard report: Patient death illustrates the importance of adhering to safety precautions in magnetic resonance environments. Health Devices 2001;30:311–4.

45. Tanaka R, Yumoto T, Shiba N, et al. Overheated and melted intracranial pressure transducer as cause of thermal brain injury during magnetic resonance imaging. J Neurosurg 2012;117:1100-9.

46. Newcombe VF, Hawkes RC, Harding SG, et al. Potential heating caused by intraparenchymal intracranial pressure transducers in a 3-Tesla magnetic resonance imaging system using a body radiofrequency resonator: assessment of the Codman MicroSensor Transducer. J Neurosurg 2008;109:159-64.

47. Shellock FG, Slimp G. Severe burn of the finger caused by using a pulse oximeter during MRI. Am J Roentgenology 1989;153:1105.

48. ECRI. A new MRI complication? Health Devices Alert 1988;1.

49. ECRI. Thermal injuries and patient monitoring during MRI studies. Health Devices Alert 1991;20:362-3.

50. Kanal E, Shellock FG. Burns associated with clinical MR examinations. Radiology 1990;175:585.

51. Keens SJ, Laurence AS. Burns caused by ECG monitoring during MRI imaging. Anesthesiology 1996;51:1188-9.

52. Brown TR, Goldstein B, Little J. Severe burns resulting from magnetic resonance imaging with cardiopulmonary monitoring. Risks and relevant safety precautions. Am J Phys Med Rehabil 1993;72:166-7.

53. Bashein G, Syrory G. Burns associated with pulse oximetry during magnetic resonance imaging. Anesthesiology 1991;75:382-3.

54. Haik J, Daniel S, Tessone A, Orenstein A, Winkler E. MRI induced fourth-degree burn in an extremity, leading to amputation. Burns 2009;35:294-6.

55. Hall SC, Stevenson GW, Suresh S. Burn associated with temperature monitoring during magnetic resonance imaging. Anesthesiology 1992;76:152.

56. Hardy PT, Weil KM. A review of thermal MR injuries. Radiol Technol 2010;81:606-9.

57. Jones S, Jaffe W, Alvi R. Burns associated with electrocardiographic monitoring during magnetic resonance imaging. Burns 1996;22:420-421.

58. Karoo RO, Whitaker IS, Garrido A, Sharpe DT. Full-thickness burns following magnetic resonance imaging: a discussion of the dangers and safety suggestions. Plast Reconstr Surg 2004;114:1344-1345.

59. Lange S, Nguyen QN. Cables and electrodes can burn patients during MRI. Nursing 2006;36:18.

60. Ruschulte H, Piepenbrock S, Munte S, Lotz J. Severe burns during magnetic resonance examination. Eur J Anaesthesiol 2005;22:319-320.

61. Teneforde TS, Gaffey CT, Moyer BR, Budinger TF. Cardiovascular alterations in Maccaca monkeys exposed to stationary magnetic fields. Experimental observations and theoretical analysis. Bioelectromagnetics 1983;4:1-9.

62. Dimick RN, Hedlund LW, Herfkens RF, et al. Optimizing electrocardiographic electrode placement for cardiac-gated magnetic resonance imaging. Invest Radiol 1987;22:17-22.

63. Damji AA, Snyder RE, Ellinger DC, et al. RF interference suppression in a cardiac synchronization system operating in a high magnetic field NMR imaging system. Magn Reson Imaging 1988;6:637-640.

64. Knies RC. Temperature Measurement in Acute Care: The Who, What, Where, When, Why, and How? Available at: http://enw.org/Research-Thermometry.htm

65. Michiaki Y. Anesthesia and body temperature: Temperature regulation under general anesthesia combined with epidural anesthesia. Journal of Clinical Anesthesia 2000;24:1416-1424.

66. Takashi M; Anesthesia and body temperature: general anesthesia and thermoregulation. Journal of Clinical Anesthesia 2000; 24:1408-1415.

67. Schubert A. Side effects of mild hypothermia. Journal or Neurological Anesthesiology 1995;7:139-147.

68. Lilly JK, Boland JP, Zekan S. Urinary bladder temperature monitoring: A new index of body core temperatures. Critical Care Medicine 1980;8:742-744.

69. Lefrant J Y, Muller L, et al. Temperature measurement in intensive care patients: comparison of urinary bladder, esophageal, rectal, axillary, and inguinal methods versus pulmonary artery core method. Intensive Care Med 2003;29:414-418.

70. Robinson J, Charlton J, Seal R, et al. Esophageal, rectal, axillary, tympanic, and pulmonary artery temperatures during cardiac surgery. Canadian Journal of Anesthesiology 1998;45:317-323.

71. Takashi A. Anesthesia and body temperature: Interoperative monitoring of body temperature and its significance. Journal of Clinical Anesthesia, 2000;24:1432-1443.

72. Gooden CK. Anesthesia for magnetic resonance imaging. Curr Opin Anaesthesiol. 2004;17:339-42.

73. Wilson TE, Sauder CL, Kearney ML, et al. Skin surface cooling elicits peripheral and visceral vasoconstriction in humans. Journal of Applied Physiology 2007;103:1257-1262.

74. Newsham KR, Saunders JE, Nordin ES. Comparison of rectal and tympanic thermometry: Discussion. Southern Medical Journal 2002; 95, 804-8

75. Greenberg KL, Weinreb J, Shellock FG. "MR conditional" respiratory ventilator system incident in a 3-T MRI environment. Magn Reson Imaging 2011;29:1150-4.

Chapter 15   Performing Sedation and Anesthesia During MRI

Debra Reinking, M.D.

Anesthesiologist
Aptos, CA

INTRODUCTION

While magnetic resonance imaging (MRI) has become the diagnostic test of choice for a variety of conditions, there are certain patients who are unable or unwilling to undergo MRI without the aid of sedation or anesthesia. Performing sedation and anesthesia in the MRI suite presents challenges that are not found in the operating room or anywhere else in the hospital or clinic setting (1). Therefore, the purpose of this chapter is to familiarize radiologists, MRI technologists, imaging nurses, and other healthcare professionals concerning the issues that are involved with administering sedation and anesthesia in the MRI environment. Importantly, it must be understood that sedation and anesthesia are part of the same continuum (2). Accordingly, when the term sedation is used, the patient may actually be anesthetized and the associated risks applied.

PATIENTS WHO REQUIRE SEDATION OR ANESTHESIA DURING MRI

Performance of an MRI examination generally requires that the patient remains motionless for each pulse sequence and the common use of multiple sequences for the MRI examination poses problems for certain individuals. Children under the age of seven years are often unable to remain motionless. However, infants under twelve-months may sometimes be scanned without sedation, especially if sleep-deprived and the scan is scheduled at a normal naptime. Patients with severe low back pain or pain from a malignancy may be unable to remain still. Back pain may be positional and the supine position can worsen the pain and elicit muscle spasms, further hindering the patient's ability to remain motionless.

A substantial segment of the population experiences extreme anxiety or claustrophobia. Others patients develop severe medical test anxiety when attempting to undergo an MRI examination. While non-pharmaceutical techniques presented in another chapter in this textbook may help manage these patients in the MRI setting, certain individuals will require sedation to complete the scan.

Patients with movement disorders such as Parkinson's disease or other uncontrollable tremors may be unable to lie motionless during MRI. Patients with torticollis may not be able to be positioned correctly or may not be able to maintain the necessary position for completion of the scan. The use of sedation or general anesthesia may be the only way to obtain a diagnostic study in the patients described above.

Patients Undergoing Intraoperative or Interventional MRI

With the advent of intraoperative and interventional MRI, patients usually require a general anesthetic for the surgical or treatment procedure. Administering anesthesia or moving an anesthetized patient into the MR system during the middle of a surgery or an intervention adds another level of complexity to what is already a complicated procedure. Designing the MRI suite to ensure safety for such advanced applications and performing anesthesia in this setting is discussed in another chapter in this textbook.

LEVELS OF SEDATION AND ANESTHESIA – A CONTINUUM

As previously stated, it must be recognized that sedation and anesthesia are part of the same continuum. Nonetheless, the terms "moderate sedation", "deep sedation" and "general anesthesia" are commonly used and their definitions should be understood. The "Continuum of Depth of Sedation: Definition of General Anesthesia and Levels of Sedation/Analgesia," from the American Society of Anesthesiologists (ASA) describes the levels, as follows (2):

Minimal Sedation/Anxiolysis is a drug-induced state during which patients respond normally to verbal commands. Although cognitive function and physical coordination may be impaired, airway reflexes, ventilatory and cardiovascular functions are unaffected.

Moderate Sedation/Analgesia (Conscious Sedation) is a drug-induced depression of consciousness during which patients respond purposefully* to verbal commands, either alone or accompanied by light tactile stimulation. No interventions are required to maintain a patent airway, and spontaneous ventilation is adequate. Cardiovascular function is usually maintained. (*Reflex withdrawal from a painful stimulus is not considered a purposeful response.)

Deep Sedation/Analgesia is a drug-induced depression of consciousness during which patients cannot be easily aroused but respond purposefully* following repeated or painful stimulation. The ability to independently maintain ventilatory function may be impaired. Patients may require assistance in maintaining a patent airway and spontaneous ventilation may be inadequate. Cardiovascular function is usually maintained. (*Reflex withdrawal from a painful stimulus is not considered a purposeful response.)

General Anesthesia is a drug-induced loss of consciousness during which patients are not arousable, even by painful stimulation. The ability to independently maintain ventilatory function is often impaired. Patients often require assistance in maintaining a patent airway and positive pressure ventilation may be required because of depressed spontaneous ventilation or drug-induced depression of neuromuscular function. Cardiovascular function may be impaired.

This document continues with the following statement (2): "Because sedation is a continuum, it is not always possible to predict how an individual patient will respond. Hence, practitioners intending to produce a given level of sedation should be able to rescue patients whose level of sedation becomes deeper than initially intended. Individuals administering Moderate Sedation/Analgesia ("Conscious Sedation") should be able to rescue patients who enter a state of Deep Sedation/Analgesia, while those administering Deep Sedation/Analgesia should be able to rescue patients who enter a state of General Anesthesia."

For an example of the continuum of sedation and anesthesia, one needs to look no further than the post-anesthesia recovery room where it is a common to see a patient complaining of post-surgical pain. When the nurse leaves the bedside to obtain pain medication (i.e., stimulation from the nurse stops), the patient often drifts into a deeper level of sedation or anesthesia, sometimes developing airway obstruction or apnea. If this respiratory problem is immediately recognized, it can usually be handled easily with vocal stimulation or by shaking the patient's shoulder. However, left unrecognized, this same scenario can cascade into prolonged respiratory arrest, hypoxemia, cardiac arrest and death. Due to the potential complications of sedation and to aid the practitioner in delivering safe sedation, standards and guidelines have been developed.

SEDATION STANDARDS, GUIDELINES, AND PRACTICE ADVISORIES

Standards and Guidelines to Improve Patient Safety During Sedation

While the American Society of Anesthesiologists (ASA) has the best known sets of standards for sedation (3), the American Academy of Pediatrics (AAP) (4), the American College of Radiology (ACR) and Society for Interventional Radiology (SIR) (5), the Department of Health and Human Services, Centers for Medicare and Medicaid (6), and the American College of Emergency Physicians (ACEP) (7) have also released standards or guidelines that apply to sedation and anesthesia.

2009 Practice Advisory on Anesthetic Care for Magnetic Resonance Imaging

In 2009, the ASA published the "Practice Advisory on Anesthetic Care for Magnetic Resonance Imaging. A Report by the American Society of Anesthesiologists Task Force on Anesthetic Care for Magnetic Resonance Imaging"(1). This Practice Advisory, acknowledging the unique physical challenges present in the MRI environment, stresses that the following components be present in an MRI facility in which anesthesia or interventional MRI will be carried out: (a) Education of anesthesia care providers and communication with the radiology team. (b) Screening of anesthesia care providers. (c) Patient screening for high-risk medical conditions, implanted devices or ferromagnetic material, imbedded foreign bodies. (d) Preparation of the MRI environment for anesthesia and a plan for each specific patient. (e) Patient management during MRI. (f) Emergency management plan. (g) Planning for post-procedure care of the patient. The content of this chapter addresses the components indicated above that specifically relate to performing sedation and anesthesia in the MRI environment.

PATIENT PREPARATION FOR SEDATION OR ANESTHESIA DURING MRI

Patient Preparation – Nil Per Os (NPO) Interval

A nil per os (NPO) interval is necessary to minimize the possibility of regurgitation with resultant laryngospasm or aspiration. NPO policies typically require that the patient fast for a minimum of two to four hours for clear liquids; four hours for breast milk; six hours for formula or a light meal and eight hours for a regular meal (3, 8). In advance of the planned sedation, instructions that emphasize the fasting period should be provided to the patient or parents. These instructions should also include the requirement for a driver to accompany the sedated patient after the procedure. **Table 1** presents an example of sedation instructions for a pediatric patient.

History and Physical - Screening for Conditions That May Impact Sedation or Anesthesia

Patient screening can detect conditions that may complicate sedation or anesthesia. A general health history should be taken, including medical conditions, allergies, medications, use of alcohol or other drugs, past surgical procedures, reactions to previous sedation or anesthesia, as well as the indication for current MRI examination. The NPO status should be verified and the person administering sedation or anesthesia should confirm with the MRI technologist that the patient has been screened for contraindications to MRI (1, 3). Some conditions that may affect sedation or anesthesia include high-risk medical conditions, including neonatal status or prematurity; patients with impaired respiratory or cardiovascular status; or patients who require equipment such as invasive monitors, or who are intubated (1). The ASA Physical Status is frequently used to document patient status (**Table 2**).

Screening of the Patient's Airway

Respiratory depression and airway obstruction are thought to be primary causes of morbidity associated with sedation (3). Airway abnormalities can both increase the likelihood of airway obstruction and can make it more difficult to deliver positive pressure ventilation, which may be needed if respiratory compromise occurs (3).

Obstructive Sleep Apnea (OSA)

Patients with OSA have periodic, partial or complete obstruction of the upper airway during sleep and are known to be particularly sensitive to the respiratory depressant and airway effects of sedatives, opioids, and other drugs. These patients are also prone to developing airway obstruction during sedation and anesthesia, making it important to screen for this disorder (9).

Focused Physical Examination

The head, neck, and mouth should be examined. Clues of potential airway problems include congenital anomalies, macroglossia, micrognathia and tonsillar hypertrophy, which are associated with an increased risk of airway obstruction during sedation (10,11). In adults,

Table 1. An example of sedation instructions for a pediatric patient. (Adapted from Reinking Rothschild, Sedation for Open Magnetic Resonance Imaging. In: Rothschild, P and Rothschild D, Editors. Open MRI. Philadelphia; Lippincott Williams and Wilkins. 2000. pp. 42-43.)

Sample Sedation Instructions - Child

Your doctor has referred your child for an MRI examination. This requires that the patient lie completely still for the duration of the exam, which may take up to 45 minutes. Many children between the ages of nine months and six years are unable to lie still and require sedation or anesthesia. Children younger than nine months usually do not require sedation and will sleep throughout the exam, provided that they are adequately sleep deprived.

Some parents prefer that their children do not receive sedative drugs. We have successfully scanned many pediatric patients with sleep deprivation alone. The parents keep the child awake until he/she is so tired that he/she simply falls asleep for the duration of the exam.

1. If your child does need sedation, it is important that he or she has an empty stomach. Generally, this means six hours without solid food or non-human milk, and at least two hours without water. The anesthesiologist will give you an exact time to stop oral intake, after taking into consideration the patient's age, weight, and exact time of day of the MRI exam.

2. Dress the child in comfortable cotton clothes. Make sure there are no zippers, snaps, or other metal objects on the clothing that could interfere with the MRI exam. Avoid t-shirts with decals, as decals have metal particles that can cause artifacts in the MR image. Your child may be required to change into a hospital gown.

3. Bring extra diapers, and juice or formula, and a snack for your child after the exam.

4. **Sleep deprivation** is helpful. Arriving at the MRI center with a sleepy child will allow the exam to be completed with a minimum of drugs. Do not let the child take his or her afternoon nap on the day before the exam. Keep the child up at least two hours past his or her usual bedtime the night before the exam, and wake him/her up an hour early on the morning of the exam. DO NOT LET THE child take a nap on the day of the procedure or fall asleep on the drive to the MRI center.

Arrive at_____ AM/PM on_____

Table 2. American Society of Anesthesiologists (ASA) Physical Status (PS) Classification System.

ASA PS 1 - A normal healthy patient
ASA PS 2 - A patient with mild systemic disease
ASA PS 3 - A patient with severe systemic disease
ASA PS 4 - A patient with severe systemic disease that is a constant threat to life
ASA PS 5 - A moribund patient who is not expected to survive without the operation
ASA PS 6 - A declared brain-dead patient whose organs are being removed for donor purposes

(Reprinted with permission of the American Society of Anesthesiologists, www.ASAhq.org.)

a large neck circumference, inability to open the mouth at least 3-cm, or a receding chin are signs of potential airway difficulties (3).

The lungs should be auscultated. The presence of rhonchi, rales, or wheezing should be noted. Auscultation of the heart for rate, rhythm, and presence of murmurs or other abnormal heart sounds should be performed.

PREPARATION OF THE MRI ENVIRONMENT FOR SEDATION OR ANESTHESIA

Whenever sedative or anesthetic drugs are used, it is imperative to monitor the patient and to have appropriate equipment and personnel immediately available to diagnose and treat complications that are reasonably anticipated to occur (12). Early recognition and treatment of complications can prevent transient problems from becoming life-threatening events. A person must be present to monitor the patient (3, 4) and monitoring should be consistent with the institution's protocol for performing physiological monitoring of similarly sedated patients elsewhere in the facility and in consideration of the available MR safe or MR conditional equipment.

In advance of the administration of sedation or anesthesia, the anesthesiologist must assure that equipment used in the MR system room (i.e., Zone IV, according to the American College of Radiology, ACR) is MR Safe or MR Conditional and work closely with members of the radiology team to determine the ideal placement of monitors or equipment for use in the MR system room (1). The presence of the electromagnetic fields used for MRI adds variables to the sedation or anesthesia plan that are not present elsewhere in the hospital. For example, the ferromagnetic attraction of the magnet can turn routine equipment into projectiles; patients have suffered burns from electrocardiogram wires and pulse oximeter cables; the static magnetic field can cause distortion of electrocardiogram tracings; and electronic monitors may introduce artifacts into the MR images (13-19).

In response to these problems, anesthesia machines and monitoring equipment have been developed specifically for the MRI environment by several companies and this information is presented in another chapter in this textbook. Ideally, equipment should be tested prior to use, with the specific MR system with which it will be used. No matter which equipment is selected, close collaboration between the anesthesiologist, nurse, biomedical engineer, MR system manufacturer, device manufacturer, MRI suite designer, radiologists, and MRI technologists is critical. The nurse or physician administering sedation or anesthesia must understand the "MR Safe" and "MR Conditional" terminology and seek answers from the radiologist or MRI technologist if there is any uncertainty regarding use or placement of devices (13). **Table 3** shows examples of emergency equipment, patient support devices, and drugs used for sedation procedures that may be used in an MRI facility performing sedation or anesthesia. All equipment for use in the MR system room (i.e., Zone IV) should be MR Safe or MR Conditional and labeled, accordingly.

Monitoring During Sedation or Anesthesia While Undergoing MRI

Patients undergoing moderate sedation, deep sedation, or anesthesia should undergo the following monitoring and preparation (1, 3): (a) Visual. This is often difficult because of the patient's position in the bore of the MR system, therefore, the provider should seek the best line-of-sight available; (b) Level of consciousness; (c) Ventilatory status, observation is difficult and generally supplemented with capnography; (d) Oxygenation status, via pulse oximetry (not a substitute for monitoring ventilation); (e) Hemodynamics via blood pressure (BP) recordings, usually every five minutes; (f) Electrocardiogram (EKG) monitoring, if feasible; (g) A healthcare professional who can recognize the complications of sedation and establish a patent airway should be present; (h) Care must be taken in positioning leads and monitoring equipment patient interfaces to avoid burns (1).

Importantly, guidelines from the ASA state that once sedation-anesthesia is established, blood pressure should be monitored every five minutes, "unless such monitoring interferes with the procedure (e.g., pediatric MRI, where stimulation from the blood pressure cuff could arouse an appropriately sedated patient)" (3). The Practice Advisory acknowledges that advisories may be "adopted, modified, or rejected according to clinical needs and constraints" (1).

Additionally, the following equipment and supplies must be present:

(a) Supplemental oxygen and a means to artificially ventilate the patient; (b) Suction equipment and appropriately-sized suction catheters; (c) Emergency resuscitative equipment such as laryngoscopes, endotracheal tubes, and a defibrillator (with pediatric capabilities if children are sedated.) All equipment must be available for the entire range of age and size of patients undergoing sedation or anesthesia.

PLANNING FOR SEDATION OR ANESTHESIA

MRI Requirements

The person administering the sedation or anesthesia must be cognizant of any procedure-specific requirements. Clear communications between the anesthesiologist, MRI technologist, referring physician and radiologist are important. The MRI technologist must inform the person administering the sedation or anesthesia of the anticipated duration of the MRI examination, the planned patient positioning, or any special or unusual circumstances regarding the scan. If breath-hold sequences or neck flexion will be needed, this must be known in advance because a controlled airway may be required. If positioning other

Table 3. Examples of emergency equipment, patient support devices, and drugs used for sedation procedures that may be used in an MRI facility performing sedation or anesthesia. All equipment for use in the MR system room (i.e., Zone IV) should be MR Safe or MR Conditional and labeled, accordingly. (Adapted from Reinking Rothschild, Sedation for Open Magnetic Resonance Imaging. In: Rothschild, P and Rothschild D, Editors. Open MRI. Philadelphia; Lippincott Williams and Wilkins. 2000. pp. 42-43.)

Equipment and Patient Support Devices

- Oxygen, wall oxygen is ideal. If cylinders must be used in the MR system room, they must be aluminum, and have MR Conditional regulators.
- Stethoscope, with minimum or no metallic parts, MR Safe or MR Conditional if feasible.
- MR Conditional gurney ; Should be large enough for the patients undergoing sedation
- Patient transfer board to facilitate moving patient from gurney to the MR system table.
- Blood pressure cuffs in sizes for all the different-sized patients who will be treated.
- Non-invasive blood pressure monitor.
- MR Conditional pulse oximeter with probes, pediatric probes if pediatric patients sedated.
- MR Conditional capnograph.
- Self inflating bags with oxygen tubing; masks in assorted sizes for the entire range of patient sizes that will be treated.
- I.V. solutions, tubing sets, microdrip tubing for pediatric use. I.V. catheters in assorted sizes 18-G, 20-G for adult use, 22-G, 24-G for pediatric use.
- Tourniquet, alcohol swabs, assorted syringes, needles, sharps containers.
- Oral airways and nasal airways in assorted adult and pediatric sizes
- Laryngeal Mask Airways (LMAs) sizes 5, 4, 3, 2 ½, 2, 1 ½, 1
- MR Conditional endotracheal tubes 7.5, 7.0, 6.5 for adult use; 6.0, 5.5, 5.0, 4.5, 4.0, 3.5, 3.0 for pediatric use. Note: LMAs and ETTs should be available in sizes appropriate for all patients sedated at the facility.
- MR Conditional suction.
- Suction catheters: rigid Yankauer catheters, as well as flexible suction catheters in various sizes for all sizes of patients who will be treated.
- MR Conditional laryngoscope handles, assorted blades, in pediatric sizes if those patients are treated. MR Conditional batteries.
- Defibrillator; Should have pediatric capabilities if pediatric patients are sedated. Must only be used outside of the MR system room
- MR Conditional electrocardiogram with accessories.

---

than supine is needed, the MRI technologist must make the sedation or anesthesia provider aware so that he or she can ensure a patent airway. The sedation or anesthetic plan cannot be formulated until all pertinent and specific radiology requirements are known.

Sedation Versus General Anesthesia

The decision whether to choose sedation versus general anesthesia will depend upon a variety of factors, including: the availability of anesthesia or sedation personnel and equipment; throughput requirements; patient factors including airway abnormalities, medical conditions; motion disorders; patient preference as well as the duration of the examination;

Table 3. Continued

Drugs
• Lubricant jelly (for use with nasal airways)
• Epinephrine 1:1,000 and 1:10,000
• Ephedrine
• Phenylephrine
• Lidocaine
• Aminophylline
• Dextrose
• Sodium bicarbonate
• Calcium chloride
• Nitroglycerin tablets
• Anticholinergics: Atropine, Glycopyrrolate.
• Diphenhydramine
• Flumazenil
• Naloxone

(Banyan Stat Kits contain emergency medications and devices such as masks, airways, endotracheal tubes and laryngoscopes in a portable, hard-sided suitcase-like container. Replacement medications and devices are available by dose or individually. For more information, visit http://www.statkit.com or call 1-888-STAT-KIT.)

the necessity of breath-hold sequences; and whether the exam is only diagnostic or part of an interventional MRI procedure.

Advantages of general anesthesia for MRI include: a quick, reliable onset and offset, which allows a busy MRI facility to maintain efficient throughput; a motionless patient; and the ability to secure the airway. Disadvantages include the necessity for anesthesia personnel and MR Safe and MR Conditional equipment including anesthesia machines, infusion pumps and monitoring equipment, as well as the inconvenience of managing such large equipment within the confines of the MRI setting, especially the MR system room.

GENERAL ANESTHESIA DURING MRI

If general anesthesia is chosen for MRI, any technique that is appropriate for the patient may be selected. Some institutions use general anesthesia for all or nearly all of their patients who are unable to complete their MRI examinations, especially children. Popular techniques for pediatric patients include an inhalational (i.e., "breathe-down") induction with sevoflurane, followed by intravenous (I.V.) line insertion. Maintenance may involve insertion of a laryngeal mask airway (LMA), allowing the patient to spontaneously breath a sevoflurane mixture, or use of an intravenous propofol infusion, while the patient spontaneously breathes with oxygen via nasal cannula or "blow by". Popular techniques for adults include intravenous induction with propofol followed by either of the two maintenance techniques listed above. Airway manipulation and intubation may need to be performed outside of the MR system room (i.e., Zone III) depending upon availability of MR Safe or MR Conditional airway manipulation equipment (1).

Since the MRI is painless (except for the possibly high auditory stimulation), it may be possible to use light levels of anesthesia, allowing the patient to awaken promptly. However, light levels may lead to patient motion, motion artifact and repeated sequences, and also render the patient more likely to experience laryngospasm (1). Because it is difficult to access a patient after he has been placed inside the MR system, the anesthesiologist may choose to control the airway, either with a laryngeal mask airway (LMA) or with an endotracheal tube (ETT) prior to placing the patient into the bore of the MR system (1). If an MR Conditional anesthesia machine is not available, inhalational anesthesia may be administered with the anesthesia machine located outside of the MR system room via an elongated breathing circuit passed through the waveguide. Similarly, if an MR Conditional infusion pump is unavailable, the pump can be located outside of the MR system room with elongated tubing passed through the waveguide (1).

SEDATION DURING MRI

Various techniques have been described for sedation during MRI. In this section, the individual who performs the monitoring, sedation teams and training, sedation adjuncts, and typical medications used for sedation will be discussed.

A Qualified Individual Must Monitor the Sedated Patient

The ASA Practice Guidelines for Sedation and Analgesia by Non-Anesthesiologists (3) and the ACR-SIR Guideline (5) both stress that a qualified individual, who is not performing the procedure, must monitor the patient under sedation. This person should understand cardiac monitoring and pulse oximetry, understand the pharmacology of medications administered, be trained in basic life support, and be credentialed by the facility. An individual with the skills to start an intravenous line and with advanced cardiac life support (ACLS) skills should be immediately available (i.e., within one to five minutes) during moderate sedation and present during deep sedation (3).

Sedation Teams and Sedation Training

Sedation teams, often under the Department of Pediatrics or the Department Anesthesia, are available at many hospitals. At some facilities, patients are screened for conditions that may complicate sedation. Patients without complicating health conditions may undergo sedation by a nurse or pediatric intensivist, while the anesthesia department may be consulted for patients who have complicated health conditions. Other sedation services are staffed and supervised by emergency medicine physicians.

The Society for Pediatric Sedation offers the "SPS Sedation Provider Course." Notably, the website, http://www.pedsedation.org, offers a wealth of information, including articles, references, educational videos and links to sample sedation regimens, sample policies as well as sedation documentation. As of the date of this writing, the syllabus from the "SPS Sedation Provider Course" is also available in its entirety on the website. The American Association of Moderate Sedation Nurses, http://www.aamsn.org, offers information about training and certification in moderate sedation for registered nurses. Articles about sedation, audio and slide presentations on airway management, and other resources are available on its website. The bookstore of http://sedationcertification.com/ offers computerized simulation training for moderate sedation, digital video discs (DVDs) on sedation, a course on capnography, as well as books on sedation and on non-pharmacologic means of sedation.

Sedation Adjuncts

While many tend to think first of medication, non-pharmacologic techniques can assist sedation. Dim lighting, calm and reassuring personnel, and quiet areas in the MRI environment can help to calm both pediatric and adult patients. Distraction, in the form of relaxing music or videos, if available, can be helpful. A special program that used Certified Child-Life specialists, a culture change within the radiology staff, MRI protocols with faster scan times, and distraction techniques including MRI video goggles, a DVD monitor, and a color light show device successfully decreased the need for pediatric sedation during MRI (20).

Sleep Deprivation

Sleep deprivation, an old and safe technique, may not be sufficient alone, but may allow lower doses of sedatives to be effective and decrease the onset time. The pediatric patient's MRI examination should be scheduled during a normal naptime. The child is kept awake two to three hours later than his normal bedtime on the night prior to the exam, and awakened one hour earlier than usual on the morning of the exam. The child should not be allowed to fall asleep in the car on the way to the MRI facility. At the facility, parents and child are placed into a darkened, quiet room to rock the child to sleep. The child is then placed onto the MR system table and secured with towels, pads and tape in order to prevent patient motion. Sleep deprivation is particularly useful for infants under the age of twelve months, the age group that is the highest risk for sedation. The success of sleep deprivation as a sole means of sedation may be influenced by the acoustic noise level generated by the MR system.

THE USE OF PHARMOCOLOGIC AGENTS FOR SEDATION

The ideal sedative drug would have a rapid, predictable onset; easy and painless administration; would be devoid of any respiratory or cardiac depression; and would cause the patient to be perfectly motionless for the exact duration of the examination and awaken completely at the conclusion of scanning. Oral, intramuscular (I.M.), intranasal, intravenous (I.V.) and rectal administration of sedation drugs have been described (21).

Considerations When Administering Sedation

The following factors should be considered when administering sedatives:

(a) *Sedation Goals May Vary From Patient to Patient.* An adult with low back pain may require primarily analgesics, while a claustrophobic patient may require only anxiolytics.

(b) *Many Sedative Drugs Are Synergistic.* When administered at the same time, many sedative drugs act synergistically, causing a much greater effect than expected from simply adding the effects of each drug. For example, narcotics are synergistic with benzodiazepines. A small dose of fentanyl plus a small dose of midazolam can cause a pronounced effect (3).

(c) *Individual Patient Response Can Vary Widely* (3).

(d) *The Route of Administration Affects Drug Absorption and Effects.* Administration of drugs via oral, rectal, or intramuscular routes can lead to erratic and or delayed drug absorption, making it difficult to predict when the drug's maximal effect will occur (21).

(e) *Sedatives Depress A Patient's Ability to Relieve Positional Airway Obstruction.* Verification of a patent airway is essential, especially after positioning of the patient. Flexion of the head and neck may lead to airway obstruction, and should be avoided if possible (21).

(f) *Sedation Should Be Administered Only Under Medical Supervision* (21).

Pharmacologic Agents

While all attempts are made to assure accuracy at the time of publication of this chapter, the practitioner should always review the package insert prior to administration of any medication.

Chloral Hydrate

Chloral hydrate has a long history of use as a sedative for pediatric patients. It is usually given orally or rectally as a 25- to 100-mg/kg dose, up to a maximum of 100-mg/kg or 2-gms, whichever is less. Chloral hydrate was popular for many years due to its ease of use, relatively lower respiratory depression than other sedatives, and relatively low incidence of complications. Disadvantages are the long and unpredictable onset time of up to 30- to 90-minutes, sedation failure rate of up to 13%, emesis from oral administration (4%), long duration of action, and concerns about toxicity and mutagenicity (21-23). As of the date of this writing, chloral hydrate has limited availability in the United States, as it was withdrawn from the market in 2012/2013 by both of its two U.S. manufacturers (24).

Barbiturates

Pentobarbital has frequently been used to sedate children, with an initial dose of 2- to 6-mg/kg intravenously (I.V.), titrated in increments, with additional doses of 1- to 3-mg/kg slowly administered up to a maximum dose of 100-mg. Advantages of I.V. pentobarbital are: the ability to titrate the drug to effect; low failure rate; rapid onset of sedative effect (one to two minutes); few patients require additional doses (4%); low, dose-dependent risk of respiratory depression; and reliability (95.5% successful sedation). Disadvantages include the necessity for intravenous access before proceeding with sedation and the prolonged duration of sedation after commonly administered doses (21,25, 26, 27). Cherry flavored oral pentobarbital, 4-mg/kg for infant sedation for radiologic procedures has also been used (26).

Propofol

Propofol (Diprivan), an intravenous sedative-hypnotic, has gained popularity for induction and maintenance of anesthesia since its U.S. introduction in the 1980s. Due to its rapid clearance, an initial bolus of propofol lasts three to five minutes, and must be followed by an infusion. The advantages of propofol are rapid onset, reliable induction of sedation or anesthesia, rapid recovery and minimal nausea and vomiting. Disadvantages are pain on injection, the need for an infusion pump, and the need for personnel who can manage an airway and provide positive pressure ventilation. Propofol can rapidly cause general anesthesia, has been associated with respiratory depression and apnea, as well as decreases in blood pressure (21). Some hospitals restrict its use to anesthesia personnel. A typical sedation dose is 1-mg/kg/min until asleep (approximately 3- to 5-mg/kg), then 50- to 150-mcg/kg/min, thereafter (21, 27, 28).

The Pediatric Sedation Research Consortium (PSRC) collected and analyzed data from 49,836 instances of propofol sedation/anesthesia. The most common complications were central apnea or airway obstruction, stridor, excessive secretions or vomiting and oxygen saturation less than 90% for more than thirty-seconds. There were no deaths and cardiopulmonary resuscitation was required twice. The authors concluded that "propofol sedation/anesthesia is unlikely to yield serious adverse outcomes …with highly motivated and organized sedation/anesthesia services," and "…safety…is dependent on a system's ability to manage less serious events" (28).

Dexmedetomidine

Dexmedetomidine is a potent alpha-2 adrenoceptor agonist with sedative, analgesic and anxiolytic effects after intravenous administration. It has been used for sedation of ventilated patients, as an adjunct to general anesthesia for surgery, and as an adjunct to post-operative analgesics. Compared to most sedatives and hypnotics, dexmedetomidine causes less respiratory depression (21). It is associated with hypotension (hypertension if loading dose is administered too rapidly) and bradycardia due to the alpha receptor effects. Dexmedetomidine should not be administered quickly as a bolus. Care should be taken when administering it to patients who are volume depleted, vasoconstricted, or have severe heart block. Dexmedetomidine can be administered intranasally, orally, submucosally, and intravenously. A typical dose when given intravenously for pediatric sedation for MRI is 0.5- to 2-mcg/kg over five to 10-minutes, followed by an infusion of 1- to 2-mcg/kg/hr (21, 29).

High dose dexmedetomidine has been used as the sole sedative for pediatric MRI with a 10-minute loading dose of 2- to 3-micrograms/kg and infusion rates of 2- mcg/kg/hr. Bradycardia (16%) and hypotension have occurred with the use of dexmedetomidine, but the deviation was not believed to be associated with adverse sequelae (30).

Midazolam

Midazolam (Versed) is a water-soluble benzodiazepine, useful for premedication and treatment of anxiety that can be administered orally, I.M., I.V. or intranasally. For pediatric premedication, a dose of 0.3- to 0.5-mg/kg orally, or 0.2-mg/kg nasally is given. Midazolam has a bitter taste and has been mixed with cola or syrup to make it more palatable. It is also available in a fruit flavored solution for oral administration. Sedation occurs within 10- to 15-minutes after nasal administration, and within 20- to 30-minutes after oral administration. Midazolam is particularly useful for brief periods of sedation due to its short duration of action (21, 31).

Local Anesthetic Cream

Local anesthetic cream containing lidocaine with or without prilocaine is helpful in diminishing pain from the placement of an intravenous line and is especially helpful to use when starting an I.V. in a pediatric patient. EMLA Cream (Astra Zeneca) (eutectic mixture of local anesthetic), containing 2.5% lidocaine and 2.5% prilocaine, and ELA-max containing 4% liposomal lidocaine are available. For optimal effect, the cream should be applied to the anticipated site and covered with an occlusive dressing 60-minutes (30-minutes for ELA-max) prior to the needle stick. Care must be taken to avoid contact of this local anesthetic cream with ocular or mucosal surfaces to prevent ocular anesthesia or ingestion (32).

Reversal Agents, Naloxone and Flumazenil

Naloxone is an opioid antagonist that should be available if narcotics are administered. For post-procedural respiratory depression in adults, 0.1-mg to 0.2-mg increments should be injected every two to three minutes and titrated to effect. Rapid reversal of opioids can result in nausea, vomiting, hypertension, tachycardia and pulmonary edema. Re-sedation is possible (3, 21, 33).

Flumazenil, a specific benzodiazepine antagonist, reverses the sedative effects within about two-minutes. The initial dose (adult) is 0.2-mgs I.V. over 15-seconds. This can be repeated at 60-second intervals up to a maximum of 1-mg (34). The half-life is shorter than that of midazolam, and re-sedation may occur (3, 21, 34).

Documentation

Pre-procedure documentation should contain a history and physical, allergies, medications, NPO documentation, informed consent and a "time-out" (i.e., a period of time to double check all important matters). The sedation record should include vital signs, oxygen saturation, respiratory function, as well as name, dosage, and time of administration of all drugs administered. A time-based anesthesia-type record is ideal.

Emergency Plans

An emergency plan should be in place addressing the specific activities and roles needed in the event of a medical emergency within the MRI facility, especially one which might occur in the MR system room (Zone IV). There must be a means to summon immediate help within the MRI department. In case of a patient cardiac arrest within the MR system room (Zone IV), while cardiopulmonary resuscitation (CPR) may be started immediately, it will be necessary for MRI personnel to immediately move the patient to a "safe location" outside of the MR system room (Zone IV) that contains a code cart, oxygen, a defibrillator and vital signs monitoring (1). Therefore, appropriate patient transfer equipment must be readily available in this setting. Furthermore, there should also be emergency plans in place to deal with environmental emergencies, including fire in the MRI suite, projectile emergencies, and a quench. Mock drills should be used to practice for each type of possible emergency event.

Post-Sedation Recovery

Once the MRI examination is completed, predetermined recovery criteria must be met before the patient who received sedation or anesthesia is released to non-medical personnel (3, 21). Before release from the facility, the following criteria should be met: (a) The patient should be alert and oriented, or returned to baseline mental status; (b) Vital signs should be stable; (c) If any reversal agents were given, adequate time should have passed so that the patient will not become re-sedated once the reversal agent wears off; (d) The patient should have sufficient muscle strength and control to maintain a patent airway; (e) A responsible adult should accompany the patient home; (f) Written discharge instructions should be sent home with the patient.

CONCLUSIONS

Performing sedation or anesthesia in the MRI setting is more challenging than it is in most other locations. Identification of high-risk patients is valuable so that a more experienced individual can care for these difficult cases. Sedation can rapidly become anesthesia and a qualified individual who can recognize and manage hypoventilation, airway obstruction, and other common problems is a necessity. Using appropriate physiological monitoring during sedation and anesthesia is essential for safety, as is the knowledge of pharmacologic principles. MRI facilities with sedation programs must meet current guidelines and should regularly review pertinent policies and procedures in order to ensure the safety of their patients. Those healthcare professionals entrusted with sedation and/or monitoring should have training and hands-on experience before attempting sedation in the formidable MRI environment

REFERENCES

1. Practice advisory on anesthetic care for magnetic resonance imaging: A report by the American Society of Anesthesiologists Task Force on Anesthetic Care for Magnetic Resonance Imaging. Anesthesiology 2009;110:459–79.

2. Continuum of depth of sedation: Definition of general anesthesia and levels of sedation/analgesia. Committee of origin: Quality Management and Departmental Administration (Approved by the American Society of Anesthesiologists, House of Delegates on October 27, 2004 and amended on October 21, 2009). Available at: http://www.asahq.org/For-Members/Standards-Guidelines-and-Statements.aspx.

3. Special article. Practice guidelines for sedation and analgesia by non-anesthesiologists. An updated report by the American Society of Anesthesiologists Task Force on Sedation and Analgesia by Non-Anesthesiologists. Anesthesiology 2002;96:1004–17.

4. American Academy of Pediatrics, American Academy of Pediatric Dentistry, Coté CJ, Wilson S, Work Group on Sedation. Guidelines for monitoring and management of pediatric patients during and after sedation for diagnostic and therapeutic procedures: An update. Pediatrics 2006;118:2587-2602.

5. American College of Radiology (ACR), Society of Interventional Radiology (SIR) Practice Guideline for Sedation/Analgesia. [online publication]. American College of Radiology (ACR), 2010. Available at: http://www.acr.org/~/media/F194CBB800AB43048B997A75938AB482.pdf

6. Clarification of the Interpretive Guidelines for the Anesthesia Services Condition of Participation. May 21, 2010. Available at: https://www.cms.gov/transmittals/downloads/R59SOMA.pdf

7. Godwin SA, Caro DA, Wolf SJ, et al. Clinical policy: Procedural sedation and analgesia in the emergency department. Ann Emerg Med 2005;45:177-196.

8. Special Article. Practice Guidelines for Preoperative Fasting and the Use of Pharmacologic Agents to Reduce the Risk of Pulmonary Aspiration: Application to Healthy Patients. Undergoing Elective Procedures. An Updated Report by the American Society of Anesthesiologists Committee on Standards and Practice Parameters Anesthesiology 2011;114:495–511.

9. Special article. Practice guidelines for the perioperative management of patients with obstructive sleep apnea. A report by the American Society of Anesthesiologists Task Force on Perioperative Management of Patients with Obstructive Sleep Apnea. Anesthesiology 2006;104:1081–93.

10. Litman RS, Kottra JA, Bekowitz RJ, Ward DS. Upper airway obstruction during midazolam/nitrous oxide sedation in children with enlarged tonsils. Pediatr Dent 1998;20:318-320.

11. Fishbaugh DR, Wilson S, Preisch JW, et al. Relationship of tonsil size on an airway blockage maneuver in children during sedation. Pediatri Dent 1997;19:277-281.

12. Standards For Basic Anesthetic Monitoring. Committee of Origin: Standards and Practice Parameters (Approved by the American Society of Anesthesiologists, House of Delegates on October 21, 1986, and last amended on October 20, 2010 with an effective date of July 1, 2011)

13. Shellock, FG. Reference Manual for Magnetic Resonance Safety, Implants and Devices, 2013 Edition. Los Angeles: Biomedical Research Publishing Group; 2013.

14. Rao CC, McNiece WL, Emhardt J, Krishna G, Westcott R. Modification of an anesthesia machine for use during magnetic resonance imaging. Anesthesiology 1988;68:640-641.

15. Kanal E, Shellock FG. Burns associated with clinical MR examinations. Radiology1990;175:585.

16. Bashein G, Syrovy G. Burns associated with pulse oximetry during magnetic resonance imaging. Anesthesiology 1991;75:382-383.

17. Knopp MV, Essig M, Debus J, Zabel HJ, van Kaick G. Unusual burns of the lower extremities caused by a closed conducting loop in a patient at MR imaging. Radiology 1996;200:572-575.

18. Jones S, Jaffe W, Alvi R. Burns associated with electrocardiographic monitoring during magnetic resonance imaging. Burns 1996:22:420-421.

19. Brown TR, Goldstein B, Little J. Severe burns resulting from magnetic resonance imaging with cardiopulmonary monitoring. Risks and relevant safety precautions. Am J Phys Med Rehabil 1993;72;3:166-7.

20. Khan JJ, Donnelly LF, Koch BL, et al. A program to decrease the need for pediatric sedation for CT and MRI. Applied Radiology 2007;4:30-33.

21. Syllabus from the SPS Pediatric Sedation Course. Presented by the Society for Pediatric Sedation. May 19, 2013.

22. Fisher DM, Zwass MS. Chloral hydrate administration to children. Anesth Analg 1993;76:668-669.

23. Vade A, Sukhani R, Dolenga M, Habisohn-Schuck C. Chloral hydrate sedation of children undergoing CT and MR imaging: safety as judged by American Academy of Pediatrics guidelines. AJR Am J Roentgenol 1995;165:905-9.

24. Drugs to be discontinued. In FDA U. S. Food And Drug Administration. In Drugs. Available at: http://www.fda.gov/Drugs/DrugSafety/DrugShortabes/ucm050794.htm. Accessed July, 2013.

25. Strain JD, Campbell JB, Harvey LA, Foley LC. IV nembutal: safe sedation for children undergoing CT. AJR Am J Roentgenol 1988;151:975-979.

26. Mason KP, Zurakowski D, Connor L, et al. Infant sedation for MR imaging and CT: oral versus intravenous pentobarbital. Radiology. 2004;233:723-8.

27. Pershad J, Wan J, Anghelescu D. Comparison of propofol with pentobarbital/midazolam/fentanyl sedation for magnetic resonance imaging of the brain in children. Pediatrics 2007;120:3e629-e636.

28. Cravero J, Beach M, Blike G, et al. Pediatric Sedation Research Consortium. The incidence and nature of adverse events during pediatric sedation/anesthesia with propofol for procedures outside the operating room: a report from the Pediatric Sedation Research Consortium. Anesth Analg 2009;108:795-804

29. Heard CM, Joshi P, Johnson K. Dexmedetomidine for pediatric MRI sedation: a review of a series of cases. Paediatr Anaesth 2007;17:888-92.

30. Mason KP, Zurakowski D, Zgleszewski SE, et al. High dose dexmedetomidine as the sole sedative for pediatric MRI. Paediatr Anaesth 2008;18:403-11.

31. Midazolam Hydrochloride Drug Summary. In: Midazolam Drug Information, PDR.net. Available at: http://www.pdr.net/drug-summary/midazolam-hydrochloride-injection?druglabelid=985. Accessed July, 2013.

32. Kundu S, Achar S. Principles of office anesthesia: Part II. Topical anesthesia. Am Fam Physician 2002;66:99-102.

33. Naloxone Drug Summary. In: Naloxone Hydrochloride Drug Information, PDR.net. Available at: http://www.pdr.net/drug-summary/naloxone-hydrochloride?druglabelid=777. Accessed July, 2013.

34. Flumazenil Drug Summary. In: Flumazenil Drug Information, PDR.net. Available at: http://www.pdr.net/drug-summary/flumazenil?druglabelid=1729. Accessed July, 2013.

Chapter 16   MRI Issues for Implants and Devices

FRANK G. SHELLOCK, PH.D.

Adjunct Clinical Professor of Radiology and Medicine
Keck School of Medicine, University of Southern California

Adjunct Professor of Clinical Physical Therapy
Division of Biokinesiology and Physical Therapy
School of Dentistry, University of Southern California

Director for MRI Studies of Biomimetic MicroElectronic Systems
National Science Foundation, Engineering Research Center
University of Southern California

Institute for Magnetic Resonance Safety, Education, and Research
President, Shellock R & D Services, Inc.
Los Angeles, CA

INTRODUCTION

An important aspect of protecting patients from magnetic resonance imaging (MRI)-related accidents and injuries involves an understanding of the risks associated with the implants, devices, and other objects (e.g., metallic foreign bodies) that may cause problems in this setting. This requires constant attention and diligence to obtain information and documentation about these items as part of the screening procedure in order to provide the safest MRI environment possible.

The standard of care for managing a patient referred for an MRI procedure with an implant or device is to positively identify the type of item that is present and then to determine the relative safety of scanning the patient. This is best accomplished by either referring to the MRI-specific labeling for the implant or device or by reviewing the *ex vivo* testing that was performed on the object and published in the peer-reviewed literature.

This chapter will discuss the important MRI-related issues for implants and devices and present information for a variety of common and not so common medical products. Notably, an annually revised textbook provides vital information for thousands of implants and devices and there is a website, www.MRIsafety.com, with pertinent content that is updated on a regular basis (1, 2). Therefore, the reader is directed to these resources when specific information is needed.

MRI ISSUES FOR IMPLANTS AND DEVICES

MRI may be contraindicated for a given patient primarily because of risks associated with movement or dislodgment of a ferromagnetic implant or device (1-4). There are other possible hazards and problems related to the presence of a metallic object or one made from conductive materials that include excessive heating, induction of currents (i.e., in materials that are conductors), changes in the operational aspects of the device, damage to the function of the device, the difficulty in interpreting MR images due to signal loss and/or distortion, and the misinterpretation of an imaging artifact as an abnormality (1-4). In consideration of the above, *ex vivo* testing is performed to assess the various MRI issues for implants and devices in order to properly characterize the possible risks (1-32).

Magnetic Field Interactions

With regard to magnetic field interactions and MRI, translational attraction and/or torque may cause movement or dislodgment of a ferromagnetic implant, resulting in an uncomfortable sensation for the patient, an injury, or even a fatality (1, 2). Therefore, both translational attraction and torque are important to evaluate for implants and devices before patients with metallic objects are allowed to undergo MRI.

The effect of translational attraction acting on an implanted ferromagnetic object is predominantly responsible for a hazard that may occur in the immediate area of the MR system. That is, as one moves closer to the scanner or as the patient is moved into the bore for the MRI examination. The predominant effect of torque (or rotational alignment to the magnetic field) as it acts on a ferromagnetic object occurs in the center of the MR system, where the magnetic field is most homogenous. Notably, torque will greatly influence implants and devices that have an elongated shape. Obviously, both translational attraction and torque combine to impact a ferromagnetic implant or device as the patient with the object moves towards the MR system and then into the center of the bore of the scanner (1, 2).

Various factors influence the risk of performing MRI in a patient with a metallic object including the strength of the static magnetic field, the level of the spatial gradient magnetic field, the magnetic susceptibility of the object, the mass of the object, the geometry of the object, the location and orientation of the object *in situ*, the presence of retentive mechanisms (i.e., fibrotic tissue, sutures, etc.), and the length of time the object has been implanted. These factors should be carefully considered before subjecting a patient with a ferromagnetic object to an MRI examination. This is particularly important if the object is located in a potentially dangerous area of the body such as a vital neural, vascular, of soft tissue structure where movement or dislodgment could injure the patient.

With respect to the potential risks for a ferromagnetic implant, in addition to the findings for translational attraction and torque, the "intended *in vivo* use" of the implant or device must be considered as well as the mechanisms that may provide retention of the object once it is implanted (e.g., implants or devices held in place by sutures, granulation or ingrowth of tissue, fixation devices, or by other means). Accordingly, sufficient counterforces may exist to retain even a ferromagnetic implant in place, *in situ*.

Numerous studies have assessed magnetic field interactions for implants and other items by measuring translational attraction and torque associated with the static magnetic fields of MR systems (1, 2). These investigations demonstrated that MRI can be performed safely in patients with metallic objects that are nonferromagnetic or "weakly" ferromagnetic (i.e., only minimally attracted by the magnetic field), such that the magnetic field interactions are insufficient to move or dislodge them, *in situ*.

Additionally, patients with certain implants or devices that have relatively strong ferromagnetic qualities may be safely scanned using MRI because the objects are held in place by retentive forces that prevent them from being moved or dislodged with reference to the "intended *in vivo* use" of the object. For example, there is an interference screw (i.e., the Perfix Interference Screw) used for reconstruction of the anterior cruciate ligament that is highly ferromagnetic. However, once this implant is implanted (i.e., screwed into the patient's bone), this prevents it from being moved, even if the patient is exposed to a 1.5-Tesla MR system. Other implants that exhibit substantial ferromagnetic qualities may likewise be safe for patients undergoing MRI under highly specific conditions as a result of the presence of counterforces that prevent movement of these objects.

In general, each implant or other item should be evaluated using *ex vivo* techniques to test translational attraction and torque before allowing a patient with the object to undergo MRI (1, 2). By following this guideline, the magnetic susceptibility for an object may be considered so that a competent decision can be made concerning possible risks associated with subjecting the patient to MRI. Because movement or dislodgment of an implanted metallic object is the main mechanism responsible for an injury, this aspect of testing is considered to be of utmost importance and should involve the use of an MR system operating at an appropriate static magnetic field strength (i.e., if the intent is to scan the patient with the implant at 3-Tesla, the implant must be tested for magnetic field interactions at that field strength).

In certain cases, there is a possibility of changing the operational or functional aspects of the implant or device as a result of exposure to the powerful static magnetic field of the MR system. For an implant that has a component that is magnetic (e.g., cochlear implants, programmable cerebral spinal fluid shunt valves, etc.), it is possible to disrupt the functional aspects of the device or to demagnetize the magnet, rendering it unacceptable for its intended use (1, 2). Therefore, this important aspect must be evaluated using comprehensive testing techniques to verify that specific MRI conditions will not alter the function of the device.

MR systems with very low (0.2-Tesla or less) or very high (9.4-Tesla) static magnetic fields are currently used for clinical and research applications. Considering that most metallic objects evaluated for magnetic field interactions were assessed at 1.5- or 3-Tesla, an appropriate variance or modification of the information provided regarding the safety of performing an MRI procedure in a patient with a metallic object may exist when a scanner with a lower or higher static magnetic field strength was used for testing. Therefore, it may be acceptable to adjust safety recommendations depending on the static magnetic field strength and other aspects of a given scanner. Obviously, performing an MRI procedure using a 0.2-Tesla MR system has different risk implications for a patient with a ferromagnetic object compared with using a 9.4-Tesla scanner.

Heating

Temperature increases produced in association with MRI have been studied using *ex vivo* techniques to evaluate various metallic implants, devices, and objects that have a variety of sizes, shapes, and metallic compositions or that are made from conducting materials (1, 2). In general, reports have indicated that only minor temperature changes occur in association with MRI and relatively small metallic objects that are "passive" implants (i.e., those that are not electronically-activated), including items such as aneurysm clips, hemostatic clips, prosthetic heart valves, vascular access ports, and similar devices. Therefore, heat generated during MRI involving a patient with a small, passive implant does not appear to be a substantial hazard. Importantly, to date, there has been no report of a patient being seriously injured as a result of excessive heat that developed in a small passive implant or device.

However, MRI-related heating is potentially problematic for implants that have an elongated shape or those that form a conducting loop of a certain diameter. For example, substantial heating can occur under some MRI conditions for objects such as elongated implants (e.g., leads, wires, etc.) that form resonant antennas or that form resonant conducting loops.

The evaluation of heating for an implant or device is particularly challenging because of the many factors that effect temperature increases in these items. Variables that impact heating include, the following: the specific type of implant or device; the electrical characteristics of the implant or device; the radiofrequency (RF) wavelength of the MR system; the type of transmit RF coil that is used (i.e., transmit head versus transmit body RF coil); the amount of RF energy delivered (i.e., the specific absorption rate, SAR); the technique used to calculate or estimate SAR that is utilized by the MR system; the landmark position or body part undergoing MRI relative to the transmit RF coil; and the orientation or configuration of the implant or device relative to the source of RF energy (i.e., the transmit RF coil).

One aspect of MRI-related heating for an implant or device that may not be intuitive is that for a given item, heating can be substantially different depending on the frequency of RF that is applied. For example, evidence from an *ex vivo* study conducted by Shellock, et al. (33) reported that significantly *less* MRI-related heating occurred at 3-Tesla/128-MHz (whole-body-averaged SAR, 3-W/kg) versus 1.5-Tesla/64-MHz (whole-body-averaged SAR, 1.4-W/kg) for a pacemaker lead that was not connected to a pulse generator (same lead length, positioning, etc.). This phenomenon whereby less heating was observed at 128-MHz versus 64-MHz has also been observed for external fixation devices, Foley catheters with temperature sensors, neurostimulation systems, relatively long peripheral vascular stents, and other implants and devices. Therefore, it is vital to perform *ex vivo* testing to properly characterize MRI-related heating to identify potentially hazardous objects prior to subjecting patients with the respective items to MRI.

Induced Currents

The potential for MRI procedures to injure patients by inducing electrical currents in implants or devices made from conductive materials such as cardiac pacemakers, neurostimulation systems, cochlear implants, and other similar items has been previously reported. The performance of *ex vivo* testing of implants and devices to assess induced currents is necessary mostly for electronically-activated devices. Recommendations have been presented to protect patients from injuries related to induced currents that may develop during MRI (1, 2).

Artifacts

The type and extent of artifacts caused by the presence of metallic implants and devices have been described and tend to be easily recognized on MR images (5, 8, 11, 18-29). Signal loss and/or image distortion associated with metallic objects are predominantly caused by a disruption of the local magnetic field that perturbs the relationship between position and frequency. In some cases, there may be areas of high signal intensity seen along the edge of a signal void or when there is an abrupt change in the shape of the item (e.g., the tip of a biopsy needle). Additionally, artifacts may be caused by gradient switching due to the generation of eddy currents.

The extent of the artifact seen on an MR image is dependent on the object's magnetic susceptibility, size, shape, position in the patient's body, the technique used for imaging (i.e., the specific pulse sequence parameters), and the image processing method. Careful selection of pulse sequence parameters can decrease the size of artifacts and this is done routinely, especially for patients that undergo MRI with implants that have large metallic masses, such as hip or knee prostheses. Additionally, several new imaging or post-processing techniques have been described that substantial reduce artifacts associated with metallic objects.

TERMINOLOGY FOR IMPLANTS AND DEVICES

With the growing use of MRI in the 1990s, the Food and Drug Administration (FDA) recognized the need for standardized tests to address MRI safety issues for implants and other medical devices (34-38). Thus, over the years, test methods have been developed by various organizations including the American Society for Testing and Materials (ASTM) International, with an ongoing commitment to ensure patient safety in the MRI environment (36-38).

The FDA is responsible for reviewing the MRI terminology and labeling that manufacturers provide for their devices. This terminology has evolved to keep pace with advances in MRI technology. Unfortunately, members of the MRI community frequently may not always understand the terms that are used and are often confused by the conditions that are specified in "MR Conditional" labeling. This lack of understanding may result in patients with implants being exposed to potentially hazardous MRI conditions or in inappropriately preventing them from undergoing needed examinations. Importantly, the current labeling terminology that exists is associated with expanded labeling information that relates to the conditions that are deemed acceptable to ensure patient safety.

Prior to implementing the current terminology, the terms "MR Safe" and "MR Compatible" were used for labeling purposes. In time, it became apparent that these terms were somewhat confusing and often used interchangeably or incorrectly. In particular, these terms were frequently used without including the conditions for which the device had been demonstrated to be safe. Therefore, in an effort to develop more appropriate terminology and, more importantly, because the misuse of the terms could result in serious accidents for patients and others in the MRI environment, a new set of MRI labeling terms was developed and released in 2005 (35). Thus, this terminology, which is currently recognized by the FDA and applied to implants and devices is, as follows: (a) *MR Safe* - an item that poses no known hazards in all MRI environments. Using the terminology, MR Safe items are non-conducting, non-metallic, and non-magnetic items such as a plastic Petri dish. (b) *MR Conditional* - an item that has been demonstrated to pose no known hazards in a specified MRI environment with specified conditions of use. Conditions that define the MRI environment may include the strength of the static magnetic field value, the spatial gradient magnetic field value, the time-varying magnetic field value, the RF field value, and the specific absorption rate (SAR) level. Additional conditions, including the specific configuration for the item (e.g., the routing of leads used for a neurostimulation system) may be required. Other possible safety issues that may be part of the MR Conditional labeling include but are not limited to thermal injury, induced currents/voltages, electromagnetic interference, neurostimulation, acoustic noise, interaction among devices, the safe functioning of the item, and the safe operation of the MR system. (c) *MR Unsafe* - an item that is known to pose hazards in all MRI environments. MR Unsafe items include ferromagnetic items such as a pair of metallic scissors.

Because of the variety of MR systems (e.g., ranging from 0.2- to 9.4-Tesla) and conditions in clinical use today, the current terminology is intended to help elucidate labeling matters for medical devices and other items that may be used in the MRI environment to ensure the safe use of MRI technology. However, it should be noted that this updated terminology has not been applied retrospectively to the many implants and devices that previously received FDA approved labeling using the terms MR Safe or MR Compatible (in general, this applies to those objects tested prior to the release of the ASTM International information for labeling in 2005). Therefore, this important point must be understood to avoid undue confusion regarding the matter of the labeling that has been applied to previously tested implants (i.e., those labeled as MR Safe or MR Compatible) versus those that have recently undergone MRI testing (i.e., now labeled MR Safe, MR Conditional)(1, 2). Notably, the specific content of the MRI labeling for an implant or device may take various forms (especially for electronically-activated implants) as the format continues to be refined by the FDA in an ongoing effort to properly communicate this information to MRI healthcare professionals.

MRI INFORMATION FOR IMPLANTS AND DEVICES

New implants and devices are developed on an on-going basis which, as previously indicated, necessitates continuous endeavors to obtain current documentation for these items prior to subjecting patients to MRI. Importantly, the labeling that ensures the safe use of MRI is highly specific to the conditions that were utilized to assess the implant or device and any deviation from the defined procedures can lead to deleterious effects, severe patient injuries, or fatalities, especially when an electronically-activated implant is present in the patient (1, 2). A selection of items evaluated for MRI issues is presented below in order to illustrate information for commonly encountered or unusual medical products (1, 2).

ActiPatch

The ActiPatch (BioElectronics, Frederick, MD) is a medical, drug-free device that delivers pulsed electromagnetic frequency therapies to accelerate healing of soft tissue injuries. The ActiPatch has an embedded, battery-operated microchip that delivers continuous pulsed therapy to reduce pain and swelling. With regard to MRI, the ActiPatch must be removed prior to performing an MRI procedure to prevent possible damage to this device and the potential risk of excessive heating.

ActiFlo Indwelling Bowel Catheter System

The ActiFlo Indwelling Bowel Catheter System (also known as the Zassi Bowel Management System, Hollister, Libertyville, IL) is intended for diversion of fecal matter to minimize external contact with the patient's skin, to facilitate the collection of fecal matter for patients requiring stool management, to provide access for colonic irrigation, and to administer medications or an enema. This system consists of a catheter, the collection bag, and the irrigation bag. The ActiFlo Indwelling Bowel Catheter System allows stool to drain directly from the rectum into a closed or drainable collection bag.

With regard to MRI issues, the ActiFlo Indwelling Bowel Catheter System was determined to be MR Conditional. Non-clinical testing demonstrated that this product is MR Conditional according to the following conditions: static magnetic field of 3-Tesla or less and highest spatial gradient magnetic field of 720-Gauss/cm or less. Important note: A metallic spring used for this device is located outside of the patient's body during the intended *in vivo* use of this product. Therefore, the only possible MRI-related issue pertains to magnetic field interactions. Heating and artifacts are of no concern. As such, the assessment of magnetic field interactions for this product specifically involved evaluations of translational attraction and torque in relation to exposure to a 3-Tesla MR system, only. Evaluations of MRI-related heating and artifacts were not conducted and are unnecessary.

Aneurysm Clips

The surgical management of intracranial aneurysms and arteriovenous malformations (AVMs) by the application of aneurysm clips is a well-established procedure (**Figure 1**). The presence of an aneurysm clip in a patient referred for an MRI procedure represents a situation that requires the utmost consideration because of the associated risks. The following guidelines are recommended with regard to performing MRI in a patient or before allowing an individual with an aneurysm clip into the MRI environment: (a) Specific information (i.e., manufacturer, type or model, material, lot and serial numbers) about the aneurysm clip must be known, especially with respect to the material used to make the aneurysm clip, so that only patients or individuals with nonferromagnetic or weakly ferromagnetic clips are allowed into the MRI environment. The manufacturer provides this information in the labeling of the aneurysm clip. The implanting surgeon is responsible for

Figure 1. Examples of aneurysm clips.

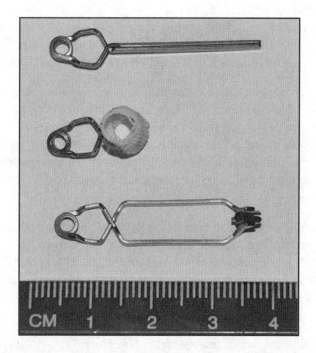

properly recording and communicating this information in the patient's or individual's records. (b) An aneurysm clip that is in its original package and made from Phynox, Elgiloy, MP35N, titanium alloy, commercially pure titanium or other material known to be nonferromagnetic or weakly ferromagnetic does not need to be evaluated for ferromagnetism. Aneurysm clips made from nonferromagnetic or "weakly" ferromagnetic materials in original packages do not require testing of ferromagnetism because the manufacturers ensure the pertinent MRI aspects of these clips and, therefore, are responsible for the accuracy of the labeling. (c) If the aneurysm clip is not in its original package and/or properly labeled, it should undergo testing for magnetic field interactions according to appropriate testing procedures to determine if it is safe. (d) The radiologist and implanting surgeon are responsible for evaluating the information pertaining to the aneurysm clip, verifying its accuracy, obtaining written documentation, and deciding to perform MRI after considering the risk versus benefit aspects for a given patient. (e) Consideration must be given to the static magnetic field strength that is to be used for the MRI procedure and the strength of the static magnetic field that was used to test magnetic field interactions for the aneurysm clip in question. Additional information for aneurysm clips may be found online at www.MRIsafety.com.

Body Piercing Jewelry

Ritual or decorative body piercing is extremely popular as a form of self-expression. Different types of materials are used to make body piercing jewelry including ferromagnetic and nonferromagnetic metals, as well as non-metallic materials. The presence of body piercing jewelry that is made from ferromagnetic or conductive material of a certain shape may present a problem for a patient referred for an MRI procedure. Risks include uncomfortable sensations from movement or displacement that may be mild-to-moderate depending on the site of the body piercing and the ferromagnetic qualities of the jewelry (e.g., size, degree of magnetic susceptibility, etc.). In extreme cases, serious injuries may occur. In addition, for body piercing jewelry made from conductive material, there is a possibility of MRI-related heating that could cause excessive temperature increases and burns.

Because of potential safety issues, metallic body piercing jewelry should be removed prior to entering the MRI environment. However, patients with body piercings are often reluctant to remove their jewelry. Therefore, if it is not possible to remove metallic body piercing jewelry, the patient or individual should be informed regarding the potential risks. In addition, if the body piercing jewelry is made from ferromagnetic material, some means of stabilization (e.g., application of adhesive tape or bandage) should be used to prevent movement or displacement.

To avoid potential heating of body piercing jewelry made from conductive materials, it is recommended to use gauze, tape, or other similar material to wrap the jewelry in such a manner as to insulate it (i.e., prevent contact) from the underlying skin. The patient should be instructed to immediately inform the MR system operator if any heating or other unusual sensation occurs in association with the body piercing jewelry.

According to Muensterer (39), even temporary or short-term piercing jewelry removal may lead to closure of the subcutaneous tract. Therefore, temporary replacement with a nonmetallic spacer may be indicated. Of course, this procedure must only be accomplished under the guidance and direction of a physician.

Contraceptive Diaphragms

A contraceptive diaphragm may have a metallic ring that maintains it in position during its intended use. Thus, certain contraceptive diaphragms with metallic components may display positive magnetic field interactions in association with exposure to MR systems and, because of the metallic parts, substantial artifacts may be found. MRI examinations have been performed in patients with these devices without complaints or adverse sensations related to movement. Furthermore, there is no danger of heating of a contraceptive diaphragm during MRI under the conditions currently recommended by the United States Food and Drug Administration. Therefore, the presence of a diaphragm is not a contraindication for a patient undergoing an MRI examination using an MR system operating at 3-Tesla or less.

Essure Device

The Essure Device (Bayer Healthcare) is a metallic implant developed for permanent female contraception. The presence of this implant is intended to alter the function and architecture of the fallopian tube, resulting in permanent contraception. The Essure Device is composed of 316L stainless steel, platinum, iridium, nickel-titanium alloy, silver solder, and polyethylene terephthalate fibers. The MRI assessment of this device involved testing for magnetic field interactions, heating, induced electrical currents, and artifacts using previously described techniques. The findings indicated that it is acceptable for a patient with the Essure Device to undergo MRI at 3-Tesla or less.

External Hearing Aids

External hearing aids are included in the category of electronically-activated devices that may be found in patients referred for MRI procedures. Exposure to the magnetic fields used for MRI can easily damage these devices. Therefore, a patient or other individual with an external hearing aid must not enter the MR system room. Fortunately, an external hearing aid can be readily identified and removed from the patient or individual to prevent damage associated with the MRI setting.

Other hearing devices may have external components as well as pieces that are surgically implanted. Hearing devices with external and internal components may be especially problematic for patients and individuals in relation to the use of MRI. Accordingly, patients and individuals with these particular hearing devices may not be allowed into the MRI environment because of the risk of damage to the components.

Glaucoma Drainage Implants (Shunt Tubes)

A glaucoma drainage implant or device, also known as a shunt tube, is implanted to maintain an artificial drainage pathway to control intraocular pressure for patients with glaucoma. Intraocular pressure is lowered when aqueous humor flows from inside the eye through the tube into the space between the plate that rests on the scleral surface and surrounding fibrous capsule. The implantation of a glaucoma drainage device is used to treat glaucoma that is refractory to medical and standard surgical therapy. For certain glaucoma drainage implants, radiographic findings may suggest the diagnosis of an orbital foreign body if the ophthalmic history is unknown, as reported by Ceballos and Parrish (40). In this case report, a patient was denied an MRI examination for fear of dislodging an apparent "metallic foreign body." In fact, the patient had a Baerveldt glaucoma drainage implant, which was mistakenly identified as a metallic orbital object based on its radiographic characteristics (i.e., due to the presence of barium-impregnated silicone).

At least one glaucoma drainage implant, the ExPRESS Miniature Glaucoma Shunt (Optonol Ltd., Neve Ilan, Israel), is made from 316L stainless steel. However, many other glaucoma drainage implants are made from nonmetallic materials and are safe for patients undergoing MRI. Commonly used devices that do not contain metal and, as such, are MR Safe include, the following: (a) Baerveldt Glaucoma Drainage Implant (Pharmacia Co., Kalamazoo, MI) (b) Krupin-Denver Eye Valve to Disc Implant (E. Benson Hood Laboratories, Pembroke, MA) (c) Ahmed Glaucoma Valve (New World Medical, Rancho Cucamonga, CA) (d) Molteno Drainage Device (Molteno Ophthalmic Ltd., Dunedin, New Zealand), and (e) Joseph Valve (Valve Implants Limited, Hertford, England).

Heart Valve Prostheses and Annuloplasty Rings

Many heart valve prostheses and annuloplasty rings have been evaluated for MRI issues, especially with regard to the presence of magnetic field interactions and heating associated with exposure to clinical MR systems operating at field strengths of as high as 3-Tesla (**Figure 2**). Of these, the majority displayed measurable yet relatively minor magnetic field interactions. That is, because the actual attractive forces exerted on the heart valve prostheses and annuloplasty rings were minimal compared to the force exerted by the beating heart

Figure 2. Examples of heart valve prostheses (a) and annuloplasty rings (b).

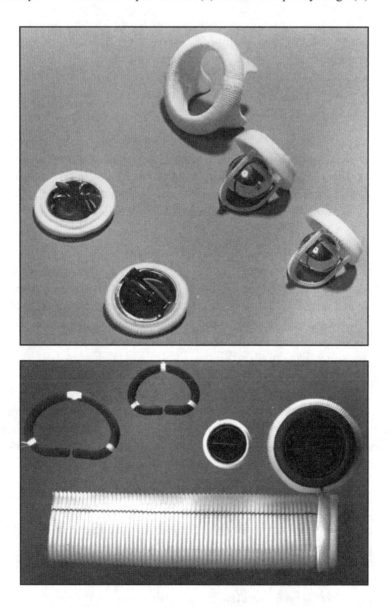

(i.e., approximately 7.2-N), an MRI procedure is not considered to be hazardous for a patient that has any heart valve prosthesis or annuloplasty ring tested relative to the field strength of the MR system used for the evaluation. Importantly, this recommendation includes the Starr-Edwards Model Pre-6000 heart valve prosthesis previously suggested to be a potential risk for a patient undergoing MRI. Heating has been reported to be relatively minor for heart valve prostheses and annuloplasty rings.

With respect to clinical MRI procedures, there has been no report of a patient incident or injury related to the presence of a heart valve prosthesis or annuloplasty ring. However, it should be noted that not all of these types of implants have been evaluated for MRI issues.

Hemostatic (Ligating) Vascular Clips

In general, it was previously believed that because virtually all hemostatic (also called ligating) vascular clips and similar devices (including "endoclips" deployed through endoscopes) are made from nonferromagnetic materials such as tantalum, titanium, and certain forms of nonmagnetic stainless steel, patients with these implants are not at risk for injury in association with MRI (1, 2) (**Figure 3**). However, there are several hemostatic clips in use today that present potential problems for patients referred for MRI procedures. Patients with these clips require special attention to ensure the safe use of MRI. In some cases, MRI is deemed "unsafe". For others, a "waiting" period is necessary and X-rays must be obtained and inspected to determine if the clips are present or not prior to performing MRI. Examples of MRI labeling statements for hemostatic clips that require further attention during the screening procedure are presented below.

Long Clip, HX-600-090L

The Long Clip HX-600-090L (Olympus Medical Systems Corporation) is indicated for placement within the gastrointestinal (GI) tract for the purpose of endoscopic marking, he-

Figure 3. Examples of hemostatic clips.

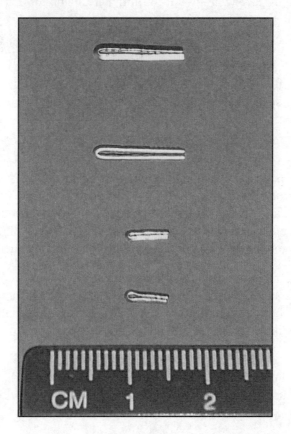

mostasis, or closure of GI tract luminal perforations within 20-mm as a supplementary method. For MRI, the Long Clip HX-600-090L labeling information is, as follows: Do not perform MRI procedures on patients who have clips placed within their gastrointestinal tracts. This could be harmful to the patient. Olympus endoscopic clips have been shown to remain in the patient an average of 9.4 days, but retention is based on a variety of factors and may result in a longer retention period. Prior to MRI, the physician should confirm there are no residual clips in the GI tract. The following techniques may be used for confirmation: (a) View the lesion under radiologic imaging. Olympus clip fixing devices are radiopaque. By using X-ray, the physician can determine if any residual clips are in the gastrointestinal tract. If no clips are evident under radiologic imaging, MRI may be accomplished. (b) Endoscopically examine the lesion. If no clips remain at the lesion, MRI may be accomplished.

QuickClip2, HX-201LR-135 and HX-201UR-135

The QuickClip2, HX-201LR-135 and HX-201UR-135 (Olympus Medical Systems Corporation) are indicated for placement within the gastrointestinal (GI) tract for the purpose of endoscopic marking, hemostasis, or closure of GI tract luminal perforations within 20-mm as a supplementary method. For MRI, the QuickClip2 (HX-201LR-135 and HX-201UR-135) labeling information is, as follows: Do not perform MRI procedures on patients who have clips placed within their gastrointestinal tracts. This could be harmful to the patient. Olympus endoscopic clips have been shown to remain in the patient an average of 9.4 days, but retention is based on a variety of factors and may result in a longer retention period. Prior to MRI, the physician should confirm there are no residual clips in the GI tract. The following techniques may be used for confirmation:

(a) View the lesion under radiologic imaging. Olympus clip fixing devices are radiopaque. By using X-ray, the physician can determine if any residual clips are in the gastrointestinal tract. If no clips are evident under radiologic imaging, MRI may be accomplished. (b) Endoscopically examine the lesion. If no clips remain at the lesion, MRI may be accomplished.

Pellets, Bullets, and Shrapnel

The majority of pellets, bullets, and shrapnel tested for MRI issues were found to be composed of nonferromagnetic materials. However, these items are often "contaminated" by ferromagnetic metals. Ammunition that proved to be ferromagnetic tended to be manufactured in foreign countries and/or used for military applications. Shrapnel typically contains steel and, therefore, presents a potential hazard for patients undergoing MRI.

Because pellets, bullets, and shrapnel are frequently contaminated with ferromagnetic materials, the risk versus benefit of performing an MRI procedure should be carefully considered. Additional consideration must be given to whether the metallic object is located near or in a vital anatomic structure, with the assumption that the object is likely to be ferromagnetic and can potentially move.

Smugar, et al. (41) conducted an investigation to determine whether neurological problems developed in paralyzed patients with intraspinal bullets or bullet fragments in association with MRI performed at 1.5-Tesla. Patients were queried during scanning for symptoms of discomfort, pain, or changes in neurological status. Additionally, detailed neurological examinations were performed prior to MRI, post MRI, and at the patient's discharge. Based on these findings, Smugar, et al. (41) concluded that patients with complete spinal cord injury may undergo MRI if they have intraspinal bullets or fragments without concern for affects on their physical or neurological status. Thus, metallic fragments in the spinal canals of paralyzed patients are believed to represent only a relative contraindication to MRI.

Eshed, et al. (42) conducted a retrospective investigation of the potential hazards of patients undergoing MRI at 1.5-Tesla with retained metal fragments from combat and terrorist attacks. Metal fragments in 17 patients ranged in size between one and 10-mm. One patient reported a superficial migration of a 10-mm fragment after MRI. No other adverse reaction was reported. The authors concluded that 1.5-Tesla MRI examinations are safe in patients with retained metal fragments from combat and terrorist attacks that were not located in the vicinity of vital organs. However, caution is advised as well as an assessment of risk versus benefit for the patient.

Dedini, et al. (30) studied bullets and shotgun pellets that were a representative sample of ballistic objects commonly encountered in association with criminal trauma using 1.5-, 3- and 7-Tesla MR systems (**Figure 4**). Findings indicated that non-steel containing bullets and pellets did not exhibit magnetic field interactions and that both steel-containing and non-steel-containing bullets did not significantly heat, even under extreme MRI conditions at 3-Tesla/128-MHz. Furthermore, steel-containing bullets were potentially unsafe for patients referred for MRI due to high magnetic field interactions, although this recommendation must be interpreted on a case-by-case basis with respect to the restraining effect of the specific tissue involved, time in place *in situ*, proximity to vital or delicate structures, and with careful consideration given to the risk versus benefit for the patient.

Penile Implants

Several types of penile implants have been evaluated for MRI issues. Of these, two (i.e., the Duraphase and Omniphase models) demonstrated substantial ferromagnetic qualities when exposed to a 1.5-Tesla MR system (1, 2) (**Figure 5**). Fortunately, it is unlikely for a penile implant to severely injure a patient undergoing MRI because of the relatively minor degree of magnetic field interactions. This is especially true when one considers the manner in which such a device is utilized. Nevertheless, it would be uncomfortable for a

Figure 4. Examples of bullets.

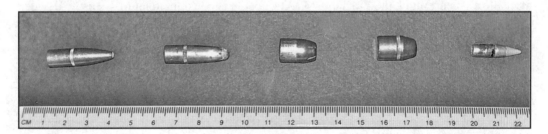

Figure 5. Examples of penile implants.

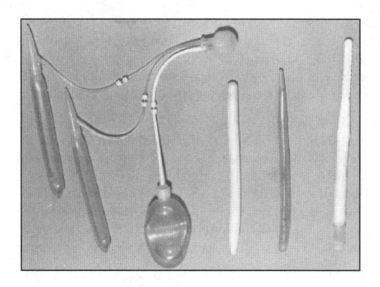

patient with a ferromagnetic penile implant to undergo an MRI examination. For this reason, subjecting a patient with the Duraphase or Omniphase penile implant to an MRI procedure is inadvisable. Findings for other penile implants indicated that they either exhibited no magnetic field interactions or relatively minor or "weak" magnetic field interactions. Heating was not observed to be substantial for any of the penile implants tested to date.

PillCam (M2A) Capsule Endoscopy Device

The PillCam (M2A) Capsule Endoscopy Device (Given Imaging Inc., Norcross, GA) is an ingestible device for use in the gastrointestinal tract (**Figure 6**). Peristalsis moves the PillCam (M2A) Capsule smoothly and painlessly throughout the gastrointestinal tract, transmitting color video images as it passes. The procedure allows the patient to continue daily activities during the endoscopic examination. The PillCam (M2A) Capsule Endoscopy Device has been utilized to diagnose diseases of the small intestine including Crohn's Disease, celiac disease and other malabsorption disorders, benign and malignant tumors of the small intestine, vascular disorders, and medication related small bowel injuries.

Undergoing an MRI while the capsule is inside the patient's body may result in serious damage to his/her intestinal tract or abdominal cavity. If the patient cannot positively verify the excretion of the PillCam (M2A) Capsule from his/her body, the patient should contact the physician for evaluation and possible abdominal X-ray before undergoing an MRI examination. Accordingly, the PillCam (M2A) Capsule is considered an MR Unsafe device.

Vascular Access Ports

Vascular access ports are implants commonly used to provide long-term vascular administration of chemotherapeutic agents, antibiotics, analgesics, and other medications. Vascular access ports are usually implanted in a subcutaneous pocket over the upper chest wall with the catheters inserted in the jugular, subclavian, or cephalic vein. These implants have a variety of similar features (e.g., a reservoir, central septum, and catheter) and may be con-

Figure 6. The PillCam (M2A) Capsule Endoscopy Device.

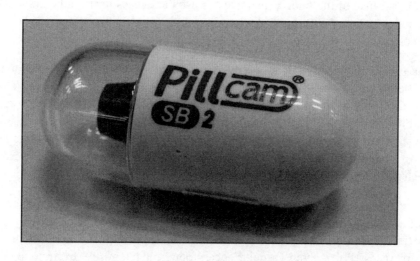

Figure 7. Examples of vascular access ports.

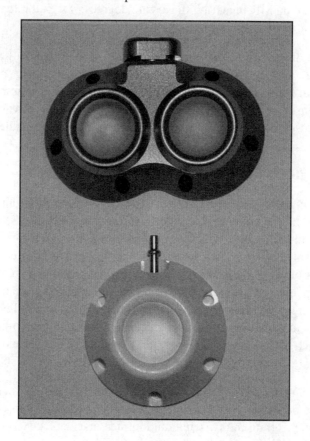

structed from different materials including stainless steel, titanium, silicone, and plastic (**Figure 7**). Because of the widespread use of vascular access ports catheters and the high probability that patients with these devices may require MRI procedures, it has been important to characterize the MRI issues for these implants.

Certain implantable vascular access ports evaluated for MRI issues showed measurable magnetic field interactions at 3-Tesla. However, the interactions were minor relative to the *in vivo* applications of these implants. For the vascular access ports tested to date, none have exhibited substantial heating during MRI at 1.5-Tesla/64-MHz or 3-Tesla/128-MHz. Therefore, an MRI procedure is acceptable when using an MR system operating at 3-Tesla or less in a patient that has one of the vascular access ports presented on www.MRIsafety.com.

With respect to MRI and artifacts, vascular access ports that will produce the least amount of artifact are made entirely from nonmetallic materials. The ones that produce the largest artifacts are composed of metal(s) or have metal in an unusual shape (e.g., the OmegaPort Access Port). Even vascular access ports made entirely from nonmetallic materials are, in fact, seen on MR images because they contain silicone (i.e., the septum portion of the port). Using MRI, the Larmor precessional frequency of fat is close to that of silicone (i.e., 100-Hz at 1.5-Tesla). Therefore, silicone used in the construction of a vascular access port may be observed on MR images with varying degrees of signal intensity depending on the pulse sequence that is used.

If a radiologist did not know that this type of vascular access port was present in a patient, the MR signal produced by the silicone component of the device could be considered an abnormality, or at the very least, present a confusing image. For example, this may cause a diagnostic problem in a patient evaluated for a rupture of a silicone breast implant, because silicone from the vascular access port may be misread as an extracapsular silicone implant rupture.

MRI GUIDELINES FOR THE POST-OPERATIVE PATIENT

There is often confusion regarding the issue of performing MRI during the post-operative (post-op) period in a patient with a metallic implant or device. Studies have demonstrated that, if a metallic object is a "passive" implant or device (i.e., there is no electronically-activated or magnetically-activated component associated with the item) and it is made from nonferromagnetic material, the patient may undergo an MRI procedure immediately after implantation using an MR system operating at 1.5-Tesla or less (or, the static magnetic field strength that was used to test the device, including 3-Tesla)(1, 2). Notably, there are several reports that describe placement of vascular stents, coils, filters, and other implants using MRI-guided procedures that include the use of high field strength (1.5- and 3-Tesla) scanners (1, 2).

For a passive implant or device that exhibits "weakly magnetic" qualities, it may be necessary to wait a period of six weeks after implantation before performing an MRI procedure. For example, certain intravascular and intracavitary coils, stents, and filters designated as weakly magnetic become firmly incorporated into tissue a minimum of six weeks following placement. In these cases, retentive or counterforces provided by tissue ingrowth, scarring, granulation or other mechanisms serve to prevent these objects from presenting risks or hazards to patients undergoing MRI. For patients with implants or devices that are weakly magnetic but rigidly fixed in the body (e.g., a hip prosthesis cemented in place; a heart valve implanted with sutures, etc.), they may be studied immediately after implantation. Specific information pertaining to the recommended post-op waiting period may be found in the labeling information or product insert for the implant or device.

If there is any concern regarding the integrity of the tissue with respect to its ability to retain the implant or object in place, the patient should not be exposed to MRI unless a radiologist gives careful consideration to the risk versus benefit aspects of the specific implant and the particular MRI conditions.

CONCLUSIONS

This chapter provided an overview of MRI issues for implants and devices and presented MRI information for several categories of medical products. Notably, there are many additional implants and devices that remain to be evaluated with regard to MRI. With the continued advances in MRI technology and the development of more sophisticated implants and devices, there is an increased potential for hazardous situations to occur in the MRI environment. Thus, all of these items require testing to determine possible risks when present in patients referred for MRI procedures.

To ensure safety for individual and patients, MRI healthcare professionals should follow the guideline whereby an MRI procedure should only be performed in a patient with a medical product that has been previously tested and demonstrated to be safe. For implants and devices with MR Conditional labeling, the specific information for a given medical product must be carefully followed to prevent patient injuries or other problems.

REFERENCES

1. Shellock FG. Reference Manual for Magnetic Resonance Safety: 2013 Edition. Los Angeles: Biomedical Research Publishing Group; 2013.

2. www.MRIsafety.com; Website devoted to MRI safety. Created and maintained by Frank G. Shellock, Ph.D.

3. Shellock FG, Crues JV. MR procedures: biologic effects, safety, and patient care. Radiology 2004;232:635-652

4. Shellock FG, Spinazzi A. MRI safety update 2008: Part 2, screening patients for MRI. AJR Am J Roentgenol 2008;191:1140-9.

5. New PFJ, Rosen BR, Brady TJ, et al. Potential hazards and artifacts of ferromagnetic and nonferromagnetic surgical and dental materials and devices in nuclear magnetic resonance imaging. Radiology 1983;147:139-148.

6. Shellock FG, Crues JV. High-field MR imaging of metallic biomedical implants: An ex vivo evaluation of deflection forces. AJR Am J Roentgenol 1988;151:389-392.

7. Shellock FG. MR imaging of metallic implants and materials: A compilation of the literature. AJR Am J Roentgenol 1988;151: 811-814.

8. Shellock FG, Schatz CJ. High field strength MRI and otologic implants. AJNR Am J Neuroradiol 1991;12:279-281.

9. Kanal E, Shellock FG. MR imaging of patients with intracranial aneurysm clips. Radiology 1993;187:612-614.

10. Shellock FG, Morisoli S, Kanal E. MR procedures and biomedical implants, materials, and devices: Update 1993. Radiology 1993;189:587-599.

11. Nogueira M, Shellock FG. Otologic bioimplants: Ex vivo assessment of ferromagnetism and artifacts at 1.5 Tesla. AJR Am J Roentgenol 1995;163:1472-1473.

12. Kanal E, Shellock FG. Aneurysm clips: effects of long-term and multiple exposures to a 1.5 Tesla MR system. Radiology 1999;210:563-5659.

13. Kangarlu A, Shellock FG. Aneurysm clips: evaluation of magnetic field interactions with an 8.0-T MR system. J Magn Reson Imaging 2000;12:107-111.

14. Shellock FG. MR safety update 2002: Implants and devices. J Magn Reson Imaging 2002;16:485-496, 2002.

15. Shellock FG. Biomedical implants and devices: assessment of magnetic field interactions with a 3.0-Tesla MR system. J Magn Reson Imaging 2002;16:721-732

16. Shellock FG, Tkach JA, Ruggieri PM, et al. Aneurysm clips: evaluation of magnetic field interactions using "long-bore" and "short-bore" 3.0-Tesla MR systems. AJNR Am J Neuroradiol 2003;24:463-471.

17. Baker KB, Tkach JA, Nyenhuis JA, et al. Evaluation of specific absorption rate as a dosimeter of MRI-related implant heating. J Magn Reson Imaging 2004;20:315-320.

18. Shellock FG, Forder JR. Drug eluting coronary stent: in vitro evaluation of magnetic resonance safety at 3 Tesla. J Cardiovasc Magn Reson 2005;7:415-9.

19. Shellock FG, Habibi R, Knebel J. Programmable CSF shunt valve: in vitro assessment of MR imaging safety at 3T. AJNR Am J Neuroradiol 2006;27:661-5.

20. Shellock FG, Wilson SF, Mauge CP. Magnetically programmable shunt valve: MRI at 3-Tesla. Magn Reson Imaging 2007;25:1116-21.

21. Shellock FG, Valencerina S. In vitro evaluation of MR imaging issues at 3T for aneurysm clips made from MP35N: Findings and information applied to 155 additional aneurysm clips. AJNR Am J Neuroradiol 2010;31:615-9.

22. Shellock FG, Bedwinek A, Oliver-Allen M, Wilson SF. Assessment of MRI issues for a 3-T "immune" programmable CSF shunt valve. AJR Am J Roentgenol 2011;197:202-7.

23. Gill A, Shellock FG. Assessment of MRI issues at 3-Tesla for metallic surgical implants: findings applied to 61 additional skin closure staples and vessel ligation clips. J Cardiovasc Magn Reson 2012;14:1-7.

24. Karacozoff AM, Shellock FG, Wakhloo AK. A next-generation, flow-diverting implant used to treat brain aneurysms: in vitro evaluation of magnetic field interactions, heating and artifacts at 3-T. Magn Reson Imaging 2013;31:145-9.

25. Escher KB, Shellock FG. An in vitro assessment of MRI issues at 3-Tesla for antimicrobial, silver-containing wound dressings. Ostomy Wound Manage 2012;58:22-7.

26. Shellock FG, Meepos LN, Stapleton MR, Valencerina S. In vitro magnetic resonance imaging evaluation of ossicular implants at 3 T. Otol Neurotol 2012;33:871-7.

27. Shellock FG, Knebel J, Prat AD. Evaluation of MRI issues for a new neurological implant, the Sensor Reservoir. Magn Reson Imaging 2013;31:1245-50.

28. Karacozoff AM, Shellock FG. In vitro assessment of a fiducial marker for lung lesions: MRI issues at 3 T. AJR Am J Roentgenol 2013;200:1234-7.

29. Sammet CL, Yang X, Wassenaar PA, et al. RF-related heating assessment of extracranial neurosurgical implants at 7 T. Magn Reson Imaging 2013;31:1029-34.

30. Dedini RD, Karacozoff AM, Shellock FG, et al. MRI issues for ballistic objects: information obtained at 1.5-, 3- and 7-Tesla. Spine J 2013;13:815-22.

31. Liu Y, Chen J, Shellock FG, Kainz W. Computational and experimental studies of an orthopedic implant: MRI-related heating at 1.5-T/64-MHz and 3-T/128-MHz. J Magn Reson Imaging 2013;37:491-7.

32. Dula AN, Virostko J, Shellock FG. Assessment of MRI issues at 7-Tesla for twenty-eight implants and other objects. AJR Am J Roentgenol (In Press)

33. Shellock FG, Valencerina S, Fischer L. MRI-related heating of pacemaker at 1.5- and 3-Tesla: Evaluation with and without pulse generator attached to leads. Circulation 2005;112;Supplement II:561.

34. Woods TO. Standards for medical devices in MRI: present and future. J Magn Reson Imaging 2007.26:1186-1189.

35. Shellock FG, Woods TO, Crues JV. MR labeling information for implants and devices: explanation of terminology. Radiology 2009;253:26-30.

36. American Society for Testing and Materials International. F2052. Standard test method for measurement of magnetically induced displacement force on passive implants in the magnetic resonance environment. American Society for Testing and Materials International, West Conshohocken, PA.

37. American Society for Testing and Materials International. F2182. Test method for Measurement of radio frequency induced heating near passive implants during magnetic resonance imaging. American Society for Testing and Materials International, West Conshohocken, PA.

38. American Society for Testing and Materials International. F2119-07, Standard test method for evaluation of MR image artifacts from passive Implants. American Society for Testing and Materials International, West Conshohocken, PA.

39. Muensterer OJ. Temporary removal of navel piercing jewelry for surgery and imaging studies. Pediatrics 2004;114:e384-6.

40. Ceballos EM, Parrish RK. Plain film imaging of Baerveldt glaucoma drainage implants. AJNR Am J Neuroradiol 2002;23:935-937.

41. Smugar SS, Schweitzer ME, Hume E. MRI in patients with intraspinal bullets. J Magn Reson Imaging 1999;9:151-153.

42. Eshed I, Kushnir T, et al. Is magnetic resonance imaging safe for patients with retained metal fragments from combat and terrorist attacks? Acta Radiol 2010;51:170-4

Chapter 17   Performing MRI in Patients with Conventional (Non-MR Conditional) Cardiac Devices

SAMAN NAZARIAN, M.D., PH.D., FHRS, FACC

Director, Ventricular Arrhythmia Ablation Service
Cardiac Electrophysiology
Johns Hopkins Hospital
Baltimore, MD

HENRY HALPERIN, M.D., M.A., FAHA

Professor of Medicine
Biomedical Engineering and Radiology
Johns Hopkins Hospital
Baltimore, MD

INTRODUCTION

Magnetic resonance imaging (MRI) provides unparalleled soft tissue resolution utilizing multiple pulse sequences, each optimized for the evaluation of particular tissue attributes. As a result, MRI is the modality of choice for numerous soft tissue conditions including various neurologic, musculoskeletal, thoracic, and abdominal abnormalities. Additionally, due to the absence of ionizing radiation, MRI is optimal for sequential imaging for disease follow-up and surveillance, as well as for diagnostic imaging in children and women of childbearing age. Parallel to the growth in use of MRI, the number of patients with permanent cardiac pacemakers and implantable cardioverter defibrillators (ICD) continues to increase. Therefore, it is inevitable that healthcare providers will face the need to perform MRI in an implantable cardiac device recipient. When performed with appropriate supervision and following a protocol for safety, many studies over the past ten years have reported the safety of MRI in patients with selected devices. However, for patients with older cardiac devices, catastrophic complications have also been reported. In this chapter, we review potential interactions of MRI with implanted cardiac devices, prior studies to assess safety, our institutional protocol for imaging, and potential effects of susceptibility artifacts.

Potential Interactions of MRI with Implanted Cardiac Devices

The electromagnetic fields used with MRI are associated with several potential risks involving implanted cardiac devices. Therefore, prior to performing clinical studies of MRI in the setting of implanted cardiac devices, our group and others performed extensive *in vitro* and *in vivo* laboratory and animal studies to understand the extent of these interactions.

Magnetic Field Interactions: Force and Torque

Ferromagnetic materials in or near the MR system are exposed to a powerful static magnetic field involving induced force (i.e., translational attraction) and torque. Therefore, a common concern among practitioners is the potential for movement of device components relative to the MR scanner. However, current lead designs contain little or no ferromagnetic components and are not likely to experience force and torque (1). Although the amount of ferromagnetic materials in cardiac device generators has substantially decreased over time and is relatively minor for modern-day systems, some ferromagnetic components remain vital to device function. The potential for movement of a pacemaker or ICD generator in the MRI environment depends upon the field strength of the static magnetic field, ferromagnetic components of the device, implant stability (i.e., how it is retained in place, *in situ*), and distance from the MR system (2). The maximal force acting upon modern permanent pacemakers (manufactured after 1996) and ICDs (manufactured after 2000) appears to be less than 0.98-Newtons (equivalent to 100-grams) in a 1.5-Tesla MR scanner. The maximum torque in our studies was not found to be substantial and, thus, is unlikely to dislodge a chronic device that is anchored to the surrounding tissue (3). These results are consistent with those of Luechinger, et al. (4) regarding modern pacemakers. However, Luechinger, et al. (4) reported that some modern ICDs may still pose problems due to strong magnetic field interactions.

Current Induction

Current may be induced within wires that are present in patients undergoing MRI examinations. Therefore, the radiofrequency (RF) and pulsed gradient magnetic fields of the MR system may induce electrical currents in leads in association with an MRI procedure. However, this is a possibility only if the lead is part of a current loop that is completed through the body (i.e., the generator must complete the current path). For cardiac pacemakers, this condition is only satisfied during specific time points within the pacing cycle and designs have been developed to overcome this limitation. The ratio of lead length versus RF wavelength and lead configurations, such as loops, are strongly associated with the extent of current induction (5-7).

We assessed the magnitude of MRI-induced current using a current recorder connected in series to single chamber permanent pacemakers programmed to sub-threshold asynchronous output during unipolar and bipolar pacing (8). Under conventional implant conditions (without additional lead loops), the magnitude of induced current was less than 0.5-mA. Current induction at greater than 30-mA resulting in myocardial capture was possible with the addition of more than four lead loops that substantially increased the total circuit area. However, the presence of so many lead loops is never observed in the clinical setting (8). Bassen and Mendoza (9) have also investigated the possibility of current induction in association with MRI and reported that unintended stimulation may occur in the setting of abandoned leads as well as leads connected to a pulse generator with loss of the hermetic seal at the connector. Additionally, Bassen and Mendoza (9) noted that pacemaker-dependent patients could receive altered pacing pulses during MRI examinations.

Heating

Another potential MRI interaction with cardiac devices is the possibility of heating and tissue damage where the lead tip contacts tissue. Metallic devices and leads can act as antennae, thus, amplifying local RF energy power deposition (10-12). In our studies utilizing clinical MRI protocols with specific absorption rates (SAR) less than 2.0-W/kg, temperature changes were limited to 1°C in an *in vitro* model and to 0.2°C in an *in vivo* model (3). However, it is important to note that due to poor correlation of heating at different SARs associated with different pulse sequences across different scanner platforms, even within the same manufacturer, the reported SAR limits from each study should not be directly applied to other MR systems. Fractured leads or lead loop configurations may increase the potential for heating even further. Epicardial leads that are not cooled by blood flow and abandoned leads may also be prone to increased heating (13, 14). The extent of heating also varies as a function of lead length and configuration, proximity to the edge of the MR system (11), proximity to the transmit RF coil (15), lead insulation thickness, and lead design (16).

Other Types of Electromagnetic Interference

Implanted cardiac devices may provide unnecessary therapies or fail to provide necessary therapies in patients are undergoing MRI procedures. Pacemakers and ICDs have the potential for receiving electromagnetic interference (EMI) in the MRI environment resulting in radiofrequency noise tracking, asynchronous pacing, inhibition of demand pacing, delivery of ICD therapies, programming changes, or loss of function. The static magnetic field of the MR system can also alter device function by inducing unexpected reed switch opening or closure. Additionally, temporary programming changes made to avoid device interaction with the scanner (such as disabling of tachycardia therapies) may lead to catastrophic results if a spontaneous arrhythmia occurs and is not recognized.

We implanted modern ICD systems (manufactured after 2000) from the three major manufacturers in the United States (U.S.) in 18 dogs, and after four weeks, performed 3- to 4-hour MRI examinations under worst-case scenario conditions (i.e., imaging over the region containing the pulse generator and using SARs up to 3.5-W/kg). No device dysfunction occurred. After 8 weeks of follow up, pacing thresholds and intracardiac electrocardiogram amplitudes were unchanged, with the exception of one animal that experienced transient (less than 12 hours) capture failure. Due to this observation, we currently do not perform MRI on pacemaker-dependent ICD patients. ICD leads are generally longer than pacemaker leads and may be more prone to heating at the lead tip. Pathological data of the scanned animals revealed very limited necrosis or fibrosis at the tip of the lead area, which was not different from controls not subjected to MRI (3). Similarly, Luechinger et al. (17) found no clear evidence of heat-induced damage on histology despite observing lead parameter changes in their *in vitro* model.

Clinical Studies of Safety

Implantable Monitors

Implantable cardiac monitors and loop recorders have been evaluated for MRI-related issues. Gimbel et al. (18) demonstrated the safety of MRI in the setting of implantable loop recorders in ten patients that underwent 11 examinations. No abnormalities were observed. Sensations of tugging or warmth at the implant site were not reported. We have also performed thoracic and non-thoracic MRI examinations on numerous implantable loop recorder recipients with similar findings of safety. Patients with an implantable loop recorder can be safely scanned under specific conditions. However, the device may record MRI-related electromagnetic interference artifacts as an arrhythmia. Therefore, care should be taken to clear episodes recorded during MRI to prevent future misinterpretation of such artifacts as clinically significant arrhythmias. The Reveal implantable monitor (Medtronic, Minneapolis, MN) received MR conditional labeling from the Food and Drug Administration (FDA) (19). Other similar devices now have labeling stating that these systems are also MR conditional (see www.MRIsafety.com for specific information pertaining to MRI labeling for implantable cardiac monitors and loop recorders).

Temporary Pacemakers

Temporary pacemakers (implanted outside of the electrophysiology laboratory) have leads that are longer and are potentially more susceptible to induction of lead currents and heating. An *in vitro* study of temporary trans-venous pacing leads showed that lead-tip heating that exceeding 15°C is common and temperature rises up to 63.1°C are possible (20). Additionally, the electronic platform of external temporary pacemakers is less sophisticated and has less filtering compared to modern permanent cardiac pacemakers. Therefore, such devices tend to be more susceptible to EMI in the MRI environment and, therefore, imaging of patients with temporary pacemakers cannot be recommended. However, we have safely performed MRI in the setting of temporary pacing utilizing an active fixation lead and externalized permanent pacemaker that had a non-conductive covering adhered to the patient's body with a pressure dressing.

Permanent Cardiac Pacemakers

Previous studies of clinical MRI in the setting of permanent cardiac pacemakers have been summarized in **Table 1**. At our institution, Johns Hopkins Hospital, we began the process of performing MRI on patients with permanent pacemakers based on findings from our *in vitro* and *in vivo* studies, which led to the development of a protocol including (a) device selection based on previous testing, (b) device programming to minimize inappropriate activation or inhibition of brady/tachyarrhythmia therapies, and (c) limitation of the specific absorption rate for the applied pulse sequences (less than 2.0-W/Kg) (21). The protocol is discussed in detail below. Using this protocol, we have now safely performed MRI on greater than 1,500 patients with implantable cardiac devices. Our latest report of safety included 237 patients with permanent cardiac pacemakers, 53 of whom were pacemaker-dependent. Pacing mode was changed to an asynchronous mode for pacemaker-dependent patients, and to demand mode for others. Blood pressure, electrocardiogram (ECG), pulse oximetry, and symptoms were monitored. The primary clinically significant event attribut-

Table 1. Clinical studies of MRI in the setting of standard permanent cardiac pacemakers.

Source	Finding
Gimbel, et al. (32)	Five patients underwent MRI. No device abnormalities were noted after MRI (0.5-Tesla). A 2-second pause was noted on pulse oximetry in the pacemaker-dependent patient whose device (with unipolar leads) was programmed to dual chamber asynchronous pacing. Patients did not report generator movement or warmth.
Sommer, et al. (33)	Eighteen patients underwent MRI. Reed switch activation and continuous pacing at a fixed rate noted in the static field. Programming changes, damage of components, dislocation/torque of the generator, and rapid pacing were not observed. Atrial and ventricular stimulation thresholds remained unchanged.
Sommer, et al. (34)	Forty-four patients were enrolled. MRI performed at 0.5-Tesla did not inhibit pacing output or cause pacemaker malfunction.
Vahlhaus, et al. (35)	Thirty-two patients underwent MRI. Lead impedance and sensing and stimulation thresholds did not change immediately or 3 months after MRI at 0.5-Tesla. However, diminished battery voltage was noted immediately after MRI with recovery 3 months later. Reed switch temporary deactivation was seen in 12 of 32 patients when positioned in the center of the bore of the MR system.
Martin, et al. (36)	Fifty-four patients underwent MRI. Cardiac, vascular and general 1.5-Tesla MRI studies were performed. Significant changes were reported in 9.4% of leads, however only 1.9% required a change in programmed output.
Del Ojo, et al. (37)	Thirteen patients underwent MRI at 2.0-Tesla. MRI was unassociated with pacemaker inhibition, inappropriate rapid pacing, or significant changes in device parameters.
Gimbel, et al. (38)	Of 10 patients that underwent imaging, seven showed a rise or fall of 0.5-V in pacing threshold values between baseline and 3-month follow-up. More patients had a decrease than a rise in pacing capture threshold.
Sommer, et al. (39)	MRI was performed in 82 patients. MRI at 1.5-Tesla was unassociated with inhibition of pacemaker output or induction of arrhythmias. However, increased capture threshold was noted post MRI. In four of 114 examinations, troponin increased from a normal baseline value to above normal after MRI (one was associated with a significant increase in capture threshold).
Nazarian, et al. (21)	In 31 patients with pacemakers (55 total patients), MRI at 1.5-Tesla was not associated with any inappropriate inhibition or activation of pacing. There were no significant differences between baseline and immediate or long-term (median 99 days after MRI) sensing amplitudes, lead impedances, or pacing thresholds.
Naehle, et al. (40)	MRI was performed in 44 patients. MRI at 3-Tesla was unassociated with changes in lead impedance, pacing capture threshold or serum Troponin-I.
Mollerus, et al. (41)	In 32 patients with pacemakers (37 total patients), MRI at 1.5-Tesla was unassociated with changes in Troponin-I levels or pacing capture thresholds.
Naehle, et al. (42)	Repetitive MRI at 1.5-Tesla (171 examinations on 47 patients) was associated with decreased pacing capture threshold and battery voltage.
Mollerus, et al. (43)	MRI was performed in 46 pacemaker recipients (52 total patients). Ectopy was observed but was unrelated to peak SAR, scan time duration, or landmark. Significant changes in pacing thresholds were not observed.

Table 1. (Continued)

Source	Finding
Mollerus, et al. (44)	MRI was performed in 105 pacemaker recipients (127 total patients). MRI at 1.5-Tesla was associated with decreased sensing amplitudes and pace impedances. Other parameters were unchanged.
Halshtok, et al. (45)	MRI was performed in nine patients with pacemakers (18 total). MRI at 1.5-Tesla was associated with 5 power-on-reset events in two patients. No other effects were reported and device replacement was unnecessary.
Strach, et al. (46)	MRI at 0.2-Tesla in 114 pacemaker recipients was unassociated with changes in lead impedance, capture threshold, or battery voltage.
Burke, et al. (47)	MRI was performed in 24 patients with pacemakers (38 total). MRI at 1.5-Tesla was unassociated with device circuitry damage, programming alterations, inappropriate shocks, failure to pace, or changes in sensing, pacing, or defibrillator thresholds.
Buendia, et al. (48)	MRI was performed in 28 patients with pacemakers (33 total patients). Temporary communication failure in two cases, sensing errors during imaging in one case, and a safety signal in one pacemaker were noted.
Nazarian, et al. (22)	MRI was performed in 237 patients with pacemakers (438 total). MRI at 1.5-Tesla was associated with two power-on-reset events. Statistically significant but clinically small (not requiring device revision or reprogramming) changes in lead parameters were observed.
Cohen, et al. (49)	MRI was performed in 69 patients with pacemakers (109 total). Decreases in battery voltage of $\geq$0.04-V in 4%, pacing threshold increases of $\geq$0.5-V in 3%, and pacing lead impedance changes of $\geq$50-Ω in 6% were observed. Clinically important differences were not observed between the MRI group and a historic control group.

able to MRI was the occurrence of power-on-reset events in up to 1.5% of device recipients. Aside from transient episodes of asynchronous pacing induced by reed switch activation in certain pacemakers, no episodes of inappropriate inhibition or activation of pacing were observed. Statistically, right ventricular sensing and atrial, and right and left ventricular lead impedances were reduced immediately after MRI. At long-term follow-up, decreased right ventricular sensing, decreased right ventricular lead impedance, increased right ventricular capture threshold, and decreased battery voltage were noted. The observed changes did not require device revision or reprogramming and there were no significant differences between baseline and immediate or long-term sensing amplitudes, lead impedances, or pacing thresholds (22).

Implantable Cardioverter Defibrillators

A summary of previous studies of performing clinical MRI in the setting of ICDs is presented in **Table 2**. During our *in vitro* testing of ICDs, we found several generators (manufactured before 2000) that were damaged by MRI. Therefore, in clinical studies, we restricted enrollment to patients with ICD systems manufactured after 2000. Based on our prior *in vitro* and *in vivo* testing, our safety protocol has now been used to safely scan more than 400 patients with ICDs. Our latest report of safety included 201 patients with ICD sys-

Table 2. Clinical MRI studies in the setting of standard ICD systems.

Source	Finding
Coman, et al. (50)	MRI was performed in 11 patients with ICD systems. One patient felt mild heating near the generator during spin echo sequences. One patient had a brief, but asymptomatic, pause in pacing during scanning. One patient with a device past the elective replacement interval had power on reset, and the device could not be interrogated after the scan. Normal device function and circuit integrity were noted at destructive testing.
Gimbel, et al. (51)	MRI was performed in seven patients with ICD systems. No changes in pacing, sensing, impedances, charge times, or battery status were observed with MRI at 1.5-Tesla. However, one implantable cardioverter defibrillator (Medtronic 7227Cx, lumbar spine MRI) experienced a "power on reset."
Nazarian, et al. (21)	MRI was performed in 24 patients with ICD systems (55 total). MRI at 1.5-Tesla was not associated with any inappropriate inhibition or activation of pacing. There were no significant differences between baseline and immediate or long-term (median 99 days after MRI) sensing amplitudes, lead impedances, or pacing thresholds.
Mollerus, et al. (41)	MRI was performed in 5 patients with ICD systems (37 total). MRI at 1.5-Tesla was unassociated with changes in Troponin-I levels or pacing capture thresholds.
Naehle, et al. (52)	MRI was performed in 18 patients with ICD systems. MRI at 1.5-Tesla was unassociated with device circuitry damage, changes in lead parameters, or Troponin-I levels. However, battery voltage decreased post MRI, and oversensing of EMI as ventricular fibrillation occurred in two devices, but therapies were not delivered.
Mollerus, et al. (43)	MRI was performed in six patients with ICD systems (52 total). Ectopy was observed but was unrelated to peak SAR, scan time duration, or landmark. Significant changes in pacing thresholds were not observed.
Pulver, et al. (53)	MRI was performed in 8 patients with ICD systems. Inappropriate pacing or significant changes in generator or lead parameters were not observed.
Mollerus, et al. (44)	MRI was performed in 22 patients with ICD systems (127 total). MRI at 1.5-Tesla was associated with decreased sensing amplitudes and pace impedances. Other parameters were unchanged.
Halshtok, et al. (45)	MRI was performed in nine patients with ICD systems (18 total). MRI at 1.5-Tesla was unassociated with any untoward effects and device replacement was unnecessary.
Burke, et al. (47)	MRI was performed in 14 patients with ICD systems (38 total). MRI at 1.5-Tesla was unassociated with device circuitry damage, programming alterations, inappropriate shocks, failure to pace, or changes in sensing, pacing, or defibrillator thresholds.
Buendia, et al. (48)	MRI was performed in five patients with ICD systems (33 total). Sensing errors during imaging in one case was noted.
Nazarian, et al. (22)	MRI was performed in 201 patients with ICD systems (438 total). MRI at 1.5-Tesla was associated with one power-on-reset event. Statistically significant but clinically small (not requiring device revision or reprogramming) changes in lead parameters were observed.
Cohen, et al. (49)	MRI was performed in 40 patients with ICD systems (109 total). Decreases in battery voltage of ≥ 0.04-V in 4%, pacing threshold increases of ≥ 0.5-V in 3%, and pacing lead impedance changes of ≥ 50-Ω in 6% were observed. Clinically important differences were not observed between the MRI group and a historic control group.

tems. All MRI examinations were completed safely and no inappropriate tachycardia therapies were delivered (22). We continue to track the safety of MRI with larger patient numbers and new cardiac pacemaker and ICD systems.

Other groups of investigators are also studying MRI safety in the setting of implanted pacemakers and ICD systems (**Table 1** and **Table 2**). A noteworthy study is the ongoing MagnaSafe Registry, a multicenter, prospective study designed to determine the frequency of major adverse clinical events and device parameter changes for 1,500 patients with standard implantable cardiac devices who undergo clinically-indicated, non-thoracic MRI at 1.5-Tesla (23-25).

Retained Leads

Retained (capped and/or cut, and abandoned) leads are susceptible to the previously described risks of heating and current induction. Depending upon the lead length and configuration, retained segments may be prone to significantly higher temperature rises than those attached to pulse generators (14). Therefore, it has been our practice to exclude patients with retained lead fragments and un-used, capped leads from MRI. However, we have performed two MRI examinations in the setting of absolute clinical necessity and retained lead segments. Both studies were completed without safety issues. More investigations on this topic are warranted to accurately delineate the risks and benefits of using MRI in this patient group.

Our Institutional Safety Protocol for MRI of Patients with Implanted Cardiac Devices

With regard to performing MRI examinations in patients with implanted cardiac devices, the safety protocol followed at our institution is based on selection of device generators previously tested under worst-case scenario (e.g., prolonged imaging over the region containing the device using SAR levels up to 3.5-W/kg) MRI conditions (3). This protocol has been summarized as a checklist in **Figure 1**.

To perform MRI on patients with implanted cardiac devices, we recommend that device generators prone to EMI (generally devices manufactured prior to 2000) be excluded. Reports of safe MRI immediately post -implantation exist in the literature (26), and the risk for lead and generator movement is extremely low. However, we recommend conservative measures to exclude patients with leads that are susceptible to spontaneous (regardless of MRI) dislodgement or that do not have chronic stable lead parameters that would allow careful measurement of safety. Therefore, we recommend avoiding MRI in patients with less than six weeks of time since the devices were implanted and those with acute parameter changes suggestive of lead malfunctions. In our experience, however, patients with mature active and passive fixation endocardial (and coronary sinus) leads of any diameter can safely undergo MRI. We do recommend avoidance of MRI when device leads are present that are prone to heating, such as nontransvenous epicardial and abandoned (capped) leads.

To reduce the risk of inappropriate inhibition of pacing due to detection of radiofrequency pulses, we program devices to an asynchronous, dedicated pacing mode in pacemaker-dependent patients. Also, given the lack of asynchronous pacing programming

Figure 1. This is the safety checklist utilized at our institution, Johns Hopkins Hospital, for performing MRI in the setting of cardiac pacemakers and implantable cardioverter defibrillators.

When was the pacemaker or ICD generator implanted?	☐ After the year 2000 ☐ Before the year 2000 • *If before the year 2000* → *cancel MRI*					
When were the leads implanted?	☐ ≥ 6 weeks ago ☐ < 6 weeks ago • *If < 6 weeks, cancel MRI*					
Are surgically placed epicardial or abandoned leads present?	☐ Yes ☐ No • *If yes, cancel MRI*					

☐ Pacemaker   ☐ ICD

Pacemaker-Dependent?	☐ Yes • *If yes, and the device is an ICD, cancel MRI* • *If yes, and the device is a pacemaker, program pacing to VOO/DOO*		☐ No • *If no, program pacing to VVI/DDI and deactivate tachycardia detection and therapies*		

• *Deactivate magnet, rate response, noise response, and all tracking and triggered pacing features*
• **Monitor blood pressure, ECG, oxygen saturation, and symptoms during MRI**

• *Device Manufacturer & model number:*	**Prior to MRI**			**After MRI**		
	Right Atrium	Right Ventricle	Left Ventricle	Right Atrium	Right Ventricle	Left Ventricle
Sensing						
Capture Threshold						
Impedance						
Battery Voltage						

• **Keep on ECG monitor after MRI until initial device programming has been restored**
• *Advise follow-up in device clinic in 3-6 months after MRI*

capability and transient loss of pacing capture after worst-case scenario (MRI involving SAR of 3.5-W/kg for 3 hours) *in vivo* testing of one of 15 animals implanted with an ICD (3), we recommend excluding pacemaker-dependent patients with ICDs.

To avoid inappropriate activation of pacing due to tracking of radiofrequency pulses, we suggest device programming in patients without pacemaker dependence to a non-tracking ventricular or dual chamber inhibited pacing mode. We also recommend deactivation of rate response, premature ventricular contraction response, ventricular sense response, and conducted atrial fibrillation response to ensure that sensing of vibrations or radiofrequency pulses does not lead to unwarranted pacing. Although asynchronous pacing for short time periods is typically well tolerated, we prefer to reduce the already minimal chance of inducing arrhythmia or causing AV dyssynchrony by minimizing asynchronous pacing in patients without pacemaker dependence through deactivation of the magnet mode when possible. We typically deactivate tachyarrhythmia monitoring to avoid battery drainage that results from recording of multiple radiofrequency pulse sequences as arrhythmic episodes. Reed switch activation in ICD systems disables tachyarrhythmia therapies. However, reed switch function in the periphery versus the bore of the MR system is unpredictable (21, 27, 28). Therefore, therapies should be disabled to avoid unwarranted antitachycardia pacing or shocks. Finally, blood pressure, ECG, pulse oximetry, and symptoms should be monitored for the duration of the MRI examination. We also favor the presence of a radiologist and cardiac electrophysiologist, or advanced cardiac life support (ACLS)-trained individual familiar with device programming and trouble shooting during all MRI examinations (21, 22, 29). At the end of the MRI procedure, all device parameters should be checked and programming should be restored to pre-MRI settings.

Figure 2. Late gadolinium-enhanced MR image obtained for planning of a ventricular tachycardia ablation procedure. Note the large susceptibility artifact due to the presence of the ICD generator. An inferior scar due to prior myocardial infarction is seen on this image.

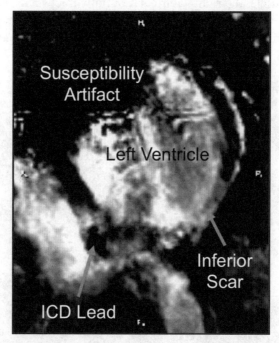

MRI Susceptibility Artifacts in the Setting of Cardiac Pacemaker and ICD Systems

The quality of the MR image is not affected when the pacemaker or ICD is located outside the field of view. However, when performing thoracic imaging, the presence of a pacemaker or ICD can cause variations in the surrounding (i.e., local) magnetic field and other issues that result in signal voids, bright areas, image distortion, or poor fat suppression. Typically, the artifacts associated with pacing and ICD leads are minimal in size. However, generator-related artifacts, particularly with ICD systems can be sizable (**Figure 2**). Such artifacts tend to be most pronounced on partial flip angle pulse sequences as well as others (e.g., inversion recovery and steady state sequences). Greater than 50% of cardiac sectors (primarily antero-apical segments) can be affected by generator susceptibility artifacts in patients with left-sided ICD systems (30). Artifacts on inversion recovery images show high signal intensity and can mimic areas of delayed-enhancement, which would otherwise indicate myocardial scar. Correlation of artifact-related bright areas on different pulse sequences can help avoid misidentification of the artifact as pathology. Selecting imaging planes perpendicular to the plane of the device generator, shortening the echo time, and using spin echo and fast spin echo sequences reduces the qualitative extent of the artifact. Using such techniques, images of sufficient quality to answer diagnostic questions can be obtained in the majority of cases (**Figure 3**).

Figure 3. MR images obtained using "TWIST" (time-resolved angiography with inter-leaved stochastic trajectories) angiography sequence in a patient with history of tetralogy of Fallot status post repair and implantation of a cardiac pacemaker. The left panel shows an enlarged right ventricle, the right ventricular outflow tract status post patch repair and mild hypoplasia of the right pulmonary artery. Minimal susceptibility artifact from the right ventricular lead is visible. The right panel shows a right-sided aortic arch with mirror image branching.

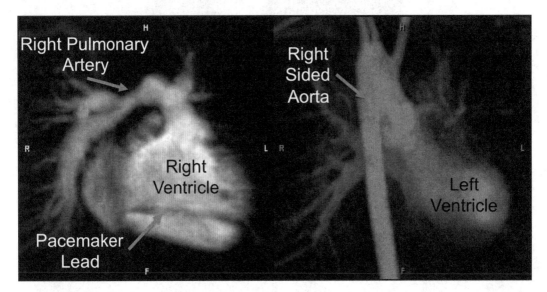

SUMMARY AND CONCLUSIONS

Magnetic resonance imaging is the favored imaging modality in many clinical scenarios. The decision to perform MRI in patients with cardiac pacemaker and ICD systems is frequently made by considering the probable benefit of MRI relative to the potential risks. Notably, it is important to conduct a systematic review of the patient's condition as well as the specific cardiac device that is present prior to proceeding with MRI. The reader is encouraged to consult other resources such as the American Heart Association Scientific Statement (31) and websites (e.g., www.mrisafety.com) that provide specific information regarding individual devices.

Disclosures

Dr. Nazarian is supported by grant K23HL089333, and Dr. Halperin is supported by grant R01-HL094610 from the National Institutes of Health. Dr. Nazarian has received honoraria for lectures from Boston Scientific, Biotronic, and St Jude Medical Inc, is on the MRI advisory panel for Medtronic Inc., and is a scientific advisor to Biosense Webster Inc. Dr. Nazarian has also received research funding from Biosense Webster. Dr. Halperin holds a patent on MRI compatible catheter technology. The Johns Hopkins University Advisory Committee on Conflict of Interest manages all commercial arrangements.

REFERENCES

1. Irnich W. Risks to pacemaker patients undergoing magnetic resonance imaging examinations. Europace 2010;12:918-920.

2. Shellock FG, Tkach JA, Ruggieri PM, Masaryk TJ. Cardiac pacemakers, ICDs, and loop recorder: evaluation of translational attraction using conventional ("long-bore") and "short-bore" 1.5- and 3.0-Tesla MR systems. J Cardiovasc Magn Reson 2003;5:387-97.

3. Roguin A, Zviman MM, Meininger GR, et al. Modern pacemaker and implantable cardioverter/defibrillator systems can be magnetic resonance imaging safe: *In vitro* and *in vivo* assessment of safety and function at 1.5 T. Circulation 2004;110:475-82.

4. Luechinger R, Duru F, Scheidegger MB, Boesiger P, Candinas R. Force and torque effects of a 1.5-Tesla MRI scanner on cardiac pacemakers and ICDs. Pacing Clin Electrophysiol 2001;24:199-205.

5. Babouri A, Hedjeidj A. *In vitro* investigation of eddy current effect on pacemaker operation generated by low frequency magnetic field. Conf Proc IEEE Eng Med Biol Soc 2007;2007:5684-7.

6. Nordbeck P, Weiss I, Ehses P, et al. Measuring RF-induced currents inside implants: Impact of device configuration on MRI safety of cardiac pacemaker leads. Magn Reson Med 2009;61:570-8.

7. Yeung CJ, Karmarkar P, McVeigh ER. Minimizing RF heating of conducting wires in MRI. Magn Reson Med 2007;58:1028-34.

8. Tandri H, Zviman MM, Wedan SR, et al. Determinants of gradient field-induced current in a pacemaker lead system in a magnetic resonance imaging environment. Heart Rhythm 2008;5:462-8.

9. Bassen HI, Mendoza GG. In-vitro mapping of E-fields induced near pacemaker leads by simulated MR gradient fields. Biomed Eng Online 2009;8:39.

10. Calcagnini G, Triventi M, Censi F, et al. *In vitro* investigation of pacemaker lead heating induced by magnetic resonance imaging: role of implant geometry. J Magn Reson Imaging 2008;28:879-86.

11. Mattei E, Triventi M, Calcagnini G, et al. Complexity of MRI induced heating on metallic leads: experimental measurements of 374 configurations. Biomed Eng Online 2008;7:11.

12. Park SM, Kamondetdacha R, Nyenhuis JA. Calculation of MRI-induced heating of an implanted medical lead wire with an electric field transfer function. J Magn Reson Imaging 2007;26:1278-85.

13. Nordbeck P, Bauer WR, Warmuth M, Hiller KH, Jakob PM, Ritter O. MRI-related heating at cardiac pacemaker leads *in vivo*. Circulation 2009;120:S371-S371.

14. Langman DA, Goldberg IB, Finn JP, Ennis DB. Pacemaker lead tip heating in abandoned and pacemaker-attached leads at 1.5 Tesla MRI. J Magn Reson Imaging 2011;33:426-431.

15. Nordbeck P, Ritter O, Weiss I, et al. Impact of imaging landmark on the risk of MRI-related heating near implanted medical devices like cardiac pacemaker leads. Magn Reson Med 2011;65:44-50.

16. Bottomley PA, Kumar A, Edelstein WA, Allen JM, Karmarkar PV. Designing passive MRI-safe implantable conducting leads with electrodes. Med Phys 2010;37:3828-43.

17. Luechinger R, Zeijlemaker VA, Pedersen EM et al. *In vivo* heating of pacemaker leads during magnetic resonance imaging. Eur Heart J 2005;26:376-83, 325-7.

18. Gimbel JR, Zarghami J, Machado C, Wilkoff BL. Safe scanning, but frequent artifacts mimicking bradycardia and tachycardia during magnetic resonance imaging (MRI) in patients with an implantable loop recorder (ILR). Ann Noninvasive Electrocardiol 2005;10:404-8.

19. Medtronic. Insertable Cardiac Monitor - Magnetic Resonance Imaging (MRI) and Reveal ICMs, http://www.medtronic.com/physician/reveal/mri.html

20. Achenbach S, Moshage W, Diem B, Bieberle T, Schibgilla V, Bachmann K. Effects of magnetic resonance imaging on cardiac pacemakers and electrodes. Am Heart J 1997;134:467-73.

21. Nazarian S, Roguin A, Zviman MM, et al. Clinical utility and safety of a protocol for noncardiac and cardiac magnetic resonance imaging of patients with permanent pacemakers and implantable-cardioverter defibrillators at 1.5 Tesla. Circulation 2006;114:1277-1284.

22. Nazarian S, Hansford R, Roguin A et al. A prospective evaluation of a protocol for magnetic resonance imaging of patients with implanted cardiac devices. Ann Intern Med 2011;155:415-24.

23. Cohen J, Costa H, Russo R. Pacemaker and implantable cardioverter defibrillator safety for patients undergoing magnetic resonance imaging (The MagnaSafe Registry). J American College of Cardiology 2009;53:A303-A304.

24. Cohen JD, Costa HS, Russo RJ. Pacemaker and implantable cardioverter defibrillator safety for patients undergoing magnetic resonance imaging (The MagnaSafe Registry). Circulation 2008;118:S778-S778.

25. Russo RJ, Costa H, Doud D, et al. Repeat MRI for patients with implanted cardiac devices does not increase the risk of clinical events or parameter changes: Preliminary results from the Magnasafe Registry. J American College of Cardiology 2012;59:E649-E649.

26. Goldsher D, Jahshan S, Roguin A. Successful cervical MR scan in a patient several hours after pacemaker implantation. Pace-Pacing and Clinical Electrophysiology 2009;32:1355-1356.

27. Lauck G, von Smekal A, Wolke S, et al. Effects of nuclear magnetic resonance imaging on cardiac pacemakers. Pacing Clin Electrophysiol 1995;18:1549-55.

28. Luechinger R, Duru F, Zeijlemaker VA, et al. Pacemaker reed switch behavior in 0.5, 1.5, and 3.0 Tesla magnetic resonance imaging units: are reed switches always closed in strong magnetic fields? Pacing Clin Electrophysiol 2002;25:1419-23.

29. Nazarian S, Halperin HR. How to perform magnetic resonance imaging on patients with implantable cardiac arrhythmia devices. Heart Rhythm 2009;6:138-43.

30. Sasaki T, Hansford R, Zviman MM et al. Quantitative assessment of artifacts on cardiac magnetic resonance imaging of patients with pacemakers and implantable cardioverter-defibrillators. Circ Cardiovasc Imaging 2011;4:662-70.

31. Levine GN, Gomes AS, Arai AE et al. Safety of magnetic resonance imaging in patients with cardiovascular devices: an American Heart Association scientific statement from the Committee on Diagnostic and Interventional Cardiac Catheterization, Council on Clinical Cardiology, and the Council on Cardiovascular Radiology and Intervention: endorsed by the American College of Cardiology Foundation, the North American Society for Cardiac Imaging, and the Society for Cardiovascular Magnetic Resonance. Circulation 2007;116:2878-91.

32. Gimbel JR, Johnson D, Levine PA, Wilkoff BL. Safe performance of magnetic resonance imaging on five patients with permanent cardiac pacemakers. Pacing Clin Electrophysiol 1996;19:913-9.

33. Sommer T, Lauck G, Schimpf R et al. [MRI in patients with cardiac pacemakers: *In vitro* and *in vivo* evaluation at 0.5 tesla]. Rofo 1998;168:36-43.

34. Sommer T, Vahlhaus C, Lauck G et al. MR imaging and cardiac pacemakers: in-vitro evaluation and in-vivo studies in 51 patients at 0.5 T. Radiology 2000;215:869-79.

35. Vahlhaus C, Sommer T, Lewalter T et al. Interference with cardiac pacemakers by magnetic resonance imaging: are there irreversible changes at 0.5 Tesla? Pacing Clin Electrophysiol 2001;24:489-95.

36. Martin ET, Coman JA, Shellock FG, et al. Magnetic resonance imaging and cardiac pacemaker safety at 1.5-Tesla. J Am Coll Cardiol 2004;43:1315-24.

37. Del Ojo JL, Moya F, Villalba J et al. Is magnetic resonance imaging safe in cardiac pacemaker recipients? Pacing Clin Electrophysiol 2005;28:274-8.

38. Gimbel JR, Bailey SM, Tchou PJ, Ruggieri PM, Wilkoff BL. Strategies for the safe magnetic resonance imaging of pacemaker-dependent patients. Pacing Clin Electrophysiol 2005;28:1041-6.

39. Sommer T, Naehle CP, Yang A et al. Strategy for safe performance of extrathoracic magnetic resonance imaging at 1.5 tesla in the presence of cardiac pacemakers in non-pacemaker-dependent patients: a prospective study with 115 examinations. Circulation 2006;114:1285-92.

40. Naehle CP, Meyer C, Thomas D et al. Safety of brain 3-T MR imaging with transmit-receive head coil in patients with cardiac pacemakers: pilot prospective study with 51 examinations. Radiology 2008;249:991-1001.

41. Mollerus M, Albin G, Lipinski M, Lucca J. Cardiac biomarkers in patients with permanent pacemakers and implantable cardioverter-defibrillators undergoing an MRI scan. Pacing Clin Electrophysiol 2008;31:1241-5.

42. Naehle CP, Zeijlemaker V, Thomas D et al. Evaluation of cumulative effects of MR imaging on pacemaker systems at 1.5 Tesla. Pacing Clin Electrophysiol 2009;32:1526-35.

43. Mollerus M, Albin G, Lipinski M, Lucca J. Ectopy in patients with permanent pacemakers and implantable cardioverter-defibrillators undergoing an MRI scan. Pacing Clin Electrophysiol 2009;32:772-8.

44. Mollerus M, Albin G, Lipinski M, Lucca J. Magnetic resonance imaging of pacemakers and implantable cardioverter-defibrillators without specific absorption rate restrictions. Europace 2010;12:947-51.

45. Halshtok O, Goitein O, Abu Sham'a R, Granit H, Glikson M, Konen E. Pacemakers and magnetic resonance imaging: no longer an absolute contraindication when scanned correctly. Isr Med Assoc J;12:391-5.

46. Strach K, Naehle CP, Muhlsteffen A et al. Low-field magnetic resonance imaging: increased safety for pacemaker patients? Europace;12:952-60.

47. Burke PT, Ghanbari H, Alexander PB, et al. A protocol for patients with cardiovascular implantable devices undergoing magnetic resonance imaging (MRI): should defibrillation threshold testing be performed post-(MRI). J Interv Card Electrophysiol 2010;28:59-66.

48. Buendia F, Sanchez-Gomez JM, Sancho-Tello MJ et al. Nuclear magnetic resonance imaging in patients with cardiac pacing devices. Rev Esp Cardiol 2010;63:735-9.

49. Cohen JD, Costa HS, Russo RJ. Determining the risks of magnetic resonance imaging at 1.5 tesla for patients with pacemakers and implantable cardioverter defibrillators. Am J Cardiol 2012;110:1631-6.

50. Coman JA, Martin ET, Sandler DA, Thomas JR. Implantable cardiac defibrillator interactions with magnetic resonance imaging at 1.5 Tesla. JAmerican College of Cardiology 2004;43:138A-138A.

51. Gimbel JR, Kanal E, Schwartz KM, Wilkoff BL. Outcome of magnetic resonance imaging (MRI) in selected patients with implantable cardioverter defibrillators (ICDs). Pacing Clin Electrophysiol 2005;28:270-3.

52. Naehle CP, Strach K, Thomas D et al. Magnetic resonance imaging at 1.5-T in patients with implantable cardioverter-defibrillators. J Am Coll Cardiol 2009;54:549-55.

53. Pulver AF, Puchalski MD, Bradley DJ et al. Safety and imaging quality of MRI in pediatric and adult congenital heart disease patients with pacemakers. Pacing Clin Electrophysiol 2009;32:450-6.

Chapter 18 MRI and Cardiac Devices: MR Conditional Pacemakers and Implantable Cardioverter Defibrillators

JEROLD S. SHINBANE, M.D., FACC, FHRS, FSCCT

Associate Professor of Clinical Medicine
Director, USC Arrhythmia Center
Director, Cardiovascular Computed Tomography/Division of Cardiovascular Medicine
Division of Cardiovascular Medicine
Cardiovascular and Thoracic Institute
Keck School of Medicine
University of Southern California
Los Angeles, CA

JOHN SUMMERS, M.D., FACC

Electrophysiology Fellow
Division of Cardiovascular Medicine
Cardiovascular and Thoracic Institute
Keck School of Medicine
University of Southern California
Los Angeles, CA

INTRODUCTION

The brisk pace of technologic evolution of magnetic resonance imaging (MRI) has led to a broad spectrum of medical applications (1). In parallel, cardiac device technologies have been developed for arrhythmia diagnosis as well as treatment of bradyarrhythmias, tachyarrhythmias and for therapy of heart failure (2). The implementation of these two technologies has reached a crossroads, as increasingly, patients with cardiac devices may require MRI but may be limited by the presence of the cardiac device (3). Assessment of the potential interactions between cardiac devices and the MRI environment are important to the current and future design of MR systems and cardiac devices in order to increase accessibility to MRI for patients with these electronically activated devices.

THE PRE-MR CONDITIONAL CARDIAC DEVICE ERA

The study of MRI/cardiac device interactions stems from known theoretical physics concerns related to the ferromagnetic content of cardiac devices, the effects of time-varying magnetic fields, and the effects of radiofrequency (RF) energy on the structure and function of cardiac pulse generators and lead systems. In the era prior to the development of MR Conditional cardiac devices (i.e., those devices specially designed to be acceptable for patients undergoing MRI examinations), these device/MRI issues had been studied through multiple means including, the following: *in vitro* assessments, *in vivo* animal models, case reports, small retrospective series of patients inadvertently or intentionally exposed to the MRI environment, and prospective series of patients intentionally exposed to MRI procedures under specified conditions. Each of these lines of research provided data regarding MRI/cardiac device interactions but had inherent limitations. *In vitro* studies allow study of the physics of cardiac device/MRI interactions but are limited because phantoms do not adequately reproduce the three-dimensional anatomy or physiology of the patient or physiologic device function. Animal models are generally limited by the lack of applicability to humans. Initial rare case reports of inadvertently scanned patients with associated mortality suffer from incomplete information on the patients, specific circumstances of the studies and a lack of physiologic monitoring (4-7). Retrospective and prospective studies of patients with preexisting devices do not serve as a true surrogate for a safety investigation.

Data from the pre-MR Conditional cardiac device era have demonstrated a small number of adverse events of variable clinical significance in patients with cardiac pacemakers and implantable cardioverter defibrillators (ICDs) who underwent MRI (**Table 1**) (5, 7-76). In regard to permanent cardiac pacemakers, prospective series of patients intentionally exposed to the MRI examinations under specified conditions have demonstrated various findings including pulse generators changing to the asynchronous mode due to activation of the reed switch in all patients (77), a decrease in battery voltage recovered at three months (23), a significant change in the pacing threshold requiring an increase in programmed output (32), a transient change to the elective replacement indicator (ERI) (43), small variances in the pacing threshold (36), statistically significant but clinically unimportant changes in the pacing capture threshold, battery voltage, and lead impedance which did not require an increase in pacing output (53, 66, 78), ventricular lead impedance rise necessitating lead replacement (76), pacing at maximum voltage at a fixed rate of 100-beats/minute (55), asystole (63), MRI-related ectopy (65), and temporary communication failures, sensing errors, and safety signals generated (79).

In regard to ICDs, some intentional scans and prospective studies have demonstrated no adverse effects (41, 46, 49, 50, 60). Other studies of patients inadvertently subjected to MRI have shown inappropriate sensing, battery voltage transient change to End-of-Life (EOL) (25), inability to communicate with the device (31), noise detected as ventricular tachycardia and ventricular fibrillation, with no therapy presumably due to magnetic mode activation and asynchronous pacing as a result of a change to the noise-reversal mode (51). Prospective studies have shown "power-on-reset" electrical reset requiring reprogramming

Table 1. Summary of MRI examinations involving patients with cardiac pacemakers and ICDs.

Author	Device	Year	Patient/Studies Report Type	MRI Condition	Findings
Iberer, et al. (12)	PPM	1987	1/1 Case Study	Unknown	No adverse effect.
Alonga, et al. (14)	PPM	1989	1/1 Case Intentional	1.5-T Brain	No adverse effect.
Inbar, et al. (15)	PPM	1993	1/1 Case Intentional	1.5-T Brain	No adverse effect.
Gimbel, et al. (18)	PPM	1996	5/5 Retrospective Intentional	0.35- to 1.5-T Cardiac, Brain, C-Spine	Two second pause.
Garcia-Boloa, et al. (19)	PPM	1998	1/2 Case Intentional	1-T Brain	No adverse effect.
Fontaine, et al. (109)	PPM	1998	1/1 Case Intentional	1.5-T Brain, C-Spine	Rapid pacing.
Sommer, et al. (77)	PPM	1998	18/18 Prospective	0.5-T Brain, Cardiac, Vascular	Asynchronous mode due to activation of the reed switch in all patients.
Sommer, et al. (21)	PPM	2000	45/51 Prospective	0.5-T Multiple	No adverse effect.
Valhaus, et al. (23)	PPM	2001	32/34 Prospective	0.5-T Multiple	Decrease in battery voltage recovered at three months.
Anfinsen, et al. (25)	ICD	2002	1/1 Case Inadvertent	0.5-T Brain	Inappropriate sensing, battery voltage transient change to EOL.
Martin, et al. (32)	PPM	2004	54/62 Prospective	1.5-T Multiple	Significant change in pacing threshold in 9.4% of leads, and 1.9% of leads requiring an increase in programmed output.
Fiek, et al. (31)	ICD	2004	1/1 Case Inadvertent	0.5-T Brain	Unable to communicate with device.
Coman, et al. (33)	ICD	2004	11/11 Prospective	1.5-T Cardiac, Vascular, General	Brief asymptomatic pause in one patient. Unable to communicate with device in one patient.
Del Ojo, et al. (35)	PPM	2005	13/13 Prospective	2-T Multiple	No adverse effect.
Rozner, et al. (43)	PPM	2005	2/2 Case Intentional	1.5-T Thorax, Lumbar	Transient change to ERI in one patient.
Gimbel, et al. (36)	PPM	2005	10/11 Prospective	1.5-T Brain, C-Spine	Small variances in pacing threshold were seen in four patients.

Table 1. (Continued) Summary of MRI examinations involving patients with cardiac pacemakers and ICDs.

Author	Device	Year	Patient/Studies Report Type	MRI Condition	Findings
Gimbel, et al. (37)	ICD	2005	7/8 Prospective	1.5-T Brain, L-Spine	"Power on reset" electrical reset requiring reprogramming in one patient.
Roguin, et al. (41)	ICD	2005	1/1 Case Intentional	1.5-T Cardiac	No adverse effect.
Wollmann, et al. (46)	ICD	2005	1/3 Case Intentional	1.5-T Brain	No adverse effect.
Sardanelli, et al. (47)	PPM	2006	1/1 Case Intentional	1.5-T Breast	No adverse effect.
Sommer, et al. (53)	PPM	2006	115/82 Prospective	1.5-T Extra-thoracic	Significant increase in pacing threshold, decreased lead impedance, and decrease in battery voltage. No inhibition of pacing or arrhythmias and no leads that required an increase in pacing output.
Naehle, et al. (49)	ICD	2006	1/1 Case Intentional	1.5-T Brain	No adverse effect.
Nazarian, et al. (50)	PPM 31 ICD 24	2006	55/68 Prospective	1.5-T	No adverse effect.
Nemec, et al. (51)	ICD	2006	1/1 Case Unintentional	Unknown Brain	Noise detected as ventricular tachycardia and ventricular fibrillation, with no therapy presumably due to magnetic mode activation. Asynchronous pacing due to noise-reversal mode.
Heatlie, et al. (55)	PPM	2007	5/6 Prospective	0.5-T Cardiac	Pacing at maximum voltage at a fixed rate of 100 beats/minute in one patient.
Mollerus, et al. (60)	PPM 32 ICD 5	2008	37/40 Prospective	1.5-T Truncal, Non-truncal	No adverse effect. No changes in cardiac troponin-I.
Naehle, et al. (61)	PPM	2008	44/51 Prospective	3-T Brain	No adverse effect. No changes in cardiac troponin-I. (Use of transmit-receive head coil).

Table 1. (Continued) Summary of MRI examinations involving patients with cardiac pacemakers and ICDs.

Author	Device	Year	Patient/Studies Report Type	MRI Condition	Findings
Gimbel, et al. (63)	PPM	2009	1/1 Case Intentional	1-T Brain	Asystole.
Goldsher, et al. (64)	PPM	2009	1/1 Case Intentional	1.5-T Cervical	No adverse effect. Scan one day after implant Pacemaker-dependent.
Mollerus, et al. (65)	PPM 46 ICD 6	2009	52/59 Prospective	1.5-T Truncal, Non-truncal	MRI-related ectopy in seven patients.
Naehle, et al. (66)	PPM	2009	47/171 Case Intentional	1.5-T General	Statistically significant but clinically irrelevant change in pacing capture threshold and battery voltage. Two or more serial scans.
Pulver, et al. (68)	PPM	2009	8/11 Prospective	1.5-T Cardiac, Non-cardiac	No adverse effect. Congenital heart disease with nine epicardial leads.
Strach, et al. (71)	PPM	2010	114/114 Prospective	0.2-T General	No adverse effect.
Millar, et al. (70)	PPM	2010	1/1 Case Study	1.5-T Brain C-spine	No adverse effects.
Burke, et al. (81)	PPM 24 ICD 10 CRT ICD 4	2010	38/92 Prospective	1.5-T Brain, Spine, Pelvis, Extremity	No adverse effects No changes defibrillation threshold (ICD).
Buendia, et al. (79)	PPM 28 ICD 5	2010	33/33 Prospective	1.5-T Cardiac, Brain, Spine, Abdominal, Extremity	Temporary communication failure in two patients. Sensing errors during imaging in two patients. Safety signal generated in one pacemaker at the maximum magnetic resonance frequency and output level.
Naehle, et al. (123)	PPM 22 ICD 10	2011	32/32 Prospective	1.5-T Cardiac	No adverse effect. Diagnostic value greater for right-sided than left-sided implants.

Table 1. (Continued) Summary of MRI examinations involving patients with cardiac pacemakers and ICDs.

Author	Device	Year	Patient/Studies Report Type	MRI Condition	Findings
Nazarian, et al. (82)	PPM 54% ICD 46% CRT System 12%	2011	438/555 Prospective	1.5-T Thoracic, Non-thoracic.	Changes in right ventricular sensing, lead impedances, increased capture threshold and decreased battery voltage were noted at six month follow-up, but did not require device revision or reprogramming. In 1.5% of patients, transient reversions to back-up programming mode were noted (power-on-reset) without long-term sequelae.
Wilkoff, et al. (98)	MR Conditional PPM	2011	226/226 Prospective	1.5-T Brain, Lumbar	No adverse effect.
Quarta, et al. (122)	MR Conditional PPM	2011	1/1 Prospective	1.5-T Brain, Cardiac	No adverse effect.
Baser, et al. (76)	PPM	2012	1/1 Prospective	Unknown Brain	Ventricular lead increased impedance and elevation of cardiac biomarkers. Ventricular lead was replaced.
Cohen, et al. (80)	PPM 85 ICD 40	2012	109/125 Retrospective Case Controlled	1.5-T Brain, Spine (All levels), Cardiac, Extremities	Decreases in battery voltage. Pacing threshold increases. Pacing lead impedance changes. Changes statistically significant but not clinically important and similar to control group.
Russo, et al. (84)	PPM 447 ICD 153	2012	600/600 Prospective MagnaSafe Registry	1.5-T Non-thoracic	No deaths, device failures, generator or lead replacements, ventricular arrhythmias or losses of capture. One or more clinically-relevant device parameter change occurred in 13% of pacemaker and 31% of ICD cases.

Table 1. (Continued) Summary of MRI examinations involving patients with cardiac pacemakers and ICDs.

Author	Device	Year	Patient/Studies Report Type	MRI Condition	Findings
Wollmann, et al. (124)	MR Conditional PPM	2012	30/30 Prospective	1.5-T Brain Lower lumbar spine	No serious adverse device effects on sensing, pacing or lead impedance. Imaging artifacts on brain diffusion weighted sequences.

Adapted and updated from Shinbane, et al. 2011 (74) with permission. Case, case report; CRT, cardiac resynchronization therapy; EOL, end-of-life; ERI, elective replacement indicator; ICD, implantable cardioverter defibrillator; PPM, pacemaker; T, Tesla

(37), MRI-related ectopy (65), a brief asymptomatic pause and inability to communicate with the ICD (33), and sensing errors during MRI (79). A retrospective case controlled study demonstrated decreases in battery voltage, pacing threshold increases, and pacing lead impedance changes that were statistically significant but clinically unimportant (80). In addition to issues related to performing MRI in patients with ICDs, whether ICD defibrillation threshold testing should be assessed after exposure to the MRI environment requires investigation (81).

In a large prospective study using MRI in patients with implanted cardiac devices, a total of 438 patients with devices (54% pacemakers and 46% ICDs) were enrolled between 2003 and 2010 (82). Of these patients, 53 (12%) had biventricular pacing systems. Patients with new devices (less than six weeks), abandoned or epicardial leads, and pacemaker-dependent patients were excluded. Pacemaker-dependent ICD patients were excluded. Of a total of 555 MRI examinations (1.5-Tesla/64-MHz), 18% of the scans were thoracic and 82% were non-thoracic. Although changes in right ventricular sensing, lead impedances, increased capture threshold and decreased battery voltage were noted at the six month follow up interval, observed changes did not require device revision or reprogramming. In three (1.5%) of the patients, transient reversions to back-up programming mode were noted (i.e., power-on-reset) without long-term sequelae.

Additionally, pacemaker and ICD data is being obtained through prospective registries. The MagnaSafe Registry is an ongoing physician initiated prospective multicenter site registry of patients with pacemakers and ICDs undergoing clinically-indicated, 1.5-Tesla/64-MHz non-thoracic scanning under specified conditions (78). Preliminary results of the first 600 cases (447 pacemakers, 153 ICDs, 1,161 leads implanted between April, 2009 and May, 2012) enrolled in the MagnaSafe Registry demonstrated no deaths, device failures, pulse generator or lead replacements, ventricular arrhythmias or losses of capture during non-thoracic MRI examinations (84). Of this cohort, 20% of the registry patients were pacemaker-dependent. One or more clinically relevant device parameter change occurred in 13% of pacemaker and 31% of ICD cases. Sub-analysis suggested repeat MRI for patients with implanted cardiac devices does not increase the risks of clinical events or parameter changes. The frequency of one or more parameter change event was 15% in those with and 18% of those without a previous MRI examination. Sub-analysis suggested repeat MRI for patients with implanted cardiac devices does not increase the risks of clinical events or parameter changes (85).

THE MR CONDITIONAL DEVICE ERA

The initial body of data related to use of MRI in patients with cardiac devices raised questions as to whether patients with important clinical issues to be resolved and no other adequate imaging options have absolute contraindications to MRI, have scanning performed based on the risk benefit ratio, or would require the engineering of cardiac devices with an MR Conditional status (57, 74, 75, 86-94). The limitations inherent in investigating and scanning patients with previous era devices has led to the development of cardiac devices, specifically designed for the MRI environment under specified conditions. Notably, a variety of MR Conditional devices are in development, testing, or released for use in the clinical setting. Each commercially available device has specified device and functional requirements as well as MRI parameters and conditions defined in the labeling and approved by the specific regulatory agency of the country where the device has been clinically released. The specifics for these cardiac devices include information, as follows: device implant site/position; limitations related to the presence of other devices/leads; acceptable lead impedance, sensing and pacing parameters for MRI; device implant timing prior to MRI; programmed mode during MRI; device identifiers or markings; type of MR system that may be used; potential limitations to landmark isocenter of the transmit radiofrequency energy (RF) coil; patient positioning within the transmit RF coil; and limitations on the specific absorption rate (SAR) to be used for the MRI examination.

MR CONDITIONAL DESIGN AND ENGINEERING

The precise use of nomenclature is extremely important to understanding and implementing technologies as it pertains to specific patient and scanning conditions in the MRI environment (95). The American Society of Testing Materials (ATSM) International designates implants and devices as MR Safe, MR Conditional, and MR Unsafe (96). An MR Safe designated device would require nonmetallic, non-conducting materials and systems with no known hazards in all MRI environments. Thus, the engineering of an MR Safe designated pacemaker or ICD is not feasible. An MR Conditional designated device refers to an item that has been demonstrated to pose no known hazard in a specified MRI environment under defined conditions of use. These defined conditions include the strength of the static magnetic field, spatial gradient magnetic field, time-varying magnetic fields, RF fields and specific absorption rate (SAR). Cardiac devices designated as MR Conditional must be used in a specified MRI environment under defined programming parameters and with close attention to the patient specific clinical factors, such as the presence of abandoned leads. MR Conditional designs have sought to take the theoretical and investigational concerns related to cardiac devices and to create designs to minimize the possibility for interactions when implanted in patients undergoing MRI examinations. Notably, the design and engineering of devices extends to all components including the pulse generator, leads, and programmer.

ELECTROMAGNETIC-RELATED ISSUES

Because MRI involves the use of static, gradient, and RF electromagnetic fields, these must be carefully considered because they can lead to substantial MRI/cardiac device interactions. Physical forces on ferromagnetic objects due to static and gradient magnetic fields can cause movement and/or vibration of these objects. Factors affecting these forces include the quantity and shape of the ferromagnetic content, proximity to the magnet, and strength of the static magnetic field (97). Studies of non-MR Conditional and MR Conditional pacemakers at 1.5-Tesla/64-MHz have not demonstrate significant clinical effects (35, 61, 98).

Conduction of electromagnetic energy through the device can occur due to pulsed RF energy or the time-varying magnetic fields, leading to heating or interference with sensing or pacing. This potential energy transfer is dependent on factors including, the following: the time-varying magnetic fields; the type of RF pulse used in the MRI sequences; the whole body averaged and local SARs; the spatial relationship and orientation of the device relative to the transmit RF coil; and the composition, length, geometry, configuration, and orientation of the lead(s) (54, 58, 59, 67, 99-102).

PULSE GENERATOR DESIGN

The reduction of ferromagnetic content of the pacemaker or ICD pulse generator can decrease magnetic field interactions. This requires the use of non-ferromagnetic materials with the appropriate characteristics including those related to conductivity, durability, and biocompatibility. The pulse generator's reed switch is susceptible to magnetic fields because this component allows the use of an external magnet to program continuous asynchronous pacing while in contact with the skin overlying the pulse generator in order to avoid electromagnetic interactions with the use of electrocautery during surgical procedures (103).

When present in the MR system, reed switch activity may be unpredictable, potentially varying with the orientation between the reed switch and magnetic field as well as with the strength of the static magnetic field (7, 17, 29, 98, 104). One option is to replace the reed switch with a solid state Hall sensor, which possesses more predictable function in magnetic fields (7, 17, 29, 98, 104). Other design changes have been formulated such as a magnetic field detection sensor that prevents reed switch issues (105). Other pulse generator design features include generator shielding and circuitry filters to inhibit or divert transference of particular electromagnetic frequencies. Importantly, ICD pulse generators are larger and more complicated than pacemaker pulse generators and have greater ferromagnetic content, circuitry hardware related to arrhythmia detection and treatment, and capacitors for cardioversion and defibrillation (106-108). Therefore, MRI issues related to ICDs versus cardiac pacemakers tend to be more problematic.

CARDIAC DEVICE LEADS

Pacemaker and ICD leads are composed of non-magnetic materials. With regard to MRI issues, leads may serve as antennas conducting electromagnetic energy impulses (30, 109). The effects of this energy transfer could potentially include pain, myocardial stimulation, heating with myocardial necrosis at the lead tip, and damage to the pulse generator. Adverse effects potentially include inappropriate sensing, increases in pacing threshold, and lead impedance changes. These factors could lead to inappropriate pacing function with associated bradyarrhythmias or tachyarrhythmias and battery depletion (7, 8, 10, 11, 13, 23, 32, 34, 36, 43, 45, 53, 55, 65, 66, 79, 109,110). These aforementioned effects can be due to the transference of MRI-related electromagnetic energies at the resonant frequency of the lead. Importantly, a resonant lead length has been associated with a greater heating effect (111).

Therefore, a focus of lead design and engineering is to avoid the resonant frequencies of the electromagnetic sources associated with MR systems through consideration of factors such a lead length, configuration, and morphology. In regard to heating, lead length, lead coiling, and the position of the lead in relation to the transmit RF coil can affect heating (59, 102, 112, 113). Lead wire coiling in a three-dimensional orientation is an important factor in transference or avoidance of the resonant frequency of electromagnetic energy (38). Decreasing the number of coiled filars, increasing the diameter of the filars and subsequent increases in the winding turns of the coils has resulted in a three-dimensional morphology for the lead that limits the conduction of MRI relevant frequencies in one design, while maintaining the strength of the lead (114). Furthermore, the use of a lead tip coating has decreased polarization. Because unipolar pacing is more susceptible to the environmental electromagnetic noise including that associated with the MR system, a bipolar lead configuration is also important to lead design (24, 45).

Since MR Conditional systems have specially designed leads, MR Conditional pulse generators cannot be simply attached to pre-existing, non-MR Conditional leads and still be considered MR Conditional. Additionally, the presence of abandoned leads can lead to conduction of electromagnetic energy and, therefore, may pose hazards when scanning a patient with an MR Conditional cardiac device (72). Therefore, abandoned leads should not be present in order to avoid lead-related issues during MRI (98). By comparison, retained epicardial wires cut short at the skin level from previous cardiothoracic surgery procedures have not been associated with significant issues during MRI (115, 116).

DEVICE PROGRAMMING

The design of an MR Conditional device requires clearly demarcated MR Conditional programming modes for the period of time when the patient undergoes an MRI examination. Programming decisions require knowledge of the patients underlying sinus rate, atrial-ventricular (AV) nodal conduction, ventricular rate and presence rate, and location of escape rhythms (**Figures 1** to **3**). These programming modes inactivate sensing and, therefore, the pacing function is either inactivated in a patient with a stable non-bradycardic rhythm or set to an asynchronous pacing mode in a pacemaker-dependent patient. Each mode possesses its own potential limitations. A patient with a non-bradycardic rhythm at the time of programming could potentially have a bradyarrhythmia while in the scanner. If a patient programmed to an asynchronous pacing mode has a ventricular rate competing with asynchronous pacing, paced beats could occur during the vulnerable period of ventricular repolarization (i.e., the R-on-T phenomenon) potentially triggering ventricular tachycardia or ventricular fibrillation (7, 117, 118). In regard to ICDs, the same pacing function issues

Figure 1. Pacemaker electrocardiograms in the setting of an intrinsic rhythm (non-pacemaker-dependent rhythm). There is an intrinsic sinus rhythm at 80-beats/min. with normal AV nodal conduction. This patient could potentially be programmed to the OOO-mode (non-functioning) for MRI. AS, atrial sensed rhythm; VS, ventricular sensed rhythm.

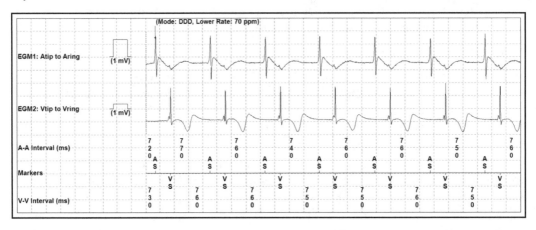

Figure 2. Pacemaker electrocardiogram in the setting of pacemaker-dependence. There is no underlying intrinsic ventricular rhythm with ventricular pacing at 35-beats/min. A patient with this rhythm would need to be programmed to an asynchronous mode (DOO or VOO) for an MRI examination. VP, ventricular paced rhythm.

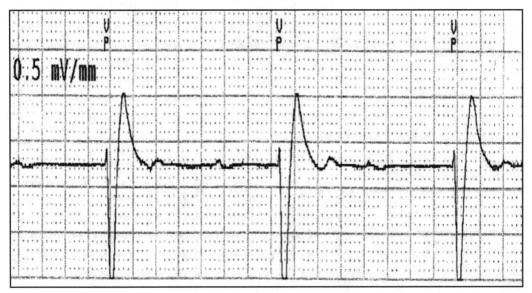

Figure 3. "Noise" in the cardiac pacing lead can result in inappropriate inhibition of ventricular pacing with ventricular pauses. Lead noise can be caused by electromagnetic interference due to operation of the MR system.

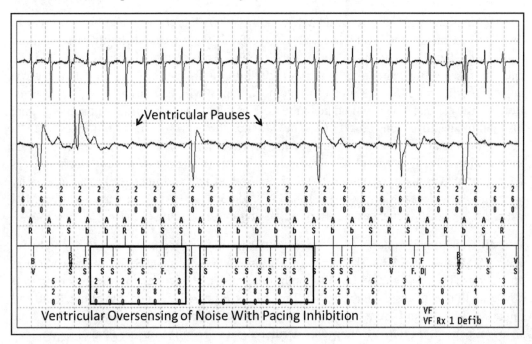

apply. In addition, antitachycardia therapies need to be inactivated during MRI. It remains unclear if ICD capacitors can properly charge in the MRI environment (49).

Given the possibilities of bradyarrhythmias or tachyarrhythmias while the patient is in an MR Conditional mode, continuous monitoring of the patient's heart rate and rhythm as well as the ability to respond to an arrhythmia is required while the patient is programmed in the appropriate MR Conditional mode for cardiac pacemakers or ICDs. As the device programmer must stay outside of the MR system room, device programming immediately before entering the MRI environment and reprogramming immediately after removal from the MRI setting can limit the amount of time that the patient is in the MR Conditional mode. Programming that permits storing pre-MRI parameters for reprogramming the device after the MRI procedure is essential.

THE MR SYSTEM AND CARDIAC DEVICES

The initial generation of MR Conditional cardiac devices has been approved by regulatory agencies for 1.5-Tesla/64-MHz scanners. Notably, performing MRI examinations using scanners greater than or less than 1.5-Tesla/64-MHz will require further design considerations and investigation (61, 63, 114, 119).

Specifically in regard to static magnetic field forces, a lower magnetic field strength and a greater distance of the cardiac device from the magnet of the MR system can decrease magnetic field interactions. The use of specialized dedicated-extremity or niche scanners used in patients with cardiac devices has been previously reported and requires further assessment (20, 120, 121)

The first commercially-released MR conditional cardiac devices had limitations with respect to the transmit RF coil isocenter, which effectively prohibited chest/thorax MRI examinations. Later regulatory-approved cardiac devices in certain countries have allowed chest/thorax imaging. The investigation of the ability to image this anatomic area is obviously important to allow the greater implementation of MR Conditional cardiac devices. Because the cardiac device would be in the field of view, imaging artifacts related to signal loss and image distortion caused by the device (i.e., the pulse generator and leads) are important factors that impact the diagnostic use of MRI, particularly for cardiac and thoracic examinations (34, 41, 50, 68, 122). Research studies involving non-MR Conditional devices with cardiac imaging have demonstrated decreased artifact and improved imaging quality with cardiac devices positioned in the right chest region (123). Artifacts can also affect MRI when certain pulse sequences are used during non-chest imaging (124).

MR Conditional systems have specific SAR limitations regarding the whole body averaged SAR and the SAR at the region of interest, such as the head SAR for brain MRI examinations. The proliferation of MR Conditional cardiac devices and future generations of devices will need to evaluate these SAR limitations, especially in regard to clinically useful ranges of SARs for different types of MRI procedures. Additionally, the impact of multiple scans on patients with MR Conditional cardiac devices requires further investigation.

MR CONDITIONAL CARDIAC DEVICE SYSTEMS

MR Conditional cardiac pacemakers are now commercially available for clinical use, under active investigation, or planned for future studies (98, 104, 124, 126-133). The MR Conditional platforms consist of an MR Conditional pulse generator, MR Conditional leads, and an MR Conditional programming device.

A randomized, unblinded, two arm multicenter study of patients with standard criteria for dual chamber pacing (484 enrolled, 464 with successful implant, 258 randomized to a single non-medically indicated MRI examination and 206 randomized to a control group) reported no significant changes in pacing parameters (i.e., sensing, threshold, or impedance changes) compared to controls (98). Both pacemaker-dependent and non-pacemaker dependent patients were studied, with devices in the asynchronous mode (n = 158) and no pacing (n = 67). The patients had continuous stable rhythms during MRI without complications reported through the one month visit including arrhythmias, electrical reset, inhibition of generator output, or adverse sensations.

A single center prospective non-randomized study of patients with standard pacemaker indications was performed in patients undergoing brain and lower lumbar spine MRI at 1.5-Tesla/64-MHz (124). Of the 30 patients scanned that were evaluated immediately pre-study, immediately after MRI, and at one and three month follow-up periods, there was no demonstration of serious adverse device effects with respect to sensing, pacing, or lead impedance.

Figure 4. Chest X-ray obtained in a patient with an MR Conditional cardiac pacemaker showing radiopaque markings identifying the pulse generator and leads as MR Conditional components.

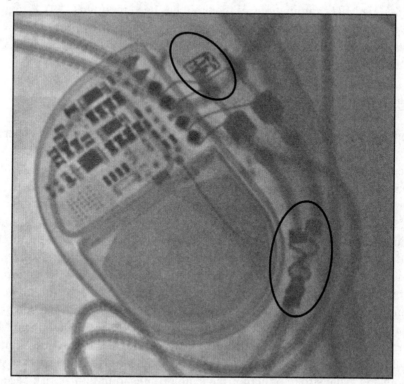

In regard to the quality of the MRI examinations, there were imaging artifacts on brain diffusion-weighted pulse sequences.

Currently, several MR conditional cardiac devices exist in the world (126-138). At the present time, there is only one Food and Drug Administration (FDA) approved MR Conditional pacing system approved in the United States (U.S.), which is the Revo MRI SureScan Pacing System (Medtronic, Inc., Minneapolis, MN)(98). Outside of the U.S., Biotronik (Berlin, Germany), Medtronic, Inc. (Minneapolis, MN), and St. Jude Medical (St. Paul, MN) all have commercially available MR Conditional pacing systems. In addition, Biotronik has received CE approval in European countries for an MR Conditional ICD. Importantly, each MR Conditional device refers to the full system consisting of an MR Conditional pulse generator, MR Conditional leads, and MR Conditional programming device. The pulse generator and leads have specific markers to indicate that these components are MR Conditional (**Figure 4**). Post market data will be important for the assessment of these cardiac devices in larger populations and over longer periods of time (114, 137).

The number of cardiac devices for diagnostic and therapeutic indications continues to increase which, in addition to standard pacemakers, there are more sophisticated ICDs and resynchronization pacemakers as well as subcutaneous ICDs, implantable arrhythmia monitors, implantable physiologic measurement devices, and temporary pacing systems. These electronically activated devices will need to be studied relative to the use of MRI as they exist in their conventional forms as well as when MR Conditional designs of these devices are developed (138). One study of an implantable loop recorder used in patients undergoing 3-Tesla/128-MHz MRI examinations of the brain has been reported (139). A total of 24 patients with the implantable loop recorder underwent 62 brain MRI procedures without adverse events or loss of data. One MRI associated artifact occurred which mimicked a narrow complex tachycardia.

CONCLUSIONS AND FUTURE DIRECTIONS

The impact of implementation of MR Conditional cardiac devices will depend on multiple factors including continued device development, demonstration of device safety and effectiveness, device approval by appropriate agencies, differences in implant practices in different patient subgroups and geographies, device costs, cost effectiveness and reimbursement. Even if MR Conditional devices become the nominal platform of cardiac devices in the future, a period of time will exist where a patient with a MR non-conditional device will need to undergo an MRI examination for diagnostic or therapeutic indications. During this transitional era, decisions regarding scanning will need to be individualized based on consideration of the following: (1) whether there are adequate non-MRI options (e.g., ultrasound, computed tomography, etc.), (2) the acuity and severity of the disease process which requires diagnosis for appropriate management, and (3) the risks and benefits of scanning with a non-MR Conditional device versus explant and placement with an MR Conditional device, including explant of abandoned leads. As the disease processes may involve potentially life-threatening conditions, including central nervous system masses, spinal cord compression, and acute stroke or hemorrhage, algorithms to minimize risk based on specified conditions in consideration of the existing literature will be helpful to guide decisions (46, 50, 57, 64, 73-75, 78, 80, 82, 84, 94, 140-141). This decision-making requires education and cooperation of the medical professionals caring for patients where device and diagnostic imaging decisions are made and implemented.

REFERENCES

1. Hundley WG, Bluemke DA, Finn JP et al. ACCF/ACR/AHA/NASCI/SCMR 2010 expert consensus document on cardiovascular magnetic resonance: a report of the American College of Cardiology Foundation Task Force on Expert Consensus Documents. Circulation 2010;121:2462-508.

2. Epstein AE, DiMarco JP, Ellenbogen KA, et al. ACC/AHA/HRS 2008 Guidelines for Device-Based Therapy of Cardiac Rhythm Abnormalities: A report of the American College of Cardiology/American Heart Association Task Force on Practice Guidelines (Writing Committee to Revise the ACC/AHA/NASPE 2002 Guideline Update for Implantation of Cardiac Pacemakers and Antiarrhythmia Devices). Developed in collaboration with the American Association for Thoracic Surgery and Society of Thoracic Surgeons. Circulation 2008;117:e350-408.

3. Kalin R, Stanton MS. Current clinical issues for MRI scanning of pacemaker and defibrillator patients. Pacing Clin Electrophysiol 2005;28:326-8.

4. Kanal E, Borgstede JP, Barkovich AJ et al. American College of Radiology white paper on MR safety: 2004 update and revisions. AJR Am J Roentgenol 2004;182:1111-4.

5. Avery JK. Loss prevention case of the month. Not my responsibility! J Tenn Med Assoc 1988;81:523.

6. Coman JA, Martin ET, Ramza BM, Margolis PD, Fair RD. Pacemaker safety during magnetic resonance imaging at 1.5 Tesla. J Am Coll Cardiol 2001;37(Suppl. A):436.

7. Irnich W, Irnich B, Bartsch C, et al. Do we need pacemakers resistant to magnetic resonance imaging? Europace 2005;7:353-65.

8. Pavlicek W, Geisinger M, Castle L, et al. The effects of nuclear magnetic resonance on patients with cardiac pacemakers. Radiology 1983;147:149-53.

9. Fetter J, Aram G, Holmes DR, Gray JE, Hayes DL. The effects of nuclear magnetic resonance imagers on external and implantable pulse generators. Pacing Clin Electrophysiol 1984;7:720-7.

10. Erlebacher JA, Cahill PT, Pannizzo F, Knowles RJ. Effect of magnetic resonance imaging on DDD pacemakers. Am J Cardiol 1986;57:437-40.

11. Holmes DR, Jr., Hayes DL, Gray JE, Merideth J. The effects of magnetic resonance imaging on implantable pulse generators. Pacing Clin Electrophysiol 1986;9:360-70.

12. Iberer F, Justich E, Stenzl W, Tscheliessnig KH, Kapeller J. Nuclear magnetic resonance imaging of a patient with implanted transvenous pacemaker. Herz 1987;7:196-9.

13. Hayes DL, Holmes DR, Gray JE. Effect of 1.5 Tesla nuclear magnetic resonance imaging scanner on implanted permanent pacemakers. J Am Coll Cardiol 1987;10:782-6.

14. Alagona P, Toole JC, Maniscalco BS, et al. Nuclear magnetic resonance imaging in a patient with a DDD pacemaker. Pacing Clin Electrophysiol 1989;12:619.

15. Inbar S, Larson J, Burt T, Mafee M, Ezri MD. Case report: nuclear magnetic resonance imaging in a patient with a pacemaker. Am J Med Sci 1993;305:174-5.

16. Amar D, Gross JN. Pacemaker interactions with transcutaneous cardiac pacing. Anesthesiology 1994;80:717-8.

17. Lauck G, von Smekal A, Wolke S et al. Effects of nuclear magnetic resonance imaging on cardiac pacemakers. Pacing Clin Electrophysiol 1995;18:1549-55.

18. Gimbel JR, Johnson D, Levine PA, Wilkoff BL. Safe performance of magnetic resonance imaging on five patients with permanent cardiac pacemakers. Pacing Clin Electrophysiol 1996;19:913-9.

19. Garcia-Bolao I, Albaladejo V, Benito A, Alegria E, Zubieta JL. Magnetic resonance imaging in a patient with a dual-chamber pacemaker. Acta Cardiol 1998;53:33-5.

20. Shellock FG, O'Neil M, Ivans V, et al. Cardiac pacemakers and implantable cardioverter defibrillators are unaffected by operation of an extremity MR imaging system. AJR Am J Roentgenol 1999;172:165-70.

21. Sommer T, Vahlhaus C, Lauck G, et al. MR imaging and cardiac pacemakers: *In-vitro* evaluation and *in-vivo* studies in 51 patients at 0.5 T. Radiology 2000;215:869-79.

22. Luechinger R, Duru F, Scheidegger MB, Boesiger P, Candinas R. Force and torque effects of a 1.5-Tesla MRI scanner on cardiac pacemakers and ICDs. Pacing Clin Electrophysiol 2001;24:199-205.

23. Vahlhaus C, Sommer T, Lewalter T, et al. Interference with cardiac pacemakers by magnetic resonance imaging: Are there irreversible changes at 0.5 Tesla? Pacing Clin Electrophysiol 2001;24:489-95.

24. Scholten A, Silny J. The interference threshold of unipolar cardiac pacemakers in extremely low frequency magnetic fields. J Med Eng Technol 2001;25:185-94.

25. Anfinsen OG, Berntsen RF, Aass H, Kongsgaard E, Amlie JP. Implantable cardioverter defibrillator dysfunction during and after magnetic resonance imaging. Pacing Clin Electrophysiol 2002;25:1400-2.

26. Dawson TW, Caputa K, Stuchly MA, et al. Pacemaker interference by magnetic fields at power line frequencies. IEEE Trans Biomed Eng 2002;49:254-62.

27. Greatbatch W, Miller V, Shellock FG. Magnetic resonance safety testing of a newly-developed fiber-optic cardiac pacing lead. J Magn Reson Imaging 2002;16:97-103.

28. Irnich W. Electronic security systems and active implantable medical devices. Pacing Clin Electrophysiol 2002;25:1235-58.

29. Luechinger R, Duru F, Zeijlemaker VA, et al. Pacemaker reed switch behavior in 0.5, 1.5, and 3.0 Tesla magnetic resonance imaging units: are reed switches always closed in strong magnetic fields? Pacing Clin Electrophysiol 2002;25:1419-23.

30. Pictet J, Meuli R, Wicky S, van der Klink JJ. Radiofrequency heating effects around resonant lengths of wire in MRI. Phys Med Biol 2002;47:2973-85.

31. Fiek M, Remp T, Reithmann C, Steinbeck G. Complete loss of ICD programmability after magnetic resonance imaging. Pacing Clin Electrophysiol 2004;27:1002-4.

32. Martin ET, Coman JA, Shellock FG, et al. Magnetic resonance imaging and cardiac pacemaker safety at 1.5-Tesla. J Am Coll Cardiol 2004;43:1315-24.

33. Coman JA, Martin ET, Sandler DA, Thomas RT. Implantable cardiac defibrillator interactions with magnetic resonance imaging at 1.5 Tesla. J Am Coll Cardiol 2004;43:138A.

34. Roguin A, Zviman MM, Meininger GR, et al. Modern pacemaker and implantable cardioverter/defibrillator systems can be magnetic resonance imaging safe: *In vitro* and *in vivo* assessment of safety and function at 1.5-T. Circulation 2004;110:475-82.

35. Del Ojo JL, Moya F, Villalba J, et al. Is magnetic resonance imaging safe in cardiac pacemaker recipients? Pacing Clin Electrophysiol 2005;28:274-8.

36. Gimbel JR, Bailey SM, Tchou PJ, Ruggieri PM, Wilkoff BL. Strategies for the safe magnetic resonance imaging of pacemaker-dependent patients. Pacing Clin Electrophysiol 2005;28:1041-6.

37. Gimbel JR, Kanal E, Schwartz KM, Wilkoff BL. Outcome of magnetic resonance imaging (MRI) in selected patients with implantable cardioverter defibrillators (ICDs). Pacing Clin Electrophysiol 2005;28:270-3.

38. Gray RW, Bibens WT, Shellock FG. Simple design changes to wires to substantially reduce MRI-induced heating at 1.5 T: implications for implanted leads. Magn Reson Imaging 2005;23:887-91.

39. Luechinger R, Zeijlemaker VA, Pedersen EM, et al. *In vivo* heating of pacemaker leads during magnetic resonance imaging. Eur Heart J 2005;26:376-83. .

40. Maldonado JG, Pereira ME, Albuquerque KR, Pires J. Magnetic resonance imaging in a patient with pacemaker. Arq Bras Cardiol 2005;84:428-30.

41. Roguin A, Donahue JK, Bomma CS, Bluemke DA, Halperin HR. Cardiac magnetic resonance imaging in a patient with implantable cardioverter-defibrillator. Pacing Clin Electrophysiol 2005;28:336-8.

42. Roguin A, Zviman MM, Halperin HR. Re.: Complete loss of ICD programmability after magnetic resonance imaging. Pacing Clin Electrophysiol 2005;28:354.

43. Rozner MA, Burton AW, Kumar A. Pacemaker complication during magnetic resonance imaging. J Am Coll Cardiol 2005;45:161-2

44. Schmiedel A, Hackenbroch M, Yang A, et al. Magnetic resonance imaging of the brain in patients with cardiac pacemakers. Experimental and clinical investigations at 1.5 Tesla. Rofo 2005;177:731-44.

45. Trigano A, Blandeau O, Souques M, Gernez JP, Magne I. Clinical study of interference with cardiac pacemakers by a magnetic field at power line frequencies. J Am Coll Cardiol 2005;45:896-900.

46. Wollmann C, Grude M, Tombach B, et al. Safe performance of magnetic resonance imaging on a patient with an ICD. Pacing Clin Electrophysiol 2005;28:339-42.

47. Sardanelli F, Lupo P, Esseridou A, Fausto A, Quarenghi M. Dynamic breast magnetic resonance imaging without complications in a patient with dual-chamber demand pacemaker. Acta Radiol 2006;47:24-7.

48. Mattei E, Calcagnini G, Triventi M, et al. MRI induced heating of pacemaker leads: effect of temperature probe positioning and pacemaker placement on lead tip heating and local SAR. Conf Proc IEEE Eng Med Biol Soc 2006;1:1889-92.

49. Naehle CP, Sommer T, Meyer C, et al. Strategy for safe performance of magnetic resonance imaging on a patient with implantable cardioverter defibrillator. Pacing Clin Electrophysiol 2006;29:113-6.

50. Nazarian S, Roguin A, Zviman MM, et al. Clinical utility and safety of a protocol for noncardiac and cardiac magnetic resonance imaging of patients with permanent pacemakers and implantable-cardioverter defibrillators at 1.5 Tesla. Circulation 2006;114:1277-84.

51. Nemec J. Suppression of implantable cardioverter defibrillator therapy during magnetic resonance imaging. J Cardiovasc Electrophysiol 2006;17:444-5.

52. Shellock FG, Fieno DS, Thomson LJ, Talavage TM, Berman DS. Cardiac pacemaker: *In vitro* assessment at 1.5 T. Am Heart J 2006;151:436-43.

53. Sommer T, Naehle CP, Yang A, et al. Strategy for safe performance of extrathoracic magnetic resonance imaging at 1.5 Tesla in the presence of cardiac pacemakers in non-pacemaker-dependent patients: a prospective study with 115 examinations. Circulation 2006;114:1285-92.

54. Babouri A, Hedjeidj A. *In vitro* investigation of eddy current effect on pacemaker operation generated by low frequency magnetic field. Conf Proc IEEE Eng Med Biol Soc 2007;2007:5684-7.

55. Heatlie G, Pennell DJ. Cardiovascular magnetic resonance at 0.5-T in five patients with permanent pacemakers. J Cardiovasc Magn Reson 2007;9:15-9.

56. Shellock FG, Fischer L, Fieno DS. Cardiac pacemakers and implantable cardioverter defibrillators: *in vitro* magnetic resonance imaging evaluation at 1.5-Tesla. J Cardiovasc Magn Reson 2007;9:21-31.

57. Shinbane JS, Colletti PM, Shellock FG. MR in patients with pacemakers and ICDs: Defining the issues. J Cardiovasc Magn Reson 2007;9:5-13.

58. Calcagnini G, Triventi M, Censi F, et al. *In vitro* investigation of pacemaker lead heating induced by magnetic resonance imaging: role of implant geometry. J Magn Reson Imaging 2008;28:879-86.

59. Mattei E, Triventi M, Calcagnini G, et al. Complexity of MRI induced heating on metallic leads: experimental measurements of 374 configurations. Biomed Eng Online 2008;7:11.

60. Mollerus M, Albin G, Lipinski M, Lucca J. Cardiac biomarkers in patients with permanent pacemakers and implantable cardioverter-defibrillators undergoing an MRI scan. Pacing Clin Electrophysiol 2008;31:1241-5.

61. Naehle CP, Meyer C, Thomas D, et al. Safety of brain 3-T MR imaging with transmit-receive head coil in patients with cardiac pacemakers: pilot prospective study with 51 examinations. Radiology 2008;249:991-1001.

62. Tandri H, Zviman MM, Wedan SR, et al. Determinants of gradient field-induced current in a pacemaker lead system in a magnetic resonance imaging environment. Heart Rhythm 2008;5:462-8.

63. Gimbel JR. Unexpected asystole during 3T magnetic resonance imaging of a pacemaker-dependent patient with a 'modern' pacemaker. Europace 2009;11:1241-2.

64. Goldsher D, Jahshan S, Roguin A. Successful cervical MR scan in a patient several hours after pacemaker implantation. Pacing Clin Electrophysiol 2009;32:1355-6.

65. Mollerus M, Albin G, Lipinski M, Lucca J. Ectopy in patients with permanent pacemakers and implantable cardioverter-defibrillators undergoing an MRI scan. Pacing Clin Electrophysiol 2009;32:772-8.

66. Naehle CP, Zeijlemaker V, Thomas D, et al. Evaluation of cumulative effects of MR imaging on pacemaker systems at 1.5 Tesla. Pacing Clin Electrophysiol 2009;32:1526-35.

67. Nordbeck P, Weiss I, Ehses P, et al. Measuring RF-induced currents inside implants: Impact of device configuration on MRI safety of cardiac pacemaker leads. Magn Reson Med 2009;61:570-8.

68. Pulver AF, Puchalski MD, Bradley DJ, et al. Safety and imaging quality of MRI in pediatric and adult congenital heart disease patients with pacemakers. Pacing Clin Electrophysiol 2009;32:450-6.

69. Shellock FG. Excessive temperature increases in pacemaker leads at 3-T MR imaging with a transmit-receive head coil. Radiology 2009;251:948-9.

70. Millar LM, Robinson AG, O'Flaherty MT, et al. Magnetic resonance imaging in a patient with a dual chamber pacemaker. Case Report Med 2010;2010:292071.

71. Strach K, Naehle CP, Muhlsteffen A, et al. Low-field magnetic resonance imaging: increased safety for pacemaker patients? Europace 2010;12:952-60.

72. Langman DA, Goldberg IB, Finn JP, Ennis DB. Pacemaker lead tip heating in abandoned and pacemaker-attached leads at 1.5 Tesla MRI. J Magn Reson Imaging 2011;33:426-31.

73. Zikria JF, Machnicki S, Rhim E, Bhatti T, Graham RE. MRI of patients with cardiac pacemakers: a review of the medical literature. AJR Am J Roentgenol 2011;196:390-401.

74. Shinbane JS, Colletti PM, Shellock FG. Magnetic resonance imaging in patients with cardiac pacemakers: era of "MR Conditional" designs. J Cardiovasc Magn Reson 2011;13:63.

75. Shinbane JS, Colletti PM, Shellock FG. MR imaging in patients with pacemakers and other devices: engineering the future. JACC Cardiovasc Imaging 2012;5:332-3.

76. Baser K, Guray U, Durukan M, Demirkan B. High ventricular lead impedance of a DDD pacemaker after cranial magnetic resonance imaging. Pacing Clin Electrophysiol 2012;35:e251-3.

77. Sommer T, Lauck G, Schimpf R, et al. MRI in patients with cardiac pacemakers: *in vitro* and *in vivo* evaluation at 0.5 Tesla. Rofo 1998;168:36-43.

78. Cohen JD, Costa HS, Russo RJ. Determining the risks of MRI at 1.5-Tesla for patients with pacemakers and implantable cardioverter defibrillators (The MagnaSafe Registry). Circulation 2010;122:A21241.

79. Buendia F, Sanchez-Gomez JM, Sancho-Tello MJ, et al. Nuclear magnetic resonance imaging in patients with cardiac pacing devices. Rev Esp Cardiol 2010;63:735-9.

80. Cohen JD, Costa HS, Russo RJ. Determining the risks of magnetic resonance imaging at 1.5 Tesla for patients with pacemakers and implantable cardioverter defibrillators. Am J Cardiol 2012;110:1631-6.

81. Burke PT, Ghanbari H, Alexander PB, et al. A protocol for patients with cardiovascular implantable devices undergoing magnetic resonance imaging (MRI): should defibrillation threshold testing be performed post-(MRI). J Interv Card Electrophysiol 2010;28:59-66.

82. Nazarian S, Hansford R, Roguin A, et al. A prospective evaluation of a protocol for magnetic resonance imaging of patients with implanted cardiac devices. Annals of Internal Medicine 2011;155:415-24.

83. The MagnaSafe Registry: Determining the Risks of Magnetic Resonance Imaging (MRI) in the Presence of Pacemakers and Implantable Cardioverter Defibrillators (ICDs). (NCT00907361). http://clinicaltrials.gov.

84. Russo RJ, Costa HS, Doud DS, et al. Determining the risks of magnetic resonance imaging at 1.5 Tesla for patients with pacemakers and implantable cardioverter defibrillators (The MagnaSafe Registry). Heart Rhythm 2012;9:S.

85. Russo RJ, Costa H, Doud D, et al. Repeat MRI for patients with implanted cardiac devices does not increase the risk of clinical events or parameter changes: preliminary results from the MagnaSafe Registry. JACC 2012;59:E649.

86. Faris OP, Shein MJ. Government viewpoint: U.S. Food & Drug Administration: Pacemakers, ICDs and MRI. Pacing Clin Electrophysiol 2005;28:268-9.

87. Smith JM. Industry viewpoint: Guidant: Pacemakers, ICDs, and MRI. Pacing Clin Electrophysiol 2005;28:264.

88. Stanton MS. Industry viewpoint: Medtronic: Pacemakers, ICDs, and MRI. Pacing Clin Electrophysiol 2005;28:265.

89. Levine PA. Industry viewpoint: St. Jude Medical: Pacemakers, ICDs and MRI. Pacing Clin Electrophysiol 2005;28:266-7.

90. Fisher JD. MRI: Safety in patients with pacemakers or defibrillators: is it prime time yet? Pacing Clin Electrophysiol 2005;28:263.

91. Martin ET. Can cardiac pacemakers and magnetic resonance imaging systems co-exist? Eur Heart J 2005;26:325-7.

92. Faris OP, Shein M. Food and Drug Administration perspective: Magnetic resonance imaging of pacemaker and implantable cardioverter-defibrillator patients. Circulation 2006;114:1232-3.

93. Wilkoff BL. Pacemaker and ICD malfunction—an incomplete picture. JAMA 2006;295:1944-6.

94. Colletti PM, Shinbane JS, Shellock FG. "MR-Conditional" pacemakers: the radiologist's role in multidisciplinary management. AJR Am J Roentgenol 2011;197:W457-9.

95. Shellock FG, Woods TO, Crues JV. MR labeling information for implants and devices: explanation of terminology. Radiology 2009;253:26-30.

96. American Society for Testing and Materials (ASTM) International. F2503, Standard Practice for Marking Medical Devices and Other Items for Safety in the Magnetic Resonance Environment.

97. Shellock FG, Tkach JA, Ruggieri PM, Masaryk TJ. Cardiac pacemakers, ICDs, and loop recorder: evaluation of translational attraction using conventional ("long-bore") and "short-bore" 1.5- and 3.0-Tesla MR systems. J Cardiovasc Magn Reson 2003;5:387-97.

98. Wilkoff BL, Bello D, Taborsky M, et al. Magnetic resonance imaging in patients with a pacemaker system designed for the magnetic resonance environment. Heart Rhythm 2011;8:65-73.

99. Park SM, Kamondetdacha R, Nyenhuis JA. Calculation of MRI-induced heating of an implanted medical lead wire with an electric field transfer function. J Magn Reson Imaging 2007;26:1278-85.

100. Yeung CJ, Karmarkar P, McVeigh ER. Minimizing RF heating of conducting wires in MRI. Magn Reson Med 2007;58:1028-34.

101. Nordbeck P, Fidler F, Weiss I, et al. Spatial distribution of RF-induced E-fields and implant heating in MRI. Magn Reson Med 2008;60:312-9.

102. Nordbeck P, Ritter O, Weiss I, et al. Impact of imaging landmark on the risk of MRI-related heating near implanted medical devices like cardiac pacemaker leads. Magn Reson Med 2011;65:44-50.

103. Driller J, Barold SS, Parsonnet V. Normal and abnormal function of the pacemaker magnetic reed switch. J Electrocardiol 1976;9:283-92.

104. Sutton R, Kanal E, Wilkoff BL, et al. Safety of magnetic resonance imaging of patients with a new Medtronic EnRhythm MRI SureScan pacing system: clinical study design. Trials 2008;9:68.

105. Shellock FG, Fischer L, Fieno D. Cardiac pacemakers and implantable cardioverter defibrillators: *in vitro* MRI evaluation at 1.5-Tesla. J Cardiovasc Magn Reson 2007; J Cardiovasc Magn Reson 2007;9:21-31.

106. Neuzner J. Clinical experience with a new cardioverter defibrillator capable of biphasic waveform pulse and enhanced data storage: results of a prospective multicenter study. European Ventak P2 Investigator Group. Pacing Clin Electrophysiol 1994;17:1243-55.

107. Brugada J, Herse B, Sandsted B, et al. Clinical evaluation of defibrillation efficacy with a new single-capacitor biphasic waveform in patients undergoing implantation of an implantable cardioverter defibrillator. Europace 2001;3:278-84.

108. Rinaldi CA, Simon RD, Geelen P, et al. A randomized prospective study of single coil versus dual coil defibrillation in patients with ventricular arrhythmias undergoing implantable cardioverter defibrillator therapy. Pacing Clin Electrophysiol 2003;26:1684-90.

109. Fontaine JM, Mohamed FB, Gottlieb C, et al. Rapid ventricular pacing in a pacemaker patient undergoing magnetic resonance imaging. Pacing Clin Electrophysiol 1998;21:1336-9.

110. Achenbach S, Moshage W, Diem B, et al. Effects of magnetic resonance imaging on cardiac pacemakers and electrodes. Am Heart J 1997;134:467-73.

111. Yeung CJ, Susil RC, Atalar E. RF heating due to conductive wires during MRI depends on the phase distribution of the transmit field. Magn Reson Med 2002;48:1096-8.

112. Mattei E, Calcagnini G, Censi F, Triventi M, Bartolini P. Numerical model for estimating RF-induced heating on a pacemaker implant during MRI: experimental validation. IEEE Trans Biomed Eng 2010;57:2045-52.

113. Bottomley PA, Kumar A, Edelstein WA, Allen JM, Karmarkar PV. Designing passive MRI-safe implantable conducting leads with electrodes. Med Phys 2010;37:3828-43.

114. United States of America Department of Health And Human Services Food and Drug Administration Center For Devices and Radiological Health Medical Devices Advisory Committee Circulatory System Devices Panel. March 19, 2010.

115. Hartnell GG, Spence L, Hughes LA, et al. Safety of MR imaging in patients who have retained metallic materials after cardiac surgery. AJR Am J Roentgenol 1997;168:1157-9.

116. Kanal E. Safety of MR imaging in patients with retained epicardial pacer wires. AJR Am J Roentgenol 1998;170:213-4.

117. Fries R, Steuer M, Schafers HJ, Bohm M. The R-on-T phenomenon in patients with implantable cardioverter-defibrillators. Am J Cardiol 2003;91:752-5.

118. Chiladakis JA, Karapanos G, Davlouros P, et al. Significance of R-on-T phenomenon in early ventricular tachyarrhythmia susceptibility after acute myocardial infarction in the thrombolytic era. Am J Cardiol 2000;85:289-93.

119. Gimbel JR. Unexpected pacing inhibition upon exposure to the 3T static magnetic field prior to imaging acquisition: What is the mechanism? Heart Rhythm 2010.

120. Shellock FG, Bert JM, Fritts HM, et al. Evaluation of the rotator cuff and glenoid labrum using a 0.2-Tesla extremity magnetic resonance (MR) system: MR results compared to surgical findings. J Magn Reson Imaging 2001;14:763-70.

121. Zlatkin MB, Hoffman C, Shellock FG. Assessment of the rotator cuff and glenoid labrum using an extremity MR system: MR results compared to surgical findings from a multi-center study. J Magn Reson Imaging 2004;19:623-31.

122. Quarta G, Holdright DR, Plant GT, et al. Cardiovascular magnetic resonance in cardiac sarcoidosis with MR Conditional pacemaker *in situ*. J Cardiovasc Magn Reson 2011;13:26.

123. Naehle CP, Kreuz J, Strach K, et al. Safety, feasibility, and diagnostic value of cardiac magnetic resonance imaging in patients with cardiac pacemakers and implantable cardioverters/defibrillators at 1.5 T. Am Heart J 2011;161:1096-105.

124. Wollmann CG, Steiner E, Vock P, Ndikung B, Mayr H. Monocenter feasibility study of the MRI compatibility of the Evia pacemaker in combination with Safio S pacemaker lead. J Cardiovasc Magn Reson 2012;14:67.

125. Forleo GB, Santini L, Della Rocca DG, et al. Safety and efficacy of a new magnetic resonance imaging-compatible pacing system: early results of a prospective comparison with conventional dual-chamber implant outcomes. Heart Rhythm 2010;7:750-4.

126. Advisa MRI Clinical Study. (NCT01110915). http://clinicaltrials.gov.

127. Clinical Evaluation of the Sorin Group's Reply MR-Conditional Pacing System. (NCT01341522). http://clinicaltrials.gov.

128. Accent MRI Pacemaker and Tendril MRI Lead New Technology Assesment. (NCT01258218). http://clinicaltrials.gov.

129. Safety and Efficacy of the Accent Magnetic Resonance Imaging (MRI) Pacemaker and Tendril MRI Lead. (NCT01576016). http://clinicaltrials.gov.

130. Safety and Performance Study of the INGEVITY Lead. (NCT01688843). http://clinicaltrials.gov

131. ProMRI AFFIRM Study of the EVIA/ENTOVIS Pacemaker With Safio S Pacemaker Leads. (NCT01460992). http://clinicaltrials.gov.

132. ProMRI Study of the Entovis Pacemaker System. (NCT01761162). http://clinicaltrials.gov.

133. Lobodzinski SS. Recent innovations in the development of magnetic resonance imaging conditional pacemakers and implantable cardioverter-defibrillators. Cardiology journal 2012;19:98-104.

134. Biotronik User's Manual: ProMRI. http//:www.biotronik.com.

135. St. Jude User's Manual: Tendril MRI, Accent MRI, Accent ST MRI, SJM MRI Activator. http://www.sjm.com.

136. Lumax 740 series ICDs with ProMRI. http://www.biotronik.com.

137. Mitka M. First MRI-safe pacemaker receives conditional approval from FDA. JAMA 2011;305:985-6.

138. Shellock FG. Reference Manual for Magnetic Resonance Safety, Implants, and Devices: 2013 Edition. Los Angeles: Biomedical Research Publishing Group, 2013.

139. Haeusler KG, Koch L, Ueberreiter J, et al. Safety and reliability of the insertable Reveal XT recorder in patients undergoing 3 Tesla brain magnetic resonance imaging. Heart Rhythm 2011;8:373-6.

140. Kanal E, Barkovich AJ, Bell C, et al. ACR guidance document on MR safe practices: 2013. J Magn Reson Imaging 2013;37:501-530.

141. Levine GN, Gomes AS, Arai AE, et al. Safety of magnetic resonance imaging in patients with cardiovascular devices: An American Heart Association scientific statement from the Committee on Diagnostic and Interventional Cardiac Catheterization, Council on Clinical Cardiology, and the Council on Cardiovascular Radiology and Intervention, endorsed by the American College of Cardiology Foundation, the North American Society for Cardiac Imaging, and the Society for Cardiovascular Magnetic Resonance. Circulation 2007;116:2878-91.

Chapter 19   MRI Safety Issues and Neuromodulation Systems

STEVEN G. MANKER, BSME

Program Director
MRI Conditionally Safe Systems
Medtronic Neuromodulation
Minneapolis, MN

FRANK G. SHELLOCK, PH.D.

Adjunct Clinical Professor of Radiology and Medicine
Keck School of Medicine
Director for MRI Studies of Biomimetic MicroElectronic Systems
National Science Foundation, Engineering Research Center
University of Southern California
Institute for Magnetic Resonance Safety, Education, and Research
Los Angeles, CA

INTRODUCTION

Magnetic resonance imaging (MRI) has been utilized in the clinical setting for close to 30 years. During this time, the technology has continued to evolve in order to improve image quality, acquisition time, and patient comfort. These changes have yielded MR systems with more powerful static magnetic fields, faster and stronger gradient magnetic fields, and improved radiofrequency (RF) transmission coils. The short-term exposures to the electromagnetic fields used for MRI procedures at the levels currently recommended in the governing MRI standard, ISO 60601-2-33, and by the United States (U.S.) Food and Drug Administration, have resulted in relatively few problems for the millions of MRI examinations performed to date (1, 2). Most reported cases of MRI-related injuries and the few fatalities that have occurred have been due to not following safety guidelines or from using inappropriate or outdated information related to the safety aspects of biomedical implants and devices (3).

The preservation of a safe MRI environment requires constant attention to the management of patients and individuals with metallic implants and devices because the variety and complexity of these objects constantly changes (3). Therefore, to guard against adverse events and other problems in the MRI setting, it is necessary to revise the safety guidelines for implants and devices according to changes that have occurred in MRI technology and based on MRI testing best practices. In consideration of the above, this chapter discusses MRI safety issues for neuromodulation systems and presents specific information for these electronically "active" devices.

STATIC MAGNETIC FIELDS

The introduction of MRI technology as a clinical imaging modality in the early 1980s is responsible for a substantial increase in human exposure to strong static magnetic fields (4). Most MR systems in use today operate with static magnetic fields ranging from 0.2- to 3-Tesla. The most common field strength is 1.5-Tesla and 3.0-Tesla is the highest field strength used in the clinical setting. Currently, ultra-high-field-strength MR systems exist in research settings, which include several 4-Tesla scanners, more than fifty 7-Tesla scanners, and an exceptionally powerful MR system operating at 9.4-Tesla (i.e., located at the University of Illinois at Chicago). The static magnetic field aligns the protons, typically hydrogen protons, to the magnetic field. These protons resonate or precess proportionally to the Larmor frequency when exposed to a powerful static magnetic field. The vector sum of the magnetic moments of all of the protons is called the bulk magnetization vector.

GRADIENT MAGNETIC FIELDS

During the MRI examination, gradient or time-varying magnetic fields switch rapidly to localize the induced signals coming from the protons in tissue to permit spatial localization. The speed and strength of the gradient magnetic fields are limited during MRI examinations because they may stimulate nerves or muscles by inducing electrical fields in patients, resulting in peripheral nerve stimulation (PNS)(5).

RF FIELDS

The RF subsystem has two phases: an excitation or transmit phase and an acquisition, or receive phase. During the transmit phase, RF energy is transmitted into the tissue of interest to tip the bulk magnetization vector out of alignment from the static magnetic field. During the receive phase, the rotating bulk magnetization vector induces current in the RF receive antenna or coil. The receive coil may be the same coil as the transmit coil (e.g., a transmit/receive RF coil) or it may be a receive-only coil that is customized for the anatomy undergoing imaging (e.g., transmit/receive RF coils exist for the head, knee, and other body parts, etc.).

The majority of the RF power transmitted for MRI or spectroscopy (e.g., carbon decoupling, fast spin echo pulse sequences, magnetization transfer contrast pulse sequences, etc.) is transformed into heat within the patient's tissue as a result of dielectric heating (6-

8). Not surprisingly, the primary bioeffects associated with exposure to RF radiation are related to the thermogenic qualities of this electromagnetic field.

Thermoregulatory and other physiologic changes that a human subject exhibits in response to exposure to RF radiation are dependent on the amount of energy that is absorbed (6, 7). The dosimetric term used to describe the absorption of RF radiation is the specific absorption rate, or SAR. The SAR is the mass normalized rate at which RF power is coupled to biologic tissue and is typically indicated in units of watts per kilogram (W/kg). The relative amount of RF radiation that an individual encounters during an MRI procedure is characterized with respect to the whole-body averaged and peak SAR levels (i.e., the SAR averaged in one gram of tissue).

Measurements or estimates of SAR are not trivial, particularly in human subjects. Notably, the calculation is even more complicated when a metallic implant is present in a patient (9-12). There are several methods of determining this parameter for the purpose of RF energy dosimetry in association with MRI procedures. The SAR that is produced during an MRI examination is a complex function of numerous variables including the frequency (i.e., determined by the strength of the static magnetic field of the MR system), the repetition time, the type of transmit RF coil used, the volume of tissue contained within the coil, the configuration of the anatomical region exposed, the orientation of the body to the field vectors, as well as other factors (6-8). Therefore, each MR system manufacturer has a slightly different approach to calculating and reporting SAR information.

MRI SAFETY AND SCREENING PATIENTS FOR MRI PROCEDURES

The establishment of thorough and effective screening procedures for patients and other individuals is one of the most critical components of a program that guards the safety of all those preparing to undergo MRI procedures or to enter the MRI environment (3). An important aspect of protecting patients and individuals from MR system-related accidents and injuries involves an understanding of the risks associated with the various implants, devices, accessories, and other objects that may cause problems in this setting. This requires obtaining accurate information and documentation about these objects in order to ensure the safest MRI setting possible. In addition, because MRI-related incidents have been due to deficiencies in screening methods and/or a lack of properly controlling access to the MRI environment (especially with regard to preventing personal items and other potentially problematic objects into the scanner room), it is crucial to set up procedures and guidelines to prevent such incidents from occurring. Importantly, many guidelines and recommendations have been developed to facilitate the screening process (see www.MRIsafety.com)(3).

MRI Procedures and Implanted Medical Devices: Neuromodulation Systems

Careful review of MRI labeling information is required if a patient referred for an MRI examination has an implant, especially if it is an "active" implant such as a neuromodulation (also referred to as a neurostimulation) system. Currently, there are three classes of implanted medical devices (13): MR Unsafe, MR Safe, or MR Conditional. If the device has known MRI safety concerns (e.g., a ferromagnetic aneurysm clip), the device is classified as MR Unsafe. If the device has no known MRI safety concerns based on its inherent design (e.g., a silicone Foley catheter) or has been proven to be safe in all MRI environments, the device is classified as MR Safe. Notably, since the MRI environment continues to evolve, there are very few MR Safe medical devices. This leaves the category of MR Conditional devices. Devices that are classified MR Conditional are acceptable for patients undergoing MRI under highly specific conditions.

To determine whether or not the device is safe for a patient in a specific MRI environment, the device and related MRI issues must be identified and properly characterized. Importantly, the labeling that documents the specific conditions for use of MRI must also be carefully followed. Identifying the device may require a review of the patient's medical records, implant identification cards, radiographic studies, or a conversation with the prescribing physician. After the device has been identified, the preferred source of MRI-related safety information is the device manufacturer. There are third-party sources for MR safety information (e.g., www.MRIsafety.com) that may also fill this critical need for information.

Interactions Between the MRI Environment and Implanted Medical Devices

Static Magnetic Field-Related Injuries or Device Damage

Magnetic field-related issues are known to present hazards to patients with certain implants or devices primarily due to movement or dislodgment of objects made from ferromagnetic materials (3). Thus, medical devices with ferromagnetic materials will be attracted to and aligned with the strong static magnetic field of the MR system (**Figure 1**) This movement could result in patient injury (e.g., torn sutures, internal bleeding, etc.) or could result

Figure 1. Example of translational attraction testing performed at 1.5-Tesla on a pulse generator used for a neuromodulation system. Note the high deflection angle indicating a relatively high translational attraction for this implant.

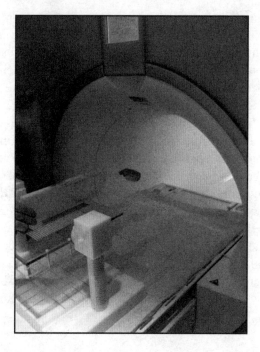

in the need for surgical revision to reposition the device to restore therapy or for patient comfort. Exposure to a power static magnetic field may also alter the device settings for an electronically activated device, requiring reprogramming or damage the device, necessitating replacement surgery (14).

Numerous studies have assessed magnetic field interactions for implants and devices by measuring translational attraction and torque associated with the static magnetic fields of MR systems. These investigations demonstrated that, for certain items, MRI procedures may be performed safely if the items are nonferromagnetic or "weakly" ferromagnetic (i.e., the object minimally interacts with the magnetic field in relation to its *in vivo* application), such that the associated magnetic field interactions are insufficient to move or dislodge the items, *in situ*. Furthermore, the "intended *in vivo* use" of the implant or device must be taken into consideration, because this can impact whether or not a particular item is acceptable for a patient undergoing an MRI examination. Notably, sufficient counter-forces may exist to retain even a ferromagnetic implant, *in situ* (e.g., fibrous encapsulation of a pulse generator used with a neuromodulation system).

Injuries or Device Damage Related to Gradient Magnetic Fields

The MRI environment may be unsafe for patients with certain biomedical implants or devices due to the induced energy and/or eddy currents related to the fast switching gradient magnetic fields that are used for spatial localization as part of the imaging process. Gradient magnetic fields used during MRI switch or "slew" between positive and negative polarity (**Figure 2**). Any circuit within these rapidly changing magnetic fields is subject to induced currents, according to Faraday's Law of Induction. The fluctuating magnetic field can be generated with a fixed magnet and moving the circuit through the magnetic field, as is done by a typical electric generator configuration or by using a stationary circuit and varying the magnetic field, as is the case with an MRI procedure.

The switching gradient magnetic field can induce a voltage along conductive structures within an MR system (**Figure 3**). With typical neuromodulation systems that utilize a lead and electrode, the circuit can be formed between the tip of an implanted electrode and the pulse generator, on metallic structures, or on individual components (specifically coiled structures like antennas or energy transfer coils). If the voltages are high enough or the resistance is low enough, current will flow. According to Faraday's Law, the larger the loop area, the greater the induced voltage. A variety of interactions can occur if current flows. For electronically activated devices like pacemakers and neurostimulation systems, there is the risk of unintentional stimulation at the switching rate of the gradient coils. Unintentional stimulation can be relatively benign as is the case with most neurostimulation scenarios, since neurostimulation pulse frequencies are similar to the gradient switching frequency associated with an MRI examination. Obviously, unintentional stimulation can have significant health risks. In addition, it should be noted that the gradient induced voltages on the antennas and recharge coils of electronic medical devices such as cardiac pacemakers and neurostimulation systems can be quite high due to the number of coils within the associated components. If the circuitry is not robust enough to shield against these high voltages, the device may sustain damage to its communication or recharge system, memory,

Figure 2. Gradient slew rate examples showing that higher speed gradients reach the maximum gradient value faster. Tesla/Meter/Second is the appropriate way to describe the gradient system's slew rate.

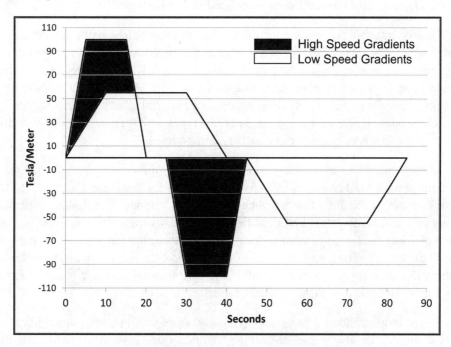

Figure 3. The switched gradients induce voltages only when slewing up or down. The induced voltage changes polarity with the slewing direction.

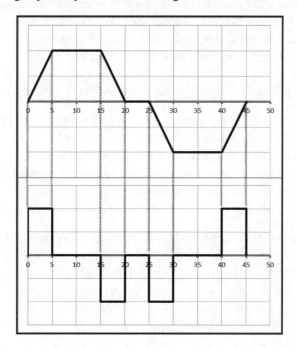

or output channels in association with an MRI examination. If the device is damaged, it may require reprogramming or surgical replacement.

Excessive Heating and Device Damage Related to RF Energy

The use of transmit RF coils, physiologic monitors, electronically activated devices, and external accessories or objects made from conductive materials has caused excessive heating, resulting in burn injuries to patients undergoing MRI procedures (3). The heating of implants and devices may also occur in association with MRI, but this tends to be problematic primarily for objects made from conductive materials that have an elongated shape such as electrodes, leads, guidewire, and certain types of catheters (e.g., thermodilution catheters with thermistors or other conducting components) (3).

In general, published reports have indicated that only minor temperature changes occur in association with MRI examinations involving relatively small metallic objects that are "passive" implants (i.e., those that are not electronically activated), including implants such as aneurysm clips, hemostatic clips, prosthetic heart valves, vascular access ports, and similar devices. Therefore, heat generated during an MRI examination involving a patient with a "small" metallic, passive implant does not appear to be a substantial hazard. In fact, to date, there has been no report of a patient being seriously injured as a result of excessive heating that developed in a passive metallic implant or device.

However, long conductive structures typically act as much better, unintentional antennas. These unintentional antennas collect the RF energy and dissipate it at the path of least resistance. For leads associated with neuromodulation systems, this typically occurs at the electrodes of the leads which are commonly found at the distal end in contact with the organ area receiving stimulation (e.g., occipital nerve, vagus nerve, sacral nerve, epidural space in the spine, etc.). Since the electrodes used with neuromodulation systems are relatively small, the dissipated energy is concentrated very close to their surface (**Figure 4**). Thus, significant heating can be generated under certain clinical conditions and there have been several reports of serious patient injuries (16-18). A variety of variables can contribute to the potential heating of a neuromodulation system (9, 10, 16-28). The critical variables that impact MRI-related heating of an implanted medical device are presented in **Table 1**.

All of these variables must be taken into consideration to create safe operating conditions for patients with neuromodulation systems undergoing MRI. It is important to appreciate the complex interactions between the variables related to RF heating. In fact, each RF frequency (i.e., 64-MHz associated with 1.5-Tesla, 128-MHz associated with 3-Tesla, etc.) needs to be tested individually for a given neuromodulation system because the resulting temperature rises may actually be less at higher frequencies (**Figure 5**)(3, 12, 15-27).

Different mitigation strategies have been employed to create MR Conditional labeling for neuromodulation products. For example, some devices exclude the RF exposure entirely by utilizing head or extremity transmit RF coils if the neuromodulation system is implanted outside of that particular transmit coil. Others use a reduced SAR limit to minimize exposure to the RF energy, while still other neuromodulation products have been specially redesigned to safely manage the RF energy so that the MR system can be operated under normal RF power levels.

Figure 4. The possible coupling of RF energy associated with an MRI procedure and a spinal cord stimulation system.

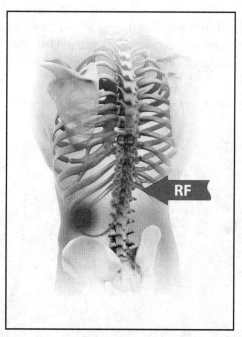

As an aside, the use of the whole body averaged SAR value reported by the MR system, itself, is especially problematic with regard to MRI-related implant heating, as reported by Baker, et al. (9, 10). The MR system reported SAR values can be considered "not to exceed" values such that each MR system manufacturer may have vastly different safety margins to ensure they do not exceed the displayed SAR value(s). Thus, it is important to understand that implant heating may differ significantly when using different MR systems of the same static magnetic field strength and frequency. The variation is due to the different methods that MR systems use to estimate and control SAR. Significant variation in implant heating for a deep brain stimulation lead in association with different 1.5-Tesla scanners (notably from the same manufacturer) was first reported by Baker, et al. (9) and further examined in other investigations (10, 11, 28). The specific concern is when MRI safety labeling is based on data generated using a particular MR system with a large SAR safety margin, because this equates to lower transmitted RF power. Subsequently, in the clinical setting, the device's safety conditions may be complied with on an MR system with a much lower SAR safety margin, equating to a higher RF power level for the same MR system displayed SAR. The result could be a much higher temperature rise for the medical implant.

As previously stated, patients with neurostimulation systems are exposed to the risks associated with the RF energy collected by the creation of unintentional antennas. Because this energy also travels in the opposite direction towards the pulse generator, device components or memory can be damaged and, thus, may require device replacement surgery in the event that the electronics are compromised by high frequency RF energy (14).

Figure 5. MRI-related heating at 1.5-Tesla/64-MHz (diamond) vs. 3-Tesla/128-MHz (circle) for a lead not connected to a pulse generator. The MR system reported, whole body averaged SAR used at 1.5-Tesla was 1.4-W/kg and 3- W/kg at 3-Tesla. Note the substantial differences in the temperature profiles during MRI-related heating of the lead, which illustrates that different resonant effects impact temperature rises for elongated implants. For an implant of a given length, different RF wavelengths will yield different heating effects (i.e., 64-MHz versus 128-MHz).

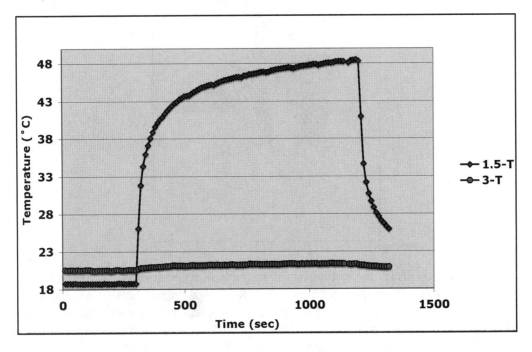

EVALUATION OF MRI ISSUES FOR NEUROMODULATION SYSTEMS

The evaluation of various MRI issues that exist for a neuromodulation system is not a trivial matter and, in fact, may be quite challenging (3, 12). The proper assessment of a medical product typically entails characterization of magnetic field interactions (translational attraction and torque), MRI-related heating, induced electrical currents, and artifacts (3, 12). Furthermore, a thorough evaluation of the impact of MRI conditions on the functional and operational aspects is also necessary. A neuromodulation system demonstrated to be acceptable for a patient according to one set of MRI conditions may be unsafe under more "extreme" or different conditions (e.g., higher or lower static magnetic field, higher or lower RF wavelength, greater level of RF power deposition, faster gradient magnetic fields, use of a different transmit RF coil, etc.). Accordingly, the specific test conditions used for a given neuromodulation system must be based on carefully conducted test procedures before making a decision regarding whether it is safe for a patient to undergo an MRI examination.

Historically, medical implants have been tested according to documents developed by the American Society for Testing and Materials (ASTM) International, including many neuromodulation systems. As MR systems have evolved, the medical device industry has come

Table 1. Critical variables that impact MRI-related heating of a medical implant.

Area	Variable	Comments
MRI Related Variables	Static Field Strength (RF Frequency)	The RF frequency is related to the static magnetic field strength of the MR system.
	RF Power Level or Whole Body Averaged Specific Absorption Rate (SAR)	In the Normal Operating Mode, the RF power is limited to 2.0-W/kg whole body averaged SAR and 3.2-W/kg average head SAR. In the First Level Operating Mode, the RF power is limited to 4.0-W/kg whole body averaged body SAR and 3.2-W/kg average head SAR. See discussion regarding SAR accuracy concerns.
	Landmark (Area of Body Exposed to RF Energy)	Depending on which area of the body is being imaged, more or less of the implanted medical device may be exposed to the RF energy.
	Transmit RF Coil Size	Transmitting with an extremity or head RF coil exposes less of the body and, therefore, potentially less or none of the implanted medical device.
	Scan Duration	Thermal injuries are based on thermal doses to tissue. Thermal dose is a function of time and temperature. It takes a shorter time to damage tissue at higher temperatures.
Medical Device Variables	Conductive Structure Design	Some design structures may be better or worse antennas.
	Conductive Structure Length	Structures may have a worst-case length depending on the resonant frequency. Short structures may not be long enough to act as a good antenna.
	Implant Location	The amount of RF energy incident on a device depends on the device location including lead routings.
	Loops/Coils of the Leads	Crossover points of the leads provided by strain relief or "slack" loops can alter the distribution of RF energy, cause some localized RF energy dissipation at the cross-over point and decrease the quantity dissipated at the electrodes.
Patient Variables	Size	Larger patients have more tissue and, therefore, more RF power is needed to excite the tissue for imaging.
	Composition	Fat is more permeable to RF energy so less energy is required penetrate it compared with a muscular patient of the same size.

to a better understanding of the possible interactions between implantable medical devices and the MRI environment, which in the case of neuromodulation systems are particularly complex. Consequently, a group consisting of representatives from medical device and MR system manufacturers, MRI scientists and engineers, and regulatory agency representatives developed a test specification specifically related to evaluating the safety of "active" implantable medical devices (or AIMDs) in the MRI environment. This work took a number of years to complete. The first edition of the document, ISO/TS 10974, was published in May 2012. This test specification is now recognized by most regulatory agencies around the globe as the preferred test methodology to generate the safety evidence necessary for MR Conditional approval (although, to date, few active implants have actually been tested according to the procedures presented in ISO/TS 10974).

Newly developed implants and devices as well as devices already on the market, are being tested for MRI issues on an on-going basis. This necessitates continuous endeavors to obtain current documentation for these devices prior to subjecting a patient to an MRI examination. In addition, the nuances of MRI testing, especially with respect to the evaluation of MRI-related heating and the identification of alteration in function for active devices, as well as the terminology applied to label implants and devices must be understood to facilitate patient management (3, 12). Importantly, for neuromodulation systems, the labeling that ensures the acceptable use of MRI typically presents many specific conditions. Any deviation from the defined procedures can lead to deleterious effects, severe patient injuries, or fatalities (3, 12, 15-18). To date, more than 5,000 objects have been tested relative to the MRI environment, while comparatively few active devices have approved MRI labeling. This information is available to healthcare professionals and others as an updated reference manual (3) and on-line at www.MRIsafety.com.

MRI PROCEDURES AND NEUROMODULATION SYSTEMS

Neuromodulation systems have been employed for a variety of neurological disorders as well as for other conditions. A typical neurostimulation system consists of an implantable pulse generator (i.e., similar to a cardiac pacemaker) and a set of wires or leads that conduct the electrical pulses to the therapeutic target via one or more electrodes. The pulse generator typically contains electronics and a single-use or rechargeable battery. The size of the pulse generator and the therapeutic target dictate the potential implant locations and lead routings through the body. With regard to current therapies approved by the U.S. Food and Drug Administration (FDA), these include spinal cord stimulation (SCS) for chronic pain; deep brain stimulation (DBS) for essential tremor, Parkinsonian tremor, dystonia, and obsessive-compulsive disorder; vagus nerve stimulation (VNS) for epilepsy and depression; sacral nerve stimulation for urinary and fecal incontinence; and gastric stimulation for gastroparesis.

During the early days of MRI, because of the inherent risks associated with neuromodulation systems relative to the MRI environment, the presence of these electronically activated implants and others was once considered a strict contraindication for patients. However, over the years, various studies have been performed that indicated the relative safety for neuromodulation systems (19-23, 25-45). In fact, many of these neuromodulation systems have received FDA approval for MR Conditional labeling for MRI. As such, if the specific guidelines are followed, MRI examinations may be conducted safely in patients with certain neuromodulation systems.

A number of tactics can be employed to allow safe MRI scans to be performed in patients with neuromodulation systems. Some constrain the static magnetic field, gradient magnetic fields, and/or the RF fields at certain levels and may also limit the landmarks or portion of the body that can be imaged. Examples of various neuromodulation systems that have criteria defined to permit safe MRI examinations are presented in this chapter. When available, labeling approved by the FDA is presented. It should be noted, however, that certain neuromodulation systems have approval outside of the United States for patients referred for MRI examinations. As previously noted, healthcare professionals are advised to contact the respective manufacturer of the device in order to obtain the latest information to ensure patient safety relative to the use of MRI.

Deep Brain Stimulation

Deep brain stimulation (DBS) is one of the most rapidly growing areas in neuromodulation. There have been well over 100,000 DBS implants worldwide since 1997. The use of DBS currently has FDA approval for the treatment of Parkinson's disease, essential tremor, and dystonia. In addition, a number of clinical trials are underway assessing the role of DBS to treat epilepsy, chronic pain, cluster headaches, obsessive-compulsive disorder, major depression, post-traumatic stress syndrome, and other indications (46-48). At the present time, only one manufacturer (Medtronic, Inc., Minneapolis, MN) has DBS systems approved for MRI procedures (head scans only).

Despite the rapid growth of using DBS for a variety of applications, there have been relatively few studies assessing the safety of MRI in patients with DBS systems (49), especially bearing in mind the many types of MRI conditions that must be taken into consideration, including MRI exams performed at different static magnetic field strengths and those using different applications (e.g., MR spectroscopy, fMRI, etc.). Healthcare professionals must only scan patients with DBS systems according to the manufacturer's specific guidelines. Unfortunately, some facilities strictly prohibit MRI examinations in patients with these neuromodulation systems because of a lack of understanding regarding this matter or due to inexperience in managing patients with electronically activated devices.

Notably, the necessity of using MRI is inherent to the use of DBS therapy in patients. MRI is frequently important for the diagnosis of hemorrhage, stroke, or other intracranial lesions, and for assessing the progression of neurodegenerative disorders as well as many other conditions. MRI-guided procedures are used to optimally position the electrodes used for DBS and, thus, substantially decrease the time required for implantation (50, 51). In addition, MRI is used post-operatively to determine DBS lead location and this information is crucial for the evaluation of patients with sub-optimal results or side effects, as well as for targeting during revision, additional DBS procedures, or other cranial surgeries. Furthermore, functional MRI (fMRI) is proving to be greatly beneficial for helping to understand the mechanisms of DBS (30, 43).

The need to use MRI in DBS patients has prompted several groups to systematically study the various safety concerns (42, 49). Investigations have been conducted to define specific conditions permitting the safe use of this imaging modality in patients with implanted DBS neuromodulation systems. Importantly, these studies have resulted in the current manufacturer's guidelines for the use of MRI in a patient with a neurostimulation system used for DBS.

DBS Systems, MR Conditional – Medtronic, Minneapolis, MN

Various investigations have evaluated MRI issues on DBS systems manufactured by Medtronic (Medtronic, Inc., Minneapolis, MN) with an emphasis on MRI-related heating (9, 10, 19, 21-23, 30, 32, 34, 37, 42 43, 45, 50, 51). This DBS system, which is FDA-approved for chronic deep brain stimulation, includes a fully implantable, multi-programmable device designed to deliver electrical stimulation to the thalamus or other brain structures. In addition to the implantable pulse generator (IPG), the basic implantable system consists of a DBS lead and an extension that connects the lead to the IPG. This neuromodulation device delivers high frequency electrical stimulation to a multiple contact electrode placed in the ventral intermediate nucleus of the thalamus or other anatomic sites. The Medtronic DBS system is branded differently for different therapies. For example, Activa DBS Systems are indicated for movement disorders (i.e., essential tremor, Parkinson's disease, and dystonia)(**Figure 6**). The Reclaim System is approved for obsessive-compulsive disorders under humanitarian use only. The Intercept System is under clinical evaluation for epilepsy.

The investigations performed on the Medtronic DBS System indicated that MRI issues are highly dependent on a number of critical factors. These investigations generally evaluated bilateral applications that used two pulse generators, extensions, and leads. Different configurations and clinically relevant positioning scenarios were assessed during *in vitro*

Figure 6. DBS system showing the Activa PC Model 37601 Neurostimulator, Model 37085 DBS extension, and Model 3389 DBS lead (Medtronic, Inc., Minneapolis, MN).

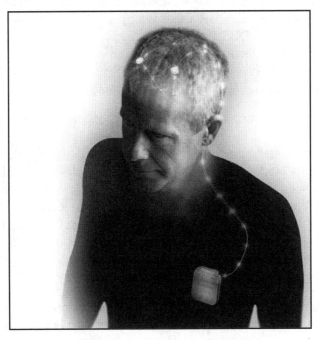

experiments. MRI procedures were performed on a gelled-saline-filled, head/torso phantom designed to approximate the head and torso of a human subject. Temperature changes were studied in association with MRI conducted in a 1.5-Tesla/64-MHz scanner at various RF energy levels using the transmit/receive RF body and transmit/receive head RF coil. The findings from these studies indicated that substantial heating occurs under certain conditions, while others resulted in relatively minor, physiologically inconsequential temperature increases (9, 10, 21-23)(**Figure 7**). Furthermore, factors that strongly influenced local temperature increases at the electrode tip of the DBS system included the positioning of the neuromodulation system (especially the electrode), the type of transmit RF coil used, the SAR used for the MRI procedure, and the method the MR system used to calculate the SAR level (9, 10, 19-23).

Figure 7. Examples of temperature changes recorded during assessment of MRI-related heating at 1.5-T.64-MHz for bilateral neurostimulation systems used for DBS. (A) Graph corresponds to the use of a transmit/receive body RF coil, an MR system reported whole body averaged SAR of 3.9-W/kg, and imaging location through the implantable pulse generators (IPG). The leads were placed in direct routes from the IPG to the deep brain positions. Note the rapid increases in temperatures recorded by fluoroptic thermometry probes on the tips of the right and left leads. (B) Graph corresponds to the use of a transmit/receive body RF coil, an MR system reported whole-body averaged SAR of 0.98-W/kg, and imaging location through the IPGs. Each lead was placed with two small loops (approximately 2.5-cm in diameter) in an axial orientation at the top of the head portion of the phantom [Rezai, et al. (22)].

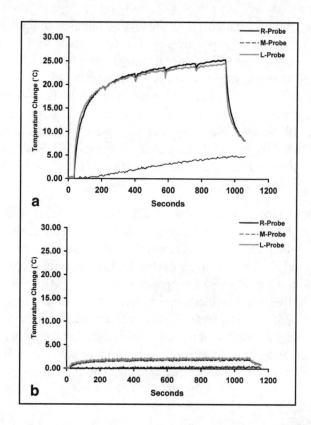

Table 2. Basic MRI information for MR Conditional DBS systems (Medtronic, Minneapolis, MN)

Device Product Names/Models		37601, 37602, 37603, 37612	7426, 7428
MR Conditions			
Static	Static Magnetic Field Strength	1.5-Tesla only	1.5-Tesla only
	Spatial Gradient Magnetic Field	Not defined	Not defined
	Configuration	Closed, horizontal bore only	Closed, horizontal bore only
RF	Specific Absorption Rate (SAR)	0.1-W/kg averaged head SAR maximum	0.1-W/kg averaged head SAR maximum
	Transmit/Receive RF Coil	T/R head RF coil only	T/R head RF coil only
Gradient	Gradient Slew Rate (dB/dt)	20-T/s maximum	20-T/s maximum
Other	Active Scan Duration	Not defined	Not defined
	Product Configuration	Stimulation Off, No broken conductors	Stimulation Off, Bipolar, Set to 0-V, No broken conductors

According to the study by Rezai, et al. (22), MRI-related heating did not appear to present a major safety concern for patients with the bilateral neuromodulation systems that underwent testing, as long as highly specific guidelines pertaining to the positioning of these devices and parameters used for MRI were carefully adhered to. Furthermore, Finelli, et al. (21) reported that MRI sequences commonly used for clinical procedures could be performed safely in patients with bilateral DBS systems at 1.5-Tesla/64-MHz with the utilization of a transmit/receive RF head coil. However, it should be noted that most high-field-strength MR systems in current operation use a body coil to transmit RF energy with a receive-only head RF coil and that a transmit/receive RF head coil may need to be specifically ordered and used for MRI. The basic MRI information for the Medtronic DBS System is presented in **Table 2** (for complete MRI labeling, visit www.medtronic.com/mri).

Note that changes in the SAR algorithm used by one MR system manufacturer prompted a revision of the MRI safety recommendations from the manufacturer (Medtronic, Inc., Minneapolis, MN), which included a recommendation to limit the average head SAR for the MRI sequences to less than 0.1-W/kg (**Table 2**). Interestingly, a study by Larsen, et al. (35) reported that following these SAR recommendations for MRI examinations appeared to be overly conservative. This investigation involved a review of the center's experience scanning 405 patients with 746 implanted DBS systems imaged using 1.5-Tesla MR systems with SARs up to 3-W/kg over a 7-year period. Many of the DBS systems were imaged multiple times, for a total of 1,071 MRI events in this group of patients with no adverse events reported. Thus, Larson, et al. (35) concluded that these findings strongly suggested that the

Figure 8. The LibraXP DBS System (St. Jude Medical, St. Paul, MN).

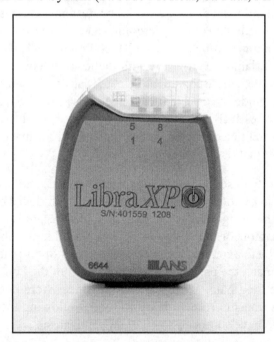

0.1-W/kg guideline for SAR may be unnecessarily low for the prevention of MRI-related adverse events.

DBS Systems, MR Unsafe – St. Jude Medical, St. Paul, MN

The Libra and Libra XP Deep Brain Stimulation (DBS) Systems (**Figure 8**) (St. Jude Medical, St. Paul, MN) are currently available outside of the U.S. and are undergoing investigational evaluation within the U.S. At the present time, the MRI labeling information for these DBS systems is, as follows: "*Magnetic Resonance Imaging (MRI).* Do not use a full body radio-frequency (RF) coil or other extremity coils on patients with a deep brain stimulation system. Because energy from MRI can be transferred through the implanted system, the potential for heat generation at the location of the electrodes exists. This isolated temperature rise may cause tissue damage at the location of the implanted electrodes, possibly resulting in severe injury or death. Injury can occur during MRI treatment whether the deep brain stimulation is turned on or off. All patients should inform their health care professional that they should not be exposed to MRI." Accordingly, the Libra and LibraXP DBS Systems are considered MR Unsafe.

Reported MRI Safety Issues with DBS Systems

This section discusses serious patient injuries that can occur in the MRI environment. Therefore, it is critically important to follow the guidelines that have been developed to ensure MRI safety for patients with DBS systems as well as all other neuromodulation systems (3, 49).

Spiegel, et al. (18) reported that a 73-year-old patient who underwent bilateral DBS lead implantation for Parkinson's disease exhibited dystonic and partially ballistic movements of the left leg immediately after undergoing an MRI procedure of the head. The scan was performed using a transmit/receive head RF coil on a 1.0-Tesla/42-MHz MR system (Siemens Healthcare, Erlangen, Germany) with the leads externalized and not connected to pulse generators. As such, these conditions deviated substantially from the manufacturer's highly specific safety guidelines, which recommend use of a 1.5-Tesla/64-MHz scanner with a transmit/receive head RF coil, only (**Table 2**). Spiegel, et al. (18) speculated that this adverse event was due to induced current in the implanted leads that caused excessive heating and subsequent thermal tissue damage.

Henderson, et al. (15) described a case of a serious, permanent neurological injury secondary to a RF lesion in a patient with Parkinson's disease produced by heating of the electrode of a DBS system during MRI of the lumbar spine. Because the patient was an avid hunter, the pulse generator for the DBS system was placed in the abdomen rather than in the subclavicular region to avoid interference with the butt of his rifle. Seven months after pulse generator placement, the patient underwent an MRI of the lumbar spine for the evaluation of back and left leg pain. Multiple scan sequences were performed using at 1.0-Tesla/42-MHz with a transmit/receive body RF coil. Following the MRI procedure, the patient was reported to have sustained a new right hemiparesis.

The patient was subsequently evaluated by his neurologist who noted the patient exhibited "obtunded aphasia with right hemiplegia, bilateral extensor plantar responses, and skew deviation, right eye below left." A computed tomography (CT) scan performed immediately following the lumbar spine MRI revealed hemorrhage surrounding the left DBS electrode. MRI of the brain performed with a 1.5-Tesla scanner two days after the lumbar MRI found "subacute hemorrhage with methemoglobin in the left thalamus, posterior limb of the left internal capsule, and left cerebral peduncle." The hemorrhage was just adjacent to the tip of the DBS electrode and there was surrounding edema seen on T2-weighted sequences (**Figure 9**). The patient was evaluated seven months following the lumbar MRI procedure and found to have severe dysarthria that made his speech nearly impossible to understand at times. He had persistent right hemiparesis with falling toward the right and clumsiness of his right hand. This patient continued to have a mild dysconjugate gaze. Tremor and bradykinesia remained improved on the left side, similar to prior postoperative evaluations (15).

Notably, this patient's neurological deficits were identified immediately upon his removal from the MR system, implicating a direct relationship between MRI and the subsequent brain lesion. In addition, the hemorrhage and edema demonstrated on subsequent brain imaging surrounded the DBS electrode circumferentially, as would be expected of a lesion generated by RF heating (15). Of further note, the patient suffered from a lesion on the left side of the brain, corresponding with the left-sided lead and the pulse generator, which was implanted in the region of the abdomen. No lesion was produced on the right side, where the lead and implantable pulse generator were in the standard infraclavicular position.

Figure 9. (A) A CT scan performed immediately after the lumbar spine MRI scan revealed evidence of a hemorrhage surrounding the left DBS electrode. (B) T2-weighted MRI of the brain showed edema around the left DBS electrode [Henderson, et al. (15)].

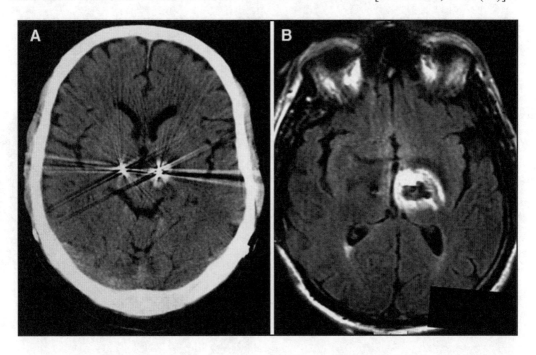

This serious accident as well as the case described by Spiegel, et al. (18) emphasize that, while MRI may be performed safely in patients with certain DBS systems with close adherence to specific safety guidelines, the generalization of these conditions to other neurostimulation system positioning schemes, scanners, and imaging scenarios can results in significant injuries (15, 16). In both of cases described here, MRI was performed under conditions that substantially deviated from the manufacturer's recommendations (**Table 2**). In order to prevent similar catastrophic incidents, the manufacturer's guidelines must be followed carefully to ensure patient safety.

Spinal Cord Stimulation Systems

Spinal cord stimulation (SCS) is commonly used to treat chronic pain of neurologic origin, as well as other conditions that are undergoing clinical investigations (49). Several types of pulse generators and many different types of leads with different electrode arrays are used to administer SCS (**Figure 10**). Thus, equipment-related factors significantly complicate MRI issues for these devices (14, 36). Importantly, the lead used for SCS varies in length depending on the spinal location targeted for stimulation, presenting particular challenges for the evaluation of MRI-related heating. While there are several different manufacturers of SCS products, currently just those from a single manufacturer (Medtronic, Inc., Minneapolis, MN) have FDA approval as being MR Conditional for MRI. One SCS neuromodulation system (Precision Plus Spinal Cord Stimulator System, Boston Scientific) has CE Mark approval MR Conditional labeling for MRI using a transmit/receive head RF

Figure 10. Spinal cord stimulation systems consist of a pulse generator attached to extensions and leads. The electrodes on the lead are typically placed in the epidural space near the spinal cord.

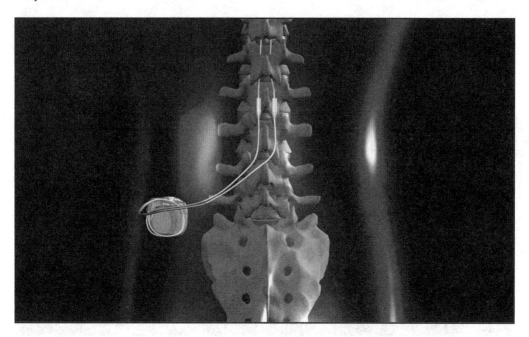

coil only at 1.5-Tesla for patients outside the U.S., for countries with applicable health authority product registrations.

Historically, SCS systems approved for patients undergoing MRI have been limited to the use of 1.5-Tesla/64-MHz scanners to image the head using a transmit/receive RF head coil, only, but in March, 2013 the first "full-body" 1.5-Tesla/64-MHz MR Conditional SCS systems were approved (Medtronic, Inc., Minneapolis), which utilize "SureScan MRI" technology. Notably, these new SCS systems required substantial redesign and still have conditions that must be complied with in order to perform risk-free MRI procedures. Nevertheless, patients with these particular SCS systems are now allowed to benefit from the additional diagnostic capabilities of MRI since other body parts can be examined.

SCS Systems, MR Conditional – Medtronic, Minneapolis, MN

Implantable SCS systems are indicated for the management of chronic, intractable pain of the trunk and/or limbs-including unilateral or bilateral pain associated with the following conditions:

- Failed back syndrome (FBS) or low back syndrome or failed back
- Radicular pain syndrome or radiculopathies resulting in pain secondary to FBSS or herniated disk
- Post-laminectomy pain
- Multiple back operations

- Unsuccessful disk surgery
- Degenerative disk disease (DDD)/herniated disk pain refractory to conservative and surgical therapies
- Peripheral causalgia
- Epidural fibrosis
- Arachnoiditis or lumbar adhesive arachnoiditis
- Complex regional pain syndrome (CRPS), reflex sympathetic dystrophy (RSD), or causalgia

MRI-related labeling for the following SCS systems (Medtronic, Inc., Minneapolis, MN) : RestoreAdvanced SureScan MRI: 97713; RestoreUltra SureScan MRI: 97712; RestoreSensor SureScan MRI: 97714 (**Figure 11**); PrimeAdvanced SureScan MRI: 97702; Restore: 37711; RestoreAdvanced: 37713; RestoreUltra: 37712; RestoreSensor: 37714; RestorePrime: 37701; PrimeAdvanced: 37702; Synergy: 7427; SynergyPlus: 7479; Synergy Versitrel: 7427V; and SynergyCompact: 7479B states that patients with these SureScan MRI devices can safely have full-body, 1.5-Tesla/64-MHz MRI examinations and the other SCS systems (i.e., those without SureScan MRI technology) can safely have 1.5-Tesla/64-MHz procedures using a transmit/receive RF head coil as long as all conditions of safety and other stated guidelines are carefully followed. The basic MRI-related labeling information is shown in **Table 3** for these SCS systems (for complete MRI labeling, visit: www.medtronic.com/mri).

Figure 11. The SCS system, RestoreSensor SureScan MRI, Model 97714 (Medtronic, Inc., Minneapolis, MN).

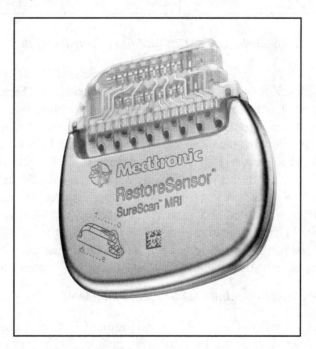

Table 3. Basic MRI information for MR Conditional SCS systems (Medtronic, Minneapolis, MN).

Device Product Names/Models		97702, 97712, 97713, 97714	37701, 37702, 37711, 37712, 37713, 37714, 7427, 7427V, 7479, 7479B
MR Conditions			
Static	Static Magnetic Field Strength	1.5-Tesla only	1.5-Tesla only
	Spatial Gradient Magnetic Field	19-T/m maximum	19-T/m maximum
	Configuration	Closed, horizontal bore	Closed, horizontal bore
RF	Average Specific Absorption Rate	Normal Operating Mode only (2.0-W/kg whole body averaged SAR maximum, 3.2-W/kg averaged head SAR maximum)	Normal Operating Mode only (3.2-W/kg averaged head SAR maximum)
	Transmit/Receive RF Coil	Transmit: Body or head coil Receive: No restriction	T/R head coil only
Gradient	Gradient Slew Rate (dB/dt)	200-T/m/s	200-T/m/s
Other	Active Scan Duration	30 minutes	Not defined
	Product Configuration	Full-body eligible, MRI mode	Stim Off, outside T/R head coil

SCS System, MR Unsafe in the U.S., MR Conditional Outside of the U.S. - Boston Scientific, Valencia, CA

The Precision Plus SCS system (Boston Scientific, Natick, MA) (**Figure 12**) is indicated as an aid in the management of chronic intractable pain of the trunk and/or limbs, including unilateral or bilateral pain associated with the following: failed back surgery syndrome, intractable low back pain and leg pain. Currently, in the U.S., this SCS system is MR Unsafe. Outside of the U.S., The Precision Plus SCS System has CE Mark approved MR Conditional labeling for MRI using a transmit/receive head RF coil, only at 1.5-Tesla/64-MHz. Thus, the Precision Plus SCS System is MR Conditional under the specific conditions defined in the supplemental manual, entitled" 1.5 Tesla MRI Guidelines to Physicians for Patients with Precision Plus Spinal Cord Stimulator System". It is important to read this information in its entirety before conducting or recommending an MRI examination on a patient with this SCS system (for complete MRI labeling, visit: www.controlyourpain.com/dfu/eu.cfm).

SCS Systems, MR Unsafe - St. Jude Medical, St. Paul, MN

The Genesis, GenesisXP, GenesisRC, Eon (**Figure 13**), EonC, EonMini and Renew SCS systems (St. Jude Medical, St. Paul, MN) are indicated as aids in the management of

Figure 12. The pulse generator used with the Precision Plus SCS system (Boston Scientific, Valencia, CA).

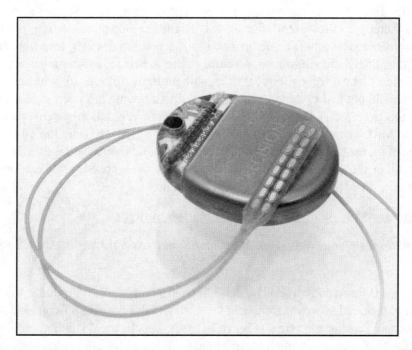

Figure 13. The pulse generator, Eon used with an SCS system from St. Jude Medical (St. Jude Medical, St. Paul, MN).

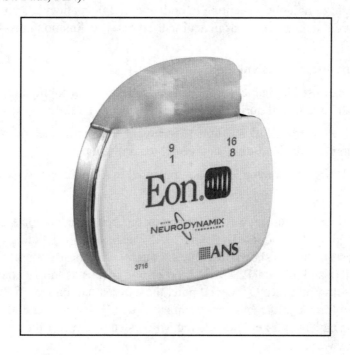

chronic intractable pain of the trunk and/or limbs including unilateral or bilateral pain associated with any of the following: failed back surgery syndrome, and intractable low back and leg pain. The labeling information for these products states: "Warnings/Precautions: Diathermy therapy, cardioverter defibrillators, magnetic resonance imaging (MRI), explosive or flammable gases, theft detectors and metal screening devices, lead movement, operation of machinery and equipment, postural changes, pediatric use, pregnancy, and case damage. Patients who are poor surgical risks, with multiple illnesses, or with active general infections should not be implanted." In addition, the following has been stated: "Magnetic resonance imaging (MRI). Patients with implanted neurostimulation systems should not be subjected to MRI. The electromagnetic field generated by an MRI may forcefully dislodge implanted components, damage the device electronics, and induce voltage through the lead that could jolt or shock the patient." Therefore, these devices are currently contraindicated, or MR Unsafe, for patients referred for MRI procedures.

Other Commercially Available Neuromodulation Systems

Argus II Retinal Prosthesis System, MR Conditional - Second Sight Medical Products, Sylmar, CA

The Argus II Retinal Prosthesis System (Second Sight Medical Products, Inc., Sylmar, CA) recently received approval for use in the U.S. and the European Economic Area. The Argus II Retinal Prosthesis System (**Figure 14**) provides electrical stimulation of the retina to induce visual perception in blind patients and is indicated for use in patients with severe-to-profound retinitis pigmentosa who meet the following criteria:

- Adults, age 25 years or older.
- Bare light or no light perception in both eyes. (If the patient has no residual light perception, then evidence of intact inner layer retina function must be confirmed.)
- Previous history of useful form vision.
- Aphakic or pseudophakic. (If the patient is phakic prior to implant, the natural lens will be removed during the implant procedure.)
- Patients who are willing and able to receive the recommended post-implant clinical follow-up, device fitting, and visual rehabilitation.

The Argus II implant is intended to be implanted in a single eye, typically the worse-seeing eye.

Comprehensive MRI testing was performed on this neuromodulation system, including the work reported by Weiland, et al. (52), in 2012. The basic MRI labeling for the Argus II Retinal Prosthesis System is shown in **Table 4**. Patients with these systems can safely have 1.5-Tesla/64-MHz and 3-Tesla/128-MHz head or body scans as long as the conditions of safety are carefully followed. Of special note, the external equipment (VPU and glasses) are not intended for use in the MRI environment (i.e., MR Unsafe) and, thus, must be removed from the patient and kept outside the MR system room (for the complete MRI labeling, visit: www.2-sight.com).

Figure 14. The Argus II Retinal Prosthesis System (Second Sight Medical Products, Inc., Sylmar, CA).

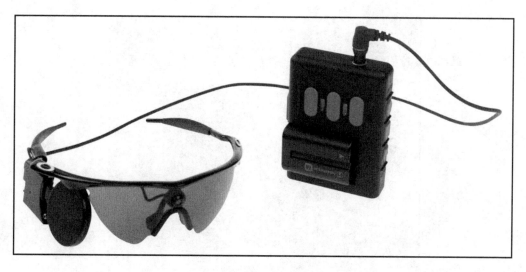

Table 4. Basic MRI information for the Argus II Retinal Prosthesis System.

Device Product Names/Models		Argus II
MR Conditions		
Static	Static Magnetic Field Strength	1.5- or 3-Tesla only
	Spatial Gradient Magnetic Field	7.2-T/m maximum
	Configuration	Not defined
RF	Specific Absorption Rate (SAR)	Normal Operating Mode only (2.0-W/kg whole body averaged SAR maximum)
	Transmit/Receive RF Coil	Not defined
Gradient	Gradient Slew Rate (dB/dt)	Normal Operating Mode only
Other	Active Scan Duration	15 minutes
	Product Configuration	Remove VPU and glasses prior to entering MR system room

Enterra Gastric Electrical Stimulation Therapy System, MR Unsafe - Medtronic, Inc., Minneapolis, MN

Gastric electrical stimulation (GES) is performed using a specialized neuromodulation system, the Enterra GES Therapy System (Medtronic, Inc., Minneapolis, MN), which is indicated for the treatment of patients with chronic, intractable nausea and vomiting secondary to gastroparesis of diabetic or idiopathic etiology (**Figure 15**). GES uses mild electrical pulses to stimulate the stomach to help control symptoms associated with gastroparesis.

Figure 15. The Enterra Therapy used for gastric electrical stimulation (GES), Model 3116 (Medtronic, Inc., Minneapolis, MN).

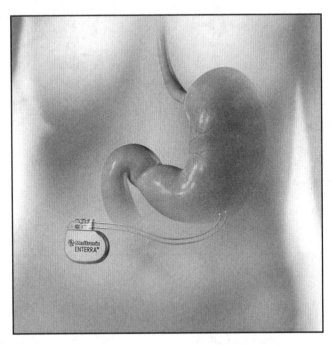

The GES system is comprised of a pulse generator, an implantable intramuscular lead, and an external programming system. Currently, the use of MRI procedures in patients with this system is contraindicated due to possible hazards related to dislodgment or heating of the pulse generator and/or the leads used for GES. Additionally, the voltage induced through the lead and pulse generator may cause uncomfortable "jolting" or "shocking" levels of stimulation. Therefore, this device is MR Unsafe.

InterStim Sacral Nerve Stimulation System, MR Conditional - Medtronic, Inc., Minneapolis, MN

The InterStim Sacral Nerve Stimulation System (InterStim, Model 3023 and InterStim II, Model 3058; Medtronic, Inc., Minneapolis, MN) is a neuromodulation system that is indicated for the treatment of urinary retention and the symptoms of overactive bladder, including urinary urge incontinence and significant symptoms of urgency-frequency alone or in combination, in patients who have failed or could not tolerate more conservative treatments (**Figure 16**). This device may also be used for bowel control and, thus, is indicated for the treatment of chronic fecal incontinence in patients who have failed or who are not candidates for more conservative treatments.

MRI labeling for the neuromodulation devices, InterStim Neurostimulator, Model 3023 and InterStim II, Model 3058, Sacral Nerve Stimulation Systems (Medtronic, Inc., Minneapolis, MN) states that patients with these devices can safely have 1.5-Tesla/64-MHz procedures using a transmit/receive RF head coil as long as all conditions of safety and

Figure 16. The InterStim II Neurostimulator, Model 3058, used for bladder or bowel control (Medtronic, Inc., Minneapolis, MN).

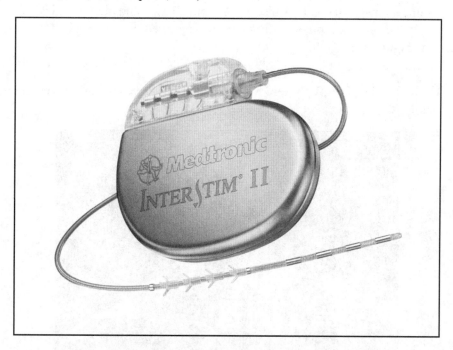

Table 5. Basic MRI information for the InterStim Neuromodulation Systems.

Device Product Names/Models		3023, 3058
MR Conditions		
Static	Static Magnetic Field Strength	1.5-Tesla only
	Spatial Gradient Magnetic Field	19-T/m maximum
	Configuration	Closed, horizontal bore
RF	Specific Absorption Rate (SAR)	Normal Operating Mode only (3.2-W/kg averaged head SAR maximum)
	Transmit/Receive RF Coil	T/R head coil only
Gradient	Gradient Slew Rate (dB/dt)	200-T/m/s
Other	Active Scan Duration	Not defined
	Product Configuration	Stim Off Outside T/R head coil

other stated guidelines are carefully followed. Basic MRI information for these systems is shown in **Table 5** (for complete MRI labeling, visit: www.medtronic.com/mri).

Vagus Nerve Stimulation System, MR Conditional – Cyberonics, Houston, TX

Vagus nerve stimulation (VNS) therapy is a technique that uses a pulse generator to deliver intermittent electrical pulses via electrodes placed on the left vagus nerve at the cervical level (28, 53-57). VNS therapy is approved in the U.S. by the FDA for treatment of epilepsy and medication-resistant depression and is under investigation as a therapy for other disorders, including anxiety, Alzheimer's disease, morbid obesity, and migraine headaches. Currently, this is the only neuromodulation system approved by the FDA for vagus nerve stimulation (**Figure 17**).

Figure 17. The VNS Therapy System with Model 102 Pulse Generator (Cyberonics, Inc., Houston, TX).

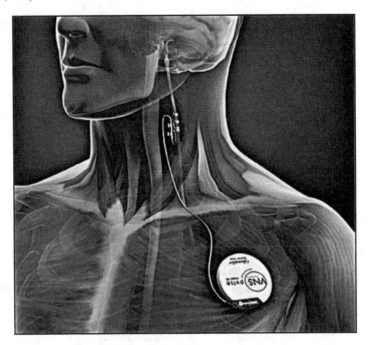

Table 6. Basic MRI information for the VNS Therapy System.

Device Product Names/Models		VNS Therapy System
MR Conditions		
Static	Static Magnetic Field Strength	1.5 or 3 Tesla only
	Spatial Gradient Magnetic Field	7.2-T/m maximum
	Configuration	Closed, horizontal bore
RF	Specific Absorption Rate (SAR)	Normal Operating Mode only (3.2-W/kg average head SAR maximum)
	Transmit/Receive RF Coil	T/R head or T/R extremity RF coils only
Gradient	Gradient Slew Rate (dB/dt)	Normal Operating Mode only
Other	Active Scan Duration	Not defined
	Product Configuration	No broken conductors, Stim Output to 0-mA, Magnet Mode to 0-mA

MRI examinations are often needed to manage patients with the VNS Therapy System, including for the purpose or elucidating the mechanisms responsible for the success or failure of this therapy (28, 53-57). The MRI testing that was utilized to expand these recommendations to 3-T/128-MHz systems as well as 1.5-T/64-MHz scanners is described in Shellock, et al. (28). Current guidelines (Cyberonics 2011) apply to 1.5-Tesla and 3-Tesla MR systems operating at the Normal Operating Mode (3.2 W/kg average head SAR). The basic MRI information for the VNS Therapy System is presented in **Table 6** (for complete MRI labeling, visit: www.cyberonics.com).

Not Commercially Available or Non-FDA-Approved Neuromodulation Systems

Atrostim Phrenic Nerve Stimulator, MR Unsafe - Atrotech Ltd., Tampere, Finland

Phrenic nerve stimulation is used to stimulate the phrenic nerves of patients to maintain respiration. Patients suffering from respiratory muscle paralysis or central alveolar hypoventilation most commonly benefit the most from this form of therapy. The use of phrenic nerve stimulation requires the normal function of phrenic nerves and diaphragm muscles. The Atrostim Phrenic Nerve Stimulator (Atrotech Ltd., Tampere, Finland) is used to stimulate the phrenic nerve (**Figure 18**). This neuromodulation system is not approved by the FDA. Furthermore, it is an MR Unsafe device.

Implantable Infusion Systems

Implantable infusion systems are used for intrathecal or intravascular administration of various medications (58-61). Targeted drug delivery with these devices provides several

Figure 18. The Atrostim Phrenic Nerve Stimulation System (Atrotech Ltd., Tampere, Finland).

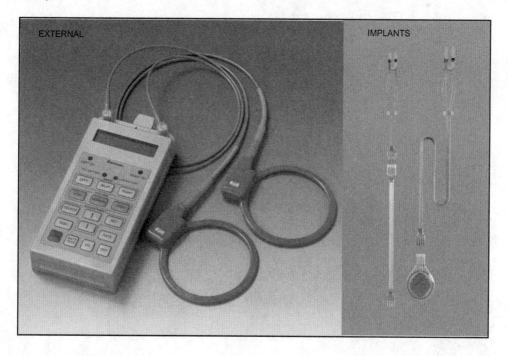

advantages including the fact that significantly decreased dosages may be used (which appears to reduce drug-related adverse events) and these devices permit increased patient mobility (58-61). Infusion pumps and associated catheters typically contain metallic components and, thus, may be impacted by MRI conditions (44, 61). For example, the MRI-related electromagnetic fields (static, gradient magnetic, and radio frequency fields) may displace this implant, generate excessive heating, alter the programmed settings, damage the device, or create substantial artifacts. Several programmable pumps have undergone comprehensive MRI testing and certain ones have FDA approved, MR Conditional labeling, including devices from the following companies: Flowonix Medical, Inc. (Mount Olive, NJ), Codman & Shurtleff, Inc., a Johnson and Johnson Company (Raynham, MA), and Medtronic, Inc. (Minneapolis, MN).

Prometra Programmable Pump, MR Conditional - Flowonix Medical, Inc., Mount Olive, NJ

The Prometra Programmable Pump (Flowonix Medical, Inc., Mount Olive, NJ) is indicated for intrathecal infusion of Infumorph (preservative-free morphine sulfate sterile solution) or preservative-free sterile 0.9% saline solution (Sodium Chloride Injection, USP) (**Figure 19**).

MR Conditional labeling for the Prometra System is shown in **Table 7** (for complete labeling, visit: www.flowonix.com). A patient with this device can safely have 1.5-Tesla MRI "full-body" scans as long as the conditions of safety are carefully followed. Of special note, the Prometra Pump's reservoir must be emptied prior to the exposure to the MRI examination.

Figure 19. The Prometra Programmable Pump (Flowonix Medical, Inc., Mount Olive, NJ)

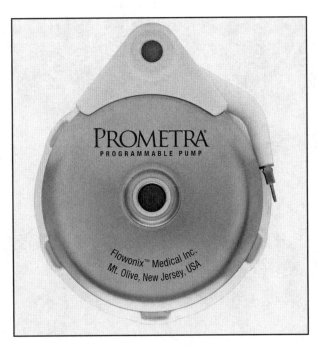

Table 7. Basic MRI information for the Prometra Pump.

Device Product Names/Models		Prometra
MR Conditions		
Static	Static Magnetic Field Strength	1.5-Tesla only
	Spatial Gradient Magnetic Field	4.1-T/m maximum
	Configuration	Not defined
RF	Specific Absorption Rate (SAR)	Normal Operating Mode only (2-W/kg whole body averaged SAR)
	Transmit/Receive RF Coil	Body or other transmit RF coil
Gradient	Gradient Slew Rate (dB/dt)	Normal Operating Mode only
Other	Active Scan Duration	20 minutes maximum
	Product Configuration	Empty drug reservoir prior to entering the MR system room, program to 0.0-mg/day

MedStream Programmable Infusion System, MR Conditional - Codman & Shurtleff, Inc., a Johnson and Johnson Company, Raynham, MA

The MedStream Programmable Infusion System is indicated for the intrathecal delivery of medication, such as Baclofen, for the treatment of severe spasticity and preservative free morphine sulfate for chronic pain (benign or malignant) (**Figure 20**).

Figure 20. MedStream Programmable Infusion System (Codman & Shurtleff, Inc., a Johnson and Johnson Company, Raynham, MA).

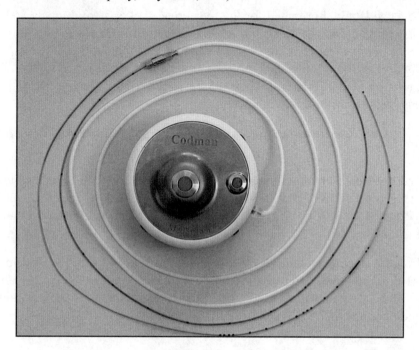

Table 8. Basic MRI information for the MedStream Programmable Infusion System.

Device Product Names/Models		Medstream
MR Conditions		
Static	Static Magnetic Field Strength	3-T and less
	Spatial Gradient Magnetic Field	7.2-T/m maximum
	Configuration	Not defined
RF	Specific Absorption Rate (SAR)	3.0-W/kg whole body averaged SAR
	Transmit/Receive RF Coil	Not defined
Gradient	Gradient Slew Rate (dB/dt)	Not defined
Other	Active Scan Duration	15 minutes maximum
	Product Configuration	Interrogate pump and restart/restart as needed.

MRI-related labeling provided for the MedStream Programmable Infusion System is presented in **Table 8** (for complete MRI labeling, visit: www.depuy.com).

SynchroMed Infusion System, MR Conditional, Medtronic, Inc., Minneapolis, MN

The SynchroMed II Infusion System (Medtronic, Inc., Minneapolis, MN) is used for chronic intrathecal infusion of Baclofen for the management of severe spasticity; chronic intraspinal (epidural and intrathecal) infusion of preservative-free morphine sulfate sterile solution in the treatment of chronic intractable pain; and chronic intrathecal infusion of preservative-free ziconotide sterile solution for the management of severe chronic pain (**Figure 21**).

MRI-related labeling provided for the SynchroMed II System, Models 8637-20 and 8637-40 (Medtronic, Inc., Minneapolis, MN) is displayed in **Table 9** (for complete MRI labeling, visit: www.medtronic.com/mri). The same labeling applies to the discontinued SynchroMed EL system, Model 8627. A patient with these devices can safely undergo an MRI examination at 1.5-Tesla/64-MHz and 3-Tesla/128-MHz as long as the safety conditions and guidelines are carefully followed.

IsoMed Constant Flow Infusion System, MR Conditional – Medtronic, Inc. Minneapolis, MN

The IsoMed Constant Flow Infusion System provides continuous, predictable drug delivery that meets the needs of patients with demonstrated stable dosing requirements (**Figure 22**). (Important Note: Medtronic, Inc. no longer sells the IsoMed Infusion Pump, Model 8472).

MRI-related labeling provided for the IsoMed Constant Flow Infusion System is shown in **Table 10** (for complete MRI labeling, visit: www.medtronic.com/mri). A patient with this device can safely undergo an MRI examination at 1.5-Tesla/64-MHz as long as the safety conditions and guidelines are carefully followed.

Figure 21. The SynchroMed II and SynchroMed EL Infusion Systems (Medtronic, Inc., Minneapolis, MN).

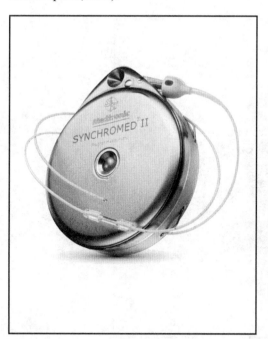
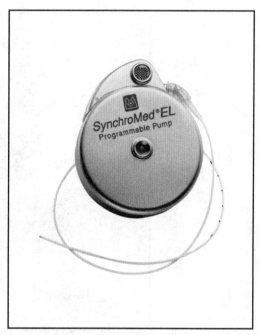

Table 9. Basic MRI information for the SynchroMed II and SynchroMed EL Infusion Systems.

Device Product Names/Models		8637-20, 8637-40, 8627
MR Conditions		
Static	Static Magnetic Field Strength	1.5- and 3.0-Tesla
	Spatial Gradient Magnetic Field	Not defined
	Configuration	Closed, horizontal bore
RF	Specific Absorption Rate (SAR)	Normal Operating Mode only
	Transmit/Receive RF Coil	No restriction
Gradient	Gradient Slew Rate (dB/dt)	Normal Operating Mode
Other	Active Scan Duration	No restriction
	Product Configuration	No perpendicular "Z-axis" orientation at 3-Tesla, Interrogate after MRI

Figure 22. The IsoMed Constant Flow Infusion System (Medtronic, Inc., Minneapolis, MN).

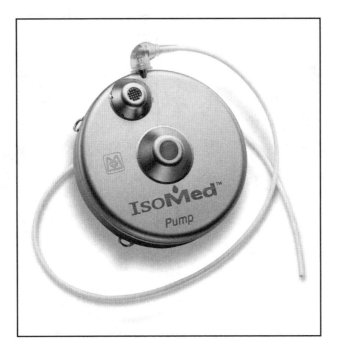

Table 10. Basic MRI information for the IsoMed Constant Flow Infusion System (Medtronic, Inc., Minneapolis, MN).

Device Product Names/Models		8472
MR Conditions		
Static	Static Magnetic Field Strength	1.5-Tesla
	Spatial Gradient Magnetic Field	Not defined
	Configuration	Closed, horizontal bore
RF	Average Specific Absorption Rate	Normal Operating Mode only
	Transmit/Receive RF Coil	No restriction
Gradient	Gradient Slew Rate (dB/dt)	Normal Operating Mode
Other	Active Scan Duration	No restriction
	Product Configuration	No restriction

CONCLUSIONS

With the continued advancements in MRI technology and the development of more so-phisticated implants and devices, there is an increased potential for hazardous situations to occur in the MRI environment. Therefore, to prevent incidents and accidents, it is necessary to be cognizant of the latest information pertaining to MRI safety and patient screening, to adhere to current guidelines to ensure safety for patients and staff members, and to follow proper recommendations pertaining to implants and devices. Fortunately, certain device manufacturers are designing and testing their devices to achieve MR Conditional labeling. In some cases, electronically activated devices that were "unsafe" previously may now have approved MR Conditional labeling. Therefore, obtaining the latest device information is critically important for patient safety as well as access to the vital use of diagnostic MRI.

REFERENCES

1. International Electrotechnical Committee (IEC). 60601-2-33 Edition 3.0, Medical electrical equipment - Part 2-33: Particular requirements for the basic safety and essential performance of magnetic resonance equipment for medical diagnostic. March, 2010.

2. U.S. Department of Health and Human Services, Food and Drug Administration, Center for Devices and Radiological Health, Guidance for Industry and FDA Staff: Criteria for Significant Risk Investigations of Magnetic Resonance Diagnostic Devices. Issued July 14, 2003.

3. Shellock FG. Reference Manual for Magnetic Resonance Safety, Implants, and Devices: 2013 Edition. Los Angeles, CA: Biomedical Research Publishing Group; 2013.

4. Schenck JF. Health Effects and Safety of Static Magnetic Fields. In: Shellock FG, Editor. Magnetic Resonance Procedures: Health Effects and Safety. Boca Raton, FL: CRC Press; 2001. pp. 1-30.

5. Schaefer DJ, Bourland JD, Nyenhuis JA. Review of patient safety in time-varying gradient fields. J Magn Reson Imaging 2000;12:20-29.

6. Shellock FG. Radiofrequency energy-induced heating during MR procedures: a review. J Magn Reson Imaging 2000;12:30-36.

7. Shellock FG, Schaefer DJ. Radiofrequency Energy-Induced Heating During Magnetic Resonance Procedures: Laboratory and Clinical Experiences In: Shellock FG, Editor. Magnetic Resonance Procedures: Health Effects and Safety. Boca Raton, FL: CRC Press; 2001. pp. 75-96.

8. Murbach M, Neufeld E, Kainz W, Pruessmann KP, Kuster N. Whole-body and local RF absorption in human models as a function of anatomy and position within 1.5T MR body coil. Magn Reson Med 2013;DOI: 10.1002/mrm.24690

9. Baker KB, Tkach JA, Nyenhuis JA, Phillips MD, Shellock FG, Gonzalez-Martinez J, Rezai AR. Evaluation of specific absorption rate as a dosimeter of MRI-Related implant heating. J Magn Reson Imaging 2004;20:315-320.

10. Baker KB, Tkach JA, Phillips MD, Rezai AR. Variability in RF-induced heating of a deep brain stimulation implant across MR systems. J Magn Reson Imaging 2006;24:1236-42.

11. Nitz WR, Brinker G, Diehl D, Frese G. Specific absorption rate as a poor indicator of magnetic resonance-related implant heating. Invest Radiol 2005;40:773-6.

12. Woods TO. Standards for medical devices in MRI: present and future. J Magn Reson Imaging 2007;26:1186-1189.

13. Shellock FG, Woods TO, Crues JV 3rd. MR labeling information for implants and devices: explanation of terminology. Radiology 2009;253:26-30

14. De Andres J, Valía JC, Cerda-Olmedo G, et al. Magnetic resonance imaging in patients with spinal neurostimulation systems. Anesthesiology 2007;106:779-86.

15. Henderson J, Tkach J, Phillips M, Baker K, Shellock FG, Rezai A. Permanent neurological deficit related to magnetic resonance imaging in a patient with implanted deep brain stimulation electrodes for Parkinson's disease: Case report. Neurosurgery 2005;57:E1063.

16. Rezai AR, Baker K, Tkach J, et al. Is magnetic resonance imaging safe for patients with neurostimulation systems used for deep brain stimulation (DBS)? Neurosurgery 2005;57:1056-1062.

17. Rezai AR, Phillips M, Baker K, Sharan AD, Nyenhuis J, Tkach J, Henderson J, Shellock FG. Neurostimulation system used for deep brain stimulation (DBS): MR safety issues and implications of failing to follow guidelines. Invest Radiology 2004;39:300-303.

18. Spiegel J, Fuss G, Backens M, et al. Transient dystonia following magnetic resonance imaging in a patient with deep brain stimulation electrodes for the treatment of Parkinson disease. J Neurosurg 2003;99:772-774.

19. Baker KB, Tkach J, Hall JD, Nyenhuis JA, Shellock FG, Rezai AR. Reduction of MRI-related heating in deep brain stimulation leads using a lead management system. Neurosurgery 2005;57:392-397.

20. Bhidayasiri R, Bronstein JM, Sinha S, et al. Bilateral neurostimulation systems used for deep brain stimulation: In vitro study of MRI-related heating at 1.5-Tesla and implications for clinical imaging of the brain. Magn Reson Imaging 2005;23:549-555.

21. Finelli DA, Rezai AR, Ruggieri P, et al. MR-related heating of deep brain stimulation electrodes: an in vitro study of clinical imaging sequences. Am J Neurorad 2002;23:1795-1802.

22. Rezai AR, Finelli D, Nyenhuis JA, Hrdlick G, et al. Neurostimulator for deep brain stimulation: Ex vivo evaluation of MRI-related heating at 1.5-Tesla. J Magn Reson Imaging 2002;15:241-250.

23. Rezai AR, Finelli D, Ruggieri P, Tkach J, Nyenhuis JA, Shellock FG. Neurostimulators: Potential for excessive heating of deep brain stimulation electrodes during MR imaging. J Magn Reson Imaging 2001;14:488-489.

24. Mattei E, Triventi M, Calcagnini G, et al. Temperature and SAR measurement errors in the evaluation of metallic linear structures heating during MRI using fluoroptic probes. Phys Med Biol 2007;21;52:1633-46.

25. Cabot E, Lloyd T, Christ A, Kainz W, et al. Evaluation of the RF heating of a generic deep brain stimulator exposed in 1.5-T magnetic resonance scanners. Bioelectromagnetics. 2013;34:104-113.

26. Gupte AA, Shrivastava D, Spaniol MA, Abosch A. MRI-related heating near deep brain stimulation electrodes: more data are needed. Stereotact Funct Neurosurg 2011;89:131-40.

27. Shrivastava D, Abosch A, Hughes J, et al. Heating induced near deep brain stimulation lead electrodes during magnetic resonance imaging with a 3 T transceive volume head coil. Phys Med Biol 2012;57:5651-65.

28. Shellock FG. Begnaud J, Inman DM. VNS Therapy System: In vitro evaluation of MRI-related heating and function at 1.5- and 3-Tesla. Neuromodulation 2006;9:204-213.

29. Benbadis SR, Nyhenhuis J, et al. MRI of the brain is safe in patients implanted with the vagus nerve stimulator. Seizure 2001;10:512-515.

30. Carmichael DW, Pinto S, Limousin-Dowsey P, et al. Functional MRI with active, fully implanted, deep brain stimulation systems: safety and experimental confounds. Neuroimage 2007;37:508-17.

31. Elkelini MS, Hassouna MM. Safety of MRI at 1.5-Tesla in patients with implanted sacral nerve neurostimulator. Eur Urol 2006;50:311-6.

32. Georgi A-C, Stippich C, et al. Active deep brain stimulation during MRI: A feasibility study. Magn Reson Med 2003;51:380-388.

33. Gleason CA, Kaula NF, Hricak H, et al. The effect of magnetic resonance imagers on implanted neurostimulators. Pacing Clin Electrophysiol 1992;15:81-94.

34. Kovacs N, Nagy F, Kover F, et al. Implanted deep brain stimulator and 1.0-Tesla magnetic resonance imaging. J Magn Reson Imaging 2006;24:1409-12.

35. Larson PS, Richardson RM, Starr PA, Martin AJ. Magnetic resonance imaging of implanted deep brain stimulators: experience in a large series. Stereotact Funct Neurosurg 2008;86:92-100.

36. Liem LA, van Dongen VC. Magnetic resonance imaging and spinal cord stimulation systems. Pain 1997;70:95-97.

37. Sharan A, Rezai AR, Nyenhuis JA, et al. MR safety in patients with implanted deep brain stimulation (DBS). Acta Neurochir 2003;Suppl. 87:141-145.

38. Gorny KR, Bernstein MA, Watson RE Jr. 3 Tesla MRI of patients with a vagus nerve stimulator: initial experience using a T/R head coil under controlled conditions. J Magn Reson Imaging 2010;31:475-81.

39. Shellock FG, Cosendai G, Park SM, Nyenhuis JA. Implantable microstimulator: magnetic resonance safety at 1.5-Tesla. Investigative Radiology 2004;39:591-594.

40. Tagliati M, Jankovic J, Pagan F, et al. and the National Parkinson Foundation DBS Working Group. Safety of MRI in patients with implanted deep brain stimulation devices. Neuroimage 2009;47 Suppl 2:T53-7.

41. Tronnier VM, Staubert A, Hahnel S, et al. Magnetic resonance imaging with implanted neurostimulation systems: an in vitro and in vivo study. Neurosurgery 1999;44:118-25.

42. Zrinzo L, Yoshida F, Hariz MI, et al. Clinical safety of brain magnetic resonance imaging with implanted deep brain stimulation hardware: large case series and review of the literature. World Neurosurg 2011;76:164-72.

43. Phillips MD, Baker KB, Lowe MJ, et al. Parkinson disease: pattern of functional MR imaging activation during deep brain stimulation of subthalamic nucleus--initial experience. Radiology 2006;239:209-16.

44. Shellock FG, Crivelli R, Venugopalan R. Programmable infusion pump and catheter: evaluation using 3-Tesla magnetic resonance imaging. Neuromodulation 2008;11:163-70.

45. Utti RJ, Tsuboi Y, et al. Magnetic resonance imaging and deep brain stimulation. Neurosurgery 2002;51:1423-1431.

46. Oluigbo CO, Salma A, Rezai AR. Deep brain stimulation for neurological disorders. IEEE Rev Biomed Eng 2012;5:88-99.

47. Taghva A, Corrigan JD, Rezai AR. Obesity and brain addiction circuitry: implications for deep brain stimulation. Neurosurgery 2012;71:224-38.

48. Taghva A, Oluigbo C, Corrigan J, Rezai AR. Posttraumatic Stress Disorder: Neurocircuitry and Implications for Potential Deep Brain Stimulation. Stereotact Funct Neurosurg 2013;91:207-219.

49. Shellock FG. MRI Safety and Neuromodulation Systems. In: Krames E, Peckham P, Hunter P, Rezai, AR, Editors. Neuromodulation. New York: Academic Press/Elsevier; 2009. pp. 243-281.

50. Starr PA, Christine CW, et al. Implantation of deep brain stimulators into the subthalamic nucleus: technical approach and magnetic resonance imaging-verified lead locations. J Neurosurg 2002;97:370-387.

51. Starr PA, Martin AJ, Ostrem JL, et al. Subthalamic nucleus deep brain stimulator placement using high-field interventional magnetic resonance imaging and a skull-mounted aiming device: technique and application accuracy. J Neurosurg 2010;112:479-90.

52. Weiland JD, Faraji B, Greenberg RJ, Humayun MS, Shellock FG. Assessment of MRI issues for the Argus II retinal prosthesis. Magn Reson Imaging 2012;30:382-9.

53. Benbadis SR, Nyhenhuis J, et al. MRI of the brain is safe in patients implanted with the vagus nerve stimulator. Seizure 2001;10:512-515.

54. Kosel M, Schlaepfer TE. Beyond the treatment of epilepsy: new applications of vagus nerve stimulation in psychiatry. CNS Spect 2003;8:515-521.

55. Groves DA, Brown VJ. Vagal nerve stimulation: a review of its applications and potential mechanisms that mediate its clinical effects. Neurosci Biobehav Rev 2005;29:493-500.

56. Narayanan JT, Watts R, et al. Cerebral activation during vagus nerve stimulation: a functional MR study. Epilepsia 2002;43:1509-1514.

57. Lomarev M, Denslow S, et al. Vagus nerve stimulation (VNS) synchronized BOLD fMRI suggests that VNS in depressed adults has frequency/dose dependent effects. J Psychiatr Res 2002;36:219-227.

58. Anderson V, Burchiel K. A prospective study of long-term intrathecal morphine in the management of chronic nonmalignant pain. Neurosurgery 1999;44:289-301.

59. Smith T, Swainey C, Coyne P. Pain management, including intrathecal pumps. Cur Pain Headache Rep 2005;9:243-248.

60. Turner M. Intrathecal drug delivery. Acta Neurchir 2003;(Suppl);87:29-35.

61. von Roemeling R, Lanning RM, Eames FA. MR imaging of patients with implanted drug infusion pumps. J Magn Reson Imaging 1991;1:77-81.

Chapter 20 Using MRI Simulations and Measurements to Evaluate Passive Metallic Implants

YAN LIU, PH.D.

Postdoctoral Fellow
Department of Electrical and Computer Engineering
University of Houston
Houston, TX

JI CHEN, PH.D.

Professor of Engineering
Department of Electrical and Computer Engineering
University of Houston
Houston, TX

WOLFGANG KAINZ, PH.D.

Research Biomedical Engineer
Division of Physics
Office of Science and Engineering Laboratories
Center for Devices and Radiological Health
Food and Drug Administration
Silver Spring, MD

INTRODUCTION

With recent advances in numerical modeling of electromagnetic fields used for magnetic resonance imaging (MRI) technology, it is now feasible to perform electromagnetic and thermal simulations to determine the maximum heating in and around passive metallic biomedical implants. The heating related to a metallic implant results from the radiofrequency (RF) energy associated with MRI (1, 2). The Finite-Difference Time-Domain (FDTD) method is generally used to compute the RF field distribution in MRI (2). In addition, the implant's surface heating pattern for various orientations of the implant relative to the incident electric field can be obtained.

Simulation studies enable the identification of worst-case heating for various implant configurations, which reduces the amount of required *in vitro* testing because only the worst-case heating configuration at the worst-case heating location on the implant needs to be experimentally verified using the technique described by the American Society for Testing and Materials (ASTM) International (3). This combined simulation or modeling and experimental approach involving temperature measurements can quickly identify, in a cost-effective and timely manner, the worst-case heating characteristics for an entire implant family. For example, for a given implant type such as an orthopedic implant, there may be different dimensions that are associated with the implant that are necessary in order to provide a proper fit of the implant due to the variances in human body sizes. By performing MRI simulations and experimental measurements to assess MRI-related heating for the metallic implant, the worst-case scenario may be identified and evaluated to ensure patient safety.

The modeling approach typically begins with electromagnetic simulations to determine the specific absorption rate (SAR) distribution and temperature rise in the vicinity of the implant placed in the ASTM phantom that is filled with gelled-saline (3). Most modeling tools have the capability to directly import engineering designs in their native computer aided design (CAD) format, which significantly simplifies the modeling procedure. By being able to use the original CAD data of the implant, it is possible to accurately represent the device in the computational tool. This representation of the implant significantly increases the accuracy of thermal heating patterns for practical medical device designs. Once simulation results are obtained, temperature measurements should be performed to validate the electromagnetic (EM) and thermal modeling.

METHODOLOGY CONSIDERATIONS

Numerical Modeling of MRI

SEMCAD X is one of several commercial full-wave electromagnetic and thermal simulation packages (4). In simulation studies, SEMCAD X is used to model the interactions between MRI-related RF signals and medical implants. In most commercial MR systems, a high pass RF transmission coil is used (also referred to as the transmit RF coil). Other types of RF coils used in scanners are low pass and band pass RF coils. For 1.5-Tesla and 3-Tesla MR systems the high pass RF coil works at two different frequencies: 64-MHz and 128-MHz, respectively. A physical RF coil is usually difficult to model because it requires the information of the detailed RF coil design, including the shape and size of the individual rungs and end-rings. These parameters often vary from one scanner to another and are difficult to obtain because the manufacturers of the MR systems consider the information to be proprietary. In addition, using a model of a physical RF coil also increases simulation time. Fortunately, it has been shown that using a simplified coil model reduces the simulation time while providing the same result as that from a physical coil model (5). Therefore, rather than modeling a real-world coil design, a simplified coil that has only eight rungs is modeled in SEMCAD for the simulation (**Figure 1**).

Figure 1. 1.5-T/64-MHz RF Coil (Top) and 3-T/128-MHz RF Coil (Bottom) models in SEMCAD.

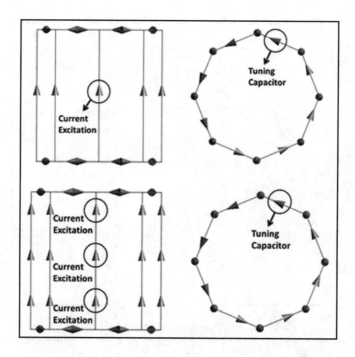

The top two models in **Figure 1** are for the 1.5-T/64-MHz transmit RF coil and the bottom two models are for the 3-T/128-MHz transmit RF coil. To ensure a uniform magnetic field inside the simplified RF coil for the 3-T system RF coil as shown in the bottom left figure of **Figure 1**, one needs to add three constant current sources for each rung and re-adjust the capacitor values on the end ring. The diameter of the RF coil is 63-cm. The height of the RF coil is 65-cm. The capacitance value is determined from several broadband simulations so that the highest resonant frequency is set to 64-MHz for 1.5-T and 128-MHz for 3-T. The detailed steps are, as follows: (1) Set an initial capacitance value for all capacitors on end rings and add a broadband pulse signal on one single rung. The other seven rungs are modeled as zero ohm resistors. (2) After the simulation, the power spectrum is extracted. If the second highest resonant frequency is not at 64-MHz, the capacitance needs to be adjusted. (3) After three to five broadband simulations, the second highest resonant frequency needs to be located at 64-MHz, as shown in **Figure 2**.

From this information, the capacitance for the end ring tuning capacitor is 7.2-pF for the 64-MHz RF coil and 1.3-pF for the 128-MHz RF coil. **Figure 3** shows the electric and magnetic field distribution at the center of the RF coil. The electric field is center-symmetric and decreases along the radial direction. The magnetic field is uniformly distributed. From **Figure 2** and **Figure 3**, it is concluded that the RF coils are operating at the right resonant mode and the field patterns are also correct. Thus, the RF coils can be used for the MRI simulation studies.

Figure 2. Spectrum of 64-MHz transmit RF coil excited by broadband signal with end ring tuning capacitance = 7.2-pF. Note the highest resonance frequency.

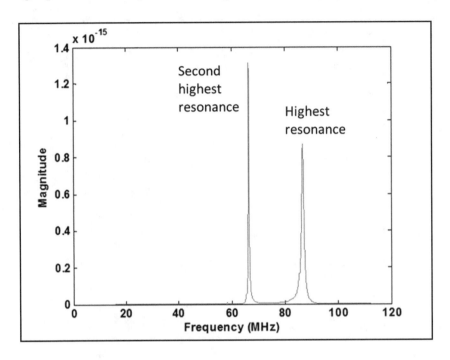

ASTM International Heating Test Procedure

Once the RF coils are developed and their operating modes are verified, it is necessary to determine the location of the maximum electric field inside the ASTM phantom that is used to assess MRI-related heating for an implant (3). To evaluate the maximum electric field inside the ASTM phantom, the phantom is placed into each RF coil, as shown in **Figure 4**. The center section of the ASTM phantom is positioned at the center of the RF coil. The bottom of the phantom is 23.85-cm above the lowest point of the RF coil, mimicking the configuration that is equivalent to an actual clinical MRI examination. The ASTM phantom consists of a plastic box that has a relative dielectric constant of $\varepsilon_r = 3.7$ and electric conductivity of $\sigma = 0$-S/m. The gelled-saline has a relative dielectric constant of $\varepsilon_r = 80.38$ and conductivity of $\sigma = 0.448$-S/m.

With this ASTM phantom positioning, electromagnetic simulations may be performed to determine the electric field distributions within the phantom. **Figure 5** shows the top view of the electric field distributions in the center plane. As shown in the **Figure 5** for 64-MHz and 128-MHz RF coils, the maximum electric field locations are near the side-walls of the phantom, along the center for both horizontal and vertical directions, as reported by Nordbeck, et al. (5). Thus, these locations are selected to place the implant or device in order to maximize the exposure and minimize the measurement uncertainty relative to RF-induced heating for a passive metallic implant. While there are other locations, such as the corners of the ASTM phantom, that have very large electric fields due to "edge effects," these electric field locations are not chosen since the regions are relatively small and, thus,

Figure 3. Electric field (Left) and magnetic field (Right) distributions at the center of the RF coil.

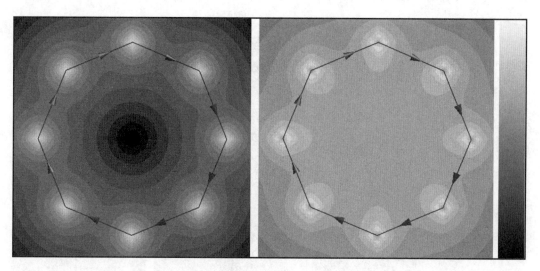

Figure 4. Simulation setup used to determine the maximum electric field location inside of the ASTM phantom that is used to assess MRI-related heating for an implant. Note the different orientations of the phantom in the RF coil (a, b, and c).

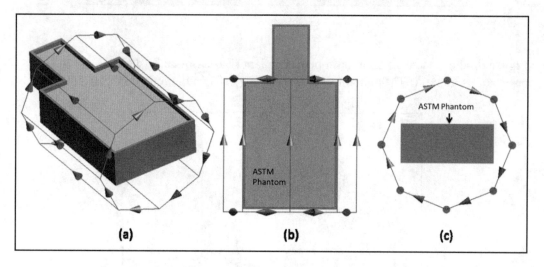

not suitable for implant placement. According to the coronal view, the electric field has a tilted angle to the boundaries of the ASTM phantom filled with gelled-saline. The tilted angle is due to the circular polarized field pattern inside the MRI RF coil.

The next step is to place implants with different dimensions inside the ASTM phantom at the location of high electric field concentration (**Figure 6**). The devices should be spaced 2-cm from the side-wall for all simulations.

Figure 5. The electric field distribution for 1.5-T/64-MHz (Left) and 3-T/128-MHz (Right) MR systems in the ASTM phantom (top view of the phantom).

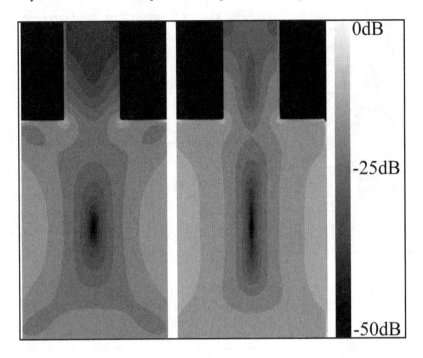

Figure 6. The placement of an orthopedic implant (Basis Spinal System) in two different orientations in the ASTM phantom: Orientation 1 (Left) and Orientation 2 (Right).

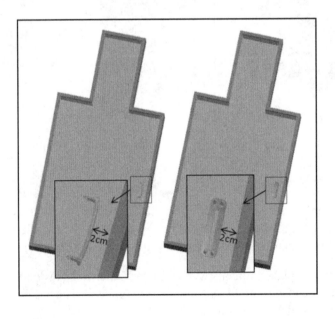

Thermal Modeling/Simulations

In most cases, SAR alone is not enough to evaluate the electromagnetic safety of patients with implanted medical devices with regard to heating. Therefore, the analysis needs to assess the temperature changes caused by the RF-induced currents. Developed in 1948 by Pennes (6), the "Bioheat Equation" (PBE) is the most commonly used model for thermal BioEM simulations. The Bioheat Equation is shown in Equation (1),

$$\rho c \frac{\partial T}{\partial t} = \nabla \cdot (k \nabla T) + \rho Q + \rho SAR - \rho_b c_b \rho \omega (T - T_b) \tag{1}$$

where k is the thermal conductivity, SAR is the specific absorption rate, ω is the perfusion rate, Q is the metabolic heat generation rate, ρ is the density of the medium, and ρ_b, c_b and T_b are the density, specific heat capacity, and temperature of blood, respectively. In the ASTM phantom, the equation can be further simplified since there is no metabolic heat generation or heat transfer by blood to Equation (2),

$$\rho c \frac{\partial T}{\partial t} = \nabla \cdot (k \nabla T) + \rho SAR \tag{2}$$

where ρ, c and k are the density, specific heat capacity, and thermal conductivity, respectively, of the gelled-saline. The maximum time step for which stability can be guaranteed is given by Equation (3),

$$dt \leq \frac{8k}{\rho c (dx)^2} \tag{3}$$

where dt is the thermal simulation time step and dx is the unit mesh size. The above equation is only valid for uniform mesh. For non-uniform mesh, the stable time-step is more complicated.

MRI-RELATED HEATING OF PASSIVE METALLIC IMPLANTS

Orthopedic implants are biomedical devices used to help heal bone fractures, replace joints, and for a variety of other purposes. Examples of common orthopedic devices include bone plates, fixation devices, and total hip replacements. Non-conductive, orthopedic implants and materials do not pose heating risks for patients undergoing MRI examinations. However, because of the length of the metallic implant or the formation of a conductive loop of a certain diameter, MRI may cause unsafe levels of heating for orthopedic implants made from conductive materials (7-10). The standard test method used to assess heating assumes that the device will be fully implanted (3). However, there are orthopedic devices,

Figure 7. Zoomed view of the SAR distribution near the orthopedic implant (Basis Spinal System) with 6.7-cm length. (Left) peak SAR distribution. (Right) 1-g averaged SAR distribution.

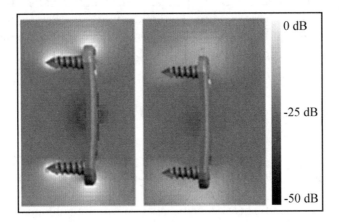

such as external fixation systems and cervical fixation devices, where the device is not entirely implanted in tissue. In addition to orthopedic devices, there are other percutaneous medical devices, such as biopsy needles, catheters, and RF or microwave ablation probes that are not entirely implanted or placed in tissue during the intended uses of these items. These partially implanted devices may result in unsafe heating during MRI due to the higher electric field intensity that exists outside the human body (10). Therefore, this chapter will present information for both types of scenarios involving passive metallic implants using an example of each type of implant (i.e., an entirely implanted device and a partially implanted device). In one section, the RF-induced heating for a spinal implant (Basis Spinal System, Medtronic, Spinal and Biologics, Memphis, TN) will be studied both numerically and experimentally. In another section, the information will be extended to the RF-induced heating of an external fixation system (i.e., a "generic" external fixation system).

Passive Implant

Based on the numerical procedure described previously, a set of electromagnetic simulations were performed on a spinal implant (Basis Spinal System) for both 64-MHz (1.5-T) and 128-MHz (3-T) transmit RF body coil conditions. In all electromagnetic simulations, the results were normalized to an input power of 1-W. However, the results can be easily normalized to a specific absorption rate (SAR) for a whole-body-averaged (WB SAR) of 2-W/kg and 4-W/kg which corresponds to the Normal Operating Mode and the First Level Controlled Operating Mode of operation for MR systems, respectively (11). The WB SAR is defined by the total absorbed power of the phantom divided by the total mass of the phantom filled with gelled-saline.

Simulation Study

To remove potential numerical errors, the 1-g averaged SAR distributions are calculated in addition to the non-averaged peak SAR distributions. The zoomed views of the local SAR distributions near the implants are shown in **Figure 7**. The length of the orthopedic implant is 6.7-cm. As indicated in **Figure 7**, the maximum peak SAR is located at the tip of a screw while the maximum 1-g averaged SAR is located at the top of the implant. Because the temperature rise is a diffusion process (6), the maximum temperature is more likely to be located close to the location where the maximum 1-g averaged SAR is observed. In order to clearly identify the maximum heating position, thermal simulations are necessary.

In **Figure 8** and **Figure 9**, the maximum local SAR as a function of implant length at 1.5-T/64-MHz and 3-T/128-MHz is displayed. As indicated in the figures, peak SAR and 1-g averaged SAR for both implant orientations (parallel and perpendicular to the electric field) are similar. As the length of the implant increases, the SAR value increases. However, for this particular implant placement, the SAR value at 1.5-T/64-MHz near the implant was higher than those at 3-T/128-MHz. Because 3-T/128-MHz systems operate at a higher frequency than 1.5-T/64-MHz scanners, more energy loss can be expected along the interface between the surface of the ASTM phantom and the implant. Therefore, the electric field incident on the implant at 3-T/128-MHz should be lower.

For the same level of input power at 3-T/128-MHz, the SAR is lower near the tip of the screw region than at 1.5-T/64-MHz, indicating that heating at 3-T/128-MHz will be less for this setup. **Figure 9** shows that the SAR values for this device at 3-T/128-MHz reach a plateau near 10-cm with regard to the length of the implant. This may be explained as the resonant wavelength effect. When the implant is longer than 10-cm, the length is less than half the wavelength at 128-MHz inside the gelled-saline. For such scenarios, the maximum heating locations will probably be close to the ends of the implants. However, as the length increases, the implant's dimensions can become comparable to the wavelength of the incident electromagnetic field. Due to the resonant effects as well as the phase variation of the incident field along the implant, the potential heating will no longer have the monotonic increment trend. These simulations were not performed because the maximum length for this particular orthopedic implant as it would be used in a patient is only 107-mm. The input power for cases shown here is at 1-W for illustration purposes. Importantly, these results need to be scaled based on local SAR values for future temperature rise evaluations.

The maximum average SAR location near the implanted device is a good indication of where the maximum temperature rise will occur. To obtain the actual temperature rise, thermal simulations need to be conducted. This can be achieved by performing additional thermal simulations based on the bioheat equation (12, 13). To determine the temperature rise as a function of time, temperature probes are placed on or near the locations on the implant where the maximum temperature rises are expected. Before starting the thermal simulations, all SAR values are scaled to the same WB SAR. For example, to determine the SAR values near the implant when the whole-body-averaged SAR is 2-W/kg, it is necessary to calculate the total energy loss within the phantom and then scale it to the total weight of the phantom.

As in the previous 1.5-T/64-MHz electromagnetic simulations, it is observed that when the input power from the RF coil is at 1-W, the total energy loss inside the ASTM phantom is 0.735-W. With the weight of the ASTM phantom at 44.86-kg, the whole-body-averaged SAR for the ASTM phantom is 0.016-W/kg. For the MR system in the Normal Operating Mode, the whole-body-averaged SAR is limited to 2-W/kg (14). Therefore, a scaling factor of 122 (2-W/kg / 0.016-W/kg) should be applied to SAR values. Using this scaled SAR value, thermal simulations should then be performed for the whole-body-averaged SAR at

Figure 8. Peak 1-g averaged SAR values as a function of implant (Basis Spinal System) length for two different orientations at 1.5-T/64-MHz.

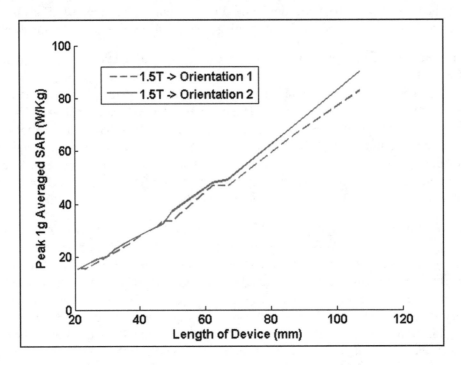

Figure 9. Peak 1-g averaged SAR values as a function of implant (Basis Spinal System) length for two different orientations at 3-T/128-MHz.

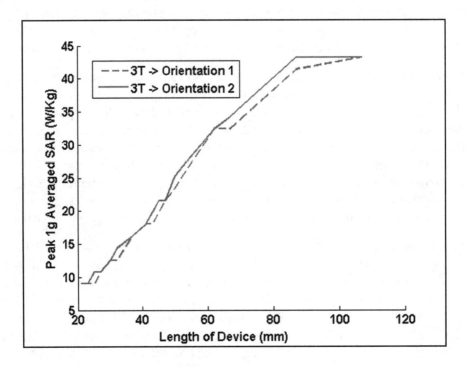

2-W/kg. Another way to perform the scaling is to use the local SAR. This requires one additional measurement of local SAR, which can be performed by measuring the local temperature rise in the gelled-saline or measuring the temperature rise of a 10-cm titanium rod (15). All results can then be normalized using this value (16).

Measurement Study

Carefully designed temperature measurements have been performed for both 1.5-T/64-MHz and 3-T/128-MHz MRI conditions. As indicated in **Figure 10**, the temperature probes were placed near the locations on the implant where maximum temperature rises were expected according to the simulation results.

Figure 11 shows the values for the simulations and the measured temperature rises over time for 15-minutes at the two temperature probe locations as a function of time for 1.5-T/64-MHz conditions. As indicated in **Figure 11**, the simulation and measurement results agree well with each other when normalized to the same whole-body-averaged SAR.

Similarly, the temperature rise simulations have been performed for 3-T/128-MHz MRI conditions based on the results obtained from the electromagnetic simulation. **Table 1** shows the temperature rise after 15 minutes for both 1.5-T/64-MHz and 3-T/128-MHz MRI conditions at the temperature probe locations obtained by the simulations and measurements. As clearly indicated in **Table 1**, a good correlation is observed.

Discussion

From the electromagnetic and thermal simulation results, it can be clearly seen that numerical techniques were able to provide a good assessment of the maximum heating location for the orthopedic implant that was evaluated. For this particular implant, the Basis Spinal System, the maximum heating locations were close to the tips of the screws and at the ends of the implant. As the length of this orthopedic implant increases, especially when the device length is comparable to the wavelength of the MRI operating frequencies, the heating patterns as well as the maximum heating location change.

From this study, the findings suggest that when this orthopedic implant's length is less than 100-mm, the maximum heating of the device is almost linearly proportional to its length. This can be explained as a wavelength effect. At 64-MHz, the electromagnetic incident wavelength is approximately 4.5-m in free space and approximately 0.52-m in the gelled-saline. When this orthopedic implant's length is less than 100-mm, the overall length is still less than a quarter wavelength. Therefore, it is not expected for the incident field to have a large phase variation or have a resonant effect for this particular orthopedic implant. However, at 128-MHz, the wavelength in gelled saline is 0.26-m. The implant's length of 100-mm approaches the half-wavelength. Therefore, the incident field will have a large phase variation along the implant, and it will exhibit resonant behavior. Thus, a monotonic relationship between the maximum heating and the implant's length will no longer be valid. For implant lengths over 100-mm, an electromagnetic/thermal simulation is performed at centimeter increments to capture the maximum heating for different lengths.

This investigation demonstrated that with numerical calculations it is possible to effectively predict which implant configuration and size will result in maximum heating as well

Figure 10. Positions for the fluoroptic thermometry probes, #1 and #2, relative to the orthopedic implant (Basis Spinal System).

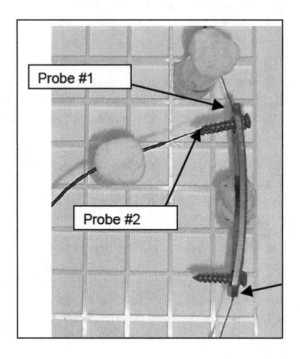

Figure 11. Simulated and measured temperature rises at temperature Probe 1 (Top) and Probe 2 (Bottom) applied to an orthopedic implant (Basis Spinal System) at 1.5-T/64-MHz.

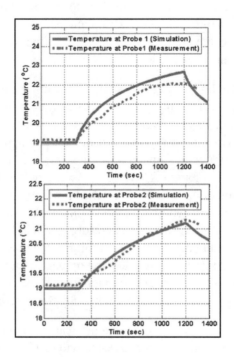

Table 1. Simulated and measured temperature changes for 1.5-T/64-MHz and 3-T/128-MHz MRI conditions after 15 minutes of RF exposure at two temperature probe locations on an implant (Basis Spinal System) normalized to the whole-body-averaged SAR.

	Simulation 1.5-T	Measurement 1.5-T	Simulation 3-T	Measurement 3-T
Probe 1	3.6°C	3.1°C	2.1°C	1.9°C
Probe 2	2.2°C	2.2°C	1.6°C	1.7°C

as the maximum heating location for the device. With this information, one can correctly place the temperature probes to record maximum temperature rises, as well as decrease the number of implants that need to be tested to ensure MRI safety. Consequently, it can significantly reduce the time and expense of testing performed to evaluate RF-induced heating for passive metallic implants. As previously indicated, using this testing strategy, one can determine the device with the worst-case heating for a particular device family.

In conclusion, electromagnetic and thermal simulations were used to determine the worst-case heating for an orthopedic implant (Basis Spinal System) with lengths ranging from 21- to 107-mm. For this particular metallic implant, it was observed that the temperature rise is related to the length of the implant. The locations of the maximum temperature rises are close to the ends of the implant or at the tips of the screws. RF-induced heating experiments were performed to record temperatures to validate the simulation results. Good correlations were observed. These findings demonstrated that electromagnetic and thermal simulations may be used as excellent tools to provide the heating pattern for passive metallic implants and to identify the maximum heating locations for the entire device family. If only the temperature measurement technique is used, temperature probes need to be placed on multiple positions on or near the device to determine the worst-case heating spot associated with the implant. Therefore, numerical modeling is an efficient way to determine the worst-case heating.

Because the maximum heating can change for different sizes or configurations of an implant, the determination of the location of maximum heating is important for a proper evaluation. MRI simulations provide the means to drastically reduce the number of measurements needed to assess the worst-case configuration and size for an entire device family. The simulation results are also the only practical way to find the location of the maximum heating on the implant and to place the temperature probe at this position during the measurements. Importantly, for validation purposes, the simulations should always be accompanied by proper temperature measurements.

External Fixation System

In this section, the MRI safety relative to heating for an external fixation system will be discussed. Indications for external fixation systems are varied and include the following treatment applications: open and closed fracture fixation; pseudoarthroses of long bones (both congenital and acquired); limb lengthening by metaphyseal or epiphyseal distraction; correction of bony or soft tissue defects; and correction of bony or soft tissue deformities. The assessment of RF-induced heating for external fixation systems is especially challenging because of the myriad of possible components, many of which are made from conductive materials, and configurations that are used for these devices. Of course, the primary concern is MRI-related heating which is dependent on the particular aspects (e.g., the lengths of the component parts) of the external fixation system. Importantly, the MRI conditions (strength of the static magnetic field, RF field, type of RF transmit coil, pulse sequence, body part imaged, position of the external fixation system relative to the transmit RF coil, etc.) directly impact the safety aspects of scanning patients with external fixation systems (18).

Importantly, the exact construct aspects of the external fixation system needs to be adjusted to fit the shape and size of the patient in consideration of the abnormality or condition that needs to be treated. A typical external fixation system is composed of bars, pins, rings, and clamps. A generic model of the external fixation system is shown in **Figure 12**. Oftentimes, larger patient body sizes require greater spacing for pins as well as deeper pin insertions to achieve good fixation or alignment. As a result, different patients will have different device configurations. Therefore, the effect of different insertion depths and pin spacing on heating of an external fixation system must be investigated to ensure patient safety in association with MRI.

Evaluation of Pin Insertion Depth and Clamp Spacing on RF-Induced Heating

According to the ASTM F F2182 (3) heating document, implanted devices need to be placed at the location of maximum exposure to electric fields in order to minimize the measurement uncertainty relative to MRI-related heating. In this investigation of an external fixation system, the pins were placed at these particular locations (17).

The external fixation system model used in this study consists of three parts, as shown in **Figure 12**. These three parts include, the following: two metallic blocks to represent the clamps, two connectors or bars to represent the rods outside the body for rigid support, and four parallel pins which are screwed into the bones during surgery. Each metallic block has the dimension of 11.4-cm × 2-cm × 3.75-cm. Each pin has a diameter of 0.5-cm and length of 16-cm. The connecting bars have a diameter of 1.1-cm and four different lengths of 31.5-cm, 36.5-cm, 41.5-cm, and 46.5-cm. When different bar lengths are used, the clamp spacing is changed to 15-cm, 20-cm, 25-cm, and 30-cm. In all the evaluations, the distance between the two connecting bars is 5-cm. Please note that this is a simplified model of an external fixation system and real-world devices are often significantly more complicated.

Simulations were repeated with four pin insertion depths of 2-cm, 5-cm, 8-cm, and 11-cm. Notably, with deep pin insertion, the spacing between the external frame and the surface of the gelled-saline filling the ASTM phantom will be reduced. There is a 2-cm space between the screws and the inner side-wall of the ASTM phantom. The bar material used in this study is carbon-fiber reinforced epoxy with a relative dielectric constant of $\varepsilon_r = 10$ and electric conductivity of $\sigma = 5.7*10^6$-S/m. The ASTM phantom consists of a plastic box which has a relative dielectric constant of $\varepsilon_r = 3.7$ and electric conductivity of $\sigma = 0$-S/m. The gelled-saline has a relative dielectric constant of $\varepsilon_r = 80.38$ and conductivity of $\sigma = 0.448$-S/m. The pins and main blocks of the device are modeled as perfect electric conductors (PEC).

Figure 12. Generic external fixation system model.

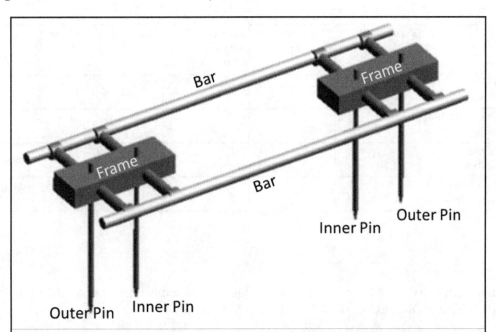

Electromagnetic simulations are first conducted to determine electric energy deposition near the pins of the device. Then, thermal simulations are carried out to estimate the temperature rise near the tips of the pins. Based on the energy deposition near the tips, the temperature rises in the ASTM phantom are calculated using the heat transfer equation given in Equation (4) [see also Equation (2)],

$$\rho c \frac{\partial T}{\partial t} = \nabla \cdot (k \nabla T) + \sigma |E|^2 \qquad (4)$$

where ρ is the gel density, 1000-kg/m^3, and c is the specific heat of the gelled-saline. The thermal conductivity, k, for the ASTM phantom, the ASTM gelled-saline, and the device are 0.2-W • m^{-1} • K^{-1}, 0.42-W • m^{-1} • K^{-1}, and 7-W • m^{-1} • K^{-1}, respectively. The specific heat capacity for gelled-saline is 4160-J • Kg^{-1} • K^{-1}. For the ASTM phantom and fixation device, the specific heat capacity is 1000-J • Kg^{-1} • K^{-1}. The electric and thermal properties of the materials in this particular evaluation are listed in **Table 2**.

For the temperature rise measurements, the ASTM International document requires an RF field producing a whole-body-averaged SAR of 2-W/Kg for approximately 15-minutes (3). Thus, for all results reported herein, the whole-body-averaged (WB) SAR of 2-W/kg is used to normalize the results.

In **Figure 13**, the maximum 1-g averaged SAR in the ASTM phantom and the temperature rises near the pins are shown for a 1.5-T/64-MHz MR system. The temperature rise

Table 2. Electrical and thermal properties for different materials used in MRI simulations for the external fixation system.

	Permittivity	Electrical Conductivity (S/m)	Thermal Conductivity (W/m/K)	Heat Capacity (J/Kg/K)	Density (Kg/m³)
ASTM Phantom Gelled-Saline	80.38	0.448	0.42	4,160	1,000
ASTM Phantom Shell	3.7	0	0.2	1,000	1,000
Device, Bar (Carbon-fiber)	10	5600000	0.2	400	1,000
Device, Other Parts (PEC)	N/A	N/A	7	400	8,000

Figure 13. Peak 1-g averaged SAR (Top) and maximum temperature rise after 15-min. MRI. (Bottom) for PEC bar in 1.5-T/64-MHz MRI condition.

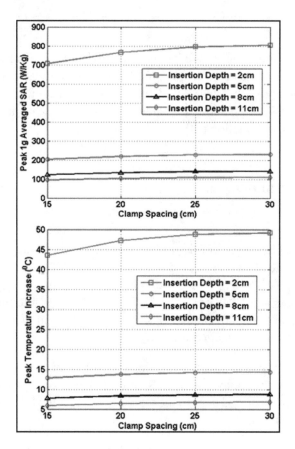

data are recorded for 15-minutes of MRI time. In each group, the environment was 1.5-T/64-MHz and the bar material was carbon-fiber. The 1-g averaged SAR and temperature rise data are shown with different clamp spacing (15-cm, 20-cm, 25-cm, and 30-cm). The four different curves in the plot represent four different pin insertion depth values: 2-cm, 5-cm, 8-cm, and 11-cm.

In the 1.5-T/64-MHz MR system, when the bars are made of carbon-fiber, increasing the insertion depth of the pins decreases the temperature rise dramatically. When clamp spacing increases, the temperature rise slightly increases.

Numerical simulation is used to study surface heating for the external fixation systems in association with a 1.5-T/64-MHz MR system. Typically, the shortest insertion depth and largest pin spacing with the conductive bar will result in worst-case heating. The heating mechanism can be explained by induced current along the device and power decay inside the ASTM phantom.

Dielectric Layer Effect on RF-Induced Heating

In **Figure 14 (a)**, the external fixation system is shown with the gelled-saline in the ASTM phantom. The four pins are defined from left to right. The maximum heating region is found to be located at the tip of the fourth pin. Variation of the dielectric constant of in-

Figure 14. (a) External fixation system inserted in a gelled-saline filled ASTM phantom. Maximum heating region is around the tip of the fourth pin from left to right; (b) Illustration of local SAR (1-g averaged) distribution inside maximum heating region for different dielectric layer material: $\varepsilon_r = 1$ (Left) and $\varepsilon_r = 9$ (Right).

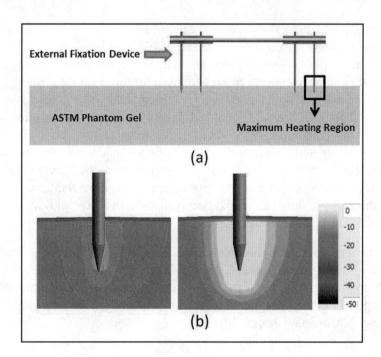

sulated layer material has a significant effect on the local SAR value at the maximum heating region. Comparison of local SAR distribution in the maximum heating region using different insulated materials ($\varepsilon_r = 1$ and $\varepsilon_r = 9$) are shown in **Figure 14 (b)**. The maximum 1-g averaged SAR values near four pin tips at different dielectric constant are shown in **Figure 15**. Maximum 1-g averaged SAR values near four pins are plotted. The 1-g averaged SAR for the external fixation system without any dielectric layer insulation (perfect electric conductor, PEC, instead of dielectric material) is plotted as a reference. From **Figure 14** and **Figure 15**, it is noticed that an insulator with high permittivity ($\varepsilon_r = 5, 7,$ or $= 9$) could lead to higher heating at the tips of the pins than those with low relative permittivity ($\varepsilon_r = 1, 2,$ or $= 3$). The dotted line in **Figure 15** is the maximum 1-g averaged SAR at the tips of the pins without an insulated layer. The maximum 1-g SAR value for the fixation device with insulated layers ($\varepsilon_r = 1, 2,$ or $= 3$) is smaller than that without an insulated layer, which shows that it is possible to reduce heating by inserting a low permittivity insulated layer between the pin and clamp. However, high permittivity materials ($\varepsilon_r = 5, 7,$ or $= 9$) could induce even higher heating than that without an insulated layer. The insulated layer between two good conductors is considered a capacitor. High permittivity material can result in high capacitance and increase the capacitive coupling between pins and clamps. Furthermore, the coupling path is found to be as efficient as a direct conducting connection between pins and clamps. Therefore, adding an insulated layer between the pin and clamp does not guarantee the decrement in RF-induced heating compared to a device configuration without an insulated layer. In this evaluation, the material with $\varepsilon_r = 2$ was found to be the most efficient way to reduce the local SAR from 649-W/kg (no insulated layer) to 209-W/kg, which is equivalent to reducing a 67.8% temperature rise at the tips of the pins.

EFFECT OF TEMPERATURE PROBE POSITIONS ON TEMPERATURE MEASUREMENTS

The placement of temperature probes on the implant may impact the integrity of the temperature recordings obtained during evaluations of RF-induced heating. Fortunately, the effect of different temperature probe positions on temperature measurements can be studied using numerical simulation. Two examples are used for this numerical study: (1) the Basis Spinal System (Medtronic, Spinal and Biologics, Memphis, TN) and (2) a generic external fixation system. The Basis Spinal System is the same implant as that mentioned in the previous section of this chapter for the study of device length effects on RF-induced heating (19). It consists of a metallic plate with a length of 65-mm and four screws perpendicular to the metallic plate near the four corners. This implant is a good representative example for a passive metallic device used in orthopedic surgery for spine fixation. The second device used in this study is the external fixation system. In this example, similar dimensions and placement of the external fixation device are used as mentioned in the previous section.

The evaluation presented in this chapter was based on prior work by Mattei, et al. (20) who studied the effect of measurement errors associated with temperature recordings using fiber-optic thermometry probes applied at different positions or orientations relative to the implant during MRI-related heating. A particular contact position was found to be useful for minimizing measurement errors (20).

Figure 15. Peak local 1-g averaged SAR at four pins (Pin1, Pin2, Pin3, Pin4) for insulated layer material ($\varepsilon_r = 1$, $\varepsilon_r = 2$, $\varepsilon_r = 3$, $\varepsilon_r = 5$, $\varepsilon_r = 7$, $\varepsilon_r = 9$) and no insulated layer (PEC).

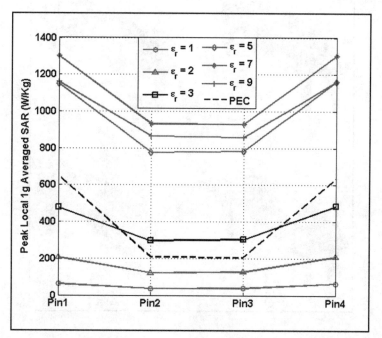

In this study, four different contact positions of fiber-optic thermometry probes are placed at the maximum heating location on each medical device. First a simulation without any probe applied to the device is used to find the worst-heating location. The probes were then placed with four different orientations at those locations near the device. Importantly, for different implants, the placement of the probes may vary due to the shape of the implant.

Four different possible probe positions are shown in **Figure 16** for the Basis Spinal System. Position 1 is a vertical orientation with the sensor side on the top; Position 2 is a horizontal orientation with probe placed tightly to the shorter edge of the device plate; Position 3 is a vertical orientation with the sensor side on the bottom; Position 4 is a horizontal orientation with the probe placed perpendicular to the shorter edge of device plate. For the four different temperature probe positions, the sensor side is located at the same location that produced the highest temperature increase according to simulation results.

Figure 17 shows four different probe positions at the tip of the pin for the external fixation system. Position 1 is a vertical orientation, with an angle of 90-degrees between probe and pin; Position 2 shows an orientation with135-degrees between probe and pin; Position 3 and Position 4 are parallel orientations with 180-degrees and 0-degrees angles between the probes and pin, respectively. Electromagnetic and thermal simulations are used to find the effect of different probe orientations relative to the implant and fixation device on the RF-induced heating. The time domain temperature increase results are obtained from the

Figure 16. Different temperature probe positions for the Basis Spinal System (Medtronic, Spinal and Biologics, Memphis, TN).

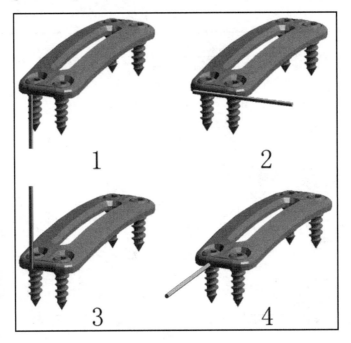

Figure 17. Different temperature probe positions for the external fixation system.

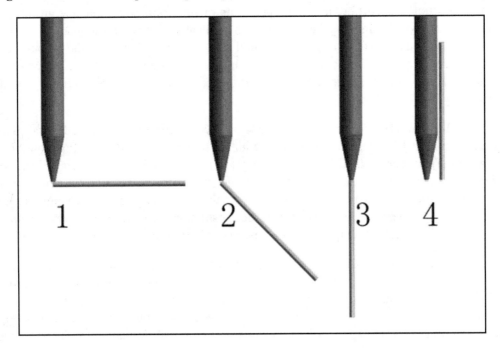

numerical simulations described above. The temperature increase curves between different probe positions and control configuration are then available for comparison.

Figure 18 and Table 3 show the results for the maximum temperature rise for the Basis Spinal System. It is found that around the edge of the metallic plate of the implant, there is less than a 1.75% temperature variation that indicates a negligible influence of the positions of the fiber-optic temperature probe on the measurements.

Figure 18. Temperature changes for different probe positions at the edge of plate for the Basis Spinal System (Medtronic, Spinal and Biologics, Memphis, TN)

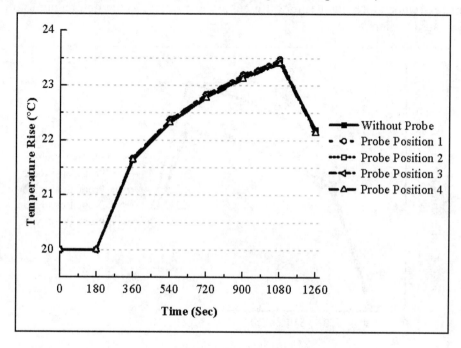

Table 3. SAR and temperature rise results for the Basis Spinal System.

	Peak 1-g Averaged SAR (W/Kg)	Error of SAR (%)	Temp. Increase After 15 min. MRI (°C)	Error of Temperature (%)
Without Probe	46.14	N/A	3.42	N/A
Probe Position 1	46.78	1.39	3.48	1.75
Probe Position 2	45.76	-0.82	3.40	-0.58
Probe Position 3	46.13	-0.02	3.46	1.17
Probe Position 4	46.01	-0.28	3.40	-0.58

Figure 19 and **Table 4** show the maximum temperature rise results for the external fixation system. Placing the probe parallel to the pins (Position 3 and Position 4) has significantly less effect on the heating than the other two positions. By placing the temperature probe 45-degrees to the pin as shown in **Figure 17**, the temperature rise could go up 27% which cannot be considered as an accurate measurement for this configuration.

From the simulation study, it is found during testing to evaluate heating for an implant or device, the position of the temperature probe position may have much more effect on the measurement accuracy on sharp and elongated structure (e.g., a pin) than on a flat structure

Figure 19. Temperature changes for different probe positions at the tip of a pin for the external fixation system.

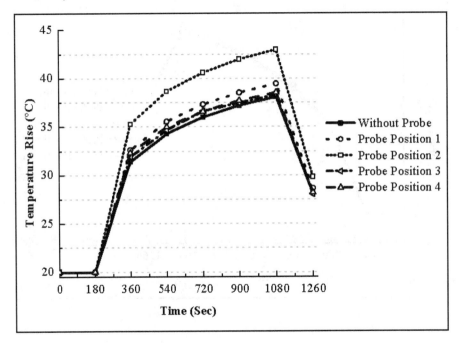

Table 4. SAR and temperature rise results for the external fixation system.

	Peak 1-g Averaged SAR (W/Kg)	Error of SAR (%)	Temp. Increase After 15 min. MRI (°C)	Error of Temperature (%)
Without Probe	313.49	N/A	18.07	N/A
Probe Position 1	323.61	3.23	19.44	7.58
Probe Position 2	381.35	21.65	22.98	27.01
Probe Position 3	293.66	-6.33	18.30	1.27
Probe Position 4	298.34	-4.83	18.54	2.60

(e.g., a metal plate). Therefore, it is recommended that the temperature probe be placed at a parallel configuration to an elongated object in order to minimize the measurement error.

CONCLUSIONS AND IMPLICATIONS FOR PATIENTS WITH PASSIVE METALLIC IMPLANTS

From the previous examples, MRI simulation is demonstrated to be an efficient tool to evaluate heating for items such as bone plates and external fixation systems. From simulation results, the following information is obtained: (1) Temperature rise distributions around devices that have an extremely large number of possible configurations can be quickly evaluated, providing reliable guidance for cumbersome laboratory or MRI-based measurements; (2) The RF-induced heating related to device dimensions (e.g., device length, diameter, etc.), device configuration and placement (e.g., insertion depth, implanted location, clamp spacing, and rod lengths for external fixation system), and non-metallic components (e.g., insulation layer, coating) can be analyzed systematically; and (3) Problems that are unclear during laboratory or MRI-based assessments, such as measurement uncertainty related to temperature probe placement, can be avoided. The measurement uncertainty caused by thermometry probes close to a metallic device is a good example for solving measurement problems using numerical modeling.

Importantly, it is valuable for physicians and researchers to understand that several factors can contribute to excessive RF-induced heating of implants in patients, including: (1) metallic components with elongated shapes; (2) sharp tips at the ends of pins or screws; (3) shallow, percutaneous insertion depths in tissue when an adequate amount of the conductive material to generate heating remains outside the body; and (4) the implanted device is close to the transmit RF coil. Thus, numerical simulations are vital for understanding RF-induced heating of metallic implants and devices in association with MRI.

Disclaimer. The mention of commercial products, their sources or their use in connection with material reported, herein, is not to be construed as either an actual or implied endorsement of such products by the U.S. Food and Drug Administration.

REFERENCES

1.   Chen J, Feng Z, Jin JM. Numerical simulation of SAR and B1-field inhomogeneity of shielded RF coils loaded with the human head. IEEE Trans Biomed Eng 1998;45:650-659.

2.   Jin JM. Electromagnetic Analysis and Design in Magnetic Resonance Imaging. CRC Press, Boca Raton, FL,1998.

3.   American Society for Testing and Materials (ASTM) International. F2182-11a. Standard test method for measurement of radio frequency induced heating on or near passive implants during magnetic resonance imaging. ASTM International. West Conshohocken, PA, 2011.

4.   SEMCAD X. Reference Manual for the SEMCAD Simulation Platform for Electromagnetic Compatibility, Antenna Design and Dosimetry, SPEAG – Schimid & Partner Engineering, 2011.

5.   Nordbeck P, Fidler F, Weiss I, et al. Spatial distribution of RF-induced E-fields and implant heating in MRI. Magn Reson Med 2008;60:312-319.

6.   Pennes HH. Analysis of tissue and arterial blood temperatures in the resting human forearm. Journal of Applied Physiol 1948:1:93-122.

7. Powell J, Papadaki A, Hand J, Hart A, McRobbie D. Numerical simulation of SAR induced around Co-Cr-Mo hip prostheses in situ exposed to RF fields associated with 1.5 and 3-T MRI body coils. Magn Reson Med 2012;68:960-968.

8. Muranaka H. Evaluation of RF heating on hip joint implant in phantom during MRI examinations. Nippon Hoshasen Gijutsu Gakkai Zasshi 2010;66:725-733.

9. Kumar R, Lerski RA, Gandy S, Clift BA, Abbound RJ. Safety of orthopedic implants in magnetic resonance imaging: An experimental verification. J Orthopedic Research 2009;24:1799-1802.

10. Luechinger R, Boesiger P, Disegi JA. Safety evaluation of large external fixation clamps and frames in a magnetic resonance environment. J Biomed Mater Res B Appl Biomater 2007;82:17-22.

11. Baker KB, Tkach JA, Nyenhuis JA, et al. Evaluation of specific absorption rate as a dosimeter of MRI-related implant heating. J Magn Reson Imaging 2004;20:315-320.

12. Brian PLT. A finite-difference method of high-order accuracy for the solution of three-dimensional transient heat conduction problem. Amer Inst Chem Eng J 1961;7:367-370.

13. Gandhi PP, Li Q, Kang G. Temperature rise for the human head for cellular telephones and for peak SARs prescribed in safety guidelines. IEEE Trans Microwave Theory Tech 2001;49:1607-1613.

14. International Electrotechnical Committee (IEC). 60601-2-33 Edition 3.0, Medical electrical equipment - Part 2-33: Particular requirements for the basic safety and essential performance of magnetic resonance equipment for medical diagnostic. March, 2010.

15. Neufeld E, Kuhn S, Szekely G, Kuster N. Measurement, simulation, and uncertainty during MRI. Phys Med Biol 2009;54:4151-4169.

16. Amjad A, Kamondetdacha R, Kildishev AV, Park SM, Nyenhuis JA. Power deposition inside a phantom for testing of MRI heating. IEEE Trans Magn 2005;41:4185-4187.

17. Fragomen AT, Rozbruch SR. The mechanics of external fixation. Hospital for Special Surgery Journal 2007;3:13-29.

18. Liu Y, Shen J, Kainz W, et al. Numerical investigations of MRI RF field induced heating for external fixation devices. Biomed Eng Online 2013 Feb 9;12:12. doi: 10.1186/1475-925X-12-12.

19. Liu Y, Chen J, Shellock FG, Kainz W. Computational and experimental studies of an orthopedic implant: MRI-related heating at 1.5-T/64-MHz and 3-T/128-MHz. J Magn Reson Imaging 2013;37:491-7

20. Mattei E, Triventi M, Calcagnini G, et al. Temperature and SAR measurement errors in the evaluation of metallic linear structures heating during MRI using fluoroptic probes. Phys Med Biol 2007 21;52:1633-46.

Chapter 21   Using MRI Simulations and Measurements to Evaluate Active Implants

JOHN NYENHUIS, PH.D.

Professor of Electrical and Computer Engineering
Purdue University
School of Electrical and Computer Engineering
West Lafayette, IN

INTRODUCTION

Active implants may pose hazards to patients referred for magnetic resonance imaging (MRI) procedures. An active implant is defined as one that relies on its function from a source of electrical energy or any source of power other than that directly generated by the human body or gravity (1). In contrast, a passive implant, such as a coronary artery stent, hemostatic clip, or hip prosthesis, does not require electrical power or other external energy in its operation or during its intended use. Some active implants have external leads and electrodes for delivery of electric current for therapy and/or for physiologic sensing. Examples of active implants include cardiac pacemakers, implantable cardioverter defibrillators (ICDs), neurostimulation systems, bone growth stimulators, and cochlear implants. Other types of active implants, such as implantable drug infusion pumps, use electrical power for operation but may not have attached metallic leads and electrodes.

IN-VITRO TESTS OF HEATING

Implants with conducting leads are referred to as "MR Critical" with respect to radiofrequency (RF) heating because of the length of the metallic materials (2). Testing in phantoms has demonstrated the potential for significant temperature rises at the electrodes of leads that are part of an active implant system (3). For example, Rezai, et al. (4) measured a temperature rise of 25.3°C on the tip of a deep brain stimulation (DBS) lead in a phantom at 1.5-Tesla/64-MHz in association with an MR system reported, whole body averaged SAR of 3.9-W/kg. Achenbach, et al. (5) reported a temperature increase of 63.1°C at the electrode tip for a cardiac pacing lead not connected to a pulse generator (PG) under 1.5-Tesla/64-

MHz conditions. Luechinger (6) measured an RF-induced temperature rise in laboratory animals (pigs). A maximum temperature increase of 15°C was measured for a passive fixation lead and a temperature rise in excess of 30°C was measured for a "cork-screw" fixation lead (6). No significant threshold or impedance changes of the cardiac pacing leads were measured nor did pathology indicate any heat-related damage under the conditions used in this investigation.

CLINICAL RELEVANCE

An understanding of heating behavior for active implant-related leads is crucial to establishing patient safety in association with the use of MRI. Excessive heating at the electrode could damage the surrounding tissue, which may be particularly serious for neurological or cardiac tissue. Active implants with lead wires are mostly contraindicated for MRI primarily because of the large temperature rises that have been reported in laboratory testing. Before an implant manufacturer can receive regulatory approval for a given product relative to the use of MRI, tests and analyses must be undertaken to document that a patient with the implant can safely undergo an MRI procedure. This is particularly important for active implants.

Several active implants have labeling approved for patients needing MRI examinations including cardiac devices, neurostimulation systems, cochlear implants, and others. For example, the first cardiac pacemaker approved in the United States (U.S.) for MRI was the Revo MRI SureScan Pacing System (Medtronic, Minneapolis, MN) (7). Patients with the Vagus Nerve Stimulation (VNS), NeuroCybernetic Prosthesis (NCP) System (Cyberonics, Inc., Houston, TX) and the Activa Deep Brain Stimulation (DBS) System (Medtronic, Minneapolis, MN) may safely undergo MRI by following highly specific conditions (8, 9).

MRI-related heating of active implants without external leads is expected to be similar for a passive implant with similar geometry and materials (10). However, interactions of the electromagnetic fields with the device circuitry could result in heating or other issues. For example, magnetic saturation of a transformer core by the static magnetic field of the scanner may result in additional power delivery by a battery.

MECHANISM OF RADIOFREQUENCY FIELD-RELATED HEATING

The radiofrequency (RF) field used during MRI induces an electric field in the patient or the phantom (i.e., in the case of evaluating heating for implants and devices). The frequency of the RF electric field is the same as that of the RF magnetic field, 64-MHz for 1.5-T and 128-MHz for 3-T. The electric field results in power deposition from the ohmic heating of tissues. The specific absorption rate (SAR) with units of W/kg is the metric for the RF power.

The mechanism for heating of an implant during MRI is coupling of the metal with the electric fields. The tangential component of the electric field along the length of the lead induces waves of electric current on the lead (11). These waves produce an electric field in the vicinity of the electrode, which produces heating of the tissue. There may also be meas-

ducting wires in a lead.

Thus, the temperature rise at an electrode is due to the tangential electric field along the entire length of the lead. This concept was quantified by Park, et al. (12) using a transfer function (TF) method. The temperature rise may be expressed as

$$\Delta T = A \left| \int_0^L E_{\text{tan}}(\tau) S(\tau) d\tau \right|^2 \tag{1}$$

In Equation (1), A is a constant with units of $°C/(V/m)^2$, E_{tan} is the tangential electric field, distance $\tau = 0$ at the electrode and $\tau = L$ at the generator, and S is the transfer function (i.e., the lead model) between the incident E_{tan} and the scattered electric field near the electrode. The dimensions of S are inverse length. Both S and E_{tan} are complex, that is, they have magnitude and phase.

Due to phase effects, it is possible to have a high or low temperature rise for different lead paths in the phantom with similar magnitude of E_{tan}. This phenomenon was demonstrated by Mattei, et al. (13) who measured temperature rises for leads in a phantom for 374 different configurations. This group reported that the observed temperature rise at the tip of a pacemaker lead depended on the path in the phantom and whether or not the pulse generator was attached to the lead. In tests conducted in a circular phantom, Langman, et al. (14) also found that heating depended on the termination conditions at the generator end of the lead. Importantly, heating of a lead will also depend on how it is constructed. Nordbeck, et al. (15) measured RF heating of unipolar and bipolar pacing lead assemblies in a rectangular phantom. It was concluded that heating could be reduced by changes in the configuration of the lead. Mattei, et al. (16) tested the role of lead structure by *in vitro* measurements on 30 commercial cardiac pacemakers and implantable cardioverter defibrillator leads in a rectangular phantom. At a whole body exposure SAR of 1-W/kg, the recorded temperature rises ranged from 2.4°C to 15°C. These tests were conducted for straight-line placement of the lead in the phantom and, thus, it is possible that greater rises would be measured for other lead paths.

CALCULATION OF RADIOFREQUENCY FIELD-RELATED HEATING

The temperature rise of a passive implant in a phantom, such as a spine prosthesis or fixation device can be accurately calculated (17) and these types of simulations are described elsewhere in this textbook. Calculation of the transfer function and consequent temperature rise for an implanted lead is difficult because of the intricate and complicated geometry of the lead. The lead conductors have a minimum feature of the order of tens of microns, which is of the order of 10^5 less than the length of the lead. Park, et al. (12) calculated S and RF-induced temperature rises for bare and insulated wires using method of moments. Neufeld, et al. (18) calculated heating for a straight insulated wire and for a helical wire using Finite Difference Time Domain (FDTD). Both groups reported agreement between calculations and measurements with a 17% uncertainty determined by Neufeld, et al. (18).

TECHNICAL SPECIFICATION ISO/TS 10974 FOR MRI AND ACTIVE IMPLANTS

A joint working group commissioned by the International Organization for Standardization (ISO) and International Electrotechnical Commission (IEC) developed a draft International Technical Specification ISO/TS 10974 that provides test methods for MRI-related hazards associated with an active implantable medical device (AIMD) including RF-induced heating (1). The technical specification (TS) presents an approach with four tiers for assessment of RF heating of active implants. Tier 1 has the simplest test and computation requirements, but also requires the most conservative assumptions on incident RF energy. Tiers 2 and 3 progressively require more measurements and simulations, but are able to use successively less overestimation of test field magnitudes. Tier 4 requires the most stringent computational analysis and utilizes the least overestimation of test field magnitudes. The committee is currently working on a second edition of the TS.

Cabot, et al. (19) evaluated RF heating of a generic deep brain stimulator in 1.5-T/64-MHz as a vehicle to test the four tiers of ISO/TSO 10974. The model implant consisted of a stainless steel "can", a dielectric header, and leads consisting of either an insulating helical copper lead or an insulated straight copper lead. Lead lengths of 50-, 100-, 150-, and 200-mm were evaluated. Simulations for this implant, which is much simpler than an actual DBS device, required as many as 500×10^6 mesh cells. Simulations were run on an accelerated cluster and it was projected that carrying out the estimated 12,000 simulations for a Tier 4 analysis would take several decades. Cabot, et al. (19) concluded with a suggestion for a procedure that follows a test strategy between Tier 3 and Tier 4.

In consideration of the above, the following information should be considered regarding MRI-related heating and active implants: (1) Heating at the electrode of an implanted lead used for a cardiac pacemaker, neurostimulation system, or other similar device that has an active lead may be significantly greater than the threshold rise of approximately 6 to 7°C for tissue injury (20). (2) Heating at the electrode is a complicated function of the magnitude and phase of the incident E_{tan} over the entire length of the lead. If only phantom tests are used to characterize lead heating behavior, a significant number of these tests may be required. (3) Current computational methods are not capable of accurately calculating the temperature rise for a clinically relevant lead wire. (4) A combined approach of innovative measurements and complementary computations will improve the accuracy and efficiency of determining the temperature rise of the lead over the clinically relevant range of incident E_{tan}.

A primary purpose of this chapter is to describe test methods and analyses to predict the heating that an active implant would undergo during MRI. The test case is a commercial neurostimulation system used for vagus nerve stimulation (Vagus Nerve Stimulation (VNS), NeuroCybernetic Prosthesis (NCP) System (Cyberonics, Inc., Houston, TX). First, the transfer function, S, is developed from electrical measurements of the response of the lead to a localized electric field and from selected phantom measurements. Second, the *in vivo* temperature rise is calculated based on the electric fields along the path of the lead in the patient during MRI and the transfer function. Thus, a focus of this chapter is on computer simula-

Figure 1. Geometry of an active implant with lead wire in the presence of a tangential electric field, E_{tan}.

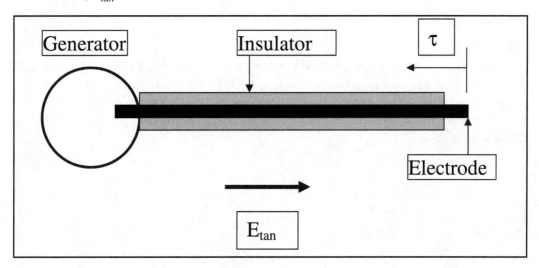

tions and laboratory tests. More clinically oriented perspectives on performing MRI in patients with active implants are presented in other chapters in this textbook.

MECHANISM AND MODELING FOR HEATING OF AN ELECTRODE AT THE END OF A LEAD

Transfer Function Concept

Heating at the electrode of a lead for an active implant occurs from coupling of the RF electric field in the body to the lead. **Figure 1** illustrates this mechanism. The tangential electric field along the length of the lead induces waves of current on the metal of the lead. The current waves propagate along the lead and are partially reflected and partially transmitted at the pulse generator and at the electrode. The transmitted current at the electrode produces power deposition in the tissue surrounding the electrode and there is a consequent temperature rise.

The relationship between electric field **E** and current density **J** in the tissue at the electrode is

$$\mathbf{J} = \sigma \mathbf{E} \qquad (2)$$

where σ is the electrical conductivity with units of S/m. The specific absorption rate (SAR) is the power deposition and is expressed as

$$SAR = \frac{\sigma E_{rms}^2}{\rho} \tag{3}$$

where E_{rms} is the root mean square (rms) value of the electric field and ρ is the mass density. For soft tissue, ρ is not too different from the value of 1000-kg/m³ for water and conductivity generally ranges from 0.1- to 1-S/m. The temperature rise at the electrode will be proportional to the power deposition P in some fixed small fixed volume surrounding the electrode,

$$\Delta T = \varsigma W \tag{4}$$

where power W is determined by the integration of the SAR around the electrode and the factor ς between ΔT and W has units of °C/W.

The background E_{tan} is the tangential electric field along the path of the lead that is present in the medium (phantom or patient) without the lead. The magnitude E_{rms} of the electric field at some location P near the electrode is due to the weighted integral E_{tan} along the length the lead.

$$E_{rms}(P) = K(P)\left|\int_0^L E_{tan}(\tau)S(\tau)\,d\tau\right| \tag{5}$$

where K is a constant that is a function of location near the electrode and S is the transfer function that reflects the degree of coupling between the tangential electric field along the length of the lead.

At a fixed position surrounding the electrode, the temperature rise is proportional to E_{rms}^2 which is expressed by Equation (1), which is repeated here because of its importance.

$$\Delta T = A\left|\int_0^L E_{tan}(\tau)S(\tau)d\tau\right|^2 \tag{1}$$

Both E_{tan} and S are complex, that is, they have both magnitude and phase. By knowing S, the temperature rise at the electrode is known for any distribution of E_{tan}.

If incident electric field is uniform in magnitude and phase along the length of the lead, E_{tan} in Equation (1) can be taken outside the integral and temperature rise ΔT_U for uniform incident electric field is

$$\Delta T_U = A \left| \int_0^L S(\tau) \, d\tau \right|^2 |E_{\tan}|^2 \equiv \gamma |E_{\tan}|^2 \qquad (6)$$

The γ factor in Equation (6) is generally what is measured in a phantom test conducted according to ASTM F2182-11a (21) on a relatively small implant that is inside a region of a uniform electric field.

The worst-case possible temperature rise ΔT_{max} is defined as the one that occurs when E_{tan} and S are conjugate in phase over the entire length of the lead. For this situation, the temperature rise depends on the magnitude of E_{tan} and S.

$$\Delta T_{max} \equiv A \left| \int_0^L |S(\tau)| \, |E_{\tan}(\tau)| \, d\tau \right|^2 \qquad (7)$$

The rise ΔT_{max} is a calculated quantity that is not directly measured. It is a consequence of constructive contribution of E_{tan} over the length of the lead. The value for ΔT_{max} can be viewed as a metric of the total input power that is applied the lead by the incident electric field.

Wave (Transmission Line) Model

A model incorporating propagation of electric current along the length of the lead and reflection of current from the pulse generator and the electrode is useful for understanding the behavior of the current waves on the lead. This model may also be useful for determination of an approximate transfer function through a spatial harmonic fit to temperature rises measured for different paths in a phantom.

Equations from transmission line theory are used to describe the behavior of the current waves on the lead. In **Figure 2**, a voltage $V_s = E_{tan} \, d\tau$ is applied at distance τ from the electrode by the tangential component of the external electric field. The current induced by V_s is

$$I_{in} = \frac{V_s}{Z_{ingen} + Z_{inelec}} \qquad (8)$$

where Z_{ingen} is the impedance from the excitation point to the generator and Z_{inelec} is the impedance to the electrode. Assume sinusoidal waves on a transmission line. Then the voltage, V, and current, I, may be written as

Figure 2. Transmission line circuit for analysis of current waves on a lead.

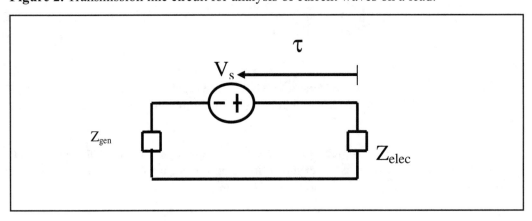

$$V(z)=V_+\left[e^{-\gamma z}+\rho\,e^{\gamma z}\right] \tag{9}$$

$$I(z)=\frac{V_+}{Z_0}\left[e^{-\gamma z}-\rho\,e^{\gamma z}\right] \tag{10}$$

where $z = 0$ is at the electrode and $z = -L$ at the generator, V_+ is an amplitude factor, and ρ is the reflection coefficient at $z = 0$. The propagation constant γ is

$$\gamma = j\beta + \alpha = j\frac{2\pi}{\lambda}+\alpha \tag{11}$$

where λ is the wavelength and α is the damping constant that arises from energy loss in the medium in which the waves propagate. The reflection coefficient at the electrode is

$$\rho_{elec}=\frac{Z_{elec}-Z_L}{Z_{elec}+Z_L} \tag{12}$$

In Equation (12), Z_{elec} is the impedance at the electrode, and Z_L is the characteristic impedance for propagation of waves along the lead. Similarly the reflection coefficient ρ_{gen} at the pulse generator is

$$\rho_{gen} = \frac{Z_{gen} - Z_L}{Z_{gen} + Z_L} \tag{13}$$

From transmission line theory

$$Z_{ingen} = Z_L \frac{e^{\gamma(L-\tau)} + \rho_{gen} e^{-\gamma(L-\tau)}}{e^{\gamma(L-\tau)} - \rho_{gen} e^{-\gamma(L-\tau)}} \tag{14}$$

$$Z_{inelec} = Z_L \frac{e^{\gamma\tau} + \rho_{elec} e^{-\gamma\tau}}{e^{\gamma\tau} - \rho_{elec} e^{-\gamma\tau}} \tag{15}$$

where L is the line length.

The electrode current due to the electric field applied over the differential length is then

$$dI_{electrode} = I_{in} \frac{1 - \rho_{elec}}{e^{\gamma\tau} - \rho_{elec} e^{-\gamma\tau}} \tag{16}$$

The voltage at the load is

$$dV_{electrode} = dI_{electrode} Z_{elec} = I_{in} Z_{elec} \frac{1 - \rho_{elec}}{e^{\gamma\tau} - \rho_{elec} e^{-\gamma\tau}} \tag{17}$$

The load voltage $dV_{electrode}$ is a function of position τ along the lead and is proportional to S.

TEST METHODS FOR MEASUREMENT OF ELECTRODE HEATING AND DETERMINATION OF THE TRANSFER FUNCTION

The objective of the tests and analysis described in this section is to determine the transfer function, S. Notably, all of the described analysis and measurement methods have been tested in this author's laboratory.

Heating Test Performed in a Rectangular Phantom (ASTM F2182-11a)

The standard from the American Society for Testing and Materials (ASTM) International, ASTM F2182-11a (21), specifies a method for testing RF-induced heating of a passive implant. It incorporates a rectangular phantom that is filled with gelled-saline and takes up much of the area of the bore of the MR system. One type of rectangular ASTM phantom is shown in **Figure 3**. The electric field induced in the phantom by the RF field used during MRI is non-uniform. Its distribution will depend on several factors including the position of the phantom in the bore, the RF frequency, and the polarization of the incident RF magnetic field. Plots of the calculated electric field for the phantom in **Figure 3** have been presented by Amjad, et al. (22). At the sides of the phantom and in the region of the landmark for MRI (i.e., the center of the body RF coil), the electric field in a vertical plane is parallel to the wall and is uniform in magnitude over a distance of approximately 20-cm. Passive implants are generally tested for heating in the region of a relatively uniform field, although the measurement accuracy may be impacted for larger implants by the variation of the electric field in the vertical direction of the phantom. The γ factor in Equation (6) may be derived from the phantom test. Since the standard specifies a fixed conductivity (i.e., 0.47-S/m) for the phantom filled with gelled-saline, the temperature rise normalized to the local background SAR will be proportional to γ.

The non-uniform distribution in magnitude and direction of electric field in the phantom can be useful for testing heating of active implants. **Figure 3** illustrates two paths for a heating test on a lead with a pulse generator. In the straight-line configuration, E_{tan} has somewhat uniform magnitude and phase over the entire lead length. The temperature rise for this configuration will be approximately proportional to γ. For the U-path, the magnitude of E_{tan} is approximately uniform along the lead, although the inner section of the loop will have smaller $|E_{tan}|$ lower than the outer. However, the phase of E_{tan} will differ by about 180° be-

Figure 3. Top views of the ASTM phantom with sample paths for testing temperature rises at the electrode for a lead attached to a pulse generator. This figure illustrates a U-path (Left) and a straight-path (Right) for the lead.

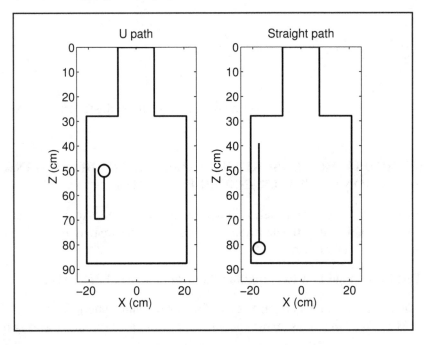

tween the two sections of the lead that are parallel to the wall. Notably, the temperature rise measured in the straight- and U-paths for the same incident RF power can be very different.

Temperature rises for a variety of E_{tan} distributions along the lead can be obtained by performing the heating tests with the lead arranged in more paths than the two that are depicted in **Figure 3**. With sufficient heating information, it is in principle possible to obtain a good approximation for the transfer function, S. For leads with S that are well fit by the transmission line model, an accurate determination of S may be possible with just a small number of tests.

Electrical Measurement of the Transfer Function

Figure 4 illustrates the principle of the measurement of the transfer function, S. A tangential electric field is applied at 64-MHz along a section of lead with a small toroidal coil. Current applied to the coil produces an electric field on its axis that launches a current wave on the lead. The scattered electric field surrounding the electrode is measured with an electric field sensor.

A typical implementation for the transfer function measurement will be for V_1 to be the amplified output from port 1 of a network analyzer. The sensor voltage V_2 is applied to port 2 and the transfer function is proportional to the S_{21} that is measured by the vector network analyzer.

The apparatus in **Figure 4** will determine the network analyzer transfer function S_{NA} which is S multiplied by a constant.

$$S = K_S S_{NA} \tag{18}$$

The constant K_S depends on the several experimental factors, including coil geometry, coil RF response, sensor geometry and location of the electrode in the sensor. K_S is determined from the temperature rise ΔT_{test}, a heating test with a known distribution of electric field:

$$K_S^2 = \frac{1}{A} \frac{\Delta T_{test}}{\left| \int_0^L S_{NA}(\tau) E_{tan}(\tau) d\tau \right|^2} \tag{19}$$

Note that K_S can be considered to be real, as adding a constant phase to the transfer function does not change the calculated temperature rise.

Foldback and Successive Length Tests in a Circular Phantom

Figure 5 shows two layouts for testing electrode heating in a circular phantom. In the foldback method, the lead with generator or other termination is placed in a circular phantom

Figure 4. Geometry for assessment of the transfer function. A tangential electric field is applied over a short length of the lead with a toroidal coil. The scattered electric field at the electrode is proportional to the voltage induced in an electric field sensor. The transfer function, S, is proportion to the ratio of the voltage, V_2, at the sensor to the input voltage, V_1, applied to the coil. The coil is translated along the lead to get the transfer function as function of position relative to the lead.

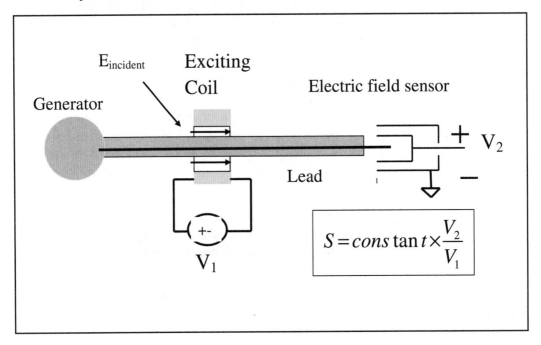

with gelled-saline of a composition that is the same or similar to that specified in ASTM F2182-11a (21). A representative phantom diameter is 33-cm. The entire length of the lead is about 2-cm from the wall of the phantom. A section of lead adjacent to the pulse generator is folded back toward the electrode. The overlapped sections of the lead should be arranged above each other, so that the entire length of the lead is at the same radial distance from the center of the phantom.

It is desired that the tangential electric field E_{tan} (ϕ component) have uniform magnitude and phase around the circumference of the phantom. This is achieved by applying the RF magnetic field B_1 perpendicular to the plane of the phantom. B_1 should be either uniform over the phantom or be circularly symmetric with respect to the center of the phantom. This geometry of B_1 could be achieved using a vertical polarized birdcage, with a single loop circular coil that surrounds the phantom, or other appropriate method.

Temperature probes are placed at the electrodes or other relevant locations. The temperature rise is measured as a function of the foldback distance (FBD) between the generator and the 180° turns in the lead. Let L_0 be the lead length. Then:

FBD = 0 means that the lead is in a straight line along the circumference.

FBD = L0/2 means that the lead is in a "U" path.

FBD = L0 means that the lead is a straight along the circumference, opposite the configuration for FBD = 0.

A possible procedure for the foldback test is as follows: (1) Measure the temperature rise for different values of FBD. A useful step size in FBD will be in the range of 3- to 5-cm. (2) Remove the lead and measure the background SAR along the path of the lead with one of the methods specified in ASTM F2182-11a (21) or other appropriate technique. (3) Determine $\Delta T_1(\text{max})$, which is the maximum rise for any of the foldback tests divided by the local background SAR. Units of $\Delta T_1(\text{max})$ are °C/(W/kg).

In the foldback test, E_{tan} has uniform root mean square (rms) intensity of E_0 and a phase of either 0 or 180°. The temperature rise is then expressed as

$$\Delta T = A E_0^2 \left| \int_0^{L_0-FBD} S \, dz - \int_{L_0-FBD}^{L_0} S \, dz \right|^2 \tag{20}$$

Potential use of the measured temperature rises for different FBD is as follows: The measurements of ΔT can be used to validate S that was obtained by calculation or a separate measurement. If we can describe S in terms of parameters in an equation, such as for the transmission line model, then we can use an error minimization algorithm to determine the fitting parameters (such as α, λ, ρ_{elec}, ρ_{gen}) based the measured temperature rises for different ΔT and FBD.

A variant on the foldback test is a progressive length ("spoke") test in which part of the lead is parallel to the radial line of the phantom. This is the diagram on the right in **Figure 5**. A portion of the lead is exposed to uniform E_{tan} and the remainder of the lead has zero E_{tan}. The temperature rise for the spoke test with a bend a distance X from the electrode and the section between the generator and the bend radially directed is

$$\Delta T = AE_0^2 \left| \int_0^X S(\tau) \, d\tau \right|^2 \tag{21}$$

For calculation of SAR and electric field in the circular phantom, let R be the radial distance of the lead from the center of the phantom, E_0 the rms value of the electric field at radial distance R, and f the frequency. In the presence of uniform B_1 with rms value B_{10}, we then have approximately

$$E_0 = \pi f R B_1 \tag{22}$$

Figure 5. Geometry for the heating tests in a circular phantom. (Left) Fold back test. (Right) The progressive length ("spoke") test.

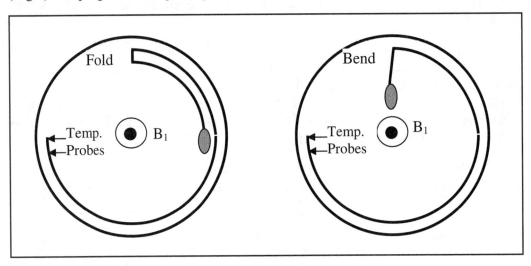

Measurement of Temperature Rise with a Locally Exciting RF Coil

The localized exciting RF coil in the TF apparatus of **Figure 4** will produce a temperature rise at the electrode. In the local coil test method, the temperature sensor in **Figure 4** is removed and the temperature rise at the electrode is measured with a temperature sensor. Assume the exciting coil is at a location away from the electrode. The temperature rise at the sensor is then

$$\Delta T = A|\Delta V|^2|S(\tau)|^2 \tag{23}$$

where ΔV is the integrated E_{tan} over the length of the exciting coil.

CASE STUDY: DETERMINATION OF LEAD MODEL AND *IN VITRO* TEMPERATURE RISE FOR A LEAD USED WITH A NEURO-STIMULATION SYSTEM

In order to illustrate the test methods and analysis for heating of an active implant, this section describes the procedure for the determination of the lead model and *in vitro* temperature rise for a commercially available neurostimulation system, the Vagus Nerve Stimulator, VNS Therapy, NeuroCybernetic Prosthesis (NCP) System (Cyberonics, Inc., Houston, TX). The methodology makes use of the afore-mentioned test methods described in this chapter. The tests and analysis were made on a system used for VNS Therapy – the Model 303 lead and either the Model 102 or Model 103 pulse generator. Results of tests of MRI-related heating for physiologic paths in a rectangular phantom have been published for this system (23). The lead contains two filars and is 43-cm long. There are two electrodes

Figure 6. Model 303 lead with the Model 102 pulse generator used in U-path configuration for a heating test. Temperature rises at the electrodes were measured with Neoptix fiber-optic temperature probes with 0.6-mm tip diameter.

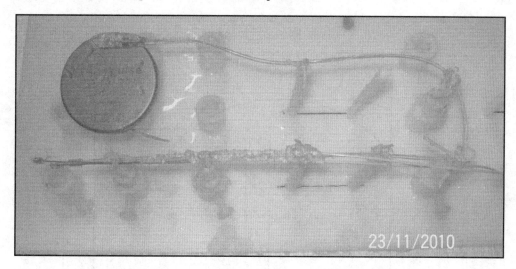

made from platinum foil that are located at the end of the lead. The evaluation was made for a lead with the pulse generator, an isolated lead (uncapped), and a lead with an insulating cap at the pulse generator connector.

Heating Tests in a Rectangular Phantom

The temperature rises were measured in a rectangular phantom with the methods specified in ASTM F2182-11a (21). The tests were made using a transmit body RF coil at 64-MHz (Signa, General Electric Medical Systems, Milwaukee, WI). The conductivity of the gelled-saline used to fill the phantom was approximately 0.5-S/m. **Figure 3** shows diagrams of the phantom and the paths of the implant for the tests. **Figure 6** shows the Model 303 lead with the Model 102 pulse generator prior to immersion into the phantom liquid. **Figure 7** shows the intensity of E_{tan} along the two lead paths. In the tests, the local background SAR near the wall of the phantom was determined with the titanium rod technique that is described in F2182-11a (21). The distribution of E_{tan} was then determined from the SAR measurement at one location and the calculated distribution of electric field induced in the phantom by the RF magnetic field. **Figure 8** shows temperature rises for the lead with the pulse generator in the straight- and U-paths. The difference in temperature rise is very much dependent on the path. For the same input RF power, the U-path produces a temperature rise that is five times greater than the rise for the straight path.

In the measurements obtained in the rectangular and circular phantoms, there is an uncertainty of about 10% in the assessment of the background SAR. The measured SAR for each test was adjusted by a factor of less than this uncertainty in order to provide the best fit between the measured and calculated temperature rises.

Figure 7. Calculated rms tangential electric fields in the ASTM phantom along the lead paths shown in **Figure 3**. The RF power was 150-W and the phantom average SAR was approximately 2-W/kg.

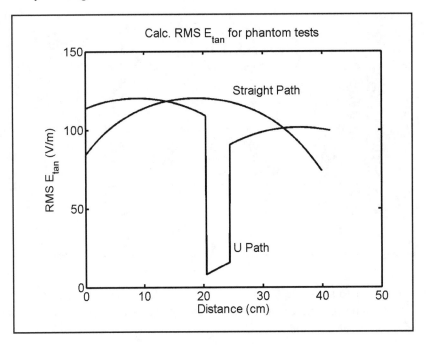

Figure 8. Temperature rises for two paths in a phantom for the Model 303 lead with Model 102 pulse generator. The rises are scaled to the same input RF power.

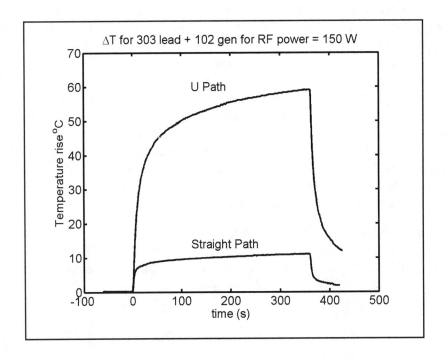

Electrical Measurement of the Transfer Function

The Model 303 lead with the Model 103 pulse generator (Cyberonics, Inc., Houston, TX) was placed in the test apparatus depicted in **Figure 4**. The output of an HP 3577 network analyzer (Hewlett-Packard) was amplified with an ENI RF power amplifier whose output was connected to the exciting coil. The toroidal exciting coil had an inner diameter of approximately 1.5-cm, outer diameter 3-cm, and height of about 2-cm. The electric field sensor was connected to port 2 of the HP3577 network analyzer. The toroidal coil was moved along the length of the lead and magnitude and phase of S_{21} were measured as a function of the location of the coil

Figure 9 shows the magnitude and phase of transfer function (TF) for the lead with an insulating cap [note, the normalizing factor A = 1°C/(V/m)² was applied for **Figure 9** and the other plots of transfer function shown in this chapter]. The points in **Figure 9** are from S_{21} measurements and the solid line is the calculation from transmission line equations presented in this chapter. There is essentially complete overlap between the measured and transmission line TF. At the capped end of the lead, the magnitude of the TF is small because the cap presents an open circuit. The TF has a maximum magnitude at about 20-cm from the cap. The maximum occurs because the impedance Z_{ingen} is small at this location because it is approximately 1/4 wavelength from the cap.

Figure 9. Transfer function (TF) for a Model 303 lead with an insulating cap over the connector to the pulse generator. Points are measurements and the solid line is a transmission line fit for wavelength λ = 80-cm and damping constant, α = 2. The TF is scaled based on the temperature measurements in the ASTM phantom and circular phantom. A=1.

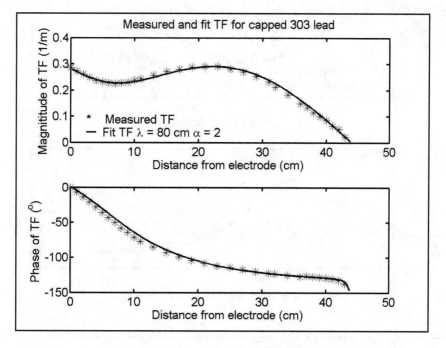

Figure 10 shows the transfer function for the lead with the pulse generator. The measured and transmission line fit TF are in reasonable overlap, but the match is not as good as for the capped lead. For this calculation, the generator impedance Z_{gen} was -30-jΩ, electrode impedance Z_{elec} was $500 - 350$-jΩ and Z_L was 100-Ω, j $= \sqrt{-1}$.   A more comprehensive analysis may result in determination of the appropriate parameters that provide a better fit to the measurements.

Foldback Tests in a Circular Phantom

Figure 11 shows the lead with the pulse generator the measured and calculated temperature rises, scaled to the local SAR versus the foldback distance. The measured rises track well with the calculated rises. The greatest rise occurs for a foldback of about half of the lead length and this configuration corresponds to the U-path in the rectangular ASTM phantom. As in the phantom tests, the temperature rise in the U-path is approximately 5 times the temperature rise in the straight path. **Figure 12** shows temperature rises measured in a foldback test on a capped lead. The measured temperature rises again track well with the calculated values. The greatest rise occurs for the lead in a straight line.

Figure 10. Transfer function for a Model 303 lead with Model 103 pulse generator. Points are measurements and the solid line is a transmission line fit for wavelength $\lambda =$ 80-m and damping constant $\alpha = 2$. The TF is scaled based on the temperature measurements in the ASTM phantom and circular phantom. A=1

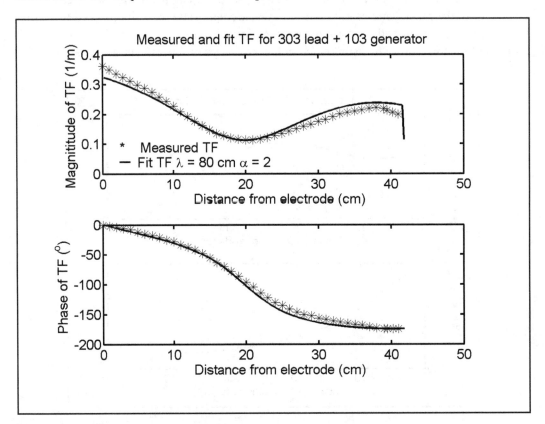

Figure 11. Temperature rises versus foldback for a Model 303 lead with Model 103 pulse generator. The points are the measurements and the line is calculation for the transfer function in **Figure 14**.

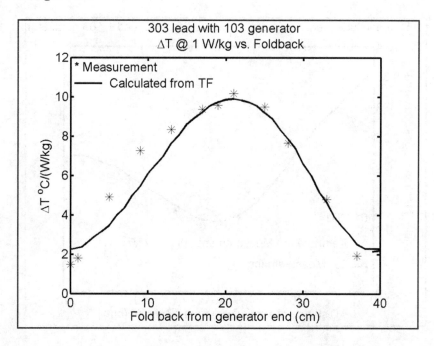

Figure 12. Temperature rises versus foldback for a Model 303 capped lead. The points are measurements and the line is the calculation for the transfer function in **Figure 14**.

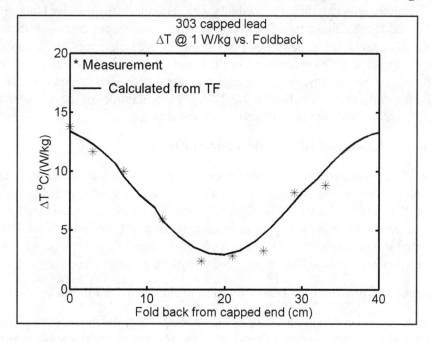

Figure 13. The solid line is the calculated magnitude of the transfer function from the S_{21} tests. The points are the transfer function magnitude measured from temperature rises at the electrodes.

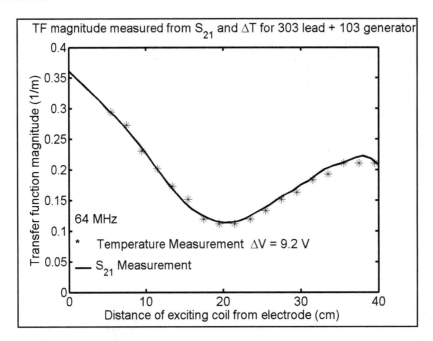

Measurement of Temperature Rise with a Local Exciting Coil

Figure 13 compares the magnitude of the transfer function obtained for the lead with the pulse generator with two different methods. The solid line is the transfer function measured by S_{21} and is normalized based on the temperature rise measurements in the circular and rectangular phantom. The points are proportional to the square root of the temperature rise at the electrode at different locations of the exciting coil, which is the same as the one used in the S_{21} measurements. For these tests, the integrated electric field over the length of the exciting coil, ΔV, is calculated to be 9.2-V. The magnitudes of the TF measured by the two different methods are in nearly complete overlap.

Comparison of Calculated Rises in the Phantom Tests

Table 1 lists measured and calculated rises for the three leads in the straight-line path in the phantom. The calculated rises are based on the transfer functions in **Figure 14** and the E_{tan} along the lead that is shown in **Figure 7**. **Table 2** lists measured and calculated temperature rises for the leads in the U-path in the rectangular phantom. The difference between the calculated and measured rises is less that 5% of the rise ΔT_{max} that would occur if the transfer function and incident electric field were in phase conjugation.

Discussion on *In-vitro* Tests for Determination of the Transfer Function

The tests described herein provide a robust assessment of the transfer function for the Model 303 lead and the three termination conditions. Three of the tests provide independent outputs that depend on both the magnitude and the phase of the transfer function: (1) The

Table 1. Measured and calculated temperature rises for the VNS lead (Model 303 lead, Cyberonics, Inc., Houston, TX) in the phantom with the lead in a straight-line path. *This measurement was made with RF power reduced 50% so the actual measured rise is half of the listed value.

Termination	Measured ΔT Straight °C	Calculated ΔT Straight °C	Calculated ΔT_{max} °C	Measured vs. Calculated ΔT % of ΔT_{max}
Capped	*77.0	76.3	109.3	0.6
Uncapped	24.8	24.5	74.6	0.4
Generator	10.8	13.9	69.6	-4.4

Figure 14. Measured transfer function for the Model 303 lead with the Model 103 pulse generator (Vagus Nerve Stimulator, VNS Therapy, NeuroCybernetic Prosthesis (NCP) System, Cyberonics, Inc., Houston, TX). These transfer functions were used to calculate the *in vitro* and *in vivo* temperature rises. The normalizing factor A is unity.

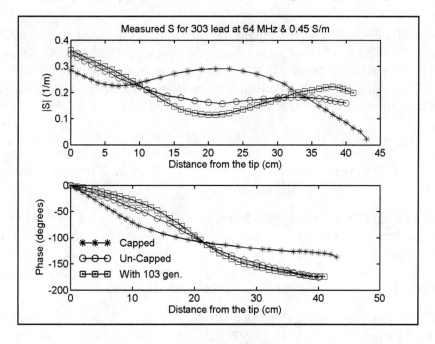

S_{21} measurement; (2) The temperature rise measurement in the circular phantom with a large RF coil; and (3) The temperature rise measurement in a rectangular phantom for different paths of the lead. In addition, the heating test with the local exciting coil provides an independent measure of the magnitude of the TF.

Notably, the transfer function derived here is specific for the medium conductivity used in the tests. The TF will be different if the electrical properties of the surrounding medium

Table 2. Measured and calculated temperature rises for the VNS lead (Model 303 lead, Cyberonics, Inc., Houston, TX) in the phantom with the lead in a U-path. *This measurement was made with RF power reduced 50% so the actual measured rise is half of the listed value.

Termination	Measured ΔT U-Path °C	Calculated ΔT U-Path °C	Calculated ΔT_{max} °C	Measured vs. Calculated ΔT % of ΔT_{max}
Capped	24.7	24.3	89.0	0.4
Uncapped	47.0	47.0	69.3	0.0
Generator	*59.0	58.6	72.6	0.5

change. However, small changes to the TF over the range of electrical properties that characterize soft tissue are to be expected.

DETERMINATION OF *IN-VIVO* TEMPERATURE RISES DURING MRI AT 64-MHZ

The transfer functions presented in this chapter and the calculated electric field in the body during MRI are used to determine the *in vivo* temperature rises at the electrodes of the VNS lead studied here. **Figure 15** shows the path that was defined for the VNS lead in the Hugo human model, which is derived from the National Library of Medicine and has been used extensively in bio-electromagnetic calculations (24).

The Finite Difference Time Domain (FDTD) method was used to calculate E_{tan} along the lead at 64-MHz inside a high pass transmit body RF coil with a circularly polarized incident RF field. The intensity and phase of E_{tan} along the lead will depend on the location of the patient in the bore of the MR system.

Figure 16 shows a plot of magnitude and phase of E_{tan} along the VNS lead path at a landmark position of 30-cm (i.e., the plane of the patient 30-cm from the top of the head is at the center of the transmit body RF coil). Similarly, **Figure 17** plots E_{tan} along the VNS lead path for the transmit/receive head RF coil. For the transmit/receive head RF coil, only the section of lead near the electrode experiences a significant E_{tan}.

The *in vivo* temperature rises are calculated for RF intensity at the normal mode limit of 2-W/kg for whole body SAR and 3.2-W/kg for head SAR. **Figure 18** shows B_{1+} that will produce a whole body SAR of 2-W/kg and/or a head SAR of 3.2-W/kg. In **Figure 18** it is assumed that the transmit RF body coil will limit B_{1+} in the Normal Operating Mode for the MR system to an amplitude of 6-μT.

Calculation of the *in vivo* temperature rises was done with Equation (1), the transfer functions in **Figure 14**, and the calculated E_{tan}. With the scaling of the TF, the temperature rises are based on the *in vitro* temperature rises after six minutes of RF power deposition. **Figure 8** shows that the *in vitro* temperature rises are effectively saturated after six minutes.

Figure 15. Path of Model 303 lead in the Hugo model. The electrodes are wrapped around the vagus nerve at the top of the path and the pulse generator is located at the bottom of the path.

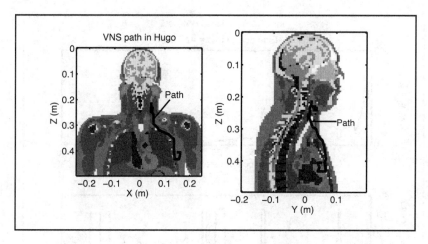

Figure 16. Magnitude and phase of the electric field along the path of the Model 303 lead for the transmit body RF coil. The landmark (i.e., center of the RF coil) is 30-cm from the top of the head and the whole body SAR is 2-W/kg.

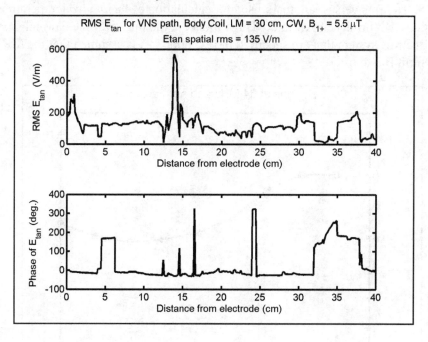

Figure 17. Magnitude and phase of electric field along the path of the Model 303 lead for the transmit/receive head RF coil. $B_{1+} = 8$ µT, which is expected to be the upper limit for the Normal Operating Mode of the MR system.

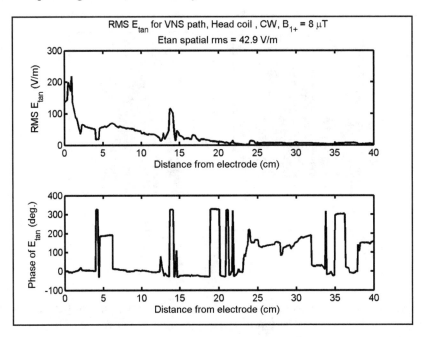

Figure 18. B_{1+} rms versus landmark used for calculation of the *in vivo* temperature rise. These values will produce SAR in the Hugo model at the limits for the Normal Operating Mode of the MR system that are specified in IEC 60601. It is assumed that the MR system will limit B_{1+} to 6-µT.

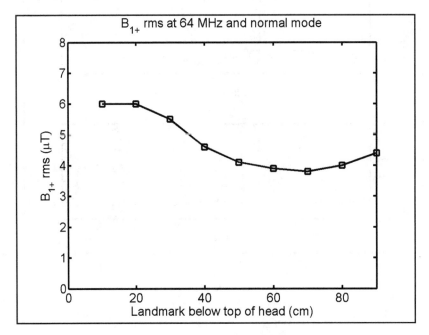

Considering as well the cooling effect of blood perfusion (25), it is expected that the *in vivo* temperature rise will reach a saturation value within six minutes after the initiation of the delivery of RF energy.

Figure 19 plots the projected *in vivo* temperature rises at the electrode versus the landmark for the Hugo model for the three types of terminations at the proximal end. The temperature rises at each landmark are the greatest of the two values calculated for clockwise (CW) and counter-clockwise (CCW) rotation. The maximum temperature rises for the three leads all occur at the landmark of 30-cm, which is approximately at the level of the clavicle. At this landmark, the whole body SAR is 2-W/kg for the applied B_{1+} of 5.5-μT. Maximum temperature rises for the capped, uncapped, and with the pulse generator leads are 45°C, 21°C, and 17°C, respectively.

Figure 19 also shows the calculated temperature rises with the RF field applied by the transmit/receive head RF coil. For this RF coil, the rise for B_{1+} of 8-μT, which is expected to exceed the maximum RF intensity with the MR system in the Normal Operating Mode, is less than 4°C.

DISCUSSION

A procedure is described in this chapter for the determination of *in vivo* temperature rises of an AIMD during MRI. Four complementary measurements for the determination of the transfer function, *S*, are presented. The overlapping results of the measurements provide confidence that the lead model presented herein has been accurately determined.

The analysis is focused on heating at 64-MHz (1.5-T). A similar methodology could be used for 3-T/128-MHz MRI conditions. The characteristics of lead heating will be different at 3-T/128-MHz because the wavelengths associated with the current waves at 3-T (128-MHz) are approximately half of those at 1.5-T (64-MHz).

The transfer function for a lead incorporates the sensitivity of the lead to the magnitude and phase of the incident field along the length of the lead. After phase and relative magnitude measurements are made with a network analyzer, as few as one measurement of the temperature rise in a phantom is needed to determine the scaling factor, K_S. However, it will be appropriate to measure the temperature rise for more than one path in the phantom in order to demonstrate the validity of the transfer function, as Equation (1) should predict the temperature rise for any path in the phantom. The procedure outlined here does not require the calculation of *S* based on the construction of the lead. Calculation of *S* for simple wire geometries is possible, as shown in **Figure 20** for a bare wire. An accurate calculation of *S* for an actual clinical lead would be extremely challenging as the wire diameter, pitch, and insulation thickness of a typical lead are several orders of magnitude smaller than the length. Nonetheless, it would be interesting to compare measured and calculated S for such a lead.

The procedure presented in this chapter does require the knowledge of magnitude and phase of the electric field in the phantom and in the human placed in the transmit RF coil of the MR system. These calculations are straightforward, being performed with FDTD and have been previously described (26). These calculations may be conducted at a modest res-

Figure 19. Calculated *in vivo* temperature rise versus landmark in the Hugo model for the Normal Operating Mode of the MR system using the B_{1+} limits in **Figure 18**. The temperature rises plotted are the maximum values for clockwise (CW) and counter-clockwise (CCW) rotation for a high pass coil. The temperature rise for the transmit/receive head RF coil (TR HC) is calculated for $B_{1+} = 8$-μT.

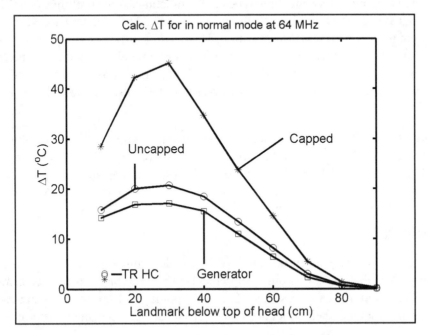

Figure 20. Measured and calculated transfer functions for a 40-cm long, 3-mm diameter aluminum rod. The transfer function was calculated with method of moments.

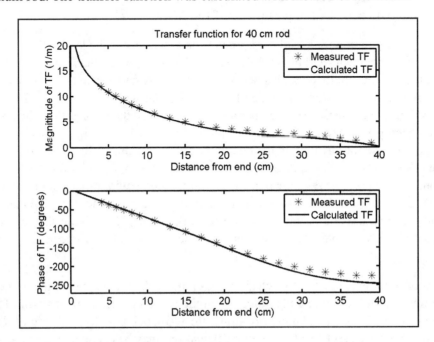

olution such as 5-mm. If needed, a locally finer resolution could be achieved in the human model with variable gridding and the Huygens box method (18).

In-vivo temperature rises presented here for the Vagus Nerve Stimulation (VNS), NeuroCybernetic Prosthesis (NCP) System (Cyberonics, Inc., Houston, TX) are shown to illustrate the overall procedure for determining RF heating. No recommendations have been made for acceptable MRI conditions. A more comprehensive assessment of the *in vivo* temperature rises would include: (1) An assessment to determine whether the electrical conductivity of the phantom materials are appropriate for the impedance conditions at the electrode; (2) An evaluation of the impact on temperature rises of the different tissue conductivities along the path of the VNS lead; (3) An assessment of the sensitivity of the temperature rises to variation in the path of the lead; and (4) A determination of *in vivo* temperature rises in additional human models, such as those in the virtual population from the IT'IS Foundation (27). Nevertheless the RF-induced temperature rises in **Figure 19** are consistent with the *Instructions for Use* for the Vagus Nerve Stimulation (VNS), NeuroCybernetic Prosthesis (NCP) System (Cyberonics, Inc., Houston, TX), which limit MRI procedures to those involving the use of a transmit/receive head RF coil and other similar RF coils (8).

The standard ISO/TS 10974 should be carefully studied when evaluating an active implant for MRI issues (1). In addition to RF heating, an assessment should be made whether other interactions associated with MRI, including magnetic field interactions, gradient stimulation, and electromagnetic interference are safe for the patient and the implant.

The calculation of the background electric field in the body during MRI and the measurement of local background SAR in the phantom are made with no implant. The calculation of temperature rise at the electrode is made assuming that the lead does not appreciably change the incident RF energy. This assumption should be fulfilled in MRI since the energy scattered by the lead should be at least two orders of magnitude less than the energy input to the RF coil. Experiments on model implants for which the measured temperature rises agree well with the calculated rises further demonstrate the validity of the computational procedure described herein (28).

Informal tests that were made with the transfer function apparatus indicate that smooth curves in the path have minimal impact on *S*. This observation is supported by results in **Table 1** and **Table 2** were the same transfer function yields calculated temperature rises that agree well with measurements for both the straight- and U-paths of the lead.

The measurements and calculations demonstrate that the temperature rise at the electrode of the VNS System (Cyberonics, Inc., Houston, TX) depends greatly on the termination state at the pulse generator. This suggests that heating of an active implant might be mitigated by optimizing the value of the termination impedance.

The methods presented in this chapter can be used to establish the SAR levels under which a patient with an active implant may undergo MRI. If the tests and analysis indicate the potential for harmful heating, then MRI may be safe only for SAR levels below the Normal Operating Mode limit of a whole body SAR of 2-W/kg or an SAR of 3.2-W/kg in the head (29). If the lead is found to heat excessively, then it may be deemed to be unsafe for

MRI. A summary of the results from the heating tests is typically presented in the MRI labeling information section of the device's *Instructions for Use* (8, 30).

In addition to safety with respect to RF heating, device and patient safety with respect to magnetic field interactions, pulsed gradient fields, and electromagnetic interference must be established before patients with the device may safely undergo MRI. Regulatory bodies such as the U.S. Food and Drug Administration review submissions by implant manufacturers prior to approval of the MRI labeling (30).

ACKNOWLEDGEMENTS

The author thanks graduate students J. Jallal, T. Mansheim, C. Miller, and N. Elder for their contributions to the measurement results presented in this chapter. In addition, the author is grateful to Dr. Sung-Min Park for his contributions to the development of the concept of the transfer function.

REFERENCES

1. International Organization for Standardization, ISO/TS 10974:2012, Assessment of the safety of magnetic resonance imaging for patients with an active implantable medical device, 2012.

2. Kainz W. MR Heating tests of MR critical implants. J Magn Reson Imaging 2007;26:450–451.

3. Nyenhuis JA, Park SM, Kamondetdacha R, et al. MRI and implanted medical devices: Basic interactions with an emphasis on heating. IEEE Trans Dev Mater Reliability 2005;5:467-480.

4. Rezai AR, Finelli D, Nyenhuis JA, et al. Neurostimulation systems for deep brain stimulation: In vitro evaluation of magnetic resonance imaging-related heating at 1.5 T. J Magn Reson Imaging 2002;5:241-250.

5. Achenbach S, Moshage W, Diem B, Schibgilla V, and Bachman K. Effects of magnetic resonance imaging on cardiac pacemakers and electrodes. Am Heart J 1997;134:467-474.

6. Luechinger RC. Safety aspects of cardiac pacemakers in magnetic resonance imaging, Ph.D. dissertation, Dept. Naturwissenschaften, Swiss Federal Inst Technol, Zurich, Switzerland, 2002.

7. Wilkoff BL, Bello D, Taborsky M, Vymazal J, et al. Magnetic resonance imaging in patients with a pacemaker system designed for the magnetic resonance environment. Heart Rhythm 2011; 6:65-73 and http://www.medtronic.com/mrisurescan

8. Vagus Nerve Stimulator, VNS Therapy, NeuroCybernetic Prosthesis (NCP) System, Cyberonics, Inc., Houston, TX; MRI with the VNS Therapy System, Cyberonics 26-0006-4200/5, 2011. http://www.cyberonics.com

9. MRI Guidelines for Medtronic Deep Brain Stimulation Systems – To the Physician. Medtronic, Minneapolis, MN; www.medtronic.com/mri

10. Nyenhuis JA, Kildishev AV, Bourland JD, et al. Heating near implanted medical devices by the MRI RF-magnetic field. IEEE Trans Magn 1999;35:4133-4135.

11. Konings MK, Bartels LW, Smits HFM, Bakker CJC. Heating around intravascular wires by resonating RF waves. J Magn Reson Imaging 2000;12:79-85.

12. Park SM, Kamondetdacha R, Nyenhuis JA. Calculation of MRI-induced heating of an implanted medical lead wire with an electric field transfer function. J Magn Reson Imaging 2007;26:1278-1285.

13. Mattei E, Triventi M, Calcagnini G, et al. Complexity of MRI induced heating on metallic leads: Experimental measurements of 374 configurations. BioMedical Engineering OnLine 2008;7:11.

14. Langman DA, Goldberg IB, Finn JP, Ennis DB. Pacemaker lead tip heating in abandoned and pacemaker-attached leads at 1.5 Tesla MRI. J Magn Reson Imaging 2011;33:426–431.

15. Nordbeck P, Fidler F, Friedrich MT, et al. Reducing RF related heating of cardiac pacemaker leads in MRI: Implementation and experimental verification of practical design changes. Magn Reson Med 2012;68:1963–1972.

16. Mattei E, Calcagnini G, Censi F, Triventi M, Bartolini P. Role of the lead structure in MRI induced heating: In vitro measurements on 30 commercial pacemaker/defibrillator leads. Magn Reson Med 2012;67:925–935.

17. Nyenhuis JA and Miller CR. Calculation of heating of passive implants by the RF electromagnetic field in MRI. General Assembly and Scientific Symposium, 30th International Union of Radio Science (URSI) Istanbul, 2011.

18. Neufeld E, Kuhn S, Szekely G, Kuster N. Measurement, simulation and uncertainty assessment of implant heating during MRI. Phys Med Biol 2009;54:4151–4169.

19. Cabot E, Lloyd T, Christ A, et al. Evaluation of the RF heating of a generic deep brain stimulator exposed in 1.5 T magnetic resonance scanners. Bioelectromagnetics 2013;34:104-113.

20. Goldstein LS, Dewhirst MW, Repacholi M, et al. Summary, conclusions and recommendations: adverse temperature levels in the human body. Int J Hyperthermia 2003;19:373–384.

21. ASTM F2182-11a. Standard test method for measurement of radio frequency induced heating on or near passive implants during magnetic resonance imaging, ASTM International, 2011.

22. Amjad A, Kamondetdacha R, Kildishev AV, Park SM, Nyenhuis JA. Power deposition inside a phantom for testing of MRI heating, IEEE Trans Magn 2005;41:4185–4187.

23. Shellock FG, Begnaud J, Inman DM. Vagus nerve stimulation therapy system: In vitro evaluation of magnetic resonance imaging-related heating and function at 1.5 and 3 Tesla. Neuromodulation 2006;9:204–213.

24. Kozlov M, Turner R. Fast MRI coil analysis based on 3-D electromagnetic and RF circuit co-simulation. J Magn Reson Imaging 2009;200:147-152.

25. Akca IB, Ferhanoglu O, Yeung CJ, et al. Measuring local RF heating in MRI: simulating perfusion in a perfusionless phantom. J Magn Reson Imaging 2007; 26:1228-1235.

26. Liu W, Collins CM, Smith MB. Calculations of B1 distribution, specific energy absorption rate, and intrinsic signal-to-noise ratio for a body-size birdcage coil loaded with different human subjects at 64 and 128 MHz. Appl Magn Reson 2005;9:5-18.

27. IT'IS Foundation. High-Resolution Human Models: Virtual Population. http://www.itis.ethz.ch/itisfor-health/virtual-population/human-models.

28. Nyenhuis J. RF Device Safety and Compatibility. Encyclopedia of Magnetic Resonance, John Wiley: 2010.

29. International Electrotechnical Commission (IEC), Diagnostic imaging equipment, publication IEC 60601-2-33 Edition 3.0, Medical electrical equipment, Part 2. International Electrotechnology Commission International Electrotechnical Commission (IEC), Geneva, Switzerland.

30. Shellock FG, Wood TO, Crues JV III. MR labeling information for implants and devices: Explanation of terminology. Radiology 2009;253:26-30.

Chapter 22   MRI Safety Policies and Procedures for a Hospital or Medical Center Setting

JOHN POSH, R.T., (R)(MR)

Director, MRI Internship and RT Continuing Education
Faculty, RT Education
Penn Medicine
Hospitals of the University of Pennsylvania
Philadelphia, PA

INTRODUCTION

No matter what the structure of the facility, be it an academic medical center, a community hospital, or a small rural hospital, the overriding mandate is to maintain a safe environment for the patients and employees. To this end, with specific regard to magnetic resonance imaging (MRI), facilities must "establish, implement, and maintain current MRI safety policies and procedures" to ensure the safety of patients, visitors, and staff members (1). These policies and procedures dictate the desires of the organization and how they are to be implemented. In consideration of the above, the objective of this chapter is to focus on policies and procedures, the nature of how these are developed, implemented, reviewed and distributed, and the legal implications with an emphasis on MRI safety in the setting of a hospital or medical center.

GENERAL INFORMATION

Policies and procedures are written for a variety of reasons. Some are designed to be the institution's response to regulatory and governing body requirements (2). This is less true with MRI than it is for modalities that use ionizing radiation (e.g., X-ray and nuclear medicine) due to differing levels of governmental oversight and regulation. Some policies and procedures are written as a means of ensuring consistency across similar entities within a larger organization, as is the case with larger academic and regional institutions with small satellite campuses and diagnostic imaging centers. Policies and procedures can also be written in response to events. For example, before 2001, few facilities had a formal policy on the use of portable oxygen cylinders or other tanks used for gases utilized in the MRI environment (3, 4). By far, the most common reason policies and procedures are written is to ensure compliance with industry best practices. Some believe that the current *de facto*, best practice standard for MRI is the American College of Radiology (ACR) Guidance Document on MR Safe Practices: 2013 (1). The ACR document rapidly changed the manner in which the clinical MRI setting operated. The MRI industry, self-governed since the beginning, suddenly had a written document to use as a template to guide MRI safety procedures. As far as written documentation was concerned, while this document had no enforceability, it almost overnight prompted significant changes.

One key concept of the ACR document, and the only element to be detailed in this chapter, is the concept of dividing the imaging facility into four discrete zones with increasingly restricted access as the zones progress from Levels I to IV. The zone model is intended to help control access to the MRI environment and, thus, facilitate safety in this setting. Zone I represents the public space and is essentially unregulated. Zone II represents the public interface and can be defined as the public space within the MRI department such as the waiting, changing, and interview areas as well as the areas for the restrooms and similar spaces. Zone III represents the limited access, technical workspace between Zone II and the MR system room. Zone IV represents the MR system room. In Zone IV, the potential problems exist whereby ferromagnetic implants, foreign bodies, and external devices will be affected. Failure to restrict access to those personnel without proper training and the use of support equipment specifically designed for use in the MRI environment can result in significant injury or death to patients, visitors, and staff members. The only other published standard, and one which dovetails nicely with the ACR guidance document, is the Sentinel Event Alert #38, published by the Joint Commission (5, 6).

When creating a policies and procedures based on industry best practices, it is important to carefully search the published literature on the topic. Drafting a policy and procedure with outdated information or improper terminology (e.g., using "MRI compatible" versus "MR Conditional" for MRI labeling purposes) offers little in the way of guidance or protection for any of the parties involved. It is also important when formulating policies based on best practices, to create a core group of policies and procedures to ensure that all aspects of operations are covered (**Table 1**).

Some MRI facilities in the hospital or medical center setting use the ACR guidance document as single blanket policy covering all general operations within the department or as a road map to drafting individual policies. While other facilities use the guidance document as a starting point and draft additional policies and procedures to narrow the focus of operational issues in key areas, as needed, or if there are persistent concerns, such as a pattern of MRI-safety related events that occur during the preparation of patients for the MRI examinations.

The scope with which policies and procedures are written can be very broad and applicable to everyone within the organization or narrowly focused to apply to a very limited target audience. Whatever the reason for writing the policy and procedure, it is vital that the policy works toward the goals of the organization without placing undue burden on operations. The global scope and application of a policy and procedure is beyond the boundaries of this chapter, which will instead focus on the basics as it pertains to radiology and, more specifically, to MRI.

In general terms, the hospital or medical center policy and procedure manuals operate on a "trickle down" approach whereby the top institutional policies and procedures apply to all those lower down the organizational and operational chain. The lower you go, the more narrow the scope of the policy. For example, an institutional policy and procedure on Infant Safe Haven Laws applies to everyone in the institution regardless of department or position, while a policy and procedure pertaining to screening patients prior to entering the MRI environment applies only to those individuals employed in and empowered to enter the MRI environment. With this in mind, the policies and procedures used in MRI are generally quite specific and require a basic understanding of the safe operation of the MR systems in use today.

POLICIES AND PROCEDURES

Policy and Procedure: Definitions

Policy and procedure manuals are an essential component of all institutions. They convey the desires of senior leadership with respect to common departmental operations. Additionally, they instruct the staff how issues are to be handled during routine operations and unexpected events. Policy and procedure manuals also set the cultural tone of the department and allow the vision of the organization's leadership to manifest itself in daily operations while protecting the institution from undue risk (7). In the broadest terms, the policy and procedure manual is the "owner's manual" for the hospital or medical center and the standard to which the facility holds itself and to which it will be held by others.

Policy and Procedure: Essential Elements

There are many formats that policies and procedures can follow. Some take the form of detailed memos, position statements, or papers that narrate how specific situations or comprehensive operations are to be handled within the department. Others utilize a formalized layout specifically optimized for hospital policies. Lastly, policies can take on the form of a clinical practice manual that governs all relevant operational items and activities within the department. Regardless of which format is selected there are a few basic needs that each should have in some form.

Policy

The "policy" is the name of the document or file pertaining to a specific situation, condition, or scenario. The following is an example:

Example 1. MRI Screening Policy – This document or file pertains to the issue of screening in MRI. This is very straightforward and names the policy precisely. This format allows no room for interpretation or debate about the information that it will contain.

Purpose: The purpose is a brief narrative of why the policy is needed. It can be as simple as "to ensure patient safety," or it can be a comprehensive rationalization of why one particular policy was written. For example, the stated purpose the MRI Screening Policy is to

Table 1. Basic policies and procedures for a hospital or medical center. This table provides a list of the basic policies and procedures needed for an MRI department, the rationale behind them, and the basic elements they should contain.

Policy and Procedure	Rationale	Basic Elements
Access Control	The MRI department represents specialized space that necessitates limiting access to specially-trained individuals, only.	This policy and procedure should detail the establishment and demarcation of a four zone system as described by the ACR, with details regarding who has access to the zones and the process for entering and leaving the area of the MR system room (Zone IV).
Personnel	The unique MRI environment requires personnel to receive specialized training.	This policy and procedure should detail the establishment of defined Level 1 and Level 2 personnel based on responsibilities and training. The type, amount, timing, and frequency of the training should be clearly defined.
Patient, Visitor, and Personnel Screening	All individuals entering the MRI environment need to be properly screened to ensure the safety of the patients, visitors, and personnel.	This policy and procedure should detail who performs the screening, how the screening is conducted, what tools are to be used, how the results are documented, and how to proceed when unsafe materials or situations are discovered. This policy should be inclusive of all individuals and patients including emergency patients, first responders, prisoners and parolees, and Level 1 and Level 2 personnel.
Device and Object Screening	Any device or equipment entering the MRI environment for use with a patient must be established as MR safe or MR conditional with the specific conditions clearly defined.	This policy and procedure is where the facility should describe how devices, equipment, and objects are to be screened, what tools should be used during the screening process, and how devices should be properly labeled.
MRI Department Staffing	The MRI department requires specialized staff with proper significant training in order to safely operate the equipment and to ensure safety.	This policy and procedure should describe and detail who is allowed to operate the MR system, what training and licensure is needed, and how the department is to be staffed during normal operations, off-hours, and emergency situations.
Pregnant Patients and Healthcare Workers	Pregnancy represents a possible risk scenario in the MRI environment.	This policy and procedure should cover pregnant patients and healthcare workers. For patients, the MRI approval process needs to be clearly defined as well as any limitation on the use of techniques and MRI contrast agents. For healthcare workers, duties should be clearly established as well as possible limitations.
Pediatric Patients	Children are not small adults. Therefore, they require the use of specialized techniques.	This policy and procedure should detail how pediatric patients are screened, scheduled, and, if needed, sedated during the MRI examination. Patient monitoring must be clearly defined as well as the role of all personnel in the process. Emergency procedures also need to be clearly defined.

Table 1. Continued

Policy and Procedure	Rationale	Basic Elements
Cryogens	Cryogens pose a unique danger in the event of a quench in the MRI environment.	This policy and procedure should detail what cryogens are, their possible risks, and what to do in the event of a quench as well as a quench with vent pipe failure.
Sedation, Anesthesia, and Pain Control	MRI facilities utilizing medications for sedation, anesthesia, and pain management need special policies regarding theses medications.	This policy and procedure should detail how patients are assessed for the need for sedation, anesthesia, and pain control medications. Patient monitoring must be clearly defined as well as the role of all personnel in the process. Emergency procedures also need to be clearly defined.
MRI Contrast Agents	MRI contrast agents are drugs and their usage needs to be clearly defined.	This policy and procedure should detail the clinical indications for MRI contrast agents, who can administer them, and what conditions prevent patients from receiving contrast agents.
Ferromagnetic Intracranial Aneurysm Clips	A patient with a ferromagnetic intracranial aneurysm clip may experience a significant risk if allowed in the MR system room.	This policy and procedure should clearly state that the pedigree for all implanted intracranial clips be established and the procedure to follow if the required information cannot be obtained.
Cardiac Pacemakers and implantable Cardioversion Defribrillators (ICDs)	Patients with cardiac pacemakers or ICDs may experience a significant risk in association with MRI.	This policy and procedure should detail the specific devices that can be scanned and the specific procedure to be followed in order to safely do so. This policy needs to be very detailed and the role of all support personnel needs to be clearly defined. Since scanning patients with many pacemakers is not FDA approved, the consent process for these patients needs to be clearly spelled out. Special directions are necessary for MR conditional cardiac devices.
Emergency Preparedness	Emergencies may occur and impact the MRI setting. All MRI facilities must have pre-planned responses in place to properly handle emergency situations.	This is a critical policy and procedure because it needs to address patient issues such as contrast reactions, cardiac situations, and seizures, etc. It also needs to cover facility issues such as water leaks, power failures, and fires both in the MRI setting and in close proximity. Lastly, this policy and procedure needs to cover natural disasters such as flooding, earthquake, tornado, and fire. This policy and procedure will reference and be intimately linked to many other policies within the hospital or medical center.

ensure that all patients, visitors, and non-MRI employees undergo comprehensive screening for the presence of contraindicated materials on or in the body that could result in injury to self or others if taken into the MR system room (i.e., Zone IV).

Scope: The section of the policy referred to as the "scope" defines the policy's intended audience. Some policies are very limited to a specific piece of equipment, room, or department, while others are all encompassing and apply to an entire organization. Accurately defining the scope helps to ensure that the policy will be followed by those who need it and not lost in the realm of non-applicable policies. If properly worded, the scope of the policy will not need to be revised when capabilities are changed, hardware is upgraded, or MR systems are added unless they involve entirely new departments.

Procedure

While the policy dictates the desires of the institution, the procedure details the methods by which the policy is carried out. Using example 1 above, the MRI Screening Policy, the procedure would detail the necessary steps to be taken to screen patients, visitors, or non-MRI personnel so that they may safely enter the MR system room. The procedure will vary in detail depending on facility type, patient mix, and level of complexity of the MRI examinations that are performed. The procedure for all MRI facilities should include the core elements of what is to be done, how it is to be done, who is responsible for performing the procedure, and what, if any, resources should be utilized.

Additionally, the procedure should contain sufficient detail so that it can be easily understood by those covered in the "scope" section of the document. It should not contain excessive details that do not provide clinical relevance. For example, a venipuncture policy that specifies the size of catheter to be used includes a detail that serves no purpose except to limit the type of departmental flexibility needed for efficient operations, since the size of catheter can vary depending on the status of the patient, size of the patient, and examination to be performed. An effective venipuncture policy should instead specify that a suitable sized catheter should be inserted based on the examination to be performed. The choice of catheter size should be at the discretion of the hospital or medical center personnel establishing the venous access. While this type of attention to detail may seem trivial and lead to frustration, we must remember that overly detailed policies make compliance difficult and lead to routine deviations. Deviations from policy are to be expected occasionally and, if clinically justifiable, do not pose a problem. On the other hand, regular deviations suggest a poorly conceived and worded policy and should be avoided.

Implementation and Revision Date for Policies and Procedures

MRI safety policies and procedures developed for MRI facilities in hospitals and medical centers should contain a minimum of two dates, one for the date of creation and/or implementation and the other indicating the date of the last revision. The implementation date can be a single date for all policies that commence on the day a new facility begins operations or the dates can vary if policies are added over time in established facilities. The implementation date should not be edited in later revisions.

The revision date indicates the date the policy was last reviewed. The preferred method for documenting revision history is with multiple date lines progressing chronologically. While this is a slightly more "busy" effect visually, it allows the full revision history to be established. A single date that changes at subsequent revisions, while satisfying the basic need to keep policies and procedures current, does not indicate any temporal frequency or periodicity with respect to the review process. The frequency of review should be annually or sooner if required by regulation. Additionally, if there is a significant change in operations such as the addition of a new MR system, new operating locations, or a major upgrade with respect to the equipment (e.g., software or hardware), this also warrants a review of the policies and procedures that specifically apply to MRI safety (1).

Signatures

All policies and procedures should be signed. The signature can be a line item on all policy and procedure documents in facilities that have numerous individual documents or a single signature on the revision page of a multi-policy and procedure manual. Exactly who signs the policies is up to each individual facility operating within a hospital or medical center. At the very least, the signature should be that of the modality, section, or department chief. Ideally, the document would claim multiple signatures from an administration representative, the MRI Safety Officer or Chairperson of the MRI Safety Committee, and the party responsible for daily operations within the department, usually the MRI Manager. The use of electronic signatures for electronic policy and procedure manuals is well established and is acceptable as long as it complies with established hospital security protocols.

Managing the Policy and Procedure Manual

The need for a comprehensive policy and procedure manual is evident. There are situations though, in which the responsibility for the manual becomes less obvious. For most hospitals and medical centers, the lines are well defined. The departmental policy and procedure manual is created and maintained by the departmental leadership. In certain cases this is not always possible, such as when MRI examinations are provided as a contracted service through a third-party company. These arrangements are overall quite common, though the service delivery model can vary considerably. Sometimes MRI service is provided one or more days per week via a visiting mobile MRI unit or the unit can be parked full-time as a lower-cost "imaging center". It is also possible to have a fully functional, fixed MRI center within the confines of the hospital that is operationalized and managed by a third-party who provides staff and operational support. Regardless of the arrangement, the policy and procedure manual needs to be agreed upon by all parties and should be discussed as a matter of course during any negotiations for provided services. Adherence to policy and procedure standards by contracted personnel should also be considered an integral part of the contracted service and any violation should be treated as a material breech of the contracted terms. It is critical to remember that the hospital or medical center is responsible for the care of their patients even if a component of the care is outsourced to a third-party.

When MRI procedures are provided via a contracted mobile service, there are additional safety policies and procedures that need to be considered. In a mobile arrangement, the zone model described by the ACR (1), while not mandatory, is less easily achieved and, therefore, it may be necessary to build docking structures, temporary shelters, or other adaptable spaces. The regulations governing the use of these spaces varies greatly from state to state with some municipalities requiring electricity, plumbing, HVAC (i.e., heating, ventilation, and air conditioning) and even fire suppression. Whatever the type of structure, it is important that the policy and procedure manual matches the delivery model.

The policy and procedure manual is also only as good as the data it contains and it is important to keep the information as current as possible, as previously stated. Regardless of MRI facility type, it is essential that the policy and procedure documents be maintained as a "living document" (1, 2). The old policies should be compared with any departmental changes and equipment upgrades to see if it still satisfies the original purpose. All facilities should be familiar with governmental, agency, or regulatory mandated review requirements, though at present few, if any exist with particular regard to MRI safety. As an example, the State of Pennsylvania mandates that all radiology policies be reviewed annually (8). Other states, recommend a two-year review while still others have no formal provision for reviewing policies and procedures (9-11). On the agency side, the Joint Commission (JC) has no formal standard, but a policy review date older than three years would raise concerns and lead the inspector to question what other areas of operations have not been reviewed or revised in greater than a three year period (Personal Communication, Joint Commission Standards Interpretation Group, December 27, 2012)

Policy and procedure review on an annual or even bi-annual basis can be time consuming but the time is well spent. There are different strategies for managing the manual. Some hospitals and medical centers use a formal committee to review, revise, and manage the policy and procedure manual. Others delegate management of specific sections of the manual (e.g., MRI, computed tomography, ultrasound, etc.) to the department managers and/or modality chiefs. Whichever technique a hospital or medical center chooses to follow, it is essential that they follow a regimented schedule of review and document the process with updated signatures and dates.

Implementing New Policies and Procedures

When developing and implementing new policies and procedures for MRI safety, it is essential that the process be based on careful research and deliberate thought as well as a focused review of industry best practices in order to be the most effective (2, 6-7). The proposed policy and procedure should be initiated as a preliminary document with an implementation date and proposed review date. The preliminary document should be revisited after the third month of implementation to assess the clinical impact and to revise, as needed. When initially written, policies and procedures tend to be either too specific or too vague. Therefore, implementing them as preliminary for a period of three months allows the department to better assess the impact of the policy and procedure on the overall operation of the department and to correct problems with the wording of the policy or the "mechanics" of the procedure. Once final and fully operationalized, there is usually no need for further revision unless mandated by departmental changes.

DISTRIBUTION OF THE POLICY AND PROCEDURE MANUAL

Once a hospital or medical center has a workable version of the policy and procedure manual, it needs to be available to all entities within the organization. For a small hospital with a single scanner this is a relatively simple task. A university-level hospital with several departments and affiliated smaller centers faces a greater challenge. Irrespective of facility type, there are two basic choices of the distribution method for the policy and procedure manual. Both have benefits and complications and the ultimate distribution choice depends on the needs of the hospital or medical center.

Hard copy distribution of the policy and procedure manual has been the standard for many years. It is basic and, once the manual is written, quite effective. The policy and procedure manual is copied and a copy is then provided to key locations where it can be accessed, such as the MRI center. Typically, there is one copy of the MRI safety policies and procedures manual provided to the MRI department and another maintained in the administrative area where it resides in a larger manual of global radiology documents covering the other imaging or therapeutic modalities. Manual distribution is low cost and requires very little time commitment. For a larger hospital or medical center with more entities and locations, or even when a few locations are geographically distant from the main facility, the manual distribution method becomes much less desirable. A major disadvantage of hard copy manuals is the intricacies of the revision process. A change in a policy and procedure, regardless of the magnitude of the change, requires that the old version be physically replaced with the newer version in all manuals. This process requires diligence and attention to detail and, thus, it is a frequent weak link in the process.

Many modern-day hospitals and medical centers and certainly most facilities with multiple clinical areas, campuses, and affiliated centers opt instead for an electronic policy manual distribution. Maintaining an electronic manual of policies and procedures offers significant benefits over hard copy manuals. For example, the master manual can be updated, as needed, and the changes applied to all subordinate documents immediately and universally. The same applies to updates for signatures and revision dates. A single source policy and procedure manual, once edited, passes through to all locations and entities ensuring consistency and minimizing the chances that an outdated document will remain in a forgotten manual. Another feature of electronic manuals is that there are few limits on what can be included. Some hospitals and medical centers include photographs that serve as visual aids for the policy and procedure or even links to videos that re-enforce certain elements of the document. Notably, the greatest benefit of an electronic policy and procedure manual is the ability of it to be linked together with other documents. In an electronic manual it is easy to include a hyperlink to another policy and procedure in the same department or any department in the organization. This is extremely important when dealing with complex policies and procedures that may contain important elements that not only directly impact the safety of the MRI department but also tie into nursing policies and those involved in safety, as well.

Examples of policies and procedures that have a high degree of commonality with other departments include any such document that discusses the administration of non-contrast medications, which relate very closely to nursing policies, or any document that discusses conscious sedation or anesthesia in the MRI department, which ties in heavily to anesthesia policies. With electronic-based policies and procedures, the referenced nursing or anesthesia policy is instantly available making the manual far more effective overall. The drawback of this increased effectiveness is that the manual requires an increased level of commitment in terms of time and resources. While it is preferred to have references to other departments, it is imperative that the reference links be maintained and that the referenced policies are current and accurate. This increased complexity requires a high level commitment at the administrative level to devote the time and resources necessary to create and maintain the electronic manual.

It is also imperative to maintain the electronic policies and procedure manual in a way that is accessible in the event of a connectivity failure, since patient care continues even in the absence of the hospital's or medical center's intranet. If the manual is copied to local computer hard drives as part of the update process, it should be readily available at all times as long as there is electrical power to the department. If the facility relies heavily on cloud-based technology the situation becomes more complicated as access to data could be compromised in the event of a connectivity failure. Generally, Information Technology departments have systems in place for maintaining data and allowing for continuation of care during a communication blackout or emergency. With respect to an electronic policy and procedure manual, it can be as simple as a periodic hard disk backup of the manual that is available in the command center or on strategically placed hard drives. The details can vary but what is important is the need to have all relevant departments involved from the beginning.

LEGAL IMPLICATIONS OF POLICIES

The rule of law is that everyone must obey the law. If people violate the law, they are subject to the consequences depending on the nature and severity of the violation. The content of the policy and procedure manual can be viewed as the "law" of the department. All employees must follow the law and no employee is exempt. As such, policy and procedure manuals are designed to clearly define the responsibilities of the healthcare professional and set the standards to which employees are held (12). Ideally, each hospital and medical center will have an up-to-date, comprehensive manual covering all aspects of departmental operations for both routine and non-routine situations. A facility without a policy and procedure manual is declaring " I cannot meet the standard of care so I have no policy for it" and, unfortunately, that facility starts on the defensive in any legal action (Personal communication, Emanuel Kanal, M.D., November 06, 2012).

In the broadest general terms, the key to any policy and procedure is its ability to be defended. The range of variation in a policy and procedure from one facility to another within the same industry may be significant. Where any facility falls within the range from conservative to liberal is based primarily on the culture of the organization. Therefore, especially with respect to MRI safety matters, it is critical that the facility constructs the policies and procedures with sound judgment and that they meet the basic standard of care set forth in the industry (1). For example, a small community hospital typically does not possess the infrastructure to scan patients with MR conditional pacemakers and, therefore, it should have a policy stating that these devices are not to be scanned at the MRI center. As the hospital grows and the level of sophistication of the department increases, the policy and procedure needs to grow as well to reflect any changes it desires. If the policy is that pacemakers are still absolute contraindications, then an exclusion policy will suffice. If the hospital or medical center decides to allow scanning of patients with MR conditional pacemakers, only, then the policy and procedure needs to be amended to reflect specifically which pacemakers can be scanned, which cannot, and the exact procedure to be followed to safely do so. This is a key point in that whatever policy and procedure the department chooses, it will remain as the standard they are held to until the document is changed.

Consider the following fictionalized example. In this example, there will be two patients with cardiac pacemakers who undergo MRI examinations at two separate, but equally capable, hospitals (Facility A and Facility B). Both MRI facilities in these hospitals are prepared to scan these complicated patients with all of the necessary collateral support from nursing and cardiology. Unfortunately, both patients experience negative consequences that require the cardiac pacemakers be replaced after the MRI examinations. Facility A has a policy and procedure detailing how pacemaker patients are to be scanned and follows that information to the letter. Therefore, Facility A's liability is limited with respect to the damaged pacemaker. Facility B performs exactly as Facility A, but their policy and procedure is outdated and states than cardiac pacemakers are an absolute contraindication to MRI and patients with these devices are not allowed into the MR system room (Zone IV). Facility B's liability is greater because, although they had the same negative outcome as Facility A, Facility B violated their own policy. This example is exaggerated to illustrate the point that each facility dictates the standards to which it will be held within the range of common practice. It is important that those standards be appropriate for the protection of patients, staff, and visitors without limiting the functionality of the department. Failing to keep policies current and accurate is like announcing, "I did not know the problem existed and, therefore, I have not thought about it" (Personal communication, Emanuel Kanal, M.D., November 06, 2012).

There is also a delicate balance between a policy and procedure that is too restrictive and one that is too vague. A policy and procedure that contains too many details can negatively impact the department on several levels. The policy will ultimately be difficult to follow, as flexibility is lost in the presence of overly tedious details. Additionally, any issues arising from failure to follow the policy and procedure place the department in a defensive posture. An overly restrictive policy and procedure, particularly in the realm of MRI safety, slows the delivery of care and will surely be violated on a regular basis, neither of which is good news for the patient, department, or facility in general.

There are times when extremely specific details are necessary for patient safety. For example, implanted devices approved for use in patients referred for MRI examinations under specific conditions are labeled MR Conditional and the specific conditions under which these devices can be safely scanned are specified in writing by the manufacturer, usually presented in the *Instructions for Use*. The difference between scanning the patient safely and risking injury relies squarely on the details, which are clearly spelled out in the product literature. Accordingly, any policy and procedure concerning the device must clearly state what needs to be done in step-by-step fashion with all possible details intact.

When drafting policies and procedures, the choice of language is also a factor. Words like "shall, "must", and "will" should be avoided as they suggest absolutes. The policy should opt for "should" instead as it allows for a bit more flexibility. Improper language, poor choice of words, absolutes, and colloquialisms are all potential problems when the policy is viewed by non-imaging professionals, opposing counsel, and in the worst case a jury.

In the event of a legal case there are a few things to be considered. First, the policies and procedures manual will be requested by opposing counsel as part of the discovery process. A good attorney knows that the manual contains the type of details that can be used to validate or discredit a witness. Second, the contents of the policy and procedure manual will be used by opposing counsel to assess fundamental knowledge during depositions and not knowing that the policy and procedure existed or what information it contains will not make the situation better. All staff members are held to the standards contained within the manual and, thus, need to know the entire content, where to find it, and what information it contains. Lastly, policies and procedures may be used during a trial. If the legal case involves a loss suffered as a result of a violation of a policy and procedure, it will certainly feature prominently in the trial process.

In the end, violating a policy and procedure of a hospital or medical center by itself is not going to result in legal action. Depending on the violation, it could result in disciplinary action as defined in the employee handbook but it is not, in and of itself, a legal issue. If the violation of the policy and procedure is determined to be the proximate cause of an injury, illness, or negative outcome for a patient, visitor, or co-worker then the situation has changed and is more likely to involve the legal system.

CONCLUSIONS

Healthcare providers must make patient, visitor, and employee safety a prime concern and take the necessary steps to create a comprehensive culture of safety within the organization. Policies and procedures serve as a sound foundation for any safety program, especially with regard to MRI safety. A policy and procedure can be a single document detailing that an industry standard or guideline (e.g., the ACR guidance document) is utilized as the *de facto* operational policy for the department, or it can be a collection of individual documents tailored to specific operational issues in the department. As long as the policies and procedures are based on industry best practices and understood by all involved parties to be the standard to which they are held, they will be an effective tool for improving safety without limiting operational agility.

REFERENCES

1.   Kanal E, Barkovich AJ, Bell C. et al. ACR guidance document on MR safe practices: 2013. J Magn Reson Imaging 2013;37:501-530.

2.   Page SB. Establishing a System of Policies and Procedures. Westerville, OH: Process Improvement Publishing; 2009

3.   Chaljub G, Kramer L, Johnson R, et al. Projectile cylinder accidents resulting from the presence of ferrous nitrous oxide of oxygen tanks in the MR suite. AJR Am J Roentgenol 2001;177:27-30.

4. Chen D. Small town reels from boys MRI death. The New York Times [online] August 1, 2001 Available at: http://www.nytimes.com/2001/08/01/nyregion/small-town-reels-from-boy-s-mri-death.html?src=pm Accessed November 2012.

5. Issue 38: Preventing accidents and injuries in the MRI suite (2008). Available at: www.jointcomission.org/assets/1/18/sea_38.PDF Accessed November 2012.

6. Gilk T, Kanal E. Interrelating sentinel event alert #38 With the ACR guidance document on MR safe practices: 2013. An MRI safety review tool. J Magn Reson Imaging 2013;37:531-543.

7. McQuate, C. Penning Effective Policies, Digital Booklet. American Society for Industrial Security: 2005

8. Pennsylvania Code Chapter 127. Radiology Services. Available at: www.pacode.com/secure/data/28/chapter127/chap127toc.html Accessed October 2012.

9. Unannotated Code of Maryland and Rules. Available at: www.lexisnexis.com/hottopics/mdcode/ Accessed October 2012.

10. State of Delaware Title 16, Health and Safety. Available at: http://delcode.delaware.gov/title16/c074/index/shtml Accessed October 2012.

11. Missouri Code of State Regulations: Title 19. Department of Health and Senior Services. Available at: www.sos.mo.gov/adrules/csr/csr.asp Accessed October 2012.

12. Judson K, Harrison C. Law and Ethics for the Health Professions, Sixth Edition. New York: McGraw Hill; 2010.

Chapter 23   MRI Safety Policies and Procedures for an Outpatient Facility

LAURA FOSTER, J.D., M.P.H.

Vice President, Regulatory Affairs
Radnet, Inc.
Los Angeles, CA

MICHAEL MANZANO, M.D.

Musculoskeletal MRI Fellow
Radnet, Inc.
Los Angeles, CA

JOHN V. CRUES, III, M.D.

Medical Director and MRI Fellowship Director
Radnet, Inc.
Los Angeles, CA
Professor of Radiology
University of California, San Diego

INTRODUCTION

A well-designed safety program to protect medical personnel and patients is mandatory for all centers performing clinical medical imaging. However, specific requirements must be stipulated for outpatient MRI procedures due to the inherent risks of MRI technology. **Table 1** lists safety concerns relevant to all medical imaging procedures, and **Table 2** lists specific concerns in the MRI environment. Because of these concerns all outpatient imaging departments must have a written safety program, which is properly implemented and maintained by management, technologists, and radiologists. This chapter will detail requirements of a safety program to help assure protection of employees, patients, and others while complying with regulatory obligations. This chapter should assist new and existing facilities in developing and/or revising safety, health, environment and loss control programs while en-

Table 1. Safety requirements shared by all diagnostic imaging modalities.

• Correctly install appropriate imaging equipment
• Adequately maintain imaging equipment
• Protect the patient and facility personnel from known risks
• Minimize patient exposure
• Ensure the correct identification of the patient
• Ensure that the correct body anatomy is properly imaged
• Protect patient health information (PHI) regarding privacy and security standards

Table 2. Specific safety concerns for an outpatient MRI facility.

• *Static Magnetic Field* – The strong static magnetic field associated with the MR system induces forces on ferromagnetic objects, which can cause dangerous movements of objects external and internal to the human body.
• *Time-Varying Magnetic Fields* – Rapidly changing magnetic fields have multiple potential biologic effects, including inducing electric currents in conductors and causing peripheral nerve stimulation.
• *Radiofrequency (RF) Energy* – RF energy can cause tissue heating, especially in conductive materials, which may result in burns.
• *Acoustic Noise* – The gradient magnetic fields associated with high field strength MR systems can produce excessive acoustic noise.
• *Superconducting Magnets* – Superconducting magnets used by high field strength MR systems are always "on", so employees and emergency personnel must maintain vigilance, especially after normal business hours. Magnet quenches are unique to superconducting magnets and require special training and procedures to ensure patient and employee safety.

suring consistency in operations and medical delivery with particular attention focused on proper policies and procedures.

PERSONNEL: RESPONSIBILITIES AND DUTIES

Staffing of the outpatient MRI facility should be carefully considered and performed. Appropriate experience and training of the management team is crucial to operating an efficient and safe imaging department. The key personnel in outpatient imaging safety include the management team, members of the MRI Safety Committee, employees, and the Chief Safety Officer. Responsibilities of the management team include, the following:

- Implementation of the Safety Program, including the policies and procedures, through motivation, training, counseling, and enforcement;

- Initiating compliance for all safety program elements;

- Identifying hazards through safety inspections and developing timely counter-measures;

- Training personnel in accident prevention and safe work habits; and

- Performing timely accident investigations and reporting, including paperwork and corrective actions.

A Safety Committee, chaired by the center's Medical Safety Officer or appropriately designated physician, should be established. The Safety Committee should be charged with the following tasks:

- Meet on a regular schedule;

- Review and approve safety programs designed to meet the goals of the center;

- Review incident reports, self-inspection results, and employee safety recommendations;

- Recommend and assist in establishing additional general safety rules as the needs are identified;

- Develop and monitor a safety improvement plan; and

- Prepare a written Safety Committee Report of its activities.

Employees are a key element that ensure a safe outpatient MRI facility. They must recognize the following obligations:

- Learn and comply with safety and health rules and regulations established by the center;

- Report all safety and health hazards to a supervisor and take all necessary actions to establish immediate or temporary control of the hazard until permanent control can be established;

- Immediately report all accidents or incidents on the job to their supervisor;

- Cooperate and assist in all investigations; and

- Use all appropriate personal protective equipment provided.

The Safety Committee should designate a Chief Safety Officer. The duties of the Safety Officer include:

- Maintaining current safety policies;

- Monitoring safety training to ensure that all new personnel are properly trained and all employees receive annual safety training;

- Reviewing incident reports and determine if appropriate corrective actions are implemented by site management;

- Conducting regularly scheduled facility safety inspections;

- Reviewing and recommend changes in the safety program as needs are identified;

- Designating the appropriate maintenance of safety record files for each facility;

- Establishing a system for providing first aid, medical emergency equipment, and personal protective equipment; and

- Serving as the Chairperson for the MRI Safety Committee.

Encouraging active communication between the different elements of the safety team is critical to long-term success. This can be facilitated by establishing a center hotline, scheduling regular meetings to discuss safety, establishing training programs, posting key responsibilities in easily accessed employee areas, and providing newsletters with relevant information.

MRI SAFETY PROGRAM

Outpatient MRI facilities should be accredited by either the American College of Radiology (ACR), the Intersocietal Commission for the Accreditation of Magnetic Resonance Imaging Laboratories, or the Joint Commission and perform services under the direct supervision of a physician, certified by the American Board of Radiology or other equivalent national medical imaging certifying body and licensed to practice medicine in the state where the center is located. Some state and local governments require additional certification. The MRI technologists should be active participants in the continuing compliance and quality assurance standards of the facility's accreditation certification. These individuals are key members of the safety team discussed above.

Patient Safety

A key component of the MRI safety program is to protect patients. This requires a comprehensive system that includes appropriate policies and procedures and begins with the patient's first interaction with the MRI facility. Scheduling of MRI studies requires an order from a licensed medical professional. The order must be provided to the facility as one of the following:

- A written document signed by the treating physician/practitioner that is hand-delivered, mailed, or faxed to the facility;
- A telephone call by the treating practitioner, with written documentation of the order by both the practitioner's office and the center; or
- An electronic communication.

Telephone orders for outpatients without a written order should be verified by a return call to the referring physician's office and the call should be documented in the medical record. The written order must be permanently maintained in the patients record. A complete order should include all of the elements listed in **Table 3**. Determination of the appropriateness of the requested examination should be performed before the patient is exposed to the MRI environment, preferably at the time of scheduling. Patients should not be scanned if the medical history does not justify an MRI examination. Appropriateness

Table 3. Order requirements for outpatient MRI services.

• Patient's name • Date of order • Exam ordered (including left or right where appropriate) • Clinical indication (including symptoms and preliminary diagnoses) • Pertinent medical history (including past difficulties with medical imaging) • Referring physician's name • Referring physician's phone number • Indication of pregnancy if appropriate
Additional items may include: • Date and time of scheduled surgery • Indicate "STAT" if requested

Criteria from the American College of Radiology can assist in this process (please see http://www.acr.org/Quality-Safety/Appropriateness-Criteria). If the patient is pregnant without the knowledge of the referring physician, then the referring physician must be notified for approval to continue before allowing the patient into the MR system room. The radiologist must approve MRI examinations on pregnant patients, and the risk versus benefits of MRI must be considered and explained to the patient by a trained healthcare professional before proceeding with the study. This process must be documented in the patient's medical record.

The MRI technologist should carefully review the examination order and confer with the radiologist if the order is incomplete, unclear, or needs amending. The MRI technologist cannot change the requested order without approval by the radiologist or authorization from the requesting physician. Any change in the original order requires documentation of an amended order including:

- Names, titles, and other identifying information for both parties involved in the amendment;
- Date and time of the amendment; and
- Specific information describing the changes made.

Importantly, Independent Diagnostic Testing Facilities (IDTFs) are required to obtain all referring physician's orders and modifications in writing.

Screening patients for the presence of implants and devices that may pose hazards in the MRI environment must begin at scheduling. Notably, the Safety Committee should provide scheduling personnel a protocol so that implants and devices contraindicated for MRI are detected before the patient is scheduled. All employees should be familiar with current MRI labeling terminology, as follows; MR Safe, MR Conditional, or MR Unsafe (1, 2). An MR Conditional device should be carefully evaluated before the patient is allowed into the scanner to ensure that it complies with the specific labeling information relative to the use of the particular MR system (e.g., static magnetic field, type of radiofrequency coil, specific absorption rate limitation, device programming changes, etc.) (2). If the scheduling personnel have questions concerning safety of specific devices, then they should have access to MRI technologists and radiologists to help them determine whether or not specific devices are unsafe or acceptable for the scanner in use at the outpatient MRI facility. A detailed list of this information can be found at www.MRIsafety.com, in an annually updated textbook (2), or from the specific device manufacturer.

Policies and procedures must be in place to ensure that patients are properly identified and the correct patient information is entered into the MR scanner and medical record.

Because of the potential risk inherent in the MRI environment (**Table 2**), the ACR recommends segmenting the MRI environment into four zones (3). In new construction, these zones can be physically separated by barriers or other appropriate means. In most outpatient MRI centers physical separation may not be practicable and, in general, has been found to be unnecessary. Outpatient MRI facilities are conceptually divided into four access zones, as follows

- Public Zone (i.e., ACR Zone I): This zone is far enough from the scanner that the magnetic field is under 5-gauss and no MR system is present. Staff and the general public and freely access this zone.

- Patient Preparation Zone (i.e., ACR Zone II): This is the area of interface between the public and imaging personnel. This is the area where patients are screened for MRI safety and medical histories obtained. In this area, patients can change into clothing acceptable for the MRI setting and be prepared for scanning. Patients should be accompanied by MRI safety-trained staff members in this area.

- Restricted Zone (i.e., ACR Zones III and IV): This area should not be accessed by unscreened individuals. This is the region where magnetic fields and equipment could cause serious injury or death. Strict control of this area by MRI safety-trained staff members is mandatory.

Regions within restricted zones where the static magnetic field exceeds 5-gauss should be clearly marked and designated as being potentially hazardous. Danger signs should be prominently displayed at the entry of the Restricted Zone, typically on and around the MR system room's door in outpatient MRI facilities.

Patients are screened for risk factors before being escorted into the Restricted Zone. This topic is covered in great detail elsewhere in this textbook. The patient (or their family, guardian, or other individual) complete a written screening form. Special diligence is required for incommunicative and critical patients. The facility can create its own screening form approved by the Safety Committee or a form can be obtained from other sources, such as the ACR (3) or downloaded from www.MRIsafety.com. Patients should fill out and sign the screening form each time the patient presents for an MRI examination. Screening of unconscious or incommunicative patients who are unable to provide a history for surgery, trauma, metal exposure, or prior MRI contrast reactions should be performed by the MRI technologist in conjunction with the patient's spouse, closest relative, guardian, or personal physician. Any accompanying individual should complete and sign the screening form designated for this purpose.

The MRI technologist performing the examination should review the completed screening form and verbally review the answers with the patient or other individual before witnessing (i.e., signing) the form. The screening form is placed in the patient's medical record. Any implants, devices, or metallic foreign bodies raising concerns relative to MRI safety should be checked with published sources or by other means (1-5), such as contacting the manufacturer of the device before allowing entry into the Restricted Zone. Consultation with the supervising radiologist or Chief Safety Officer is recommended if any concerns of safety cannot be clearly resolved by referring to standard resources or if there is any confusion regarding the information. The MRI technologist should perform a final visual and verbal safety check of each patient (or accompanying individual) prior to entering the MR system room.

Sedated, anesthetized, incommunicative or high-risk patients should undergo appropriate physiologic monitoring throughout the MRI examination. This may include checking the patient's vital signs, such as respiratory rate, heart rate, blood pressure, monitoring the electrocardiogram and/or using pulse oximetry as clinically indicated and as deemed appropriate by the MRI facility and responsible radiologist (2).

A critical component of the outpatient MRI facility's safety program is planning for attending to patients who may have medical emergencies in the MR system room. Appropriately trained personnel and supervisory physician shall be available at all times to provide emergency medical treatment to patients with cardiac and respiratory arrest. Mock emergency or "code blue" drills are recommended to ensure that the emergency team can efficiently manage medical emergencies. In the setting of a serious emergency such as a cardiopulmonary arrest, the patient should be rapidly and safely removed from the scanning room and immediate basic or advanced life support or other appropriate treatment should be initiated. Emergency medical equipment and medications should be readily available and accessible to emergency personnel.

Pregnant Patients

Special consideration should be given to the pregnant patient. Pregnant patients can be scanned at any stage of pregnancy if the patient's physician and radiologist determine that the risk versus benefit warrants performing the study. This topic is covered in another chapter in this textbook. The indications and other information should be documented in the patient's medical record and should include, the following:

- The information from the MRI study cannot be acquired via non-ionizing means (such as ultrasound);

- The diagnostic imaging information is medically indicated to diagnose either the mother or fetus during pregnancy;

- The referring physician does not believe that it is prudent to wait to obtain the information until a later stage of pregnancy or after pregnancy; and

- The patient agrees to have the examination, completes and signs a Pregnancy Consent Form approved by the Safety Committee. (It should be noted that this step is currently not recommended by the latest MRI safety document from the ACR).

MRI contrast agents should not be routinely administered to pregnant patients. This is a decision that should be made on a case-by-case basis by the MRI-trained radiologist in consideration of the risk versus benefit.

Specific Patient Risks

The time-varying magnetic fields applied during image acquisition create current in conductors in the field's influence and, when applied in the presence of a large magnetic field, create torque on the gradient coils, producing acoustic noise in the bore of the MR system (2-5). Because of the intensity of the noise induced by gradient switching in high field strength MR systems, it is recommended that patients be instructed to wear hearing protection when undergoing MRI (3, 6). Typical hearing protection devices include earplugs, headphones with music, or headphones with noise reduction technology. These protections may also be available to patients undergoing low field strength MRI, as needed.

Table 4. Adverse events leading to emergency room visits from Radnet, Inc. outpatient MRI centers (2010 and first half of 2011; Presented to the Food and Drug Administration on 10/15/11).

Exams	Burns	Shock	Metal-related	Hearing-related	Pace-maker	MRI Contrast	911 Calls	Deaths	Total
785,584	10	4	4	2	1	57	44	0	122
100%	.0013	.0005	.0005	.00025	.00012	.00725	.0056	0	.015

The radiofrequency (RF) fields used in MRI examinations produce currents in electrical conductors (2, 7, 8). Therefore, all unnecessary electrical conductive materials should be removed from the MR scanner before initiating acquisition sequences in order to prevent excessive heating or burns. All electrical connections, such as on surface RF coils, leads, monitoring devices, and others should be checked by the MRI technologist prior to each usage to ensure the integrity of the electrical connection, and that the thermal and electrical insulation is intact. Damaged cables and exposed wires should be immediately reported to the service engineer and the equipment taken out of service until it is repaired.

For electrical conductive material, such as wires, required to remain in the bore of the MR system with the patient during MRI, the wires must be configured so that no loops are formed in order to avoid patient burns. Adequate thermal insulation (i.e., using air, pads, etc.) should separate the patient's skin from all conducting material and the transmit RF coil (e.g., the body RF coil) during MRI. Procedures to prevent excessive heating and burns in patients during MRI have been previously presented (2) and should be closely followed for patients undergoing MRI examinations.

Many outpatients require sedation in order to complete a successful MRI examination (9-11). Notably, the Safety Committee should have written policies and procedures detailing how adult and pediatric patients should be sedated in the MRI environment. For example, for pediatric patients, these policies and procedures should be based on national standards, facility-specific policies defined by the referring pediatrician and the pediatric radiologist, the age of the patient, the mental capacity of the patient, the time duration of the MRI examination, and the depth of sedation needed.

Written sedation policies for adult sedation are also needed in the safety policies. Adults typically require sedation to overcome claustrophobia or extreme anxiety. Facility-specific policies determine the type of sedation that is utilized. These can be orally administered by the referring physician, or intravenously administered at the MRI facility. Sedation should always be administered in accordance with national guidelines and state and local laws (9-11). Separate sedation consent forms must be approved by the Safety Committee and explained to the patient by an appropriate healthcare professional before the patient or parent signs the document.

The most common adverse event leading to emergency room visits from outpatient MRI facilities is an adverse reaction to intravenous administered MRI contrast agents (**Table 4**). No patient should be given an intravenous contrast agent without the written prescription of a licensed physician or in accordance with state laws. MRI contrast agents should only

Table 5. Screening questions for determining risk for nephrogenic systemic fibrosis (NSF).

• Are you on dialysis? • Do you have known kidney failure? • Do you have a history of kidney disease (including solitary kidney, kidney transplant, kidney surgery, and kidney tumor)? • Do you have diabetes controlled by insulin or oral medication? • Do you have severe liver disease, prior liver transplant, or pending liver transplant? • Do you have hypertension requiring medical therapy?

be administered when the medical information requested justifies use in accordance with national guidelines and the interpreting radiologist. Depending on state regulations, either a radiologist, registered nurse, or IV-qualified MRI technologist may start and attend to the peripheral intravenous access line and administer the contrast agent as a bolus or continuous injection.

Before administering an intravenous an MRI contrast agent, preferably at the time of study scheduling, a history must be obtained from the patient or patient's guardian concerning prior contrast injections and possible adverse reactions (12-15). A history of asthma or allergic-type respiratory reaction not associated with MRI contrast agents is a risk factor for adverse reactions to MRI contrast media, but does not require premedication in most circumstances. Monitoring the cardiovascular and/or respiratory status (i.e., via careful visual monitoring of the patient and using an MR Conditional pulse oximetry) is prudent during and following administration of intravenous gadolinium-based MRI contrast agents in high-risk patients. If the patient has a history of adverse reaction to a gadolinium-based contrast agent, then the patient should be considered for premedication prior to receiving the contrast dosage according to recommendations by the ACR (12). The patient's cardiovascular and respiratory status should also be carefully monitored using appropriate techniques during MRI and for 30 minutes following contrast administration.

In addition to obtaining a history of adverse contrast reactions, screening questions designed to determine the patient's risk for nephrogenic systemic fibrosis (NSF) should be asked at the time of scheduling and when the MRI technologist obtains the patient's history during the time the patient presents for the MRI examination (16-25). **Table 5** lists screening questions that we recommend to be asked of all MRI patients before administrating gadolinium-based contrast agents relative to the issue of NSF. A positive answer to any of these questions requires calculation of the patient's glomerular filtration rate (GFR) to determine risk for NSF before administering gadolinium-based contrast agents in the outpatient setting.

If the patient is on dialysis, has an estimated GFR less than 30 mL/min/1.73-m^2 (stage 4 or stage 5 renal disease), or has acute renal injury, then injection of a gadolinium-based contrast agent should be given cautiously only after the following information is documented:

- The referring physician and radiologist must confer and decide that use of the gadolinium-based contrast agent is essential for diagnosis and no other reasonable means is available;

- Written orders from the referring physician and the responsible radiologist must be obtained, which include the name of the patient, the name and brand of the MRI contrast agent used, dose, route and rate of administration, the date and signature of the radiologist;

- Written informed consent from the patient; and

- The lowest possible dose of a low-risk gadolinium-based contrast agent (e.g., Multihance, Bracco Diagnostics, Inc.) should be used. (For 15<GFR<30, we use a 0.5 or 0.25 dose of MultiHance. For GFR<15 we use a 0.25 dose of Multi-Hance.)

We do not believe that outpatients need to be screened for NSF unless they have the known risk factors stated above. Specifically, we do not consider age alone to be a risk factor. However, the ACR Manual on Contrast Media, Version 8, considers age greater than 60 years of age to be a risk factor (12).

If the patient is on dialysis, the patient should undergo hemodialysis as soon as possible after the administration of the gadolinium-based contrast agent, preferably within a few hours of the study. Some investigators recommend that dialysis should be repeated 24 hours later. Interestingly, peritoneal dialysis has not been shown to protect against NSF.

Visitor Screening

At times it is necessary for visitors to enter the Restricted Zone. All visitors entering the Restricted Zone must first be screened for MRI risk factors. The visitor should fill out a specific screening form designed for those not undergoing and MRI examination (2). The visitor must fill out and sign this form in the Patient Preparation Zone and undergo screening by the MRI technologist. If the patient is deemed safe to enter the Restricted Zone by the MRI technologist, then the visitor may be allowed access to the Restricted Zone under direct supervision of an MRI technologist. Prior to entering the Restricted Zone, pockets must be emptied of hairpins, removable hearing aids, jewelry, analog watches, and any other devices, which are ferromagnetic or could be damaged in the presence of a high static magnetic field.

Emergency Personnel

All emergency (e.g., first responders), firefighters, police, and security personnel must be fully screened as a visitor and cleared by an MRI technologist before being allowed access to the Restricted Zone. It is prudent for outpatient MRI facilities to inform their local police and firefighter organizations of the risks of the powerful static magnetic field of the MR system and the 24-hour presence of the magnetic field for superconducting magnets before emergencies arise so that emergency personnel will be cognizant of the risks before responding to emergencies. Security personnel must remove all metal objects from their possession, including guns and ammunition, electronically-activated restraint devices, radios, cell phones, badges, name tags, jewelry, coins, wallets, keys, pocket knives, nail clippers, steel-toed boots or shoes, and similar items before entering the Restricted Zone. If the patient is a detainee and requires a restraining device, then in the Restricted Zone, then a plastic restraint device must be used.

Employee Safety

The outpatient MRI facility is a dynamic environment where personal and work related frustrations, difficulties, and issues often arise and are intimately intertwined. It is important to establish policies and procedures for proper behavior and etiquette because a worker's frustration or difficulties can translate into unnecessary patient stress on top of an anxiety-provoking examination. Personal conversations of work related difficulties should not be discussed in the presence of the patient. Technologists should only discuss results of patient examinations with the interpreting radiologist. Center personnel who interact with patients should properly identify themselves and explain their roles in medical care to instill confidence in their patient-related abilities. Food and beverages should not be consumed in the hallways or at workstations.

All employees in an outpatient MRI center must be screened for MRI risk factors, and any employees who are deemed to be unsafe for the MRI environment must be restricted from the Patient Preparation and Restricted Zones. Employees with access to the Restricted Zone must complete and pass an MRI safety training course which should be repeated on an annual basis.

If an equipment malfunction occurs, then the chief MRI technologist, facility manager, or radiologist should be informed in a timely manner. Only certified and qualified MRI technologists and MRI-trained radiologists should be permitted to operate an MR system and have unrestricted access to the Restricted Zone. These individuals must be extensively trained and educated in the broader aspects of MRI safety, including issues related to the potential for attraction of ferromagnetic devices, burns, peripheral nerve stimulation, and other potential risk factors described elsewhere in this chapter and in **Table 2**.

In order to minimize errors, it is recommended that the primary MRI technologist indicated in the patient's medical record should be the responsible for screening the patient and performing the MRI examination. Only certified MRI technologists should be authorized to perform MRI screening. Non-MRI personnel should be accompanied by and/or under the immediate supervision of an MRI technologist while they are in the Restricted Zone.

Pregnant Personnel

Pregnant healthcare workers should be permitted to work in and around the MRI environment throughout all stages of their pregnancy (2, 3). This includes, but is not limited to, positioning patients, scanning, archiving, injecting MRI contrast agents, entering the scan room in an emergency, etc. However, pregnant workers should not be allowed or required to work in the Patient Preparation and Restricted Zones if the worker is uncomfortable with exposure to the static magnetic field of the MR system. Pregnant healthcare workers should not remain within the bore of the scanner during the operation of the MR system. Additional information on this topic is covered in another chapter in this textbook.

Equipment

Proper installation and maintenance is necessary for the safe operation of the MR system. All ancillary equipment used in the Restricted Zone must be deemed safe or otherwise acceptable for use in the MRI environment. Oxygen tanks must be non-ferromagnetic throughout the imaging facility. Fire extinguishers must be MR Conditional models and must be placed in a conspicuous place in or near the scanner room. Monitoring equipment, such as pulse oximeters and anesthesia equipment, must be MR Conditional in order to be used in the MR system room. All other equipment such as IV poles, step stools, stretchers, and other patient support items must also be MR Safe or MR Conditional.

There are risk factors unique to the powerful magnets associated with an MR system. For example, if an individual is "trapped" against the magnet by a large ferromagnetic object, then the magnetic field may need to be shut down immediately. If the magnet is resistive, then the power can be shut off. If the magnet is a superconducting magnet, then the field must be quenched using the emergency shut down button, which should be located in a conspicuous place. Special training and education is important for all staff members working in the outpatient MRI facility with regard to specific procedures to follow involving a quench.

Preventive maintenance is mandatory to ensure high performance of the scanner in order to minimize down time and to maximize image quality. Preventive maintenance should be performed according to the manufacturer's recommendations and should be properly documented.

CONCLUSIONS

Optimal MRI safety in outpatient imaging centers requires a well-organized plan that includes the center's management, employees, an MRI Safety Committee and a committed Chief Safety Officer. A written safety plan that includes policies and procedures that address the risks uniquely associated with the MRI environment must be developed and explained to all employees, along with the assignment of specific responsibilities for execution of the plan. Since few lay people understand the risks associated with high static magnetic fields and other potential hazards associated with MRI, screening must begin at scheduling and strict adherence to patient safety management must be practiced. Visitors, emergency personnel, and others must be screened and prohibited from entering the MR system room with unsafe devices to ensure their safety as well as that of patients and staff members. Fortunately, extensive experience with MRI in outpatient facilities worldwide during more than twenty-five years has shown that outpatient MRI is extremely safe if proper policies and procedures are in place and the precautions discussed herein are rigorously enforced.

REFERENCES

1. Shellock FG, Woods, Crues JV. MR labeling information for implants and devices: Explanation of terminology. Radiology 2009;253:26-30.

2. Shellock FG. Reference Manual for Magnetic Resonance Safety, Implants, and Devices: 2013 Edition. Los Angeles, CA: Biomedical Research Publishing Group, Los Angeles, CA, 2013.

3. Kanal E, Barkovich AJ, Bell C, et al. ACR guidance document on MR safe practices: 2013. J Magn Reson Imaging 2013;37:501-530.

4. Shellock FG, Crues JV. MR procedures: Biologic effects, safety, and patient care. Radiology 2004;232:635-52

5. Shellock FG, Spinazzi A. MRI safety update 2008: Part 2, screening patients for MRI. AJR Am J Roentgenol 2008;191;1140-9.

6. Lauer AM, El-Sharkawy AM, Kraitchman DL, Edelstein WA. MRI acoustic noise can harm experimental and companion animals. J Magn Res Imaging 2012;36:743-7.

7. Zikria JF, Machnicki S, Rhim E, Bhatti T, Graham RE. MRI of patients with cardiac pacemakers: A review of the medical literature. AJR Am J Roentgenol. 2011;196:390-401.

8. Jacob ZC, Tito MF, Dagum AB. MR imaging-related electrical thermal injury complicated by acute carpal tunnel and compartment syndrome: Case report. Radiology 2010;254:846-50.

9. Berlin L. Sedation and analgesia in MR imaging. AJR Am J Roentgenol 2001;177:293-9.

10. Bluemke DA, Breiter SN. Sedation procedures in MR imaging: Safety, effectiveness, and nursing effect on examinations. Radiology 2000;216:645-52.

11. Finn JP. Sedation in MR imaging: What price safety? Radiology 2000;216:633-4.

12. ACR Manual on Contrast Media: Version 8. American College of Radiology, 2012.

13. Sena, BF, Stern JP, Pandharipande PV, et al. Screening patients to assess renal function before administrating gadolinium chelates: Assessment of the Choyke questionnaire. AJR Am J Roentgenol 2012;195:424-8.

14. Jung J, Kang H, Kim, M, et al. Immediate hypersensitivity reaction to gadolinium-based MR contrast media. Radiology 2012;264:414-22.

15. Prince MR, Zhang H, Zou Z, et al. Incidence of immediate gadolinium contrast media reactions. AJR Am J Roentgenol 2011;196:402.

16. Altun E, Martin DR, Wertman R, et al. Nephrogenic systemic fibrosis: Change in incidence following a switch in gadolinium agents and adoption of a gadolinium policy – Report from two U.S. universities. Radiology 2009;253:689-96.

17. Juluru K, Vogel-Claussen J, Macura KJ, et al. MR imaging in patients at risk for developing nephrogenic systemic fibrosis: Protocols, practices, and imaging techniques to maximize patient safety. Radiographics 2009;29:9-22

18. Wang Y, Alkasab TK, Narin O, et al. Incidence of nephrogenic systemic fibrosis after adoption of restrictive gadolinium-based contrast agent guidelines. Radiology 2011;260;105-11.

19. Leiner T, Kucharczyk W. Special issue: Nephrogenic systemic fibrosis. J Magn Res Imaging 2009;30:1233-5.

20. Perez-Rodriguez J, Lai S, Ehst BD, Fine DM, Bluemke DA. Nephrogenic systemic fibrosis: Incidence, associations, and effect of risk factor assessment – Report of 33 cases. Radiology 2009;250:371-7.

21. Sieber MA, Lengsfeld, P, Walter J, et al. Gadolinium-based contrast agents and their potential role in the pathogenesis of nephrogenic systemic fibrosis: The role of excess ligand. J Magn Res Imaging 2008;27:955-69.

22. Wang Y, Alkasab TK, Narin O, et al. Incidence of nephrogenic systemic fibrosis after adoption of restrictive gadolinium-based contrast agent guidelines. Radiology 2011;260:105-11.

23. Wertman R, Altun E, Martin DR, et al. Risk of nephrogenic systemic fibrosis: Evaluation of gadolinium chelate contrast agents at four American universities. Radiology 2008;248:799-806.

24. Wiginton CD, Kelly B, Oto B, et al. Gadolinium-based contrast exposure, nephrogenic systemic fibrosis, and gadolinium detection in tissues. AJR Am J Roentgenol 2008;190:1060-8.

25. Shellock FG, Spinazzi A. MRI safety update 2008: Part I, MRI contrast agents and nephrogenic systemic fibrosis. AJR Am J Roentgenol 2008;191:1129-39.

Chapter 24   MRI Policies and Procedures for a Children's Hospital Setting

CHRISTINE HARRIS, R.T. (R) (MR)

MRI Safety Officer
Radiology Manager
Department of Radiology/MRI
Children's Hospital of Philadelphia
Philadelphia, PA

INTRODUCTION

In all aspects of life, children are provided with a different set of rules and regulations than adults to help keep them safe and this is no different in the medical field, particularly in radiology. Currently, a major initiative in radiology is to reduce exposure to ionizing radiation in the pediatric population. In 2008, the *Image Gently Campaign* was created by the Alliance for Radiation Safety in Pediatric Imaging to help the medical community change their practice by increasing awareness of the opportunities to promote radiation protection in the diagnostic imaging of children. While there is presently no similar group leading the effort with regard to the use of magnetic resonance imaging (MRI) in the pediatric population, it is this author's hope that we will continue to share best practices within the MRI community which will help ensure safety in pediatric patients relative to the utilization of MRI procedures.

The objective of this chapter is to provide information pertaining to best practices of the Children's Hospital of Philadelphia (CHOP), as well as to present policies and procedures as they relate to MRI safety in the pediatric patient. Notably, in the MRI environment, children can present many challenges in imaging and safety (1). Trying to establish safety policies and guidelines in the use of equipment (e.g., radiofrequency coils, monitoring systems, anesthesia equipment, etc.) and the development of MRI techniques can be difficult. To help guide us through this process, CHOP established an MRI Safety Committee and safety enhancement program.

WHY HAVE AN MRI SAFETY COMMITTEE

Within the Children's Hospital of Philadelphia (CHOP), it can be challenging to impose the concept of MRI safety upon those not directly involved with it on a daily or otherwise routine basis. Before we instituted an MRI safety committee, the involvement from our ancillary teams (e.g., nursing, anesthesia, etc.) was tenuous because members of our MRI department projected an image that we worked independently on developing rules and regulations that could greatly impact the workflow of others involved in patient care. We found that, by not seeking the advice or input from the other healthcare professionals at our institution, the implementation of new policies and procedures was less acceptable.

Developing an MRI safety committee composed of vital representatives from ancillary departments, such as anesthesia, the intensive care unit (ICU), respiratory care, and nursing staff members has proven beneficial over the years because it provided a path by which the members of the committee become the liaison between radiology/MRI and the individual disciplines and departments. Importantly, the team members became more knowledgeable as we educated them about critical aspects of the MRI environment, the challenges with MRI safety, and the how's and why's of new policies and procedures.

FUNCTION OF THE MRI SAFETY COMMITTEE

Before developing an MRI safety committee, careful thought should be given to how the committee will function, as well as to the development of the roles and responsibilities of the various committee members. There are several avenues the group can take when forming an MRI safety committee. The committee can be one of three basic types: (1) Advisory, (2) Policy Making, or (3) a Combination of the two.

(1) The Advisory Committee investigates MRI safety issues within the department and hospital, offering guidelines, as needed. This committee does not make policies, but rather, offers opinions to those that do develop the rules that will impact the MRI environment.

(2) The Policy Making Committee is entrusted with the power to make or change policies and procedures based on their safety findings or in response to a need to address an accident or incident. Similar to the Advisory Committee, the Policy Making Committee may have to investigate or research topics and issues, but this committee is also granted the further discretion to formulate new policies and procedures.

(3) The Combination Committee takes into account recommendations from both the Advisory Committee and the Policy Making Committee. This committee should be given specific guidelines on its authority. In some instances, its authority may be advisory, while other issues may require the latitude to develop and implement new policies and procedures (2-4).

The goal of the MRI safety committee at CHOP, along with our overall safety program, is to promote awareness and understanding of MRI safety issues by collaborating and actively soliciting information that will provide a safer and more secure MRI environment. At CHOP, our MRI safety committee functions effectively as a Combination Committee. Our MRI safety committee is collaborative, with standing membership and participation from the following groups:

(1) Radiology Leadership including the Radiologist-in-Chief, Associate Radiologist-in-Chief, Radiology Patient Safety Officer/MRI Safety Committee Medical Director, Radiology Administrative Director, Radiology Manager and MRI Safety Officer, Neuroradiologist, and MRI Safety Committee Co-Director

(2) Anesthesia, including personnel from Cardiac Anesthesia and General Anesthesia

(3) Environmental Health and Safety, Director of Environmental Health and Safety

(4) Radiology Sedation, General Pediatric Anesthesia, and Medical Director of Sedation Services

(5) MRI Technologists including the MRI Team Leader, MRI Quality and Safety and Co-MRI Safety Officer, and the Cardiac MRI Team Leader

(6) Radiology Quality and Safety Manager

(7) Cardiology including the Cath Lab Director, MRI Cardiologist, and Cardiac Nursing Director

(8) Radiology and Sedation Nursing including the Radiology Nursing Manager, Radiology Nursing, and Radiology Nursing Quality Assurance

MRI SAFETY ENHANCEMENT PROGRAM

The MRI enhancement program at CHOP allows us to plan the activities for each coming year. While the goals may change, they usually include the following:

- An education and communication plan
- Environmental enhancement needs
- Budgeting for new safety equipment, devices, and software

Essentially, this program has adopted the same philosophy as the Institute for Magnetic Resonance Safety, Education and Research (IMRSER.org) which is, as follows (5):

- To promote awareness and understanding of MRI safety
- To disseminate information regarding current and emerging MRI safety issues
- To develop and provide materials and resources to facilitate MRI safety-related education training
- To respond to critical MRI safety issues with a sense of urgency

Education

The education program at CHOP promotes MRI safety by providing training in the form of the following:

(1) Road trips to nursing units. This is a 15-minute slide presentation covering
- Basic MRI
- MRI safety concerns
- The purpose and importance of family members filling out the MRI screening forms
- Images of accidents highlighting the importance of MRI safety
(2) On-line courses. These courses provide general knowledge about MRI safety, present accidents that have occurred at CHOP MRI facilities, and discuss basic rules and regulations to know before arriving in the MRI suite.

(3) One-on-one education with the MRI technologist. All personnel who need access to the MRI environment must take the on-line course and must meet with the MRI technologist in the MRI environment in order to discuss the policies and procedures.

(4) Yearly education is provided to the ancillary teams who frequent the MRI environment, including:

- Security officers and first responders receive training on MRI polices to maintain a level of competency regarding MRI safety.
- Pediatric Intensive Care Unit (PICU) nursing staff members who accompany all ICU patients to the MRI suite and stay during their MRI examinations. MRI staff members are part of their orientation program and provide a tour and general information on MRI safety and policy and procedures.
- Anesthesia personnel who are in the MRI environment on a daily basis. Everyone interested in access to the MRI environment must complete both the on-line course as well as the one-on-one educational component on an annual basis.

(5) Education via other avenues within the Children's Hospital of Philadelphia. This includes:

- Patient safety day
- Patient safety evening forum

MRI safety is usually misunderstood by those not working in the MRI environment and therefore, these avenues of education provide an opportunity to remind all hospital personnel of the dangers inherent in the MRI setting and to provide our ancillary staff members knowledge to keep our children safe. The pursuit of MRI safety is also part of the overall safety program of the hospital via posters, games, newsletters, and lectures.

SIMULATION AND ITS ROLE IN MRI SAFETY

Hospitals, including the Children's Hospital of Philadelphia, now offer variations of simulation-based training whereby medical and other personnel have the opportunity to develop skill sets on mannequins and to use other tools in specific settings before actually performing the skills on patients. While these programs have been developed to improve skill sets, such as venipuncture and responses to emergencies, CHOP has begun to utilize our simulation center as a way to improve the culture of safety at every level, including relative to the MRI environment. Within the realm of MRI, CHOP uses the simulation center to help review current policies and procedures by simulating real life situations. The objectives of these simulations are to ensure that the policy and procedures are clear and that all involved can perform the critical tasks at hand, as needed. The following is an example of one of our MRI simulations as it relates to the policies and procedures involving a quench of the MR system (i.e., the emergency shut-down of a superconducting magnet):

Scenario and Background: Accident Related to Large Metallic Projectile

It is Thursday evening, approximately 9 pm. An authorized contractor who was performing minor work-related activities throughout the main hospital was looking for a particular sprinkler and entered the unoccupied MR system room. The contractor has an acetylene tank with him that was attracted by the powerful static magnetic field of the MR system and, now, cannot be removed (**Figure 1**).

Figure 1. An MRI accident simulation in which a construction worker enters the MR system room with an acetylene tank that subsequently was attracted by the powerful static magnetic field of the MR system and, now, cannot be removed.

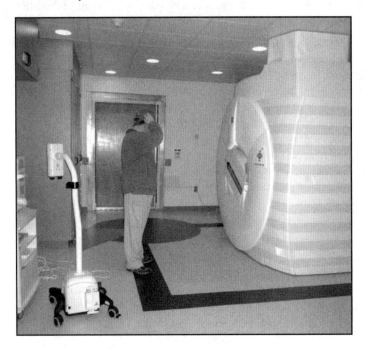

Learning Objectives

At the end of the MR system-related emergency simulation session, the participant should be able to do the following:

1. Articulate the roles and personnel needed for this emergency event involving a steel tank
   a. Facilities Operations
   b. Security
   c. Environmental Health and Safety
   d. Radiology Technologist and/or MRI Technologist
   e. Nursing Supervisor
2. Demonstrate the method used to determine the severity of the event
3. Display the decision-making process to quench the magnet of the MR system
4. Perform the safety measures necessary to ensure the safety of all personnel

Feedback

- Notifications

a.   The contractor experienced difficulties finding the phone numbers to call Facilities Operations, however, once he did, Facilities Operations was notified along with Security to respond to the MRI facility. The Philadelphia Fire Department was notified but was told not to respond because this was a simulation.

- Initial Survey of Scene

a.   Facilities Operations performed an initial assessment of the scene to determine whether the tank contained a hazardous material (i.e., the acetylene) and could be a safety threat to the immediate area or hospital. The inspection determined that the tank was hazardous but not an immediate safety threat because there was no obvious damage or leak affecting the tank (personnel from Facilities Operations performed a "soap test" on the tank valve assembly and detected no leaks in the system). After completing the inspection and performing the test to detect leaks, it was determined that the tank was in good condition. However, Environmental Health and Safety was not contacted until after the above maneuvers were performed. Although, they were contacted and arrived to the scene 20-minutes after the original phone call, they should have undergone initial MRI screening, even via telephone. Upon arrival to the scene, Environmental Health and Safety and Facilities Operations did a reassessment of the scene and acetylene tank. Facilities Operations attempted to call the MRI Supervisor multiple times via her pager and cell phone but struggled because the telephone number from the hospital operator was the wrong contact number. The correct number was finally obtained from another source. Suggestions were made to post a list of emergency contacts in each MRI facility and the outer entry area of each MR system room in order for personnel to quickly locate important phone numbers and beeper numbers in the event of an emergency. The contact list contains a chain of command, including a call to the MR system manufacturer's service technician. Although, the MR system manufacturer's service technician was not on the initial contact list, it was decided by the group that he or she could be an asset to emergency situations in the initial assessment.

b.   There was great concern regarding the security and safety of personnel entering the MRI environment, particularly the MR system room. Notably, there was minimal to no MRI screening performed in the area and the yellow guard-chain in front of the door to the MR system room remained down during the entire event. Importantly, the MRI technologist was never contacted. MRI technologists are considered the "gatekeepers" of MRI and are responsible to ensure that all staff members entering the MRI environment are screened and deemed safe. The current practice is that MRI technologists are the only personnel who can grant access to the MR system room. Furthermore, it was determined that the MRI technologist should be a first responder with their sole job and responsibility being safety surveillance of personnel entering and/or leaving the MR system room.

c.   Security personnel secured and monitored the outside area in order to ensure safety. They removed all unnecessary personnel and manned the front entrance of the MR system room. However, two other potential entrances/exits to this area exist which did not have controlled access (i.e., from the operating room, OR, and the sedation room). Thus, it was determined that there should be only one entrance/exit to ensure proper safety and security in the area. Additionally, if there is more than one entrance/exit to an MR system room, it was suggested to have extra security to secure the other entrances/exits.

Decision to Quench the MR System

a.   Since the acetylene tank was determined to be hazardous material that could not be emptied or physically pulled from the magnet of the MR system, the decision from the team was to quench the magnet. There was chaos in the area due to presence of numerous personnel and a disconnection in communication between the MRI technologist, Environmental Health, and Safety and Security staff members. A suggestion was made by the team to include a "time out" in the process in order to make sure that all steps have been completed, all questions have been answered, and all personnel are removed from the area. Although a simulated quench was performed, the MR system manufacturer's service technician stated that in a real situation, he would have attempted to remove the tank without quenching the magnet (important note: removing a large ferromagnetic object from the magnet is not advised).

b.   In order to safely quench the magnet, the team needed to perform these additional steps:

- Precautions should be taken to secure the tank with cushions to prevent it from falling during the quench. This procedure was performed.

- Additional perimeter security was needed by Security on the top of the roof of the MRI facility near the quench vent.

- Facilities needed to increase the air condition system to 100% exhaust. Although this occurred, several of the Facilities Operations personnel voiced that they did not know where to find the control to perform this action. Suggestion was made to better label the control mechanism for the exhaust system.

- Security notified the command center for Transport/PENNSTAR to alert them of the impending quench and keep helicopters from landing on the roof. The fire department was notified as well to ensure that the venting gases were not interpreted as "smoke" related to a fire.

- Security directed the roof-mounted camera to the area of quench.

- All staff removed from the immediate area were notified of the impending event. This helps to determine the scheduling of the actual quench time due to the fact that this was not an emergent event.

- The MRI Technologist, Environmental Health and Safety personnel, and the Senior Security Officer are the group members who determine the timing of the quench.

Recovery

The MRI Technologist should confirm loss of the static magnetic field of the MR system after 15-minutes. This timeframe is documented in the Policy and Procedure labeled, "Quench and Emergency Shut Down".

Changes Needed

- Environmental Health and Safety are part of the initial screening process even if it takes place by phone.

- The MRI Technologist should be contacted in the initial phone calls because they are the gatekeepers of the MRI environment and are the only personnel who can grant access to the area, especially the MR system room.

- Add an emergency phone number contact list to be posted in the preparation area and outer entryways of all MR system rooms.

- The emergency phone contact list should contain information regarding a "chain of command".

- The MR system manufacturer's service technician should be added to the emergency contact list.

- Additional security should secure the other entrances in order to ensure safety.

- Create and/or update the quench decision and procedure tree and post this information in the control areas of the MR system rooms, as well as in the security office and other key offices, detailing the steps to be taken in an emergency quench event.

- The procedure for quench should be posted in all MRI preparation control areas.

- Add a "time out" procedure prior to quenching the magnet.

- Make sure the participants realize the time of day of the simulation event. This event was supposed to take place at 9 pm but the participants responded as if it were 2 pm. This made it difficult to suspend disbelief because there would be limited personnel available on site at 9 pm.

- Suggestions to limit the number of observers to the simulation in order to decrease confusion associated with the event.

Following simulations at CHOP, the teams have a follow up meeting with all departments in attendance to review the lessons learned and suggestions for changes to ensure that proper procedures are in place and to plan additional simulations for the following year. As a result of the simulation presented above, CHOP has developed a more focused quench policy to replace our former policy. Additionally, we have formulated procedures for the two different types of quenches (i.e., controlled quench and uncontrolled quench) and an appropriate decision tree has been created.

QUALITY MEASURES OF THE MRI SAFETY PROGRAM

Evaluation of the MRI safety program helps to determine whether the strategies, policies and procedures, and implementation of new technology are effective in improving MRI safety. Three methods of evaluation are, as follows:

- Consultation

- Transparency and Awareness

- Monitoring and Data Collection

Consultation

Since the beginning of our MRI safety program in 2008, we have invited a prominent MRI Safety Leader, Dr. Frank Shellock from the University of Southern California, to CHOP to review and critique our program. The role of the MRI Safety Leader is to:

- Review the current policies and procedures

- Provide suggestions for new polices

- Give advice on additional policies and procedures that are needed

- Tour the various MRI facilities to evaluate current safety equipment and suggest additional enhancements that may be needed
- Provide comprehensive presentations to hospital staff about current MRI safety topics
- Meet with members of the MRI safety committee to present findings on the current safety status and provide suggestions.

Transparency and Awareness

In order to ensure that staff members are aware of all policies, procedures, and job aids, all documents are reviewed and updated annually and kept publicly available on CHOP's intranet.

Monitoring and Data Collection

To verify that we understand and are compliant with current policies and procedures, members of the MRI safety committee monitor, collect, and evaluate data pertaining to MRI safety issues on a monthly basis. The following are representative data that are collected:

Time Out and Visual Check of the Patient and Equipment

1.   *Properly identify patient and MRI exam*

- Two patient identifiers
- Confirm type of MRI exam and body part undergoing the MRI procedure
- Two-way communication with registered nurse, nurse practitioner, physician, and/or parent
- Ancillary Staff - remove jackets, squeeze pockets to identify items, etc.
- Review the MRI screening form

2.   *Visual check of patient and equipment*

- For the patient - lift blankets, sheets and gowns
- Confirm the stretcher or wheelchair are MR safe or MR conditional and what the conditions are that are stated for proper use
- Check the stretcher and/or wheelchair for unsafe items
- Confirm the O2 tank is acceptable for use in the MR system room

3.   *All staff members entering MR system room remove all unsafe items*

4.   *Removal and replacement of yellow guard-chain*

The yellow guard-chain (**Figure 2**) is the tool utilized as a visual and physical barrier to remind staff members to stop before entering the MR system room. The yellow chain should be in place at all times, except upon entering and exiting the room. All staff members are instructed to replace the yellow chain after entering, even if remaining in the scanner room. This simple concept has been an effective and inexpensive means to help ensure safety in the MRI environment. Initially it was challenging to get compliance from ancillary staff. Often, the members of the anesthesia team felt that the time needed to remove and replace the yellow chain would delay them in getting to the patient quickly, in the event of an

Figure 2. The use of the yellow guard-chain across the door is an additional tool to remind staff members to stop before entering the MR system room.

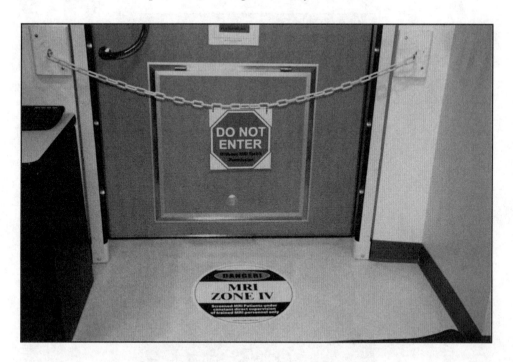

emergency. However, the MRI safety committee was very instrumental in helping the anesthesia team to balance both patient safety and MRI safety by convincing the anesthesia team that reaching the patient quickly could result in a hazard for the patient if they accidently brought in an item that was not acceptable for use in the MR system room (i.e., an MR unsafe item such as a laryngoscope).

5.   *The prep room door is locked at all times*

The cardiac and fetal MR system at CHOP is actually part of an operating room/Cath Lab environment where there is no office or administration area and the induction bay goes directly from a freely accessible environment into the MR system's control room (i.e., Zone III), off of a main, active hallway. This particular physical setting makes it especially challenging to keep unwanted metallic objects out of the MR system's control room. Therefore, to prevent metallic items from entering this area, we installed a door to this room and have taken the necessary steps to ensure that it is locked at all times (**Figure 3**).

POLICIES, PROCEDURES, AND JOB AIDS

Now that some of the important MRI safety policies and procedures at CHOP have been presented, what actually is a policy, a procedure, or even job aid to facilitate a safe working environment? For the purpose of this chapter, the discussion of policies, procedures, and job aids are defined by the Children's Hospital of Philadelphia.

Figure 3. This door, which is locked at all times, was installed to prevent unwanted metallic items from entering the area of the MR system room.

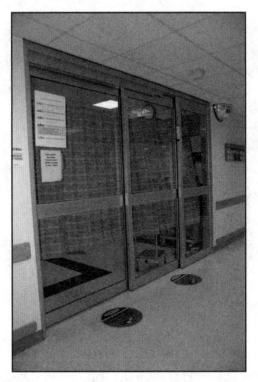

In early 2011, as part of our patient and safety culture assessment, CHOP engaged a "Focus and Simplify" format. During the assessment, it was learned from staff members and leaders that many of the existing policies and procedures had various shortcomings. For example, they lacked important information, they were informal and not clearly stated or defined, they were not easily accessible, and they needed more specificity in order to be understandable.

A "policy", as defined by CHOP, is a non-negotiable requirement of a regulatory agency or a self-imposed governing rule to ensure safety, quality, compliance, or cost-effectiveness. The policy should be written clearly and concisely, in a few sentences. Language in the policy statement should mirror the language of the regulation itself. Policies should be fewer in number in the "Focus and Simplify" format. A key point is that if procedures and job aids are well-written, a policy may only need to be accessed infrequently as the associated documents help one to adhere to the policy (6).

A "procedure", as defined by CHOP, outlines a step-by-step process to carry out a work process, much like a recipe. It outlines the steps an employee needs to follow, in order, from start to finish. A procedure may be related to a policy, or it may be a stand-alone procedure. In the new format, there should be many more procedures than policies (6).

A "job aid", as defined by CHOP, is any informational tool or supplement used to carry out a policy or procedure. It is important to note that a single policy or procedure may have multiple job aids associated with it. Information contained in job aids is guidance-oriented, rather than action-oriented. Examples of job aids include, but are not limited to, the following: checklists, flowcharts, pictures or diagrams, and lists. In the new format, there should be many more job aids and procedures than policies (6).

Guidance Documents

The Children's Hospital of Philadelphia uses three types of documents to communicate workflow expectations – policies, procedures, and job aids. Remember, if a procedure or job aid is well written, the user doesn't need to read the policy, since performing in a way that is consistent with the policy is self evident. The three types of documents are defined below:

(1) Policy

- **Purpose** - Defines a governing rule or a non-negotiable requirement
- **Volume** - Few in number
- **Source** - Regulatory agency or self-imposed to ensure safety, quality, compliance or cost effectiveness
- **Structure** - Written clearly and concisely in a few sentences
- **References** - Included on the document
- **Use** - Accessed only when needed and for informational purposes

(2) Procedure

- **Purpose** - Provides step-by-step actions to carry out a work process or to achieve an outcome, usually based on a policy
- **Volume** - Many
- **Source** - May be related to a policy or may stand-alone. May also have multiple procedures for a single policy.
- **Structure** - Includes steps in a process (e.g., think about a recipe). Two-column or three-column format. Minimum level of detail for the experienced person and supplementary.
- **References** - Not usually included in the document
- **Use** - Can be reference or a continuous use document

(3) Job Aid

- **Purpose** - Any informational tool or supplementary information used to carry out a policy or procedure
- **Volume** - Many
- **Source** - May be related to a policy or procedure or may stand-alone
- **Structure** - Not defined. Could be a form checklist, decision aid, reference guide, list, or sign
- **References** - Not usually included
- **Use** - Can be reference or a continuous use document

Importantly, when writing policies and procedures, make sure that they are evidence-based and not just based on the way things have always been done.

EXAMPLES OF POLICIES AND PROCEDURES

Now that the CHOP's definition of polices, procedures, and job aids have been presented, let's look at the special concerns that children bring to the formulation of these matters for MRI safety (7-10).

Screening Policies

Most pediatric patients are unable to speak for themselves and rely on parents and guardians to speak for them and to ensure their safety. If you are a parent, you know that when you take your child to the hospital for an examination or procedure, you are focused on the child getting diagnosed or treated and may not always remember the answers to all the questions being asked. At CHOP, we have found that parental anxiety plays a major role in how screening questions for MRI are answered and, therefore, having multiple tools and or interviewing sessions provides parents with the opportunity to remember something they didn't before.

MRI Screening Process for In-Patients

Pediatric in-patients rely heavily on ancillary personnel to support them during MRI procedures. Monitoring the ancillary staff, allowing a family member in the MR system room, performing the scan, answering telephones, and other tasks can be overwhelming for the MRI technologist due to the sheer numbers of support staff involved and the duties that are required. To help us monitor the large number of staff members in the MRI environment, we greatly depend on our screening policies and procedures.

The MRI Screening Form

Currently, the various MRI sites at CHOP keep a supply of MRI screening forms readily available and we require that a family member or responsible guardian fill out the screening form for the pediatric patient. In the event that there is not a parent or guardian available before the MRI procedure, then a nurse or physician can fill out the form. Notably, the MRI screening form includes the parent or guardian's cell phone number in the event that it is necessary to ask questions so that we can reach these individuals directly and not delay their child's MRI examination. Once the screening form has been completed, the MRI technologist will review it for the following information:

- Any item or device that is of concern
- Follow up on any questions on the form answered "yes" or "unknown"
- A list of prior diagnostic imaging procedures

The MRI technologist then signs the screening form, which verifies that the form was reviewed and the information was verified. In addition, if the pediatric patient has an implant or device, this information is documented with respect to the name, model, and warnings, if applicable, in CHOP's Radiology Information System. The patient is then approved to be scheduled for the MRI examination. Upon arrival to the MRI department, the patient is screened again by an MRI technologist - once in the department and then again at the final "Time Out and Visual Check" procedure, described below (**Figure 4**). This is a five-step process that includes, the following:

1. ***Proper identification of the patient and the MRI examination***

   a. We verify that we have the correct patient, utilizing the two patient identifier as suggested in the Joint Commission's goals (i.e., name, date of birth, medical record number, etc.) (6)

   b. We verify that we are performing the correct examination and that the correct body part is undergoing the MRI procedure

2. ***Review of the MRI screening form***

   a. This is performed to ensure that all questions and concerns have been addressed

3. ***Visual inspection of ancillary staff***

   a. To ensure that staff members remove jackets and other clothing articles that may hide ferromagnetic objects in the pockets

   b. All pockets are to be squeezed, not simply patted, to identify objects

Figure 4. This figure shows the "Time Out and Visual Checklist" procedure during which the final checking of the patient is performed before entering the MR system room. During this time, healthcare staff members confirm that the correct patient will undergo the MRI examination, all unsafe items are identified and removed, the MRI screening form is reviewed again, and a visual check is made of the patient transport device (i.e., the gurney) and the patient to ensure that there are no hazards present.

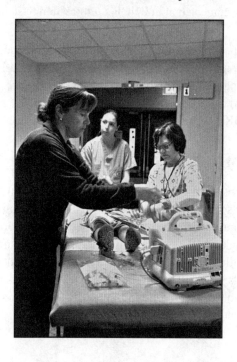

4.   *Visual check of equipment*

a. For the patient, we lift blankets, sheets, and gowns to look for ferromagnetic items or other unsafe objects

b. Confirm that the stretcher is MR safe or MR conditional and labeled as such

c. Check the stretcher or other patient transport device for unsafe items

d. Confirm that the O_2 tank and IV pole are acceptable for use in the MRI environment

5.   *Remove the yellow guard-chain*

a. Enter the MR system room (i.e., Zone IV) and replace yellow chain, immediately

MRI Screening Process for Out-Patients

Of course, the MRI screening process is different for out-patients versus in-patients. While it is our goal to screen all patients before being placed on the MRI schedule, the following is our current process for all but our cardiac or fetal MRI patient referrals. The pediatric patient and parent are asked five brief questions during the scheduling process that should trigger any concerns. If there is a concern, an email is sent to the MRI safety group (a team of six MRI technologists) whose responsibility is to investigate implants, devices, or safety issues before the patient arrives to the MRI facility. All details of the investigation are documented with the scheduled visit.

We like to perform a preliminary MRI screening procedure before the patient arrives for the appointment, but if this does not occur during this time, then it will be conducted on the day the patient arrives and before the next screening step is performed. In order to facilitate this process, the MRI technologist may evaluate, the following:

- Review the most recent X-rays and report for implants or devices
- Review medical documentation in CHOP's Information System for the presence of implants or devices

On the day of the appointment, the patient is prescreened and, upon arrival, a more in-depth documented screening process is conducted before the patient is sent to the nursing station to ensure that the patient is safe to have the MRI procedure. Once the patient is ready for the MRI examination, we will perform an official "Time Out and Visual Check" procedure at the door to the MR system room.

PROTECTION FROM ACOUSTIC NOISE

Acoustic noise can pose a threat to a child's psychological and physical health. This includes interference with speech and language, impaired learning and hearing difficulties. Therefore, the use of proper hearing protection in pediatric patients is an important part of ensuring safety. Modern-day MR systems can generate acoustic noise from 78 to 130-decibels, or even higher. While certain MR scanners may have reduced the maximal acoustic noise levels to 90-decibels, it is still recommended that all patients utilize hearing protection. In addition, healthcare workers who remain in the MR system room during the MRI procedure should likewise wear hearing protection.

Hearing protection is utilized to minimize the risk of hearing impairment in association with the MRI examination. At CHOP, we currently use special noise attenuation devices, MiniMuffs (Natus Medical, Seattle, WA), for children 1 day to 6 months of age (**Figure 5**). These devices may be used in conjunction with soft ear putty (silicone- based). We also try to add additional protection such as sponges (that are provided with the MR system's head RF coil) to help prevent acoustic noise-related problems for pediatric patients. In the MRI setting, we chose the combination of MiniMuffs and ear putty over other types of earplugs because they provide the best type of noise reduction and help to avoid the difficulty of inserting earplugs into relatively small ear canals. This strategy also prevents the possibility of small children swallowing or choking on tiny earplugs. At CHOP, we are in the process of further refining this protocol and have partnered with our audiology department to ensure that we have the right level of protection for the level of noise generated by the MR system, particularly with respect to the length of time the child is exposed to high noise levels.

MRI SAFETY ISSUES RELATED TO THERMOREGULATION IN PEDIATRIC PATIENTS

Thermoregulation is the ability to maintain body temperature independent of the outside environment. Infants rely on their mothers to regulate their temperatures, *in utero*. Once born, the infant has somewhat limited ability to regulate body temperature in response to exposure to cold environments primarily due to the inability to shiver. While an infant can sweat, only the glands in the head, neck, hands and feet are active (being about 25 to 30% of their total body size). To keep warm, a baby may try to curl up into the fetal position,

Figure 5. MiniMuffs (Natus Medical, Seattle, WA) are noise attenuation devices that are used to protect hearing in pediatric patients undergoing MRI examinations.

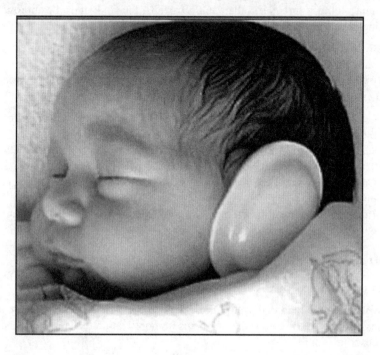

move, or cry. However, a baby's main source of heat production is the special body fat, known as brown adipose tissue, or BAT. BAT starts developing at 26 to 30 weeks of gestation and makes up about 2 to 7% of the baby's total body weight at birth. BAT is similar to the fat tissue found in hibernating animals (8).

BAT plays an important role in providing body heat for the infant. Unfortunately, a disadvantage of using BAT to stay warm is that the metabolism associated with utilizing this type of fat to produce heat requires extra oxygen and glucose. This can result in the newborn becoming physically stressed, as the infant attempts to maintain a proper body temperature. If allowed to become too cold (the baby's temperature should be no lower than 36°C), the infant may be reluctant to feed in an effort to conserve energy, thus, compounding the problem (8).

The following is the procedure at CHOP for ensuring newborn patient temperatures are maintained at an acceptable level during the MRI examination. Importantly, once a patient from the neonatal intensive care unit (NICU) is ready to travel to the MRI facility, we follow a checklist composed of three sections: (1) Pre-Study, (2) Arrival at MRI, and (3) Post-Scan Instructions.

Pre-Study

This checklist is followed in the NICU and before arrival to the MRI facility.

- A decision is made regarding how we will keep the patient still and comfortable during the MRI examination. The choices are sedation or feeding combined with an immobilization technique.

- A pre-scan body temperature is recorded to determine if it is safe to take the infant out of the NICU environment.

- If the infant's temperature is less than 36.5°C axially, the study must be approved by the attending physician.

-If the baby is approved to travel to the MRI facility, certain items must come with the patient, including those items required before traveling (e.g., items needed to care for patient outside of the NICU) as well as the following items specific to the MRI environment. The following must be considered:

   • Confirmation that the MRI screening form has been completed and sent to the MRI facility
   • The hard copy of the MRI screening form comes with the pediatric patient
   • The infant is placed in clothing with no snaps (hospital issued clothing, only)
   • Confirmation that there is a need for extra intravenous tubing for patients on infusion pumps
   • If patient has a metal-based tracheostomy tube in place, it must be changed to a silicone tube before going to the MRI facility

Arrival at MRI

   • Hand-off care from NICU staff to MRI nursing staff
   • Body temperature recorded again, if less than 36.5°C axially, the NICU attending physician is informed to discuss sedation versus immobilization technique or cancelation of the MRI examination.

- MRI nursing staff will check for the following:

  -The hard copy of MRI screening form is available
  -Clothing has no metallic parts (e.g., snaps, zipper, etc.)
  -Need for "cozy bunting" or other immobilization device
  -Hearing protection is in place
  -Change over or remove unsafe items such as electrodes, monitoring devices, etc.
  -Placement of an acceptable (i.e., MR conditional) temperature probe

(Note: If the temperature recorded using the MR conditional temperature probe does not correlate with the axially acquired temperature, document both readings and leave the temperature probe on for trending purposes. Furthermore, if the body temperature appears to begin a downward trend, add extra blankets and/or hot packs. If temperature drops by 1°C during the MRI examination, the procedure must be discontinued and rescheduled.) The infant must be returned to a warmed environment (Isolette and/or warming bed) as soon as possible.

Post-Scan Instructions

- Documentation of post-scan body temperature

  -If less than 36.5°C axially, determine the need to transport the infant in a Transwarmer or Isolette.
  -If the infant is on oxygen delivered by a source in the MR system room, the infant should be weaned off of oxygen and then transferred to oxygen delivered via a tank.
  -Each infant travels with a checklist of the above information and this checklist is kept in the MRI facility. Each month, we review the checklist to trend changes in temperature associated with the MRI procedure and work closely with NICU staff members to ensure the maintenance and stabilization of body temperature for the infants.

CONCLUSIONS

The physiology of children and adults is different and these differences can impact MRI safety issues. The safety of the MRI environment for a pediatric patient relies on the proper training and education of healthcare professionals, ancillary staff, family members, and others. One component of this process involves developing and implementing specialized policies and procedures that are collaborative, evident-based, and supported by the MRI safety committee.

REFERENCES

1. SMRT Educational Seminars. MR Safety in the Pediatric MR Environment. In: Update: Safety in MR Examinations. 2005;8:20-30. http://www.ismrm.org/smrt/homestudy/0803.htm

2. Advisory Committee. In: The Office of the United States Trade Representative Available via Web Article. http:// www.ustr.gov/about-us/intergovernmental-affairs/advisory-committees. Accessed May, 2013.

3. Committee Types and Roles. In: the Congressional Research Service. Available via Web Article. http:/ /www.judiciary.senate.gov/legislation/upload/CRS-CommitteeTypes.pdf November 10, 2010. Accessed May, 2013.

4. Building an Effective Advisory Committee. In: The Mentoring Resource Center. Available via Web Article. http://educationnorthwest.org/webfm_send/232 April 21, 2008. Accessed, May 2013

5. Institute for Magnetic Resonance Safety, Education, and Research (IMRSER.org), MRI Safety Guidelines. In: IMRSER Available via Web Article http://www.imrser.org/PaperPDFlist.asp?pgname=Guidelines 2012. Accessed May, 2013.

6. Focus and Simplify. In: Office of Patient Safety and Quality CHOP Employee Intranet. http://intranet.chop.edu/sites/patient_safety/focus-and-simplify/index.html January 27, 2011. Accessed May, 2013.

7. Hospital National Patient Safety Goals. In: The Joint Commission. Available via Web Article http://www.jointcommission.org/assets/1/6/2013_HAP_NPSG_final_10-23.pdf. Accessed May, 2013.

8. Labour and Birth. In: From Bellies to Babies and Beyond. Available via Web Article http://www.birth.com.au/Your-baby-soon-after-birth-what-you-need-to-know/Body-temperature-regulation?view=full. Accessed, May 2013.

9. Hallowell LM, Stewart SE, de Amorim e Silva CT, et al. Reviewing the process of preparing children for MRI. Pediatr Radiol 2008;38:271–79.

10. Kanal E, Barkovich AJ, Bell C, et al. ACR guidance document for safe MR practices: 2013. J Magn Reson Imaging 2013;37:501-30.

11. Temperature Measurement in Acute Care: The Who, What, Where, When, Why, and How? In: Emergency Nursing World via Web Article   http://enw.org/Research-Thermometry.htm. Accessed, May 2013.

Chapter 25   MRI Safety Policies and Procedures for a Research Facility

ANNE MARIE SAWYER, B.S., R.T.(R)(MR), FSMRT

Manager, MR Whole Body Research Systems
Radiological Sciences Laboratory
Richard M. Lucas Center for Imaging
Stanford University School of Medicine
Stanford, CA

INTRODUCTION

Maintaining safety in the magnetic resonance imaging (MRI) environment is a never-ending challenge, whether it is in relation to a clinical facility or one that is restricted to research studies. There are, however, specific concerns that are generally only encountered in a research facility due mainly to the variety of individuals allowed to access the MRI environment, including for the development of software, hardware, and ancillary equipment. This calls for specific policies and procedures that are vigilantly maintained by those managing and supporting MRI laboratories in the research setting.

It has been reported that the number of reported MRI safety incidents is increasing. There are many theories as to why this is happening including an increase in the number of MR systems worldwide, the increase in the number of MR systems with higher static magnetic fields being installed especially at research facilities, the improvement in the reporting of such incidents, the increase in the number of MR systems being installed in departments and facilities outside of the traditional radiology department, an increase in the overall number of MRI procedures performed, or possibly more incidents are actually occurring.

In consideration of the above, an investment is required to ensure that the utmost is being done to maintain safety for patients and volunteer subjects, researchers, and staff members. Realizing that this investment requires both time and money, paves the way for a successful MRI safety program. In addition, it is critical to remember that all it takes is one mistake for the freedom that an MRI research facility currently enjoys to be changed. As Peter Marshall (Scots-American preacher, 1902 to 1949) said, "May we think of freedom, not as the right to do as we please, but as the opportunity to do what is right." Therefore, we must act responsibly and out of concern for all.

DESIGN AND ACCESS OF THE MRI ENVIRONMENT

Zones of the MRI Environment

Since the early developments of interventional or intra-operative MR systems, the areas associated with the MRI department have been divided into specific sections as a method to clearly identify who and what instruments are given access, and under which conditions. This was further reinforced by the American College of Radiology (ACR) document on MRI safety, first published in 2002 and updated in 2004, 2007, and 2013, thus, identifying and demarcating the four "zones" of an MRI department (1-4).

Basically, the four zones described by the ACR include as follows, the area typically accessed by the public (Zone 1); the dressing room, bathroom and patient preparation room (Zone 2); control room (Zone 3); and the MR system room (Zone 4). The MRI suite of rooms should include specific areas separated by locked doors using card key access or other means to control access, but not combination locks. Combination information can be easily communicated to many individuals and forgotten, requiring multiple changes.

The initial design of the MRI suite includes important details such as, the following: card key locked access from the hallway, lobby, or reception area into the MRI suite; easy visual access from the control room to the MR system room door and the path leading from the dressing room and patient preparation room towards the MR system room door; visual access from the control room into the MR system room, emergency exhaust fan controls located inside and outside of the scanner room; quench button for a superconducting magnet located immediately inside or outside of the MR system room door; and video observation of the inside of the bore of the MR system.

For many, it may be problematic to move walls due to cost and space issues when planning to renovate an MRI suite for enhanced safety. Therefore, it is critical to focus on what can be done to ensure maximum safety through reduced and controlled access to the various areas of the MRI environment (1-4). Doors with locked access should be in place between general access areas such as main hallways, waiting rooms and reception areas (i.e., Zone 1), as well as Zones 2, 3, and 4. Only individuals, appropriately screened and accompanied by trained MRI staff members are allowed to access the dressing room and patient preparation room (Zone 2), MRI technologist/radiographer (note, these designations are synonymous) control room (Zone 3), and the MR system room (Zone 4) (1-4). Patients and volunteer subjects should never be allowed unaccompanied access past Zone 1 into Zones 2, 3, or 4 and should never be left unattended in Zones 2, 3, or 4.

Access

Policies and procedures must be in place that clearly identify which kind of access is given to each of the MRI staff members as well as MRI physicians, other healthcare professionals supporting patients or volunteers undergoing the MRI examination, clinicians, and family members. For example, technologist's aides may be allowed to initially review the completed screening form with patients or volunteer subjects, and accompany them to the dressing room and give initial preparation instructions. The MRI technologist conducts the final review of the completed screening form and accompanies the patient or volunteer

Figure 1. An example of signs, rugs, placards, and stanchions used to warn individuals of the dangerous environment of the room in which the MR system resides. Signs on the wall next to the MR system room door are important if someone leaves the door open, in which case, the signs on the door would then not be visible.

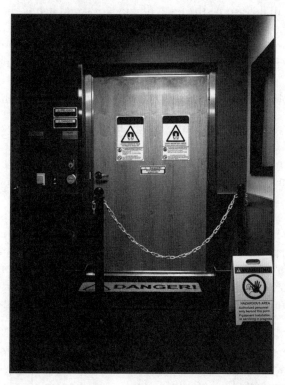

subject into the MR system room, positions and immobilizes, and gives instructions immediately before and during the examination.

Signage

Current and appropriate signage, especially immediately before entering the MR system room, (Zone 4) is an absolute requirement (1-4). Other forms of warning to individuals entering the area of the dangers of the MRI environment are also recommended. These include MRI warning rugs, stanchions, placards, or gates placed in front of the door leading into the MR system room (**Figure 1**). Frequently, something more three-dimensional or that provides a tactile experience is extremely helpful in reminding all individuals about the potential danger of entering the MR system room.

PERSONNEL

Assigned Responsibilities, Education, and Training

Depending upon the number and type of MR systems present in the research facility, an adequate number of appropriate staff should be present to support the various research studies and patient examinations (1-4). This includes but is not limited to: MRI technologists, nurses, receptionists, assistants and/or technologist aides, radiologists and/or clinicians, administrative support, and/or research associates (e.g., doctoral, Ph.D., scientists). Current policies and procedures must include the assigned level of responsibility for each staff member. This will determine the level of education and hands-on training required for each. In addition to the staff previously listed, limited but appropriate training will also need to be provided to other individuals including, the following: housekeeping and maintenance personnel, ancillary staff (nursing, respiratory therapy, etc.), physicians, firefighters, police and security officers, and first responders. It will be beneficial to invite firefighting personnel to discuss safety issues, while acquainting them with the dangers of the MRI environment.

In order to properly support scientific research studies, the MRI technologists must possess a thorough working knowledge of MRI. Using research software, hardware, radiofrequency (RF) coils, and prototype accessory devices can result in a variety of artifacts and other imaging challenges including safety. Possessing a clear understanding of the principles and physics of MRI allows the MRI technologists to quickly address MR system difficulties resulting in the efficient completion of research studies. Competency lists are excellent tools to determine the educational needs of each staff member. At a minimum, these lists should include anatomy and physiology, MRI physics and principles, scan parameters and imaging options, safe and appropriate use of RF coils and other ancillary equipment including physiologic monitoring systems, patient and volunteer subject preparation, instruction and communication, positioning and immobilization, sterile technique, and emergency procedures.

On-going education is a must in the rapidly changing world of MRI especially in the research facility. Time and financial support must be provided to ensure that all staff members maintain a comprehensive knowledge in order to competently support the research MRI studies being conducted. Continuing education can be obtained through attendance at educational seminars, completion of on-line webinars, and video taped training. Subscription to the MRI technologist society, the Section for Magnetic Resonance Technologists, (www.ismrm.org/smrt/) Educational Seminars and MRI automatic email list servers play a valuable role in keeping current with knowledge shared by their peers and other experts in the field. The investment in continuing education for MRI technologists results in knowledgeable, concerned healthcare professionals. Understanding MRI physics and principles is necessary to comprehend the issues in MRI safety and screening. It also clearly communicates to the staff that they are a valued part of the team resulting in responsible, interested individuals. In addition, enlisting the faculty at the research facility to use their specific expertise to provide training to the MRI technologists increases their overall comprehension. This results in the successful completion of their research studies because the staff understands the faculty's priorities and needs. Both didactic and hands-on training are equally as valuable in this comprehensive training program.

MRI Safety Committee

A most critical asset for a research MRI facility is that of a Safety Committee (1-4). The safety officers who sit on this committee are responsible for setting MRI safety and screening policies and procedures. They must be afforded time and resources to maintain their MRI safety and screening expertise. The safety officers are selected from those with an advanced knowledge in MRI and MRI safety. To ensure comprehensive safety support, the committee should include an MRI technologist, a radiologist or MRI clinician, and an MRI scientist (e.g., typically a doctoral level person, Ph.D.). The MRI technologist and radiologist/MRI clinician are primarily responsible for making all decisions concerning MRI pre-procedure screening of patients, volunteer subjects and researchers.

Research MRI Procedures Conducted by MRI Technologists

MRI research examinations that involve the administration of MRI contrast agents, interventional procedures, the introduction of intra-cavitary coils, and patients or volunteer subjects with special concerns such as paralysis require the presence of an MRI research technologist (2, 3). Proficiency in sterile technique and intravenous (IV) set up procedures is part of the competency required by the MRI technologist. As healthcare professionals are trained in the skills of medical procedures and patient communication, this background is extremely valuable to ensure patient comfort and safety during IV placement, positioning of the patient or volunteer subject with the IV line in place, resuscitation procedures in the event of a reaction to the IV placement or injection, extravasation issues, and/or insertion of an endo-rectal RF coil.

The IV administration of contrast media requires the presence of a minimum of two healthcare professionals. In addition to the MRI technologist, either a nurse or physician is required to ensure safety for the patient or volunteer subject during IV placement. For example, if the patient should suddenly lose consciousness, it will require two trained healthcare professionals to safely and successfully address the situation (i.e., to slowly lower the subject's head to the same level as the body while maintaining control over the IV site). A physician (i.e., trained in emergent care) is required to be present in the MRI suite during the injection of the contrast media and for a short period thereafter (approximately 15-minutes) to ensure there are no resulting reactions or complications (1, 2).

It is extremely beneficial that an MRI technologist be present for more complex animal model research studies. In addition to the operation of the MR system, this individual's responsibility includes maintaining a safe environment for people and equipment. Research studies commonly involve multiple individuals (researchers, clinicians, surgeons, veterinarians, and veterinary technicians) who are present in the MRI environment but engaged in their specific roles, focusing on their particular research needs and outcomes of the research study. In addition to protecting the many individuals working in the research study, the MRI technologist is responsible for preventing expensive damage to the MR system and maintaining cleanliness standards required for human MRI examinations (patients and volunteer subjects).

MRI Procedures Conducted by Researchers

Researchers may be allowed to conduct research studies on phantoms and human subjects without an MRI technologist present. The researchers must have completed their requirements for MR system access and use, first including MRI safety and policy and procedure training, hands-on scanner training, RF coil training, and Health Insurance Portability and Accountability Act (HIPAA) training (3-5). In addition, it is policy that any MR system, equipment or accessory issues, or human subject screening question issues be reported immediately to the appropriate support staff or the MRI Safety Committee for resolution.

All new MRI accessories, equipment, devices, RF coils, furniture, and patient support equipment are required to be reviewed by the MRI Manager (MRI technologist on the MRI Safety Committee) before being taken into the MR system room. If the device has an electronic component, then it must undergo comprehensive testing to ensure that it does not add noise (i.e., electromagnetic interference) to the images or other data being acquired (6).

Imaging accessories, devices, and RF coils are often designed and developed for use as prototypes during research MRI examinations. In addition, these same prototype components may be purchased from third party vendors. If an investigational device is a "nonsignificant risk device", an investigator does not need to submit an investigational device exemption (IDE), the IDE will be "considered approved" under Food and Drug Administration (FDA) regulations. Such devices do not have to comply with FDA premarket approval and performance standards prior to use in research studies (7). With regard to such equipment, to ensure safety for the patients and volunteer subjects as well as the MR system, and that it will function properly with the MR system in use, early contact with the members of the MRI Safety Committee is recommended to prevent inappropriate designs that could result in costly mistakes, wasted resources, and/or potential safety issues.

Other Personnel Responsibilities

Combining the responsibilities of conducting weekly quality assurance (QA) or quality control (QC) on the MR systems with stocking supplies and linen is recommended because they can be done simultaneously. Although human subjects must be visually and verbally monitored on a continuous basis, phantom scans do not. Therefore, it is recommended that an MRI technologist or technologist aide complete these responsibilities to ensure the medical supplies present are not only correct, but also not expired when they are needed. Along with sterile technique, importance of cleanliness in the medical imaging environment is stressed during didactic and hands-on training to ensure human subject safety as long-term consequences can prevail without this. Maintenance and stocking of the crash cart located in the MRI suite is required by a healthcare professional, either MRI technologist or nurse due to the presence of drugs.

An important part in maintaining patient and volunteer subject safety is routine monthly preventative maintenance conducted by the MR systems' manufacturer field service engineer. In addition to poor image quality, poorly maintained MR systems can result in serious patient injuries (e.g., burns). Frayed cables of RF coils or monitoring equipment cables and/or fractured housing on RF coils or connector boxes are just a few potentially dangerous scenarios if left unrepaired.

Regular preventative maintenance of all ancillary equipment directly involved with human MRI examinations must be performed annually, at a minimum. This includes automatic injectors, infusion devices, and physiologic monitoring equipment to ensure that compromised function of any equipment does not affect the patient or volunteer subject or the MR system.

MRI SAFETY: POLICY AND PROCEDURE TRAINING

To access and/or use any of the research MR systems, completion of an initial MRI Safety Policy and Procedure Training conducted by the MRI Manager (MRI technologist member of MRI Safety Committee) is required. All researchers are required to complete this training despite any previous experience working on or around MR systems at other facilities, either clinical or research. Typically this review is a ninety-minute comprehensive yet interactive presentation that includes all aspects of MRI safety and human subject screening, in addition to covering the research facility's policies and procedures. Annually, each of the approved researchers is required to complete an online renewal that is similar to the initial training but includes quizzes spaced throughout the tutorial. It also includes completion of the MRI pre-procedure screening form. The results of each completed quiz is automatically emailed to the members of the MRI Safety Committee.

A commitment for a minimum of six months' use of the research MR systems is required by researchers to attend the initial MRI Safety Policy and Procedure Training and to subsequently be given access to the MR systems. In addition, if a researcher has completed this training and then is absent from conducting or participating in research scans for a period of three months or longer, completion of the online version of the MRI Safety and Policy and Procedure Training is required prior to accessing the MR systems. A database is maintained with all of the trained researchers' names and contact information that allows automatic reminders to be sent instructing them to take the required annual training, and automatic removal from accessing the MR systems if the training is not completed within a designated time period. Other databases are maintained for the purpose of distribution of information to researchers.

The presence of a whole body 7-Tesla (T) MR system highlights the need for an additional and highly specific MRI safety training. This focuses on not only the challenges present in working around such a high static magnetic field MR system for both researchers, patients, and volunteer subjects but also the significantly high fringe field associated with this setting. Currently, at most facilities housing high field MR systems such as 1.5-T or 3-T, the five gauss line is contained within the MR system room itself. However, the fringe field present in the control room, equipment room, or other nearby rooms of a 7-T scanner can often exceed 100-gauss. Careful thought must be given to the type of access allowed to each individual and specifically where the MRI pre-procedure screening form is completed by a patient or volunteer subject to prevent any inappropriate access.

All researchers are provided cards to carry that contain the names and phone numbers of the individuals who support their research studies being conducted at the MR systems. This includes the MRI Safety Committee members (i.e., the MRI Manager, lab director, and radiologist or clinician), MRI research technologists, and the building manager. The cards also include the phone numbers for each of the MR system suites, security services, and the local law enforcement agency.

MRI SYSTEM TRAINING

After completion of the initial MRI Safety Policy and Procedure Training, each researcher undergoes additional required training at the scanner with an MRI research technologist. This hands-on training includes emergent MR system cradle and table removal, location and operation of the quench button and exhaust fan, safe and appropriate use of RF coils, presence and operation of research devices, insulation and separation of the human subject using positioning pads and sponges (i.e., to prevent excessive heating and possible burns), room temperature and MR system bore fan operation, research support equipment and accessories, scanner software, and support information (3, 5). An important policy for all those accessing the MRI suites is to keep the MR system room door closed at all times. A scanner room door should only be allowed to remain open if an MRI safety-trained individual is actively monitoring all equipment and persons attempting to pass through.

Emergent MR System Cradle and Table Removal

In the event of a suddenly unconscious or unresponsive patient or volunteer subject, researchers must be fully trained in the safe removal of the individual from the MR system and the room, itself, into the patient preparation room prior to the arrival of paramedics or other resuscitation (code blue) team members. Emergent care of the patient or volunteer subject must never be conducted within the MR system room due to the unmonitored devices carried and used by first responders to revive the subject and the time required to properly complete screening procedures for those individuals (3, 5). This requires the utmost preparation and speed to complete certain procedures prior to the arrival of the resuscitation team or first responders.

The number of researchers required to be present for MRI procedures conducted on human subjects, whether patients or normal volunteers, is determined by the day and time of the examination. MRI examinations conducted in the evening (after 6:00 pm), early morning (12:00 am to 7:00 am), and weekends require a minimum of two researchers to be present. This is to ensure the necessary emergent procedures can be completed successfully in the event of a safety issue with the patient or volunteer subject. Even if only "normal" volunteer subjects are being scanned, there is always a risk, albeit small, that these individuals could experience a stroke, heart attack or syncope. Being thoroughly prepared for this type of situation demonstrates to university officials that the researchers conducting MRI examinations are as prepared as any clinical facility to adequately deal with any human frailties. Importantly, these training and preparation procedures can successfully prevent liability for the academic institution.

Quench Button and Exhaust Fan

The location and operation of the quench button and exhaust fan is also part of the comprehensive MR system training for researchers. In the event an individual would be pinned against the MR system requiring release of the magnetic field of a superconducting magnet to prevent further injury or death, researchers must be fully trained as to when quenching is necessary and when it is not. In addition, all of the potential resulting issues from a quench should be addressed in proper training including the formation of a helium cloud in the MR system room, lack of an exhaust fan that may prevent the opening of the door to the MR system room, and liquid helium dripping from the exhaust pipe. Training in the operation of the quench button should only be given to appropriate researchers, never to housekeeping or maintenance personnel. Instructions that clearly and quickly direct researchers on quench procedures are posted in convenient locations in the MRI suite.

Safe and Appropriate Use of RF Coils

Instruction in the safe and appropriate use of RF coils specific to each research study is given to all researchers. This instruction in the prevention of potential risks associated with RF coils includes the operation and safe utilization of these devices, and correct RF coil selection in the MR system software. Basic knowledge is reviewed in the appropriate use for specific anatomy, positioning of the RF coil as well as the associated cable and connector box, and immobilization of the coil relative to the human subject. Additionally, training should encompass the prevention of coiling of cables upon themselves, having the cables coming into contact with other cables, devices, human subjects and/or the bore the MR system (1-3, 5, 8). First-time use of any RF coil at the research facility requires training by the MRI Manager (MRI technologist on Safety Committee), MRI research technologist, or Scientific Center Director (e.g., the Ph.D. on the MRI Safety Committee).

All RF coils and devices should be thoroughly checked before use in any MRI examination for signs of damage including fraying cables, cracked housing and/or loose contents in the coils or connector boxes in order to prevent risk of burns to the patient or volunteer subject, or damage to the MR system. RF coils used to image anatomy other than its designated use must be referred to the MRI Manager or MRI research technologist for approval. For example, wrapping a cardiac RF coil around an elbow and positioning it next to the MR system's bore is a mistake that could easily result in injury to the patient and/or MR system. Imaging pediatric brains using a knee coil may be an acceptable alternative to the indicated anatomy, and should not result in any potential dangers for the patient or MR systems.

Presence of Research Devices

Research MRI examinations may involve additional devices to be placed in the magnet with the patient or volunteer subject, or in the MR system room. This is especially true of functional MRI (fMRI) research studies. Some of these devices include response boxes and cables, electroencephalography (EEG) cap and cables, transmagnetic stimulation (TMS) coil and cables, eye tracker video camera and cables, thermode (this provides heat for pain stimulation) and cables, plethysmograph sensor (or pulse oximetry) and cable, galvanic skin response (GSR), and electrocardiography (ECG) electrodes and cables. Many of these items may not have been FDA approved for use within the confines of an MR system. All prototype designs must be used with equal care as product devices to prevent loops in their cables, prevent loops with other devices present and their cables, and prevent secondary interaction with the human subject and the MR system's bore (1-3, 5, 8).

Insulation and Separation using Positioning Pads and Sponges

Positioning sponges and pads in a multitude of sizes and shapes are available in the MR system room to be used to immobilize and provide comfort to the patient or volunteer subject. In addition, the sponges and pads are used to provide separation and insulation for all cables and devices to prevent areas of excessive heating to the patient or volunteer subject and/or damage to the MR system (1-3, 5, 8, 9). The necessary insulation space between cables and devices, between cables, devices and the human subject, and between cables, devices and the MR system's bore is a minimum of 1-cm (9).

In any scan in which the RF is transmitted by the body coil that is housed within the shroud or cover of the MR system, the risk for inducing a substantial current is greater as a larger area is exposed as opposed to that of a much smaller transmit-receive head RF coil or knee RF coil (1-3, 5, 8). Many RF coils in use are receive-only in which the body coil is used for the transmission part of the MRI scans. These receive-only RF coils are not only used to image large anatomical areas such as the chest, abdomen and pelvis, they may also be smaller coils designed to image the brain, knee, or wrist but still use the much larger RF body coil to perform the RF transmission. Therefore, it is critically important for the researchers to clearly understand how the RF coil(s) they are using operates to ensure necessary insulation is provided for the human subject, coils, cables and devices present in the bore of the MR system.

If there is not 1-cm of insulation guaranteed and maintained using pads and sponges between the subject's arms, chest or abdomen and the bore wall of the MR system, the patient should not be scanned because the risk of burns is far too great. Faulty RF coils including the body RF coil can also be the cause of burns. Positioning sponges or pads between the subject's arms and other body parts that come into close proximity to the bore walls is, therefore, a requirement for all imaging that utilizes the body coil to transmit RF energy (**Figure 2**). The cost of positioning sponges and pads for use in the MRI environment is expensive, especially those that are durable, and maintain their position without slipping. However, the issues surrounding a patient or volunteer subject burn in the MRI environment results in a far greater financial liability.

Figure 2. An example of placement of sponges or pads between the volunteer subject and the bore of the MR system to prevent issues related to direct contact with the transmit RF body coil.

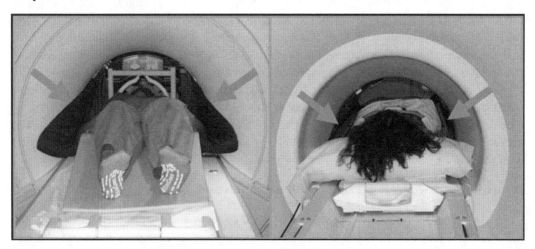

Room Temperature and Bore Fan Operation

Understanding the potential issues with ambient room temperature is another topic to be reviewed with all researchers. The MR system room temperature should not exceed 65 to 68°F given the ease with which temperature may increase in the MR system's bore and subsequently, the MR system room, due to rapid imaging sequences with multiple RF pulses.

The operation of the scanner's fan is to be used to prevent an increase of temperature inside the bore and to maintain patient and volunteer subject comfort during the procedure (1-3, 5, 8). There are anecdotal scenarios in which individuals experienced severe heating and/or a burn during an MRI examination where profuse sweating was present. While no concrete evidence exists relating to the presence of perspiration and a burn from an MR system, it is recommended that patients or volunteer subjects not be exposed to extreme heat or any situation that challenges their innate ability to regulate their body temperature during MRI examinations.

Research Support Equipment and Accessories

Non-magnetic carts are available in all of the MRI suites to allow easy transport of the larger RF coils, IV and contrast media supplies, and various supplies and equipment employed in the research MRI examinations. Before moving any non-magnetic carts into the MR system room, the researchers are required to check all shelves for any potential projectiles. These carts or shelves do not have drawers or cupboard doors in order to prevent the accidental introduction of hidden projectiles.

A wide variety of support equipment and accessories are available in the MRI setting and MR system room, and all must be verified to be safe to use. Audio systems, projectors, mirror systems, and screen-mirror combinations for RF coils are available for fMRI studies. MR conditional physiologic monitoring systems are available that provide a variety of data including: heart rate, electrocardiography (ECG), oxygen saturation, end tidal CO_2, body temperature, non-invasive blood pressure, invasive blood pressure, and automatic identification of anesthesia agent(s). Water blankets for body temperature maintenance are also available for animal model MRI examinations.

MR Safe or MR Conditional plastic chairs, step stools, aluminum IV poles, aluminum ladders, and plastic containers are available for use by researchers in the MR system room. In addition, a wide variety of accessories are available including, earplugs, earphones, and disposable earphone covers, table pads and immobilization straps for human subjects and RF coils, phantoms of various sizes and contents (e.g., water, saline, agar, peanut oil, copper sulfate, etc.).

MR System Software

Hands-on training is provided to all researchers using the MR system to ensure maximum efficiency and ultimately successful studies. Training should be tailored specifically to the type of study each individual researcher will be conducting. This will include selection of imaging sequences (research and product), scan parameters and options, graphic scan prescription, high order shimming, advanced scan control variables, post-processing, monitoring of the raw data directory, accessing the service error log, trouble-shooting system errors and artifacts transfer and/or archival of raw and image data, completion of the online scanner reports, and a request for immediate support.

Support for Researchers Using MR Systems

Support is provided to all researchers using the MR systems during all operational hours, which at a research MRI facility is twenty-fours a day, seven days a week (24/7). This support includes safety and screening questions [answered only by the MRI Manager [MRI technologist] or radiologist (clinician) from the Safety Committee] and MR systems' difficulties or artifacts. The MRI Manager is on call twenty-four hours a day and seven days a week (24/7). The radiologist/MRI clinician and research scientist (Ph.D.) from the MRI Safety Committee provide additional support 24/7.

MRI PRE-PROCEDURE SCREENING

Each research MRI facility should configure a list of basic MRI safety rules on which all researchers are encouraged to focus every time they are working in the MRI environment. These should be simple, thereby, making them easy to remember. For example:

1 - Make no assumptions

2 - Trust no one

3 - Ask questions

4 - Screen four times

5 - Know your RF coils

6 - No loops in cables or humans

7 - Keep the MR system room door closed

8 - Remain vigilant at all times

Patients and Volunteer Subjects

All patients and volunteer subjects undergoing research scans must be ambulatory (i.e., possess the ability to walk into the MR system room unassisted and climb up on to the table). If they are not fully ambulatory, the MRI Manager must be consulted to provide procedures that are safe for the patients and volunteer subjects, as well as for the researchers.

If the research facility is not licensed by the state, in-patients from any healthcare facility cannot undergo an MRI examination at that location. In addition, no scans can be conducted in which patients or volunteer subjects pay for the scans or their insurance pays for the scans.

Injection of drugs or the administration of gases to patients and volunteer subjects is not allowed at any time unless approved by the Institutional Review Board (IRB) and the members of the MRI Safety Committee at the research facility. Sedatives, sedation (full, moderate, or conscious) is not allowed unless an anesthesiologist is present for the entire examination.

Scans of human subjects are never to be conducted for health issues that are not part of an IRB-approved research study. In addition, patients and volunteer subjects are not allowed to receive complete or incomplete sets of their image data from the researchers. If the image data has been transferred to the picture archiving and communication system (PACS) and an interpretation by a radiologist has been conducted, then the patient or volunteer subject can obtain their report and images through the radiology department at the hospital.

MRI Pre-Procedure Screening

Safety screening of patients and human subjects is conducted routinely before each and every MRI examination (1-5). Screening is done to ensure safety upon entering the MR system room, entering the MR system and residing in the scanner during the examination. Potential dangers are due to the presence of the static main magnetic field (B_0), radiofrequency (RF) electromagnetic fields (B_1), and the varying gradient magnetic fields ($G_{x,y,z}$).

Metals and conductors are the main concerns but other issues will be discussed as well including the sound levels attributed to the time-varying magnetic fields. It is helpful to remember that metal can exhibit one or more behaviors when exposed to an MR system including it can become a projectile or missile by being pulled into the magnet due to the change in static main magnetic field (B_0) over distance (dB/dZ), rotate or attempt to align with the static main magnetic field lines (i.e., torque), heat, and/or cause artifacts in the image and raw data (1-5). Translational attraction is strongest at the ends of the MR system and zero at the center whereas torque is strongest at the center of the scanner. Due to the additional magnetic shielding added to an MR system allowing it to have a reduced fringe field, the compressed field lines of the magnet result in projectiles experiencing attraction to the sides of the bore as well as to the center of the bore in the Z-direction.

In 2005, the American Society for Testing and Materials (ASTM) International published new terminology for use in describing or labeling implants and devices as well as items under consideration to enter the MR system room and to potentially be present in the scanner during the examination. The labeling terms are MR Unsafe, MR Safe, and MR Conditional (6).

MR Unsafe describes an item that poses hazards in all MRI environments. MR Safe describes an item that poses no known hazards in all MRI environments. MR Conditional describes an item that has been demonstrated to pose no known hazards in a specified MRI environment with specified conditions of use. Field conditions that define the specified MRI environment include field strength, spatial gradient, dB/dt (time rate of change of the magnetic field), radio frequency (RF) fields and specific absorption rate (SAR). Additional conditions, including specific configurations of the item, may be required (6). In view of the above, implants, devices, and other items should be labeled with proper terminology and researchers engaged in performing investigations using MRI technology should carefully consider this information in the realm of MRI screening policies and procedures.

Researchers are required to screen each patient and volunteer subject four times including: conducting a telephone interview or email screening, completing the screening form on site at the MRI facility on the day of the scheduled examination (followed by a review of the completed form by the researcher with the patient or volunteer subject), a visual and verbal screening at dressing room, and a visual and verbal screening immediately before entering the MR system room.

MRI Pre-procedure Screening Forms

Two MRI screening forms should be available (**Figure 3**). One form is used for patients and volunteer subjects undergoing MRI to complete prior to entering the MR system room (1-5). A shorter version is available for individuals who wish to enter the MRI environment but that will not be scanned. This second form is used for family members when it is necessary or useful for them to be present in the MR system room with the patient or volunteer subject. It is also used for maintenance and housekeeping personnel, visiting researchers, clinicians, nurses, and others. It is important to routinely check with all researchers to ensure they are using the most current MRI pre-procedure screening forms. This is especially important for researchers from departments other than the one in which the MR system is located.

The screening process is an interactive one between the researcher and the patient or volunteer subject. The researcher conducting the screening must be trained and, therefore, qualified to do so (1-5). They must have completed the required MRI Safety Policy and Procedure Training and be current with their online safety training. All screening questions regarding biomedical devices and implants, and/or any other condition which may prevent the patient or volunteer subject from undergoing the MRI examination is forwarded to the MRI Manager or radiologist/MRI clinician from the MRI Safety Committee. Always a good rule of thumb in MRI safety is that "a previous MRI procedure does not guarantee safety" for any subsequent MRI examination. In addition, researchers are required to consult with the MRI Manager, or radiologist/MRI clinician from the MRI Safety Committee if the patient or volunteer subject mentions any previous surgeries. Further investigation is then necessary to obtain additional information in order to make the decision for the patient or volunteer subject to undergo the research MRI examination. This includes the date of the surgery, city, state and country in which surgery was conducted, the physician's and/or surgeon's name, name of hospital, anatomical location, reason for surgery, and devices or implants present (1 5).

Researchers are required to complete the patient and volunteer subject MRI pre-procedure screening form once a year when they complete their MRI Safety Policy and Procedure Training tutorial online. If a researcher has surgery, or acquires a biomedical device or implant then they are required to report to the MRI Manager to determine if it is safe for them to enter the MR system room, to work around the MR system and/or be scanned. Pregnant patients and volunteer subjects may undergo research MRI examinations if approved by the Institutional Review Board (IRB) and the MRI Safety Committee. The decision to allow pregnant researchers to enter the MR system area is made by the MRI Safety Committee for that particular research facility.

In research studies, it may be the case that more than one MRI examination will take place during the course of the investigation. In this situation, the participant undergoes the informed consent process and signs the consent form once. However, the MRI pre-procedure screening form is completed for each and every time the participant is scanned, even if the scans are only one day apart (1-5). Much can happen in twenty-four hours that would not be immediately noticeable to the researcher conducting the study (e.g., having a pacemaker implanted). It is also critical that the screening form be completed on-site at the research facility on the day of the scan. Researchers are required to conduct a telephone interview or email pre-screening for major issues such as the presence of biomedical devices or implants, pregnancy, presence of acupuncture needles, body piercing, etc. These are issues that would need to be resolved by those responsible from the MRI Safety Committee before the patient or volunteer subject would be allowed to undergo the MRI examination.

It is critical that the researcher conveys to the patient or volunteer subject the seriousness of the screening form and how important it is to provide accurate, complete answers to ensure safety. After the patient or volunteer subject completes the MRI pre-procedure screening form, the researcher sits down with the individual to review the information on the form. This is to ensure that the patient or volunteer subject has not missed or forgotten any information, surgeries, or conditions that might prevent them from undergoing the MRI examination. After the review is complete, the researcher prints his or her first and last name at the bottom of the completed form. This ensures that a record is kept of which individual reviewed the completed screening form with the patient or volunteer subject before taking this individual into the MR system room. The completed screening form goes on file with the completed consent form in the office of the principal investigator (PI) as evidence that everything was done to ensure safety for the patient or volunteer subject during the MRI examination.

As with a clinical MRI department, it should be clearly documented in the research facility's policies and procedures, to which the responsibility falls to make the decision for the patient or volunteer subject to undergo the MRI examination if there is a potential safety issue present such as a biomedical device or implant. As the patients and volunteer subjects undergoing MRI research scans are enrolled in a research study, there is typically no benefit versus risk evaluation conducted as is done in a clinical facility. In addition, frequently there is not a formal image or data interpretation by a board-certified radiologist with a report entered into the radiology department database (i.e., the Radiology Information System, RIS). Research studies are conducted on groups of people, typically not done to provide diagnoses on individual patients. Because of this, pre-procedure screening becomes much more conservative than what is practiced in the clinical MRI department. Pregnant women and volunteer subjects with pacemakers, even MR conditional pacemakers, are not scanned unless approved by the IRB and the MRI Safety Committee. If there is any risk at all, the radiologist makes the final decision (1-5, 10). If neither the MRI Manager nor the radiologist/MRI clinician can be contacted for approval, the patient or volunteer subject is not to enter the MR system room nor undergo the research MRI examination.

Most biomedical devices and implants are considered "MR Conditional" unless they are made completely from nonmetallic and non-conducting components such as plastic or nylon (1, 3, 4, 6). Each manufacturer of a biomedical device or implant determines the spe-

Figure 3. Example of an MRI Pre-Examination Screening Form that is used for patients and volunteer subjects (a).

MRI PRE-EXAMINATION SCREENING FORM

Xxxxx Xxxxxxx Center for Imaging
Department of Radiology, Xxxxxx University School of Medicine
1200 Smith Road, MC 1234, Room P900, Xxxxxx, XX 90900-1234
(xxx) xxx-xxxx, (xxx) xxx-xxxx

Date _____   Magnet ❑ 3T1   ❑ 3T2   ❑ 3T3   ❑ 7.0T

Name _____ Height_____ Weight_____
        Last name   First name   M.I.
Date of Birth _____   ❑ Female ❑ Male   Ethnic Origin _____
Address_____ City_____
State_____ Zip Code_____ Phone (H)(_____)_____ (W)(_____)_____
Physician's name & address_____

1. Have you ever had surgery or other invasive procedures?   ❑ Yes ❑ No   If yes, please list below.
   Type:_____   Date: ____ / ____ / ____
   Type:_____   Date: ____ / ____ / ____
2. Have you had any previous MR studies?   ❑ Yes ❑ No   If yes, please list most recent below.
        Area of Body   Date   Facility Name & Location
   _____ ____ / ____ / ____ _____
3. Have you ever worked as a machinist, metalworker, or in any profession or hobby grinding metal?   ❑ Yes ❑ No
4. Have you ever had an injury to the eye(s) by a metallic object (metallic slivers, shavings, or foreign body)?   ❑ Yes ❑ No
5. Are you pregnant, experiencing a late menstrual period, or having fertility treatments?   ❑ Yes ❑ No
6. Are you currently taking or have recently taken any medication? ❑ Yes ❑ No   Please list:_____
7. Do you have drug allergies or have you had an allergic reaction? ❑ Yes ❑ No   Please list:_____
8. Have you ever had an allergic reaction to a MR contrast media injection?   ❑ Yes ❑ No
9. Do you have or previously had kidney problems? ❑ Yes ❑ No   Please list:_____

Some of the following items may be HAZARDOUS to your safety and some may interfere with the MRI examination. Do you have any of the following:

❑ Yes	❑ No	Cardiac pacemaker or defibrillator	❑ Yes	❑ No	Ocular implant (eye)
❑ Yes	❑ No	Implanted cardiac pacing wires	❑ Yes	❑ No	Artificial limb or joint
❑ Yes	❑ No	Aneurysm clip or brain clip	❑ Yes	❑ No	Electrodes (body or brain)
❑ Yes	❑ No	Carotid artery vascular clamp	❑ Yes	❑ No	Shrapnel, buckshot, or bullets
❑ Yes	❑ No	Neurostimulator or DBS	❑ Yes	❑ No	Metal fragments (eye, head, ear, skin)
❑ Yes	❑ No	Spinal fusion stimulator	❑ Yes	❑ No	Tattoos: body, eyeliner, eyebrows or lips
❑ Yes	❑ No	Implanted drug infusion device	❑ Yes	❑ No	Body piercing(s) *(Remove before scan)*
❑ Yes	❑ No	Heart valve prosthesis	❑ Yes	❑ No	Ear tubes
❑ Yes	❑ No	Aortic or vascular clips	❑ Yes	❑ No	Implant held in place by a magnet
❑ Yes	❑ No	Cochlear, otologic, or ear implant	❑ Yes	❑ No	Facelift or other cosmetic surgery
❑ Yes	❑ No	Stents, filters, or coils (vascular or other)	❑ Yes	❑ No	Metal or wire staples, sutures, mesh implants
❑ Yes	❑ No	Shunt (spine or ventricles)	❑ Yes	❑ No	Metal rods in bones; joint replacements
❑ Yes	❑ No	Vascular access port or catheters	❑ Yes	❑ No	Bone/joint pin, screw, nail, wire, plate
❑ Yes	❑ No	Swan-Ganz catheter	❑ Yes	❑ No	Wig, toupee, or hair implants, extensions
❑ Yes	❑ No	Harrington rods (spine)	❑ Yes	❑ No	Hearing aid *(Remove before scan)*
❑ Yes	❑ No	Intrauterine Device (IUD)	❑ Yes	❑ No	Dentures *(Remove before scan)*
❑ Yes	❑ No	Pessary or bladder ring	❑ Yes	❑ No	Asthma or breathing disorders
❑ Yes	❑ No	Transdermal drug delivery patch	❑ Yes	❑ No	Seizures or motion disorders
❑ Yes	❑ No	Prosthesis (eye/orbital, penile, etc.)	❑ Yes	❑ No	Claustrophobia

PLEASE REMOVE ALL METAL OBJECTS before the MR examination including: Cell Phone, Keys, Hair Pins, Barrettes, Jewelry, Watch, Safety Pins, Paperclips, Money Clip, Coins, Pens, Belt, Pocket Knife, Metal Buttons & Clothing with Metal. HEARING PROTECTION is required during the MRI examination.

_____   ____ / ____ / ____
     Signature of Person Completing Form   Date

Form Completed by: ❑ Patient / Volunteer   ❑ Relative:_____
                    ❑ Physician:_____ ❑ Other:_____

Form Reviewed by (please print name clearly & attach to consent form):_____

Rev. 11_0912

Figure 3. (continued) Example of a Visitors MRI Screening Form that is used for individuals who are not going to be scanned but will enter the MR system room including family members, physicians, healthcare professionals, maintenance, and housekeeping personnel, and others (b).

VISITORS MR SCREENING FORM (3T1, 3T2, 3T3 & 7T)

Xxxxx Xxxxxxx Center for Imaging
Department of Radiology, Xxxxxx University School of Medicine
1200 Smith Road, MC 1234, Room P900, Xxxxxx, XX 90900-1234
(xxx) xxx-xxxx, (xxx) xxx-xxxx

WARNING: THE MAGNET IS ALWAYS ON

Note: If you are going to be scanned, you are required to complete a different form.

Date_____/_____/_____   Magnet ❑ 3T1   ❑ 3T2   ❑ 3T3   ❑ 7.0T

Name _____
                  Last name   First name   M.I.

Age_____   Telephone (H)(_____)_____ (W)(_____)_____

Address_____ City_____

State_____ Zip Code_____

1. Have you ever had surgery or other invasive procedures?   ❑ Yes   ❑ No   If yes, please list:

   Type:_____ Date: _____/_____/_____

   Type:_____ Date: _____/_____/_____

2. Are you pregnant, experiencing a late menstrual period, or having fertility treatments? ❑ Yes ❑ No

Some of the following items may be hazardous to your safety due to the proximity of the MR system and the strong magnetic field. Do you have any of the following:

❑ Yes	❑ No	Cardiac pacemaker or defibrillator
❑ Yes	❑ No	Aneurysm clip or brain clip
❑ Yes	❑ No	Neurostimulator or Deep Brain Stimulator (DBS)
❑ Yes	❑ No	Insulin or infusion pump
❑ Yes	❑ No	Implanted drug infusion device
❑ Yes	❑ No	Spinal fusion stimulator or spinal cord stimulator
❑ Yes	❑ No	Cochlear, otologic or ear implant
❑ Yes	❑ No	Implant held in place by a magnet
❑ Yes	❑ No	Artificial or prosthetic limb or prosthesis
❑ Yes	❑ No	Heart valve prosthesis
❑ Yes	❑ No	Aortic or vascular clips
❑ Yes	❑ No	Stents, filters or coils (vascular or other)
❑ Yes	❑ No	Shunt (spine or ventricles)
❑ Yes	❑ No	Metal fragments (eye, head, ear or skin)
❑ Yes	❑ No	Hearing aid
❑ Yes	❑ No	Other implants in body or head

PLEASE REMOVE ALL METALLIC OBJECTS before entering the magnet room: keys, pager, cell phone, paperclips, coins, hair pins, barrettes, safety pins, money clip, computer jump drive, credit cards, hearing aid, pocket knives, tools & analog watches.

_____   _____/_____/_____
        Signature of Person Completing Form   Date

Form Completed by: ❑ Researcher / Scientist   ❑ Visitor

Form Reviewed by (please print clearly):_____

Rev. 2013_0122

cific conditions under which their product can safely undergo an MRI examination. In research studies, the scan parameters are selected and maintained across all scans of all individuals participating in that particular research study. Modification of scan parameters in research protocols to adjust conditions include but are not limited to the static main magnetic field strength, maximum spatial magnetic field gradient the patient can access, specific absorption rate (SAR), and/or slew rate and maximum amplitude of the time-varying magnetic fields.

One family member (i.e., parent, spouse, adult child, etc.) is allowed to accompany the patient or volunteer subject into the MR system room. The shorter screening form for visitors and other similar individuals is completed first and reviewed by the researcher. All metals and potential projectiles including jewelry, watches, hair accessories, hearing aids, and other related items are removed and secured in a locker. If the family member is going to remain in the MR system room with the patient or volunteer subject, then hearing protection is required.

MRI pre-procedure screening forms should be comprehensive but the information contained should be easily understood, therefore, not too technical nor should it contain too much medical jargon. The MRI Safety Committee reviews and updates these forms on a regular basis, typically every six months. Any new changes due to information from the FDA, ASTM International, manufacturers of medical implants and devices, and other entities, should be reviewed by the MRI Safety Committee which subsequently determines if changes or additions should be made to the screening forms.

Examples of MRI pre-procedure screening forms can be obtained at: http://www.mrisafety.com (created and maintained by Frank G. Shellock, Ph.D.) and at the website for the Institute for Magnetic Resonance Safety, Education, and Research, http://www.imrser.org (11, 12).

Static Magnetic Field

Metallic items that are attracted to a magnet are referred to as ferromagnetic (1-7, 13). Examples of ferromagnetic materials include iron and certain types of steel. Some examples of nonferromagnetic materials include aluminum, copper, brass, lead, nickel, titanium, cobalt, mercury, chromium, platinum, and gold. It is important to remember that often metals are a mixture (or alloy) that makes it difficult to easily determine if a given item is ferromagnetic even if the percentage of each element present is known. Testing by very strong handheld magnet is typically the only way to determine if a specific item will be attracted to the magnet of the MR system, remembering that handheld magnets are generally never as strong as the MRI, such as 1.5-T or 3-T (1-5).

Every precaution must be taken to ensure that ferromagnetic items are not taken into the MR system room. Given the shielding present in most MR systems, the spatial gradient of the static magnetic field is quite steep. Therefore, the distance traversed between a ferromagnetic item feeling no attraction, to quickly being pulled into the MR system is quite small. This translational attraction is dependent upon several conditions including the strength and spatial gradient of the static magnetic field, magnet design (e.g., long-bore ver-

Figure 4. MRI labeling system showing the icons as defined by the ASTM International that is used to mark implants, devices, and equipment.

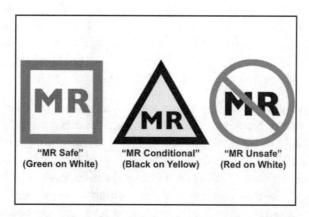

"MR Safe"
(Green on White)

"MR Conditional"
(Black on Yellow)

"MR Unsafe"
(Red on White)

sus short-bore), the degree of attraction due to mass and geometry of the object, the type of retention, location, orientation, and time in place (i.e., for implants), and other factors.

Items in the patient preparation room or any rooms located close to the scanner room must be clearly identified with labels indicating that they may not be taken into the MR system room at any time for any reason (1-4). Some of these items may include crash carts, laundry carts, storage cabinets, and chairs. It is recommended that items that reside in the patient preparation room be identified and labeled as MR Safe or MR Conditional. However, it is more realistic that some items that reside in the control room as well as the patient preparation room will not fit into either of those categories meaning they may be MR Unsafe. This is especially true in the research environment with hardware and devices that are under development. Therefore labels indicating MR Unsafe are absolutely necessary for such items. It is recommended that the labels used for this purpose are those defined by the ASTM International (1-4, 6). **Figure 4** shows the proper labels for marking purposes related to MR Safe, MR Conditional and MR Unsafe.

RF Electromagnetic Fields

The specific absorption rate (SAR) is a means of characterizing the absorption of radiofrequency (RF) energy in human tissue and is typically reported in watts per kilogram (W/kg) (1-4, 8, 14). SAR is primarily dependent on the following parameters: imaging frequency, type of RF pulses, repetition time (TR), type of transmit RF coil, anatomy exposed to the transmitting RF coil, and patient weight (and height on some MR systems). The measurement of SAR is typically reported on MR systems as whole body averaged and peak values. In general, as SAR increases, the number of slices available in a given imaging sequence is reduced in order to decrease the whole body averaged SAR level. Realistically, the only modifiable parameters available to the MRI operator are the repetition time and/or number of slices, unless the researcher can change the transmit RF coil or move to a lower static magnetic field MR system. Entering the incorrect weight of the patient or volunteer subject is risky and could result in increased RF energy being deposited into the patient, potentially resulting in a burn (8).

Risks surrounding the RF electromagnetic fields (B1) include the heating of metallic objects or devices, associated components, and/or the surrounding tissues. The increased heating that can potentially result in burns to the patient or volunteer subject, and/or damage to the MR system and RF coils may occur in a variety of scenarios. These include the exposure or close proximity to a transmit RF coil, focus of RF energy in a specific area (i.e., the antenna effect), currents being induced in conductors (e.g., cables, metallic devices of certain lengths and human beings), and an inappropriate use of an RF coil (1-5, 8).

Procedures to prevent currents being induced in connectors, and the proper positioning and insulation of cables, RF coils, devices and human subjects must be utilized for all MRI examinations especially those using the RF body coil to transmit RF energy, as previously described. In addition, loop formation must be prevented including cables forming loops, cables forming loops with other cables, and cables forming loops with human subjects (1-5, 8). Loops can be defined as crossing and/or touching, or changing direction within the MR system (e.g., a cable runs through the bore, then turns and runs back through the bore a second time) (1-5, 8, 9). Loops in cables present in the MR system's bore become a greater risk as the loop becomes larger. For example, if an ECG cable is attached to a patient or volunteer subject via electrodes, the cable then runs out the back of the magnet, turns and returns through the scanner to its electrical connection at the front of the MR system. This forms a very large and potentially dangerous loop. Cables on RF coils are sometimes too long. Placing a sponge or pad to separate the smaller unpreventable loops of the cable should prevent induced currents.

Attention must be given to the potential for patient burns occurring due to the human body acting as a conductor. A gap 1-cm of air must be guaranteed between anatomy within the confines of the transmitting RF coil using sponges and pads to separate and insulate (1-5, 8, 9). For example, during any scan in which the RF body coil is used as the transmit RF coil, hands should not be clasped together, hands should not rest on forehead during breast MRI examinations, hands should not rest against hips, and calves (i.e., lower leg) should not touch. In addition to the potential for peripheral nerve stimulation due to time-varying magnetic fields, these types of contact or any other combinations should be avoided due to the risk of providing an easy route for induced currents to flow.

In the research environment, many prototype devices are designed and constructed to be used while imaging patients and volunteer subjects. These are either used alone or simultaneously with other product or prototype devices. Individuals possessing the appropriate expertise must complete extensive testing to ensure these prototype devices can be used safely within the magnetic environment. The device design and safety risks, if present, are described in the human study protocol to be approved by the IRB prior to use. In addition, consultation with the MRI Manager is required before use in the MR system room.

Utilizing different static magnetic field strengths within the same research facility necessitates the possession of knowledge regarding RF bandwidth, its dependence upon the static magnetic field, and interaction with certain lead lengths (as applicable) as well as the human body. This is critical in the prevention of not only image artifacts but also potential risks for burns. For example, imaging the brain at 3-T versus that of 1.5-T means the RF frequency is 128-MHz versus 64-MHz. The brain then encounters more "half wavelengths" at 3-T resulting in a B_1 inhomogeneity (dielectric resonance) that is seen as brightness in the center of the axial brain images (1-8, 15, 16). While SAR (RF energy deposited into the human body) increases at 3-T versus that at 1.5-T, there may be conflicting issues. For example, dependent upon a given lead length, there may be less resultant heating at 3-T/128-MHz versus 1.5-T/64-MHz, as reported by Shellock et al. (17).

Due to the many different designs of RF coils from major MR system manufacturers and third party vendors, it is critical that specific instructions be followed when utilizing these coils. This is especially true of the so-called "array" coils available as product versions since the early 1990s. Various designs of RF array coils include coupled, isolated, or phased. Some of these designed to image large areas of the body (e.g., cardiac, torso and abdomen coils) are manufactured as two parts, one to be positioned anteriorly and the other, posteriorly. Preventing these particular RF coils from overlapping at the sides of the patient or volunteer subject may be a requirement to prevent interactions resulting in excessive heating and possible burns. Sponges or pads must always be present or placed between the RF coil and the anatomy being imaged, some of which are provided by the manufacturer. This is to prevent inappropriate loading that can potentially result in malfunction of the RF coil and subsequent disproportionate heating.

Positioning one RF coil inside of another for MR imaging is generally something that should never be done unless the coils are specifically designed by the manufacturer to do so safely. For example, an earlier version of the endorectal coil was used to image the prostate in conjunction with a pelvic phased array coil. To proceed safely, researchers must first consult the MRI Manager, MRI research technologist, or lab director of the research facility. Finally, an RF coil should never be left unplugged and in the bore of the scanner during an MRI examination.

Time-Varying Magnetic Fields

Risks associated with the time-varying magnetic fields are due to the rapid switching to spatially localize during MR imaging (1-5, 18). This rapid switching is made up of two parts, the size [maximum amplitude measured in millitesla per meter (mT/m)] and the speed [slew rate measured in millitesla per meter per millisecond (mT/m/msec)]. As a current is made to flow in a conductor moving through a static magnetic field, a flowing current can also be induced in a static conductor when exposed to a rapidly changing magnetic field.

Other risks include peripheral nerve stimulation and auditory effects that are associated with the time-varying magnetic field (1-5, 18). While peripheral nerve stimulation due to the slew rate is a reality, it is subjective and, therefore, difficult to tell exactly which patients and volunteer subjects will experience this sensation. While it can be perceived as painful or extreme pressure, it has not been reported to result in residual effects. Some of the MR systems offer options to image under reduced slew rates, thereby minimizing the risk.

Manufacturers of MR systems continue to devise methods to reduce the acoustic noise generated by gradient magnetic fields and this topic is covered in detail in another chapter in this textbook. New imaging sequences, especially those being designed in research facilities are more rapid, increasing the noise level. Therefore, it is essential to use earplugs or other hearing protection accessories and devices rated appropriately by the (noise reduction ratings (NRR). In addition, it is of equal importance that the earplugs be placed correctly within the ear canal. Headphones are recommended for use in conjunction with earplugs to provide maximum protection during scans of the body and extremities. Researchers are required to instruct their patients and volunteer subjects to notify them using the squeeze bulb or verbally through the intercom system if the earplugs become loose, fall out, or if the noise of the MR system is bothersome or painful so that the examination can be immediately stopped. Posters demonstrating the procedure for correct placement of earplugs should be posted within each of the research MR system rooms for easy referral for researchers and their patients and volunteer subjects. If earplugs cannot be positioned appropriately, the patient or volunteer subject should not be scanned. If headphones are used alone, the NRR should be at least 30-dB of protection that is provided including any earplugs that fit inside of the headphones, some of which deliver audio instructions during research studies.

Presence of Biomedical Implants or Devices

The risks of allowing human subjects with MR Unsafe or MR Conditional (when conditions have not been met) biomedical implants or devices into the MRI environment to undergo an MRI examination include the objects being moved or dislodged, induction of a current in the device or associated lead wires, excessive heating, altered function of the device, de-magnetization of the device, temporary or permanent damage to the device, and other problems (1-5, 7, 8, 10, 14, 19-21).

Having general policies for managing individuals with biomedical devices and implants are never a good idea because testing has not been conducted on all implants, there tend to be exceptions, new devices are being developed on an on-going basis, and implants and devices are affected differently by different MR system conditions (4, 5).

Risks are dependent upon many criteria including the static magnetic field strength, spatial gradient of the static magnetic field, ferromagnetic properties of the implant or device [composition, mass and geometry, passive versus active, and method of activation (electrically, magnetically, or mechanically)], and/or location and orientation of the implant or device [type of tissue, retention means (scarring, sutures, cement, etc.)], adjacent vital anatomic structures, and other factors (1-5, 7, 8, 10, 14, 19-21).

To accurately evaluate acceptability under which a patient or volunteer subject with an implant or device can undergo an MRI examination, specific information must be obtained including the name of the manufacturer of the device or implant, composition of the material, date surgically placed, anatomical location, name of surgeon and hospital, and/or reason for placement of implant or device (1-5, 7, 8, 10, 14, 19-21). The more information that can be obtained about the implant or device, the easier it will be to make a knowledgeable and accurate decision. Patients are sometimes given cards to carry with information from the manufacturer about the implant or device. In addition, contacting manufacturers or reviewing their website can provide the necessary information. The decision to undergo the MRI examination, however, should never be made from a verbal reply only (e.g., "The surgeon said it was ok to scan."). Dependent upon the type of implant or device, the MRI Manager or, more appropriately, the radiologist/MRI clinician from the MRI Safety Committee should make the decision for the patient or volunteer subject to undergo the MRI procedure. For more serious or complex devices such as cardiac pacemakers and neurostimulation systems, it is the radiologist/MRI clinician who must make the final decision not the MRI Manager or MRI facility manager (1-5, 7, 8, 10, 14, 19-21). As stated earlier, the patients and volunteer subjects undergoing MRI procedures are enrolled in a research study, therefore, they are considered "volunteers" for the research study. Thus, there is typically no benefit versus risk evaluation conducted as is done in a clinical facility.

If the implant or device is identified to be MR Conditional, then the set of MRI scan parameters and other conditions as set down in the research protocol must be reviewed to ensure it is capable of being modified to ensure that the specific conditions are met without affecting the outcome of the research study (and acceptable by the Principal Investigator of the research study).

All individuals must remove metallic body piercing and cosmetic jewelry before being involved in research MRI examinations. As there is no benefit versus risk evaluation conducted for research scans, even the smallest amount of risk must be removed. Patients and volunteer subjects with cosmetic jewelry or piercings that cannot be removed cannot undergo MRI.

Screening Tools

A list of common projectiles that have made their way into MR systems should be provided to researchers to ensure that they remember what items could be problematic. For example, paper clips, staples, hairpins, barrettes and other hair accessories, jewelry and watches, keys, hearing aids, scissors, pocketknives, tools, flashlights, metal pens, clipboards, notebooks, money clips, cell phones, and other similar objects.

Quality handheld magnets are another valuable investment to be made for checking equipment, imaging accessories, and hair accessories and jewelry (worn by researchers) (1-5). To check any of these items, they must be removed from the body and placed on a hard surface over which the handheld magnet is placed. Handheld magnets should never be used to detect the presence of ferrous metal in or on the body (1-5). Strong handheld magnets are available in several forms. The most valuable is a neodymium magnet (1200-gauss or higher). The use of a handheld magnet of a lower strength is discouraged.

Reference materials including books and websites can be very helpful in information gathering concerning many aspects of MRI safety and screening. The recent publication from the American College of Radiology (ACR) is a comprehensive document that should be carefully reviewed by the MRI Safety Committee members (1). Utilizing reference materials and websites are especially helpful for the evaluation of biomedical devices and implants. It should be remembered, however, that these are for reference only and should never be used as the sole piece of evidence to decide whether the patient or volunteer subject should undergo the MRI examination.

Websites to consult are those from the manufacturer of the biomedical device or implant which provide information and conditions under which a particular device can safely be exposed to all parts of the MRI examination involving the respective electromagnetic fields. Websites such as www.mrisafety.com (created and maintained by Frank G. Shellock, Ph.D.) provide educational documents and testing results for thousands of biomedical devices and

Figure 5. Participation in a worldwide MRI technologist or radiographer automatic list server is helpful in adding to one's arsenal of knowledge in MRI safety.

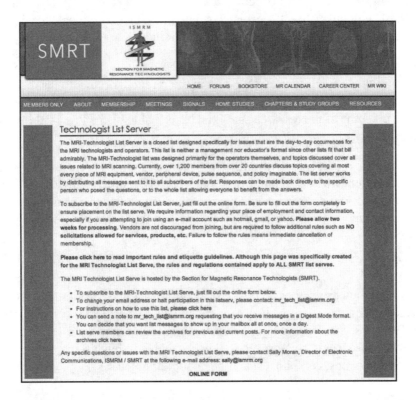

implants (11). In addition, other websites such as www.imrser.org, provide a wealth of information about safety and pre-procedure screening in the MRI environment that can be used by those on the MRI Safety Committee to keep their knowledge of MRI safety current (12). A textbook entitled, "Reference Manual for Magnetic Resonance Safety, Implants, and Devices", is an information resource that is fully updated on an annual basis (3). This is an extremely valuable yet inexpensive investment for all MRI departments, both research and clinical.

Participation in a worldwide MRI technologist automatic email list server is also helpful in adding to one's arsenal of knowledge in MRI safety and screening (**Figure 5**). Questions are answered, suggestions made, and issues discussed on a daily basis. In this manner, a wealth of information is being shared freely without cost to the participants. However, time is required to triage the emails and read the ones particularly valuable to a given research facility.

Ferromagnetic detections systems (FMDS), devices that identify ferromagnetic materials, have recently replaced the metal detectors initially thought to be an important part of the fully equipped MRI department in the 1980s. Conventional metal detectors quickly became viewed as a waste of funds given the many issues surrounding them including over-dependence by users, the generation of false-positives and false-negatives, the function-related dependence upon size and mass of the metallic object, the sensitivity setting of the device, and other issues. Currently there are several different companies manufacturing a variety of designs for FMDS and a chapter is devoted to this topic in this textbook.

These devices can be very helpful in preventing injuries from larger ferromagnetic objects such as oxygen tanks, IV poles, infusion machines, gurneys, hospital beds, and many other items that have found their way into MRI environments over the years. Most of these situations resulted in expensive damage to the MR systems and RF coils. Others resulted in injuries to healthcare workers and patients and at least one death involving a patient. A recent report by Shellock and Karacozoff (25) indicated that a FMDS may also be used to identify ferromagnetic implants and foreign bodies.

However, there is a tendency for all of us, as human beings, to fully embrace machines to do our work, which lessens the necessity for us to think and make critical, conscious decisions. As long as we remember to do our job and remain vigilant, then and only then, will a FMDS become a valuable adjunct to MRI pre-procedure screening. Finally, we must always remember that no one part of the screening process stands alone in making the decision to allow an individual access to the MR system room or for a patient or volunteer subject to undergo an MRI examination. All of the necessary questions must be asked, and all of the resources must be checked to make an accurate decision.

Visitors, Tours, Classes, and Video Taping

Visitors to the MRI suite are allowed if an individual who has completed the required MRI Safety Policy and Procedure Training accompanies them. Visitors are not allowed to enter the MR system room except when absolutely necessary and then an approval must be obtained from the MRI Manager (the MRI technologist from the MRI Safety Committee). If approved to enter the MR system room, the visitor completes the appropriate screening form that is then reviewed by an MRI safety-trained individual. The visitor then checks all pockets by placing their hands inside of each and removes all potential projectiles in addition to jewelry, watches, hair accessories and hearing aids.

Due to the extremely high fringe field associated with a 7-Tesla MR system, the control and scanner room are treated the same with regards to screening visitors and other individuals. Thus, the screening form is completed in the lobby or in the patient preparation room, reviewed, and approved before the visitor may enter the control and/or MR system room of the 7-Tesla scanner.

The performance of tours, classes, and video taping sessions in the MRI suite must obtain approval from the MRI Manager prior to scheduling. Classes and video taping sessions are scheduled through the MRI Manager to ensure the availability of an MRI research technologist. This has proven to be valuable as the technologist scans while the faculty member (i.e., scientist or physician) delivers instruction to the class. Having an MRI technologist present not only ensures safety for individuals present and the MR systems, it prevents modifications from being made to the MRI suite and its contained equipment (e.g., relocating computers and monitors spontaneously and randomly, relocating audio and video equipment in the control room, removing cables from waveguides in penetration panels, removing lights and doors, etc.). It also ensures that the MRI suite that appears in a video shown on

TV or in media pictures will be represented appropriately and that any scanning and human subjects that are participating are only filmed according to departmental policy.

Housekeeping and Maintenance Staff

The MRI Manager and Building Manager are responsible for training the housekeeping and maintenance staff in the basic aspects of MRI safety (1-4). Specifically, this includes in which rooms they can access and which they are never allowed to access. Complete agreement and support must be obtained from housekeeping management to ensure that, in the event of sick leave or vacation, the MRI Manager and/or Building Manager gets notified immediately and that replacement housekeeping staff is fully trained before entering any of the MRI suites. Housekeeping and maintenance staff is never to enter the MR system rooms at any time. Cleaning and maintenance are scheduled for each of the MRI suites when the MRI Manager, Building Manager, or MRI technologist is available to provide full time monitoring.

PREPARATION OF PATIENTS AND VOLUNTEER SUBJECTS

During the scheduling process for patients and volunteer subjects, it should be communicated clearly that many items should be left at home including all jewelry, body piercing, hair accessories, and undergarments with metal fibers. Facial makeup should not be worn as some can result in an irritation to the skin from tiny metallic components. The same can be said for some hair products that may contain a component of metallic glitter. Artificial hair extensions have proven to be problematic for imaging of the brain due to the resulting lack of homogeneity and failure of magnetic field shimming due to the presence of the synthetic material that is present. Wigs and hairpieces should be removed or closely checked underneath for any hairpins that may be in place.

Having all patients and volunteer subjects change out of street clothes into scrubs or gowns that do not have pockets is required for all MR systems (1-4). This policy takes pockets out of the equation and allows easier visual access to ensure that items that may be problematic have been removed. It is also a way to remind the patients and volunteer subjects that preparation for entering the MRI environment is a serious issue and that their safety is considered paramount by the researchers conducting the MRI investigations. Compare the costs associated with the purchase of disposable scrubs and those provided by a laundry service. It can be the case that disposable scrubs are less expensive over time. Disposable foot covers are also a requirement for patients and volunteer subjects. Whether placed over bare feet or socks, it ensures some additional cleanliness in the MRI area but, more importantly, the dots on the bottom of the foot covers assist in the prevention of slipping and possible injuries.

All personal items belonging to patients and volunteer subjects must be secured in a locker within the MRI suite. This process facilitates a conversation between the researchers and the patient or volunteer subject to store all items and objects in the locker. Additionally, it acts as a reminder that nothing should be taken into the MR system room. Leaving personal items of any kind out on counters, especially jewelry or wallets, can be problematic. This can lead to a patient or volunteer subject making a claim that "something is missing".

Glasses can be worn into the MR system room but should never be worn by the patient or volunteer subject into the bore of the MR system due to the metallic components (small screws) that will result in artifacts in images and data acquired. Pillows or toys from home should never be allowed in the scanner room unless fully checked with a strong handheld magnet first. Items such as these can easily hide the presence of a piece of ferromagnetic material.

It is valuable to have a checklist present or a "stop, look, and feel" policy and procedure before entering the MR system room with the patient or volunteer subject (1-4). This is especially important in research facilities that may have patients and volunteer subjects arriving by wheelchair or gurney, and/or with IV poles and/or infusion devices. If the MR system table does not undock to be moved to the patient preparation room for transfer of the patient or volunteer subject, an acceptable (i.e., MR Safe or MR Conditional) wheelchair and/or gurney should also be available. All of these items should be included on the checklist to ensure none from the outside make their way into the MR system room. In addition, checking under sheets and blankets is also a requirement before entering the scanner room.

Policies and procedures must also be in place for patient and volunteer subject transfers from wheelchairs and gurneys to the MR system table. Only those individuals trained in the proper techniques should perform lifts and transfers of human subjects in order to prevent injuries. Depending on the number of patient/volunteer transfers necessary, purchasing a patient lift sling may prove to be indispensible.

Patients and volunteer subjects participating in a research study that requires the administration of a contrast media intravenously undergoes the intra-catheter placement in the patient preparation room immediately prior to the MRI examination. This prevents using valuable MR system time for this type of preparation that can be time consuming in the event that veins are not easily accessed.

As previously mentioned, specific instruction for the preparation and placement of earplugs or other hearing protection must be given as well as checking to ensure necessary hearing protection will be provided (1-4). If the MRI examination includes audio delivery via headphones (e.g., fMRI), sanitary covers are required. As hearing damage from exposure to loud noise is cumulative and typically irreversible, this procedure should be given adequate time to complete successfully.

Research MRI studies may involve more than one individual in a family. There may be times when an entire family is present for the MRI examination. If there are small children being imaged, the entire family may be waiting in the patient preparation room or control room in the MRI suite. Therefore, researchers must be on constant alert, monitoring the whereabouts of each of the family members, especially the children. It is helpful to point out to each family member the areas they can and cannot access. For example, "that is the door into the MR system room, so no one enters that room without one of the researchers taking you in." It is also a good idea to remind parents and spouses who are not going into the MR system room that they cannot enter the area without being properly screened and prepared even if their child or spouse calls out for them. Keeping the scanner room door closed during these studies is always important to ensure that family members are not accidentally "lured" in by the sight of their child or spouse on the table of the MR system.

They should be reminded they are to wait in the patient preparation room or in the control room and not wander about the MRI suite.

POSITIONING AND IMMOBILIZING OF PATIENTS AND VOLUNTEER SUBJECTS

An explanation pertaining to the MR system and the planned examination is highly recommended for all patients and volunteer subjects. This is the critical first step in securing their trust and compliance. This should include a brief explanation describing the MR system, the room, lighting, fan control, intercom system, and use of the emergency squeeze ball.

Instructions should also include the value of maintaining position of the anatomy plus control of breathing and swallowing, if pertinent to the anatomy being imaged. Patients and volunteer subjects should be reminded not to rearrange any of the devices or accessories placed in the MR system (**Figure 6**). If modifications are necessary, the researchers should be immediately notified via the intercom system or squeeze ball to make the requested changes for the patient or volunteer subject. This is especially important for many items including cables and RF coils, mirrors and/or screens used in fMRI studies, and GSR (galvanic skin response) cables, eye trackers, EEG caps and cables, and TMS coils.

Pads and sponges are strategically placed to immobilize and comfort the patient or volunteer subject. They are also used to provide safety and prevent burns as previously de-

Figure 6. To prevent unwanted interactions and possible excessive heating, patients and volunteer subjects should be reminded that they should not rearrange any devices or accessories placed in the MR system bore with them. This includes all monitoring devices, visual aids, and RF coils.

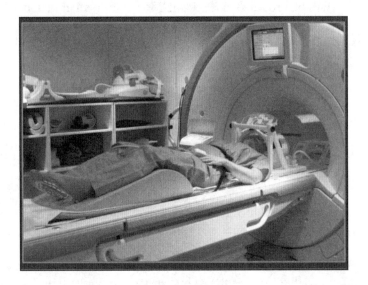

scribed (1-4). These procedures are especially critical if the RF body coil is being used to transmit RF energy.

Whenever the patient or volunteer subject is moving into or out of the MR system, the researchers are to closely observe the process to ensure it is completed without injury to the person being scanned or damage to the equipment or accessories. Furthermore, the patients and volunteer subjects should be instructed to notify the researchers via the intercom system and/or squeeze ball if they feel or experience anything uncomfortable or painful. They should be reminded that the fan can be turned on or the speed increased if they become too warm, or blankets can be added if they become too cold.

After leaving the MR system room and returning to the control room, the researcher is to immediately check in with the patient or volunteer subject using the intercom system to inquire about their present state. Notifying the individual of the upcoming scan time, table (cradle) motion, and pre-scan (tuning) procedure is very important as part of maintaining communication. This will reassure the individual that he or she has not been left alone or abandoned. This communication should take place at the end of each scan to inquire about the patient's or volunteer subject's condition as well as immediately before each subsequent scan, coaching the individual to remain still, breathe quietly, and to relax.

EMERGENCY PROCEDURES

Instruction in emergency procedures is provided to researchers as part of the training for the MRI Safety Policies and Procedures. This includes fire and earthquake training but is particularly focused on emergent removal of the patient or volunteer subject from the MR system and the room, itself (e.g., in the event of a magnet quench).

The researchers are instructed in the proper evacuation techniques to follow if the patient or volunteer subject should become unresponsive. This includes removing the cradle from the MR system using the emergency handle that releases it (i.e., the table top) from the "trolley unit" that pulls and pushes the cradle in and out of the scanner. Importantly, for some MR system with detachable tables, the cradle must be in the "home" position before the table can be undocked from the front of the MR system and moved out of the room. If the research MR system does not have a patient table that undocks and rolls away from the scanner, an appropriate gurney (i.e., MR Safe or MR Conditional) must be readily available in the MRI suite as well as an appropriate transport board or roller system. The transport board or roller system allows the researchers to safely and quickly move the patient or volunteer subject from the table onto the gurney without experiencing possible injuries.

Selecting the appropriate pedal at the foot end of the table undocks the MRI patient table. On some MR systems, there exists a backup release handle typically located under or near the docking unit at the housing of the scanner. Arm rails should be raised to prevent the patient or volunteer subject from falling off of the table during the transport out of the room to the patient preparation room.

In the case of a serious emergency, one researcher is responsible for calling first responders (e.g., 911) if the MRI research facility is a stand-alone building and not attached to a hospital. This researcher then promptly goes to the front door of the MRI research facility to receive the paramedics and quickly direct them to the appropriate MRI area. The second researcher is responsible for moving the patient or volunteer subject out of the MR system, undocking the table and moving the table into the patient preparation room, closing the MR system room door, and monitoring the individual until the paramedics arrive. Emergent care must never be conducted in the MR system room due to the increased risk of metal objects being brought into the MRI environment, as previously stated. The MRI pre-procedure screening form that was completed by the subject should be made available to the paramedics when they arrive as they will need information regarding current conditions and medications.

For a quench, the procedures include information for a deliberate/controlled quench (e.g., in a 'life or death' situation) and a spontaneous quench (e.g., in the event of an earthquake or substantial problem with the magnet of the MR system) (1-4). Researchers would be responsible to deliberately activate a quench if an individual, for example, is pinned to the magnet by a large metal object and is unable to get loose, and/or has experienced life-threatening injuries. A comprehensive set of instructions with easy-to-follow bullets is posted in the MRI suites with regard to instructions to follow for a quench. During hands-on training, the location and function of the quench button is reviewed with researchers. In the event of a spontaneous quench, researchers are instructed to quickly remove the patient or volunteer subject from the MR system and turn on the emergency exhaust fan in the room to remove any collection of helium gas that may form.

POTENTIAL ABNORMALITIES

Researchers are required to evaluate all MR images reconstructed at the MR system during the examination and those reconstructed off-line as soon as possible to identify motion artifacts, artifacts from other sources, and potential abnormalities. If the majority of images acquired during an MRI research study are not transferred to PACS for an interpretation by a radiologist, then specific procedures must be in place for researchers to follow in the event of a possible abnormality. Anything that is observed in the images that is suspected of being a potential abnormality is reported to the MRI research technologists. A medical record number and accession number should be generated, and forwarded to PACS. Results are forwarded to the PI and researcher who conducted the scan. The PI or representative then discusses the report with the patient or volunteer subject, and forwards the results to the individual's physician.

The researchers are also required to report to the MRI Manager, MRI research technologists, or lab director any suspicious artifacts present in the images. It is then determined if these fall under potential abnormalities, presence of metal in the body or biomedical implants, system software or hardware issues, or subject-generated (e.g., from motion) artifacts.

EXIT FORM

All patients and volunteer subjects are required to complete an Exit Form immediately after the scan concludes and before leaving the MRI research facility (**Figure 7**). This form is designed so that the researcher completes the top half of the form while the subject is

Figure 7. An example of an Exit Form that should be completed by the patient or volunteer subject immediately after the MRI examination. This information provides a conduit to provide feedback to the researchers and those individuals managing the MRI research facility. Additionally, these completed forms provide evidence to the level of safety that is being maintained at the MRI research facility.

EXIT FORM for SCAN SUBJECTS
Xxxxx Center MR Research Studies

☞ PLEASE PRINT LEGIBLY
☞ PLEASE COMPLETE ALL SECTIONS BEFORE EXITING MAGNET SUITE

Researcher completes this section

Magnet: ☐ 3T1   ☐ 3T2   ☐ 3T3   ☐ 7T

Date_____ Researcher name_____ PI name_____

Anatomy scanned: ☐Brain ☐Chest ☐Abdomen ☐C Spine ☐T Spine ☐L Spine
                  ☐Neck ☐Breast ☐Pelvis   ☐Shoulder ☐Knee ☐Other:_____

Coil: ☐ 8 channel Head ☐ 8 channel NeuroVascular ☐ 32 channel Nova Head ☐ Cardiac 8ch Array
      ☐Other_____

Scan subject name_____ Date of Birth_____

Gender: ☐Female ☐Male   Phone #_____

Scan subject completes this section

Current medical conditions?_____

Medications currently using?_____

Current medical treatments?_____

On a scale from 1 (**most** comfortable) to 5 (**least** comfortable):

	most				least
How comfortable were you **before** the scan?	☐1	☐2	☐3	☐4	☐5
How comfortable were you **during** the scan?	☐1	☐2	☐3	☐4	☐5
How comfortable were you **after** the scan?	☐1	☐2	☐3	☐4	☐5

During the MR exam did you experience any of the following:

Nervousness	☐ Yes	☐ No	Sleepiness	☐ Yes	☐ No
Muscle Stimulation	☐ Yes	☐ No	Dizziness	☐ Yes	☐ No
Heat Sensation	☐ Yes	☐ No	Headache	☐ Yes	☐ No
Changes in vision	☐ Yes	☐ No	Nausea	☐ Yes	☐ No
Unusual Taste	☐ Yes	☐ No	Pain	☐ Yes	☐ No

Other_____
_____
_____

Signature of Scan Subject_____

Questions: Xxxxx Xxxxxxx, (111) 111-1111, Xxxxx Center for Imaging, Xxxxxx University School of Medicine, xxxxxxxx@xxxxx.edu

Rev. 10 2/7/13

being scanned, and then the individual completes the bottom half. The top half of the form includes the MR system at which they were scanned, RF coil used and anatomy scanned, date, researcher and PI name, and patient/study subject information. The bottom half includes questions regarding medical conditions, medications and treatments, a comfort scale for before, during, and after the MRI examination, and questions regarding nervousness, muscle stimulation, vision changes, unusual taste, dizziness, headache, nausea and pain.

The Exit Form provides the patient and volunteer subject with a conduit to provide feedback to the researchers and those individuals managing the MRI research facility. Importantly, this is valuable information concerning many aspects of the research examinations and the respective MR systems. All completed forms are entered into a secure database. This database also provides evidence to the level of safety that is being maintained at a specific MRI research facility. Since the early 1990s, regulatory agencies, primarily in Europe, have sought to limit exposure of humans to MRI. Due to concerns on the part of researchers and staff at MRI facilities, discussions initiated during the International Society for Magnetic Resonance in Medicine's (ISMRM) MRI Safety Committee meetings identified methods to provide data to ensure that accurate regulations were implemented. These included the collecting of data from patients post-examination in association with different MR systems.

CONCLUSIONS

Potential risks exist in the MRI environment for, not only the patient or volunteer subject, but also for MRI technologists, other healthcare professionals, physicians, and others who only intermittently access the MR system room. This becomes a more complex issue in the research setting because there is often more freedom for a wide variety of individuals present in the facility including researchers and scientists, research assistants, students and post-docs, physicians, visiting scholars, and research and administrative staff. Intermittent but routine visitors to the research MRI facility include manufacturer representatives and scientists from various companies developing products, camera and photography personnel taping for television programs and documentaries, and other specialized healthcare professionals from nursing, anesthesia and respiratory therapy. Insofar as many of these individuals may not be healthcare professionals but investigators engaging in a systematic activity to acquire knowledge, it is often difficult to successfully manage all MRI safety policies and procedures that are set down by the MRI Safety Committee. This requires ongoing monitoring of all those using the research MR systems including regular verbal and written reminders. This continued one-on-one communication should convey to the researchers a genuine interest in their safety, as well as the patients and volunteer subjects, and the MR system, ancillary equipment, and ultimately, an interest in the successful completion of the research study.

As George Bernard Shaw (Irish playwright and a co-founder of the London School of Economics, 1856 to 1950) said, "The single biggest problem in communication is the illusion that it has taken place." Continuing communication, both facilitated and offered, is a critical tool in maintaining safety in the MRI environment. In addition, any and all assumptions must be entirely removed, as they are certainly the beginning of a dangerous and risky path for all present.

REFERENCES

1. Kanal E, Barkovich AJ, Bell C. et al. ACR guidance document on MR safe practices: 2013. J Magn Reson Imaging 2013;37:501-530.

2. Kanal E, Barkovich AJ, Bell C, et al. ACR guidance document for safe MR practices: 2007. Am J Roentgenol 2007;188:1447-74.

3. Shellock FG, Spinazzi A. MRI safety update 2008: part 2, screening patients for MRI. Am J Roentgenol 2008;191:1-10.

4. Shellock FG. Reference Manual For Magnetic Resonance Safety, Implants, and Devices: 2013 Edition. Los Angeles, CA: Biomedical Research Publishing Group; 2013.

5. Shellock FG, Crues JV. MR procedures: biologic effects, safety, and patient care. Radiology 2004;232:635-652.

6. American Society for Testing and Materials (ASTM) International, Designation: F2503-08. Standard Practice for Marking Medical Devices and Other Items for Safety in the Magnetic Resonance Environment. ASTM International, West Conshohocken, PA, 2008.

7. Woods TO. Standards for medical devices in MRI: present and future. J Magn Reson Imaging 2007;26:1186-1189.

8. Shellock FG. Radiofrequency energy-induced heating during MR procedures: a review. J Magn Reson Imaging 2000:12:30-36.

9. Schaefer DJ. Safety aspects of radiofrequency power deposition in magnetic resonance. Magn Reson Imaging Clin N Am 1998;6:775-89.

10. Shellock FG. Guest Editorial. Comments on MRI heating tests of critical implants. J Magn Reson Imaging 2007;26:1182-1185.

11. http://www.mrisafety.com

12. http://www.IMRSER.org, website for the Institute for Magnetic Resonance Safety, Education, and Research.

13. Schenck JF. Safety of strong, static magnetic fields. J Magn Reson Imaging 2000;12,2-19.

14. Baker KB, Tkach JA, Nyenhuis JA, et al. Evaluation of specific absorption rate as a dosimeter of MRI-Related implant heating. J Magn Reson Imaging 2004;20:315-320.

15. Kuhl CK, Träber F, Schild HH. Whole-body high-field-strength (3.0-T) MR imaging in clinical practice. Part I. Technical considerations and clinical applications. Radiology 2008;246:675-96.

16. Kuhl CK, Träber F, Gieseke J, et al. Whole-body high-field-strength (3.0-T) MR imaging in clinical practice. Part II. Technical considerations and clinical applications. Radiology 2008;247:16-35.

17. Shellock FG. MRI Safety and Neuromodulation Systems. In: Krames ES, Peckham PH, Rezai AR, Editors. Neuromodulation. New York: Academic Press/Elsevier; 2009.

18. Schaefer DJ, Bourland JD, Nyenhuis JA. Review of patient safety in time-varying gradient fields. J Magn Reson Imaging 2000;12:20-29.

19. Shellock FG. Biomedical implants and devices: assessment of magnetic field interactions with a 3.0-Tesla MR system. J Magn Reson Imaging 2002;16:721-732.

20. Levine GN, Gomes AS, Arai AE, et al. Safety of magnetic resonance imaging in patients with cardiovascular devices: an American Heart Association scientific statement from the Committee on Diagnostic and Interventional Cardiac Catheterization. Circulation 2007;116:2878-91.

21. Shinbane J, Colletti P, Shellock FG. MR in patients with pacemakers and ICDs: defining the Issues. J Cardiovascular Magnetic Resonance 2007;9:5-13.

22. Armstrong ML, Elkins L. Body art and MRI. Am J Nurs 2005;105:65-6.

23. DeBoer S, Fishman D, Chwals W, Straus C, Amundson T. Body piercing/tattooing and trauma diagnostic imaging: medical myths vs. realities. J Trauma Nurs 2007;14:35-8.

24. Muensterer OJ. Temporary removal of navel piercing jewelry for surgery and imaging studies. Pediatrics 2004;114:e384-6.

25. Shellock FG, Karacozoff AM. Detection of implants and other objects using a ferromagnetic detection system: implications for patient screening prior to MRI. Am J Roentgenol (In Press).

Chapter 26   Safety Issues for Interventional MR Systems

Daniel F. Kacher, M.S. - 1
Janice Fairhurst, B.S., R.T. (R)(MR) - 2
Ramon F. Martin, M.D., Ph.D. - 3
Lawrence P. Panych, Ph.D. - 2
Angela Kanan, R.N., BSN, CRN - 2
Ehud J. Schmidt, Ph.D. - 2
Nobuhiko Hata, Ph.D. - 2
Ferenc A. Jolesz, M.D. - 2

1 - Biomedical Engineering Department
2 - Radiology Department
3 - Anesthesiology Department
Brigham and Women's Hospital
Harvard Medical School
Boston, MA

INTRODUCTION

During the last two decades, interventional and intraoperative uses of magnetic resonance imaging (MRI) have evolved into important applications for image-guided therapy and surgical procedures (1, 2). These two unique uses of MRI technology will be referred to as "iMRI" in this chapter. Because iMRI involves toolsets not used in diagnostic MRI, it presents multiple challenges in designing a safe work environment (3). The complex and unique workflow of therapy and surgical procedures may involve anesthesia and new approaches for perioperative and intraoperative care. Various clinical applications have to be translated to the MRI environment, adapted from the interventional suite and the operating room (OR) (4, 5). For example, percutaneous needle-based procedures (6), percutaneous thermal ablations (7), catheter-based intravascular interventions (8), endoscopies (9), and open surgeries (10-12) have special instrumentation and access requirements. The therapy-related armamentarium for each type of procedure can introduce not only difficult requirements for integration with the MRI technology (13, 14), but also an increasing need for safety. In this more active and potentially chaotic environment, assuring safety for the patient and staff members is a priority. This chapter presents the most important aspects of safety in the interventional and intraoperative environments based on more than twenty years of experience using multiple types of MR systems and with a large number of clinical applications at the Brigham and Women's Hospital.

The design of interventional suites and ORs requires consideration of various workflow paradigms related to the procedures. If image-guidance is involved, the imaging systems should be closely integrated with the procedural workflow (15). However, since imaging systems potentially can cause injuries and harm to the patient and personnel, safety issues are of paramount importance. Safety issues in the iMRI environment are inherently unique. These factors must be considered when an MRI interventional suite is designed and built (16). Furthermore, when an intraoperative MR system is located in an OR environment, the requirements are even more complex, since MRI safety has to be combined with other patient safety measures (5). If an MR system is co-located with an X-ray (XMRI), positron emission tomography (PET), or computed tomography (CT) system, then MRI safety issues are compounded with concerns regarding system interactions and the use of ionizing radiation (17).

The Advanced Multimodality Image Guided Operating (AMIGO) Suite at the Brigham and Women's Hospital (BWH) is comprised of three procedure rooms: a central OR with a ceiling-mounted, single-plane x-ray machine flanked by a positron emission tomography (PET)/computed tomograph (CT) room on one side and an MR system on the other. Sliding doors adjoin the three rooms (18). Each room has a separate entrance to the control corridor and support spaces (**Figure 1**). This area contains every safety challenge experienced by other iMRI sites. Minimally invasive procedures done in the MR room involve an in-and-out approach, in which the patient is scanned at isocenter then withdrawn partially from the bore of the scanner for continued intervention. All devices and instruments used in this setting must be MR Safe or MR Conditional. In the center OR, a combination of conventional MR Unsafe ferromagnetic devices and instruments are used for a variety of procedures but are moved outside of the five-gauss line or removed from the room before the ceiling-mounted, mobile 3-Tesla MR system enters the room for the imaging portion of the procedure (19). To acquire a PET/CT scan during an OR procedure, the patient is shuttled along a removable bridge that connects the OR table with the PET/CT table, through the sliding doors that adjoin the rooms, and into the adjacent stationary PET/CT scanner. Although the MRI risks are absent, the hazards associated with moving an intubated patient with intravenous access are present. The AMIGO Suite will be used in this chapter as an example to illustrate the safety issues for iMRI systems and to propose solutions. The valuable perspectives of other groups related to this topic have also been published (20- 24).

Various competing paradigms have emerged for suite design and procedural workflow (25). Additionally, the procedure types are expanding (20). The facilities built to support iMRI are unique and often reflect the designer and the specific purpose of the space. Although safety issues related to iMRI can be challenging, they can be minimized and managed through effective policies, procedures, staff training, access controls, and facility design to promote best practices and the correction of safety lapses.

Figure 1. (Top) Floor plan showing the size of each room and its respective control room as well as the equipment in each room and its maneuverability. (Bottom) Panoramic cutaway rendering of the areas (courtesy of Balazs Lengyel M.D.).

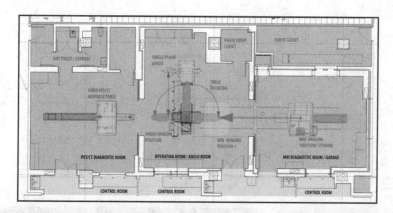

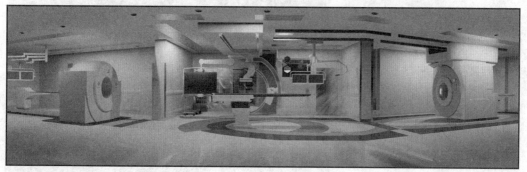

DESIGNING FOR SAFETY

Architectural design is one useful means of facilitating desired behaviors for MRI safety. Selecting a space remote from the main OR enables personnel to enter the mindset that they are not in their usual working environment and need to adapt their habits to the MRI environment. A remote location further limits the flow of personnel not involved with the procedure. In a code or other emergency situation, it affords the opportunity to post a healthcare professional at the door to ensure only personnel trained to be in the space are responding. The disadvantage of a remote location is the impaired rapid response by additional anesthesiologists and other healthcare professionals. Because the AMIGO Suite is located near a cardiology recovery room, anesthesia personnel from that space, rather than from the OR, would respond.

The AMIGO Suite was laid out in accordance with recommendations from the American College of Radiology (ACR) document pertaining to the MRI environment by which the first layer of swipe-card access enables personnel to enter from Zone I (public space) into Zone II (a restricted personnel gowning area) (27) (**Figure 2**). A second swipe-card access point is located at the entrance to Zone III (the control room corridor).

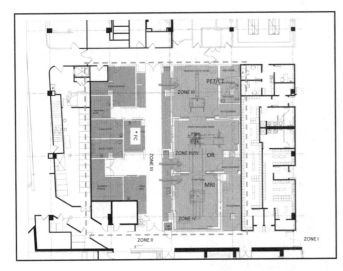

Figure 2. The floor plan for the AMIGO Suite. (Left) Procedure space is to the right of the central corridor and support space is to the left. The ACR designed zones are labelled. The position of the flow coordinator (* FC) is central to the suite. The dashed lines show the boundary of the suite. The arrows indicate the doors into the three procedure rooms.

(Right) Cutaway rendering of the three procedure rooms (courtesy of Balazs Lengyel, M.D.).

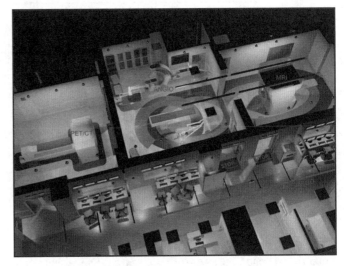

The MR system room is in Zone IV, where all personnel must be MRI safety-trained or under direct supervision, and no ferrous objects are allowed. Depending on the location of the MR system, the OR shifts between Zone III, where ferromagnetic objects are permitted, and Zone IV. As a policy decision, all personnel entering the OR are required to make themselves essentially ferrous-free, meaning no analog watches, pagers, cell phones, wallets, and other similar items regardless of the location of the MR system.

Before the MR system enters the OR, the sliding door that adjoins the OR and MR rooms opens to create one large shielded room and enables the MR scanner to move along the ceiling-mounted rails into the OR. Upon opening the sliding doors, the MRI control room door automatically locks to prevent personnel from entering while the MRI technologist prepares the patient for the scan. The control room is considered Zone III and is under the control of AMIGO Suite's Flow Coordinator, a post that is continuously manned during business hours. All access points are monitored by security cameras connected to the Flow Coordinator's desk and hospital security.

This layout mandates that non-ambulatory patients be wheeled into the control corridor before entering the appropriate procedure rooms, a practice not consistent with interventional spaces such as cardiac catheter labs, which have a hallway parallel to the control corridor at the rear of the procedure room with a second door into each procedure room for patients to enter and exit. If another entry point like this were to be added to an iMRI suite, a proper line-of-site from the control corridor to the door would not be possible, and the desired restriction of personnel access would be compromised. The complexity of controlling access into the MR system room (Zone IV) also increases at sites (i.e., unlike the AMIGO Suite), where a single MR system services multiple ORs.

The doors into the procedure rooms can be activated by a push plate or set to a mode requiring a keypad code. The keypad code is held by only a few core staff members. Controlling or eliminating pathways for personnel flow helps to ensure that no MR Unsafe devices or instruments are brought into the room with the MR system.

With regard to the AMIGO Suite, a ferromagnetic detection system was installed in the Zone III control corridor (**Figure 3**). Since completion of our project, the use of such a device has become a standard Facilities Guideline Institute requirement for all future MRI projects. A single ferromagnetic detection system services both the OR and MRI rooms. Due to space constraints, the ferromagnetic detection system was not installed at the entrances to the OR and MRI procedure rooms because the width of the doors would mandate a wider system, lowering the sensitivity of ferromagnetic detection. Moreover, devices with ferrous metallic components (e.g., the surgical microscope or ultrasound machine) are routinely brought into the OR in a controlled manner. It was determined during the design phase that alarm fatigue would cause personnel to disregard the alarms from the ferromagnetic detection system when a true issue arose. Personnel use the ferromagnetic detection system after checking in with the Flow Coordinator and removing unwanted items that are placed in day lockers where cell phones, pagers, or other similar problematic objects are deposited before entering Zone IV rooms.

MRI danger signs were posted on doors and conspicuous mats that read "Stop Magnet Always On" were placed on the floor. Indicator lights above the doors inform personnel in which room the MR system is "parked", and when X-ray or the laser is in use (**Figure 3**). Importantly, while signage is necessary, in reality, it is seldom effective. Physical barriers such as locked doors and limited entrances are crucial to mitigate risk in the iMRI environment.

SAFETY POLICIES AND PROCEDURES

Policies and procedures, which can be difficult to standardize, are tailored for site appropriateness. An issue all facilities have in common is the daunting risk inherent to combining medical procedures and iMRI. It has now been many years since the patient fatality (28-29) that galvanized the MRI community to deal with safety issues centered on diagnostic MRI. Despite policy recommendations and raised awareness since that event (30), it has been suggested there has been an increase in the number of reported accidents related to the MRI environment (31). Risks tend to be greater in the iMRI environment. Frequently, ferrous materials and devices are knowingly introduced into the environment to accomplish

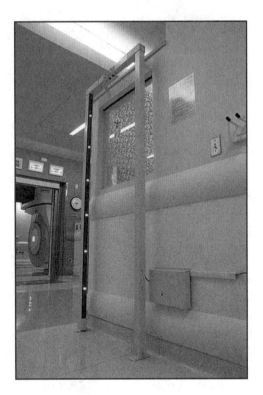

Figure 3. (Left) Ferromagnetic detection system. The LEDs will depict the location on the body where a ferromagnetic object may be detected. Illuminated signage is seen in the background above the door to the MRI procedure room.

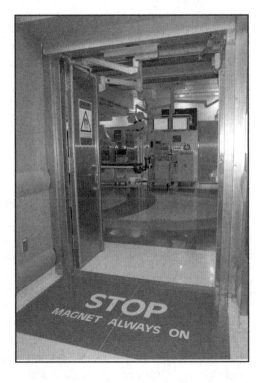

(Right) Safety mat at entrance to the OR and fringe field values marked on the floor.

certain tasks. Furthermore, the use of necessary interventional devices and monitoring equipment can increase the risk of patient burns associated with imaging if not properly used.

Whereas suite design can facilitate acceptable behavior from personnel by limiting or directing flow within the suite, the department policies are meant to establish a desired set of behaviors and are subject to the fallibility of the individual. A clear and effective safety policy is a valuable tool to reduce risk. Establishing a dedicated multidisciplinary core team assigned daily to the iMRI environment is an important factor to formalize, promulgate, and enforce policies and procedures that help ensure safety within the suite. Primary issues that should be addressed by all iMRI sites include training, access, and safety checklists. Policy governing site-specific issues such as the shared use of space for clinical and research purposes as well as the management of tour groups and vendors should be considered. Other centers have site-specific issues such as the shared use of the installation for interventional and/or intraoperative use and diagnostic imaging (32).

Training and Testing

All personnel who work in or have duties that require them to have access to the AMIGO Suite must complete AMIGO safety training prior to receiving unrestricted access to the area. Training and testing ensure that all individuals working in the suite have a clear understanding of policy and procedures and fully comprehend the potential risks associated with MRI and radiation hazards in the AMIGO environment. Training modules include: a general suite orientation, MRI safety, and general radiation safety. Staff members must pass a written exam on MRI safety and have no contraindications to working in the MRI environment, as documented on an MRI safety screening form that is reviewed by the MRI Technologist or Flow Coordinator. Upon successful completion of training, a visual indicator is added to the hospital badge.

Procedure Vetting Process

All procedures in the AMIGO Suite are performed under Institutional Review Board (IRB) approval. An application describing the procedure, focusing on the impact that image guidance is likely to have on patient outcomes, is required. An internal and external panel reviews the application and refines the proposed procedure. This process forces clinicians to invest their time learning about the MRI environment.

The next step in preparation for new iMRI procedures is to conduct multiple mock procedures to refine workflow, decrease procedure time, and to do a gap analysis on devices and instruments. All personnel who will be involved in the case must be present for these sessions. The sessions are videotaped and analyzed. Failure Mode and Effects Analysis can be applied to identify and address areas of concern. Volunteer imaging and MRI protocol development is typically done outside of these sessions for the sake of brevity. Team building and cohesion as well as the creation of a culture of safety occur during this crucial period. In these mock sessions, procedure specific MRI safety checklists are developed and tailored to include both equipment and work flow. These safety checklists are reviewed in the OR before the MR system enters the room.

Tailored Checklists and Tailored Roles

Typically, the MRI technologists are the primary personnel tasked with ensuring MRI safety in the diagnostic imaging area. In the iMRI setting, safety challenges require the expertise of a more diverse group. In addition to our core team members who have specific roles for each procedure, it has been necessary to create two new roles whose focus is entirely on safety and compliance within the suite during a procedure.

The first new role is a Safety Nurse, who is neither scrubbed into the procedure nor circulating, and is responsible for knowing the roles and background of all personnel in the procedure and adjoining space (and ensuring unnecessary personnel are ejected from the space). The Safety Nurse is charged with tracking items and when and why each piece of equipment is introduced into the procedure (and ensuring unneeded equipment is not admitted). He or she administrates the safety checklists in conjunction with the MRI technologist.

Figure 4 shows the safety checklists used to mitigate risks prior to bringing the patient into the iMRI room or the adjoining OR as well as the safety checklists used between procedures in the OR prior to each time the MR system is moved into the room via tracks on the ceiling. Each procedure has a checklist tailored to the equipment and instruments used and modified to adapt to changes in the procedure as it evolves. The MRI status of each device is noted and appropriate actions are taken to ensure safety and artifact free imaging.

Ceiling-mounted booms, lights, and monitors are pivoted towards the walls where rails have been installed as tether points. For the patient, it is confirmed that he or she has hearing protection and the monopolar electrosurgical unit return electrode is removed, which may be a risk for an MRI-induced patient burn due to the conductive foil backing. The checklist mandates an accurate instrument count, since consequences of an inaccurate count are increased in the iMRI environment. A ferrous tool can become projectile when the patient enters the bore of the scanner. If the tool is touching the patient, an image artifact or even a burn can occur. Consistent with our institution-wide policy, the World Health Organization Surgical Safety Checklists are also used before inducing anesthesia, before skin incision, and before the patient leaves the OR (33).

The MRI technologist is the *de facto* MRI Safety Officer for the suite, in charge of screening the patient prior to the procedure. The MRI technologist may reference literature and established criteria to confirm that an implant can be safely imaged. Another role of the MRI technologist is to collect MRI data, sometimes in conjunction with an MRI physicist, and to gather vendor claims about a new device for review by an internal committee before it is used in proximity to the MR system.

Another new role is that of the Flow Coordinator who sits at a central location in the suite. He or she has camera views of the Zone I to Zone II transition as well as the Zone II to Zone III transition. The Flow Coordinator is responsible for maintaining a sign-in list of all personnel present for a procedure and ensures each team member has undergone all necessary training, is properly attired, has removed ferrous items from their person, and has undergone screening using the ferromagnetic detection system. The watchful eyes and constant communication involving the Safety Nurse, Flow Coordinator, MRI technologist and other personnel associated with the procedure have prevented many potential errors in the two years of operation of the AMIGO Suite.

Emergency Response

Personnel including anesthesiologists, nurses, surgeons, interventionalists, radiologists, and MRI technologists should be trained to respond to cardiopulmonary emergencies that may occur either in the MR scanner room or in the OR with the MR system present. Mock emergency code drills (e.g., code blue) are important for refining the processes and to gain comfort levels surrounding the different situations. Policy and education should exist to prevent responders from other areas from bringing ferrous materials and equipment into the scanner room.

Figure 4. (a) Checklist used during "pause" before the patient is brought into iMRI room or the adjoining OR.

BRIGHAM AND WOMEN'S HOSPITAL
AMIGO CHECKLIST

Date/Time _____

Pre-Procedure MRI Safety Checklist – Before Entering OR or MRI Room

ACTION		Verified
Confirm patient is on MR Safe stretcher	MR Tech/RN	
MRI patient screening form completed	MR Tech/RN	
Jewelry & ferrous items removed	MR Tech/RN	
Eyeglasses ___ Dentures___ Hearing-aid ___ Medication Patch ___ removed	MR Tech/RN	
All staples/paperclips removed from chart/forms that will enter room	MR Tech/RN	
Self pat-down completed; ferrous items removed (pager, phone etc)	MR Tech/RN	

Signature: _____RN Circulator

Signature: _____MRI Tech

Last edited on 9/26/2013

(b) Checklist used during "pause" prior to bringing the ceiling mounted mobile 3-T MR system into the OR.

BRIGHAM AND WOMEN'S HOSPITAL
AMIGO CHECKLIST

Date/Time _____

Checklist for Moving Magnet into OR prior to surgery

	Pre-Op Image	Intra-op Image	Post-op Image
SELF PAT DOWN PERFORMED BY EACH TEAM MEMBER			
• Patient placed in final position for procedure and imaging			
• Safety straps in place			
• Pressure points are padded			
• Bair Hugger blanket in place (if needed)			
• Teds or (SCD) sleeves applied (if needed)			
• Earplugs inserted and secure			
• MRI coil has no loops and is not touching patient			
• No direct skin to skin contact			
• Foley catheter is draining; metal clamp removed from tubing & *replaced with orange plastic clamp*			
• Surgical clipper and head is removed from room			
Confirm Surgical Counts are done			
• Remove all instruments, needles, sharps, small accessories/countables from surgical field			
• Perform counts *of above ferrous items* & verbally report and document that counts correct			
• Patient cleared by RN/MRI tech			
Move ALL equipment outside 5 gauss line			
• *All equipment tethered*			
• *All booms tethered*			
• *All lights moved*			
• *Ferrous Angio foot pedal TIE down *** remove from room*			
• *Remove Dosimeter/lead aprons*			
Patient Safety Check			
• Confirm earplugs in place			
• Remove ESU return electrode (grounding pad) and cord			
• Remove ESU pencil and cord			
• Remove bipolar forceps and cord			
• Remove suction tubing and suction tips			
Anesthesia counts completed and correct			
Patient draped for scan			
Check to make sure Sliding door pathways have been cleared			
MR/OR doors opened by MRI Technologist			
Final safety check completed: RN & MRI Tech			
Verbal OK & Initials			
• RN #1 MRI Tech			

Signature: _____RN

In the AMIGO Suite, the emergency code button has a different meaning from the code button in other areas of the hosptial. A special MRI-trained team with swipe-card access responds to the emergency. Currently, there is no equipment available that is MR Conditional to resuscitate a patient. Therefore, the patient undergoing an intervention in the MR system room is immediately removed from the room and brought to a designated code area within the suite. Some scanners have break-away tables that can serve as a transport table. Scanners with fixed tables require that the patient is transferred to an MR Safe or MR Conditional stretcher. A designated team member should be responsible for shutting and locking the MRI room door and maintaining access restrictions, while other personnel expeditiously move the patient to the location outside the MR system room (Zone IV) where resuscitation will be performed. The area should have adequate space, oxygen, suction, and electrical outlets for to facilitate resuscitation and management of a patient.

If the MR system is in the OR when an emergency occurs, the MR system is removed from the OR, and then the doors to the MRI room are closed and locked. Once the magnetic field has been removed from the OR, the crash cart, defibrillator, and other rescusitation equipment can then enter the OR area.

Although known difficult intubation or prior history of allergic reaction to medication or a contrast agent can be addressed prior to entering the MR system room (Zone IV), unanticipated difficult intubation or an anaphylactic reaction requires quick action and exit from this area. The oxygen used in the OR setting as well as therapeutic heat sources (e.g., laser) increase the risk of fire. Non-ferrous fire extinguishers are available for management of small fires. In the rare event of a quench, boiling off cryogens can displace the oxygen in the room. Sites should have a plan for rapid removal of patients in these life-threatening situations, even when there is no time to close a surgical wound.

Screening

Patient screening must be conducted by an MRI safety-trained staff member (34, 35). The screening form combined with a verbal interview will help to rule out contraindications for MRI procedures such as cardiac pacemakers, ferromagnetic aneurysm clips, and certain electronically-actived implants. Personnel who work in the iMRI suite should be subjected to the same screening procedure. However, since the personnel will not be imaged, some contraindications (e.g., ferromagnetic aneurysm clips, pacemakers, etc.) do not need to be considered. Screening forms designed for patients and other individuals (i.e., staff members, visitors, etc.) may be obtained from the website, www.MRIsafety.com. Patients should change into a hospital gown as per surgical standard of care. External hearing aids, hairpins, barrettes, jewelry (including body piercings), analog watches, and similar items should be removed prior to entering the iMRI room or OR.

Patient Positioning

There is often a compromise between the ideal imaging position and the ideal surgical or interventional position. The ideal positioning centers the anatomy in the "sweet spot" of the magnet to enable imaging without distortion artifacts related to off-isocenter positioning. Sweet spot dimensions vary across MR systems but are typically 30- to 50-cm ellipsoids. Body habitus, rather than the patient's weight limit, can be an exclusion for an iMRI procedure. A patient with a large shoulder girth should be scheduled for a 'fit test' prior to booking the procedure.

In many iMRI cases, the patient will be under general anesthesia and unable to move. Therefore, it is essential that the patient be positioned properly and placed in proper alignment. All pressure points should be appropriately padded to maintain good circulation. Padding must be used to eliminate closed loops created by skin-to-skin contact or contact between the skin and an electrocardiogram (ECG) cable or the cable used with the RF coil. The integrity of the insulation and/or housing of all components, including RF coils, leads, cables, and wires need to be regularly checked.

SAFETY STANDARDS AND TESTING

Labeling

The American Society for Testing and Materials (ASTM) International has designated definitions (i.e., terminology) for labeling devices, including MR Safe, MR Conditional, and MR Unsafe (36). At our institution, handheld instruments that are too small for a label are color-coded: green for safe, yellow for conditional, and red for unsafe. Commercially available labels are used for larger devices. Any new instrument introduced to the procedure room is tested with a powerful handheld magnet by the AMIGO charge nurse, MRI technologist, or MRI physicist before being brought into a procedure room. Equipment used in the MR system room is either MR Safe or MR Conditional. Much of the equipment used in the OR is MR Unsafe, but is appropriately managed before the MR system enters the room. In the MRI room, an RF enclosure recessed in the wall houses MR Unsafe equipment. Waveguides in this enclosure enable IV tubing and temperature control hoses to be passed through from this area to the patient.

Another ASTM International standard (37) may be useful for creating a pass/fail criteria for determining if a handheld instrument or device has the potential to become a projectile in the presence of the magnetic field and involves testing for translational attraction (37). While the worst-case location is specific to the model of the MR system, even for scanners operating at the same field strength (e.g., Siemens 3-Tesla Trio versus Siemens 3-Tesla Verio), this position tends to be in the proximity of the opening of the bore of the MR system. Other ASTM International standards are used to test biomedical implants for torque (38), radiofrequency (RF)-induced heating (39), image artifact (40), and safety for active implants (41).

Although these standards are useful for implants, specific standards are needed for the task of evaluting items used in iMRI (e.g., robotic actuators, head fixation systems, infusion pumps, AC/DC power adaptors, biopsy trajectory devices, patient positioning devices, and others) but, at the present time, they do not exist. The MR system manufacturers have their own sets of tests for device evaluation. Accordingly, the end-user is largely reliant on the vendor for providing information for a given device. This information may be distributed by various means including the device user manual, vendor-issued bulletins, and labels on the device itself. As always, the term "MR Conditional" has specific meaning on a per device basis, requiring the user to be sophisticated enough to understand the meanings.

In the AMIGO Suite, dedicated anesthesia technologists manage the anesthesia equipment and appropriately position MR Conditional and MR Unsafe devices. As an example of the complexity, a device may have different maximum permissible field strengths where it can be safely used that is different from the AC/DC adaptor that powers it. It is the nature of some surgeries that the anesthesia set-up may be at the patient's left or right based on the surgical approach. As such, equipment is regularly moved. Human vigilance is essential for preventing error. If this process were managed by a larger non-dedicated group of personnel, the likelihood of error would substantially increase.

Claims are often specific to tested conditions, such as the strength of the static magnetic field, the spatial gradient of the magnetic field, imaging gradient slew rate and amplitude, specific absorption rate (SAR), and configuration or position of the device (e.g., parallel or perpendicular to the bore, proximity to the wall of the bore, routing for cables, etc.). Notably, after an equipment upgrade or change to the environment, testing results may no longer be applicable.

The ACR takes the position that, "… users need to recognize that one should never assume MR compatibility or safety information about a device if it is not clearly documented in writing" (27). Practices at the AMIGO Suite reflect an amplification of this recommendation but verify even written vendor claims, because some claims are inaccurate or nonapplicable. If in-house expertise exists, a set of tests can be performed to confirm vendor claims or establish the level of safety of an instrument or device (42).

Static Magnetic Field-Related Issues

Although the adverse events associated with diagnostic MRI that are most frequently reported in the Food and Drug Administration's (FDA) Manufacturer and User Facility Device Experience (MAUDE) database and in the United Kingdom (43) are due to burns, the greatest safety concern in environments where MRI-guided open surgeries (e.g., breast, brain, and spine) are performed are those related to the static magnetic field. Such procedures may require the use of MR Unsafe items such as surgical microscopes, electrosurgical units, and light sources.

The effect of the static magnetic field drastically increases with proximity to the bore of the MR system. This sudden change in translational attraction gives little warning to a staff member holding a ferrous object as he or she approaches the scanner. Lines indicting the fringe field levels associated with the MR system can be marked on the floor around the scanner to serve as a visual reminder to staff members. In the AMIGO Suite, the five-gauss fringe field is marked on the floor. The 400-gauss field line is also shown to indicate the limit for the particular anesthesia machine utilized in this setting. The MR system used in the AMIGO Suite can be offset and rotated 180-degrees to enable additional procedural workflows in the MRI room. Therefore, the fringe field markings on the floor are a superposition of the lines for the two different imaging locations. A second set of lines is present in the OR to depict the fringe field when the scanner is at its third imaging location.

Translational attraction and torque constitute the greatest risks in MRI. An object may become a projectile as it accelerates in the direction of the spatial gradients of the static magnetic field. Large objects can generate incredible force as they are rapidly drawn into the magnet. As previously stated, our practice is to test all devices, even with MR Safe labels, using a powerful handheld magnet. Additionally, we cautiously introduce such items into the MR room with a tether, if necessary, and follow other appropriate procedures to conduct a proper evaluation of magnetic field interactions.

For facilities performing surgery very close to the MR system or with the patient's head protruding from the rear of the scanner, MR Safe or MR Conditional instruments are necessary. Titanium, titanium alloy, and ceramic materials are not subject to magnetic field interactions and cause relatively small artifacts that are the direct result of their non-negligible magnetic susceptibilities. Various vendors at points in time produced instruments for the iMRI market (44). Understandably, costs and lead times for these instruments are higher than for conventional instruments. Some conventional off-the-shelf instruments are constructed from titanium, with the advantage of being lower in weight compared to steel.

Image Artifacts Caused by a Device

Electromagnetic interference (EMI) emanating from an active device can manifest in the MR image as a zipper artifact or increased noise across the whole image, depending on the bandwidth of the noise and of the MR system's receiver bandwidth. Vendors may erroneously assume that because their device passes EMI tests at a higher field strength/frequency, the test results can be extended to lower field strengths/frequencies. However, EMI harmonics may be present in the imaging bandwidth at one field strength, but not another. The user may learn this when a patient is undergoing MRI and a zipper artifact obscures the critical anatomy of interest.

EMI testing may be performed by running the MR system manufacturer's quality assurance scans for noise with and without the device present. The device can be activated, in a stand-by mode, or off but plugged in, depending on its state in the clinical setting during imaging. The particular frequency of the zipper can be identified and can be useful in tracing the source in the electronics. A zipper drifting in frequency usually indicates the source of EMI is the electronics associated with a digital clock in the device. The EMI revealed by such scans may have low enough energy as to not be clinically relevant, so scans from a clinical protocol should also be tested. Variations in shielding of MR Conditional devices has yielded one instance of a device that does not emit EMI and another that is problematic. A complicated issue, however, is the interactivity of multiple devices. EMI from one device can be carried or amplified by another device resulting in image artifacts when the devices used individually are not problematic. Moreover, EMI from a device may be a function of position within the room. The device may pick up and amplify EMI from a leaky penetration panel, window, or other vulnerable point in the radiofrequency (RF) shielding. A device placed in the line-of-site to the receive RF coil may induce a zipper artifact, whereas the same device placed on the side of the scanner may not be problematic. A spectrum analyzer with a sniffer loop is a valuable tool in identifying EMI sources. These analyzers are not MR Safe, so long cables are required.

Image artifacts can be assessed in phantoms by imaging with and without the test object present. Distortion or signal void due to susceptibility mismatch between the object and the surrounding medium can evaluated (45). Artifact is a function of field strength/frequency, pulse sequence parameters (mainly receiver bandwidth and echo time), and the orientation of the object to the static magnetic field of the MR system (46). Artifacts can change the apparent location of the device, which for example can give rise to inaccurate or unsafe needle targeting associated with a biopsy procedure (47). In open surgery, the susceptibility mismatch between air and tissue can appear as a region of hyperintensity that can mimic contrast-enhanced tissue (48). For this reason, it is our group's practice to fill surgical cavities with saline prior to imaging to move the artifact away from the region of interest.

Currents induced by the imaging gradients can interact with the static magnetic field and cause vibrations in a device, which can create ghosting in the image. The coupling of electrically conductive structures with the electromagnetic field can result in signal shielding. Such RF artifacts can compromise visualization of the lumen in the presence of a vascular stent (49).

Artifacts can lead to image misinterpretation due to distortion of geometry, or regionally obscuring or obliterating the signal from tissue. The degree of acceptable artifact is subject to the judgement of the physician performing the procedure and the radiologist interpreting the images. If contrast administration during brain tumor resection is repeated, images may be difficult to interpret due to the continued spread of contrast throughout the edematous brain. This problem is not experienced in the comparatively brief diagnostic MRI sessions. To avoid this problem, some centers reserve the administration of intravenous contrast until the tumor has been resected (50).

Unintentional Output and Operational Inhibition of Devices

It should be confirmed that the static magnetic field, imaging gradients, and RF pulses do not impact the function of the device. For example, one MR Conditional physiological monitor had design issues with the motor that inflates the blood pressure cuff. Long-term exposure to the static magnetic field impacted the motor performance of this and resulted in the feature being unusable.

The imaging gradients create a field switching at about 100-Hz to several kilohertz. The worst-case scenario location for testing is not at isocenter of the MR system. The fields due to the imaging gradients increase proportional to the distance from isocenter and then fall off outside of the field of view. The peak field is about 30-cm from isocenter and varies across different scanners. The time-varying magnetic field can induce eddy currents in the patient and in conducting materials, but is generally not a concern for heating. However, the induced currents in devices can interact with the static magnetic field, creating forces and torques on the device. If the device vibrates and is in contact with the patient, image artifacts can occur. If the device is a part of a positioning stage and the gradients cause vibrations in a component of the device, inaccuracies may occur.

Heating

Devices and instruments that are left in contact with the patient during scanning must be tested for MRI-induced heating. Current safety guidelines limit temperature increases in the torso to 2°C or a peak specific absorption rate (SAR) of 8- to 10-W/kg. The whole-body-averaged SAR is limited to 4-W/kg in the body, and 3.2-W/kg in the head over a 15-

minute period (51, 52). RF energy associated with MRI is a concern for heating due to ohmic heating. Most MRI-related adverse events are due to RF-induced patient burns (53).

The transmit body RF coil runs almost the entire length of the bore of the MR system. The worst-case locations occur where the electric field (as opposed to the magnetic field used to create the MR image) is highest. The field tends to be highest closest to the conductors and is impacted by coil geometry. Any conductor in or near the transmit RF coil, including the patient, is subject to RF-induced heating.

Cables should be padded to eliminate contact with the patient's skin or, if possible, removed during scanning. As a preventive measure, a cold compress or ice pack can be applied to sites subject to heating. Skin-to-skin contact points should be avoided, since these have been reported to be associated with burns (54). Precautions to prevent excessive heating are of particular importance for patients under sedation or general anesthesia who are unable to notice or report pain. Heating may be minimized with the use of a local transmit RF coil (e.g., quadrature head coil) instead of the body RF coil and judicious selection of pulse sequences and parameters to limit the specific absorption rate (SAR) (55).

A fiber-optic temperature measurement device with multiple probes is necessary to accurately test for heating. Probes should be placed near corners and tips and other discontinuities where the electric field tends to be the highest (56). The design that is used for the phantom to simulate the patient is critical. A device in free space will behave differently than a device that is in contact with the patient. For example, our team assessed a carbon-fiber Jackson table used for positioning patients undergoing spine surgery. No heating was measured with the square piece of material in isolation. When a tissue equivalent load was placed at the corner, a notable temperature elevation was observed.

Temperature elevations that occur in long conducting wires can be sudden and extreme, especially at the tip of the wire. Our team observed a 50°C temperature elevation after five seconds of MRI in the cable of an RF ablation probe that is not marketed for MRI. Solutions to this problem are needed to enable the use of devices for vascular interventions and other procedures (57-59).

Occupational Considerations

Some personnel have reported that while moving their heads close to the bore of the scanner or having their heads in the bore of the scanner during activation of the gradients, they experience reversible side effects such as nausea, vertigo, magnetophosphenes (flashes of light), or metallic taste. Therefore, clinicians planning to perform iMRI procedures should be assessed for these possible issues to determine if such sensations will be problematic.

SAFETY IMPLICATIONS FOR ROOM CONFIGURATION

Approaches for the iMRI suite layout include a dual room environment in which the MR system room and procedure room are separated and a single room where the the imaging and procedural environments are co-located. The advantage of the dual room solution is that the procedure room is a more familiar setting to the proceduralist. In the absence of the magnetic field, conventional MR Unsafe equipment like a surgical microscope, ultra-

Figure 5. The IMRIS MR system moving into the AMIGO Suite OR area on the ceiling-track. (**A** and **B**).

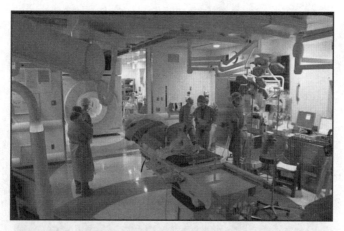

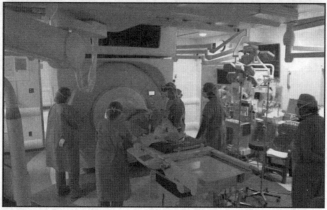

sound system, and steel instruments can be used. Great care must be taken into account to manage all devices and instruments before imaging. As in the AMIGO Suite (20), before the mobile MR system (i.e., IMRIS) enters the procedure room (i.e., the MR system that moves in and out of the room on a ceiling track), ceiling-mounted booms, lights, and monitors are pivoted to the walls and other MR Unsafe items are either brought out of the room or moved outside the five-gauss line (**Figure 5**).

Alternatively, the patient can be moved from the OR into the MR system room. In addition to the risk of unaccounted for items becoming projectiles when the patient is moved, there is a risk of extubation or extravasation due to tension on the breathing circuit or intravenous lines, respectively. The anesthesia machine and physiological monitor equipment are tethered by interfaces to the patient and, therefore, these devices must move as a unit with the patient table. A work-in-progress approach by MedTrak integrates the patient table with the anesthesia devices via tracks on the ceiling (60). A commonality with MedTrak and other two-room solutions is that the patient stays on a rigid transfer board for the entire procedure. The transfer board is MR Safe and is integrated with both the MR system platform and the surgical table platform. One solution from General Electric Healthcare (GE) utilizes a modified MRI table that end-docks with the surgical table, collects the transfer

Figure 6. A solution by General Electric Healthcare for the iMRI setting in which the MR system table end-docks to the OR table, collects the transfer board and patient, and delivers them to the MR system.

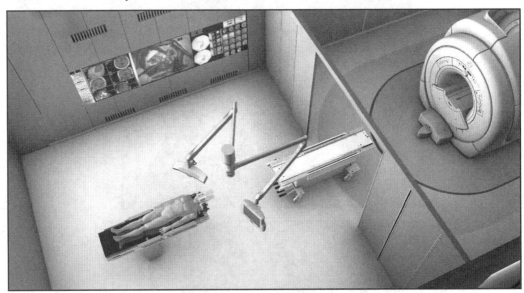

Figure 7. A solution by General Electric Healthcare for the iMRI setting in which the OR table travels to the MR system on floor tracks. The table top and patient move into the scanner as a unit.

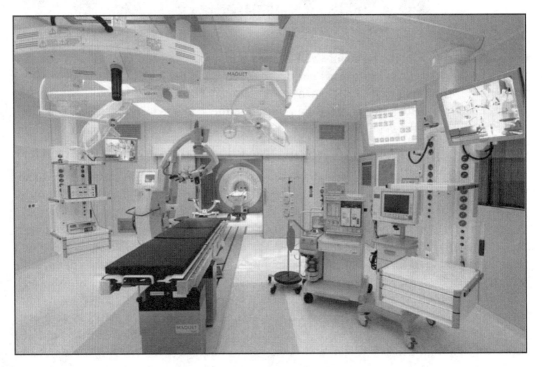

board/patient, moves into the MR system room, and docks with the scanner for imaging (**Figure 6**). The Miyabi solution is similar and is offered by Siemens and Brainlab. The Miyabi solution as well as an offering by Philips (61) can be used as a long linear shuttle system that can be encapsulated into a single room, if it is large enough, to permit a working space in the fringe field. Another solution developed by GE is to move the OR table on floor tracks into the MR system room, where the OR table will then undock from the MR system table for patient transfer (62) (**Figure 7**). Efforts have been made to couple a defeatured anesthesia machine (63) and physiological monitor to the table to avoid cable tension. The GE solution has been leveraged by in-house efforts with another manufacturer's scanner (32).

The advantage of the single room solution is the rapid turn around between imaging and intervention. This gain comes at the expense of using MR Safe or MR Conditional equipment and regaining needed functionality through ingenuity, or omitting the functionality, potentially compromising the procedure. Alternatively, MR Unsafe devices can be used while managing the risk. Brainlab offers a solution to pivot the patient out of the bore of the MR system and into the fringe field for surgery/intervention (**Figure 8**). Neurosurgical procedures can be performed with the in-and-out paradigm, in which the patient's head extends from the back of the bore of a high field scanner to permit the surgical procedure and then back into the MR system for MRI. Imaging can be achieved by moving the patient approximately one-meter to isocenter (64). Similarly, abdominal interventions can be performed with this same in-and-out paradigm. An ultra-low-field dedicated MR system (Medtronic, Inc.) mitigates risks associated with MRI by two means: the field is so low (i.e., 0.15-T) that projectile risk is almost nonexistent and the scanner drops out of the way for surgery so the patient does not need to move (**Figure 9**) (65). Procedures can also take place in the gap of a horizontal, "open" scanner with iMRI offerings by Symbow Medical Technologies, Hitachi, and Philips (**Figure 10**). A 0.5-Tesla vertically-open MR system (GE) was able to support a multitude of procedures without moving the patient, while enabling good support for the patient (4), however, this product was discontinued. Morrison, et al. (66) reviewed the interventional use of open scanners. Each of the above iMRI approachs has its advantages and disadvantages.

Multimodality environments are emerging in which and MR system is coupled with other imagers in the vacinity to complement capabilities. The AMIGO OR is flanked by an MR system room and PET/CT scanner (**Figure 11**). MR Conditional ECG electrodes, physiological monitoring equipment, and the anesthesia machine are used in the PET/CT room to avoid MR Unsafe devices from entering the suite as well as to obviate logistics regarding which devices can be used during MRI.

ANESTHESIA DELIVERY IN THE MRI ENVIRONMENT

All of the anesthesia concerns in the diagnostic MRI environment are present in the interventional/intraoperative environment. A patient receiving anesthesia in the iMRI environment is at a higher risk than a patient undergoing anesthesia in a conventional setting (67-69). Therefore, a facility planning member from the Department of Anesthesia is critical for identifying and minimizing risks in the iMRI setting (70).

Figure 8. A single room solution by Brainlab for the iMRI setting in which the patient table pivots out of the scanner to a safe point in the fringe field for surgery.

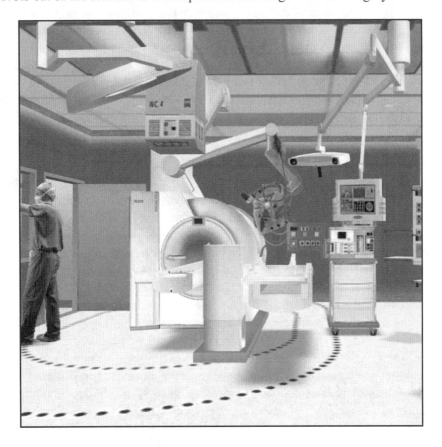

Figure 9. An ultra-low-field dedicated MR system (Medtronic, Inc.) single room solution for iMRI. This scanner drops out of the way for surgery so the patient does not need to move.

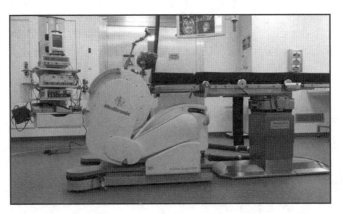

Figure 10. Example of an "open" MR system used for iMRI.

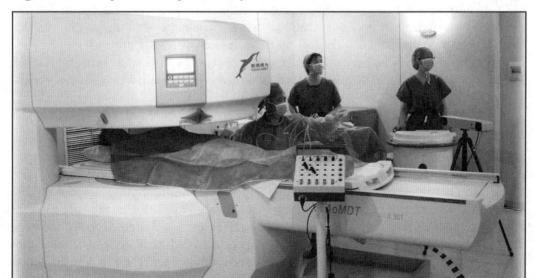

Figure 11. Bridge and transfer board solution used between the AMIGO OR table and the PET/CT scanner.

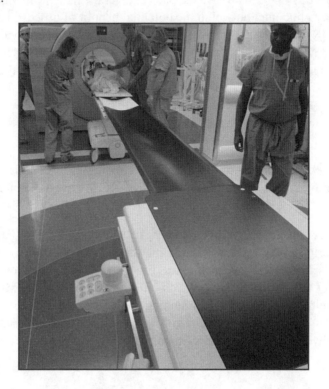

The electromagnetic fields used with MRI necessitates that all monitors and devices be MR Conditional. Not all available devices used in the conventional setting are mirrored in the iMRI environment. It is critical that anesthesia personnel cycle through the area frequently enough to maintain competancy on these devices which are not encountered elsewhere in the institution, as well as to maintain awareness of MRI safe practices. Backup devices should be available in the event that the primary devices fail, which increases costs.

MR Conditional Equipment

Although MR Conditional anesthesia machines, ventillators, drug infusion pumps, and physiological monitors are available, the development of MR Conditional anesthesia support equipment is not keeping pace with the development of new procedure enabling devices. While simultaneous electroencephalography (EEG) monitoring during functional MRI (fMRI) is now common (71), there is no commercially available MR Conditional bispectral index device for assessing the depth of anesthesia. It is not practical to use an MR Unsafe device in the dual room setting for neurosurgery because it is difficult to remove the equipment for imaging while maintaing a sterile field, and the equipment is difficult to reposition after imaging. Similarly, there is no commercially available MR Conditional peripheral nerve stimulator for assessing the depth of anesthesia. Futhermore, at present time, there is no external defibrillator that is MR Conditional. If either cardiac arrhythmias or cardiac instability are noted during an iMRI procedure, the patient must be removed from the MR system room (i.e., Zone IV) before using an external defibrillator. In situations where there is the likelihood of cardiac instability or arrhythmia in non-MRI environments, external defibrillator/pacing pads may be placed on the patient before the induction of anesthesia. This cannot be done in the MR system room because the metallic foil backing on the pads increases the chance of skin burns where the pads contact the patient. In this case, the risk of instability or arrhythmia may outweigh the potential benefit of proceeding with the procedure. Although MR Conditional core body temperature measurement devices are now available, there are no MR Conditional temperature control devices for patients. For example, at BWH, the air blower is removed prior to the MR scanner entering the OR. In the MR system room, a blower is positioned in an RF shielded closet built into the room. MR Safe extension hoses are used to replaced the MR Unsafe hoses packaged with the device. Although there is some loss due to heat transfer through the hose, it is still possible to warm or cool the patient.

Laryngoscope handles require MR Conditional batteries. Steerable endoscopes have been constructed by several research groups (72, 73). However, commercially available scopes for visualizing the vocal cords during difficult intubations are MR Unsafe.

The inadvertent placement of a certain type of endotracheal tube (Fast Trach ETT) at our institution during a diagnostic MRI examination of a patient with a difficult airway resulted in images with substantial signal losses (**Figure 12**). No injury occured to the patient. The packaging for this particular ETT had no indication of its level of MRI-related issues. This ETT has a reinforcing metallic coil running the length of the tube, which is magnetic. This incident led to an appraisal of this and other items in the conventional armamentarium for anesthesia delivery, some of which are listed in the *Reference Manual for Magnetic Res-*

onance Safety, Implants, and Devices: 2013 Edition (74) and posted online at www.MRIsafety.com.

Cardiac Issues

Patients that are candidates for intervention and intraoperative procedures often have cardiac comorbidities. The poor quality of continuous ECG tracings when the patient is in the MR system is the most serious limitation in monitoring an anesthetized patient. Imaging gradients can induce characteristic field frequency-based artifacts in the ECG that can mimic malignant arrhythmia. Additionally, the static magnetic field can induce apparent ST-segment abnormalities (75). The benefit of image-guidance, therefore, should be weighed against the risk of anesthetizing a patient at risk of further cardiac injury during ischemic stress.

There are multiple efforts underway to develop an iMRI treatment for arrhythmias using ablation catheters (76-79). This procedure, and others, will benefit from enabling developments to overcome current limitations. Historically, cardiac pacemakers and implantable cardioverter defibrillators are considered contraindications for MRI (80). Several groups are challenging this assertion and an MR Conditional device has been FDA cleared. There are efforts to improve ECG monitoring.

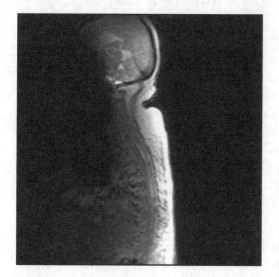

Figure 12. (Left) MR image depicting signal void created by Fast Trach endotracheal tube.

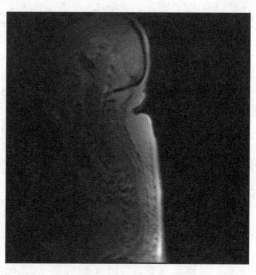

(Right) image with MR Conditional Sheridan endotracheal tube.

Adaptive filters have been shown to be successful in removing noise induced by the imaging gradients, which are present only during scanning (81). ECG monitoring in the static magnetic field, however, is problematic even when images are not being acquired. A dominant QRS complex and undistorted S-T segment are important for both cardiac-gated MRI examinations and to permit physiological monitoring for cardiac ischemia, especially during cardiac interventions (82). The magnetohydrodynamic (MHD) effect arises when blood, which is conductive, flows in the presence of a static magnetic field. The MHD effect generates a voltage that distorts the "real" electrocardiogram, especially with respect to the S-T segment when blood flow occurs from the left ventricle into the aorta (83). It is possible to remove the MHD artifact by processing ECG signals using a baseline ECG collected outside the bore of the MR system in conjunction with an adaptive filter (84).

Concerns of imaging a patient with a cardiac implant include triggering of arrhythmias, inhibition of pacing output and triggered stimulations, and RF-related heating of the pacing leads with potential thermal damage at the electrode-tissue interface. In the United States, commercially available MR Conditional cardiac pacemakers are now available but presently have limitations on what body parts can be imaged due to restrictions on positioning of the implanted device in the bore of the MR system (74, 85). It has been recently shown that imaging without positioning restrictions can be achieved at 1.5-Tesla/64-MHz (86). Furthermore, patients with cardiac implants previously considered MR Unsafe are now being imaged without consequential adverse events at 1.5-T/64-MHz (87). Additional information pertaining to MRI and patients with cardiac devices is covered in two chapters in this textbook.

Remote Monitoring

Acoustic noise from the gradient magnetic fields, especially at 3-Tesla, can prohibit the anesthesiologist from hearing the physiological monitor's alarms and ECG tones when more than a few feet from the equipment. Although developing technologies with active noise cancellation will allow transmission of monitoring equipment alarms and tones into the anesthesiologist's headphones, this technology is not widely available. As an alternative, remote monitoring is routinely performed.

Primarily because of the acoustic noise associated with MRI, the anesthesiologist in the AMIGO Suite remotely monitors the patient after the onset of anesthesia and the patient is stable. Remote monitoring is accomplished with a "slave" physiological monitor placed in the control room that displays information for the patient's vital signs and end tidal gases; a view of the anesthesia machine's ventilator and its settings by either direct line-of-site or remote camera; and a camera view of the patient in the bore of the MR system. Line-of-site to the patient is limited when the patient is inside the bore, even when the anesthesiologist is at the bedside. If an intervention by the anesthesiologist is needed during imaging, the scan is halted until the issue is resolved.

SAFE USE OF MRI PULSE SEQUENCES FOR IMRI

The type of pulse sequence that is used during iMRI is generally more constrained than it is for diagnostic imaging. Real-time interactive imaging can be employed, which demands high acquisition rates, while sacrificing some contrast and resolution. Special fast-imaging pulse sequences used in iMRI are more likely to make use of fast gradient switching and/or may employ RF pulsing rates that are substantially greater than those used in routine clinical imaging and, thus, are more likely to push the limits of safe use. Safety concerns related to pulse sequence choice are also heightened in iMRI because of the possibility of interaction with implants or interventional devices that are in place during the MRI procedure and result in a greater potential for dangerous levels of heating from RF fields or induction of currents from gradient switching.

As previously indicated, the primary biological effects in MRI are tissue heating due to RF exposure, nerve stimulation due to currents induced by gradient switching and sensations such as vertigo caused by rapid movement in the static magnetic field (88-90). Pulse sequences that tend to cause the greatest heating due to RF exposure are those with a high temporal density of RF pulsing, such as fast (or turbo) spin-echo sequences, which employ multiple high-flip-angle refocusing pulses as well as steady-state sequences such as FIESTA (or True FISP), which have very short repetition times (91-95). These sequence types are commonly used in iMRI and may be referred to as "high-SAR" pulse sequences. Pulse sequences that involve very rapid gradient switching (such as echo-planar sequences) (96-98), which induce currents that can cause peripheral nerve stimulation or interfere with the operation of devices such as cardiac pacemakers, are also used in iMRI and may be referred to as "high-dB/dT" sequences. Safety concerns in iMRI, as with MRI in general, involve the use of high-SAR and/or high-dB/dT pulse sequences. Artifacts such as signal loss and distortions caused by imaging in the presence of objects such as biopsy needles can also be considered a safety issue as they diminish or confuse MR-guidance capabilities during interventional procedures. Gradient-echo pulse sequences (especially multi-echo sequences such as echo-planar imaging) are especially likely to exhibit artifacts caused by the susceptibility effects due to the presence of metallic objects in tissues. High bandwidth spin-echo sequences and special sequence adaptations may be employed to minimize such artifacts (99, 100).

Regulatory bodies such as the FDA have placed limits on the allowable exposures for patients to RF energy and gradient magnetic fields. MR system manufacturers include monitoring software and hardware to ensure that these exposures are not exceeded when their MR scanners are running in routine operating modes. In the absence of implants, devices, or foreign objects present during the scanning, MR systems are set in routine operating modes (i.e., the Normal Operating Mode or First Level Controlled Operating Mode) should not be of concern. Even when high-SAR or high-dB/dT sequences are used, limitations by the MR system on the setting of parameters such as the number of slices or the repetition time will ensure that exposures remain within the defined limits. It may possible to supercede the limits as set by regulatory bodies, although Institutional Review Board approval and informed patient consent is required in such cases. As long as system SAR and dB/dT monitoring remains in place, the degree of exposure can be assessed and a decision whether or not to proceed based on risk versus benefit analysis can be made. Involving an MRI physicist to assess these risks would be advisable in such cases.

Of greater concern when using high-SAR or high-dB/dT sequences is when implants catheters, needles or other foreign objects are present during scanning because heating can be enhanced by the presence of the device, and it is much more difficult to predict the degree of the effects. Ideally, information is available from the manufacturer of the device in terms of specifying conditions of use. For example, perhaps a given device is limited with respect to the strength of the static magnetic field and/or the Normal Operating Mode must be used.

CONCLUSIONS

The use of MRI is not inherently safe, therefore, the possibility of accidents should not be underestimated. In the iMRI environment, the potential risk is even higher due to the extra complexity of interventions or surgeries and the presence of less experienced personnel from outside of radiology. However, safe behavior can be encouraged by measures such as suite layout and restriction of access. Furthermore, a safe behavior can be engrained in personnel by training and policy enforcement. These two means must act in concert to ensure safety.

Since the early 1990s when iMRI was first introduced, it has rapidly developed and the number of users and procedures have increased. iMRI expanded through the introduction of new surgical approaches and/or techniques in open surgery, vascular and cardiac applications, and minimally-invasive endoscopies. Efforts now focus on the development of new, more advanced imaging methods, navigational techniques, surgical instruments and devices, the more efficient use of computing technologies, and the integration of diagnostic and therapy devices with navigational tools to expand iMRI applications.

Safety measures must keep pace with this increasingly complex environment as the number of installations also increases. Patient and personnel safety is the concern of a large multimodality and multidisciplinary infrastructure like that which exists in the BWH's AMIGO Suite, where iMRI is complemented with newly developed, multiple molecular probes (e.g., nuclear, optical, mass spectrometer, etc.) that also must be used safely. A chief concern for the operation of the suite is how to provide a safe environment for clinical and research activity in iMRI that incorporates multimodal imaging. The workflows in the suite should be designed to suit the way that multidisciplinary teams work while understanding and mitigating safety risks.

Most of the centers involved in iMRI report no serious adverse incidents. In our 20-years of experience with a 0.5-Tesla iMRI (23) and, more recently with 3-Tesla, we also have a major incident-free operation. Hushek, et al. (22) reported another perfect safety record over more than five years with more than 400 surgeries performed at 0.5-Tesla. According to these data, with appropriate control, a strong safety record can be maintained. The main reason for this successful and safe operation is continuous vigilance, policy enforcement, and a serious attitude towards safety.

REFERENCES

1. Jolesz FA, Blumenfeld SM. Interventional use of magnetic resonance imaging. Magn Reson Q 1994;10:85-96.

2. Jolesz FA. Interventional and intraoperative MRI: a general overview of the field. J Magn Reson Imaging 1998;8:3-7.

3. Kettenbach J, Silverman SG, Schwartz RB, et al. Design, clinical suitability and future aspects of a 0.5 T MRI special system for interventional use. Radiologe 1997;37:825-34.

4. Kettenbach J, Kacher DF, Koskinen SK, et al. Interventional and intraoperative magnetic resonance imaging. Annu Rev Biomed Eng 2000;2:661-90.

5. Jolesz FA. Neurosurgical suite of the future. II. Neuroimaging Clin N Am. 2001;11:581-92.

6. Silverman SG, Collick BD, Figueira MR, et al. Interactive MR-guided biopsy in an open-configuration MR imaging system. Radiology 1995;197:175-81.

7. McDannold NJ, Jolesz FA. Magnetic resonance image-guided thermal ablations. Top Magn Reson Imaging 2000;11:191-202.

8. Kandarpa K, Jakab P, Patz S, Schoen FJ, Jolesz FA. Prototype miniature endoluminal MR imaging catheter. J Vasc Interv Radiol 1993;4:419-27.

9. Hsu L, Fried MP, Jolesz FA. MR-guided endoscopic sinus surgery. AJNR Am J Neuroradiol 1998;19:1235-40.

10. Schwartz RB, Hsu L, Wong TZ, et al. Intraoperative MR imaging guidance for intracranial neurosurgery: experience with the first 200 cases. Radiology 1999;211:477-88.

11. Nabavi A, Mamisch CT, Gering DT, et al. Image-guided therapy and intraoperative MRI in neurosurgery. Minim Invasive Ther Allied Technol 2000;9:277-86.

12. Woodard EJ, Leon SP, Moriarty TM, et al. Initial experience with intraoperative magnetic resonance imaging in spine surgery. Spine 2001;26:410-7.

13. Jolesz FA, Morrison PR, Koran SJ, et al. Compatible instrumentation for intraoperative MRI: expanding resources. J Magn Reson Imaging 1998;8:8-11.

14. Jolesz FA, Nabavi A, Kikinis R. Integration of interventional MRI with computer-assisted surgery. J Magn Reson Imaging 2001;13:69-77.

15. Jolesz FA. Designing a safe work environment. 1996 RSNA Eugene P. Pendergrass New Horizons Lecture. Image-guided procedures and the operating room of the future. Radiology 1997;204:601-12.

16. Silverman SG, Jolesz FA, Newman RW, et al. Design and implementation of an interventional MR imaging suite. AJR Am J Roentgenol 1997;168:1465-71.

17. Colen RR, Kekhia H, Jolesz FA. Multimodality intraoperative MRI for brain tumor surgery. Expert Rev Neurother 2010;10:1545-58.

18. Hushek S. Systems for Interventional MRI. Interventional Magnetic Resonance Imaging. In: Kahn T, Busse H, Editors. Interventional Magnetic Resonance Imaging (Medical Radiology/Diagnostic Imaging). Berlin Heidelberg: Springer-Verlag; 2012. pp. 3-15.

19. Kahn T, Busse H, Editors. Interventional Magnetic Resonance Imaging (Medical Radiology/Diagnostic Imaging). Berlin Heidelberg: Springer-Verlag; 2012.

20. Kacher DF, Whalen B, Handa A, Jolesz FA. The Advanced Multi-Modality Image Guided Operating (AMIGO) Suite. In: Jolesz FA, Editor. Intraoperative Imaging and Image Guided Therapy. New York: Springer Science; (In Press).

21. Sutherland GR, Kaibara T, Louw D, Hoult DI, Tomanek B, Saunders J. A mobile high-field magnetic resonance system for neurosurgery. J Neurosurg 1999; 91:804–813.

22. Hushek SG. Safety protocols for interventional MRI. Acad Radiol 2005;12:1143–8.

23. Kettenbach J, Kacher DF, Kanan AR. Intraoperative and interventional MRI: recommendations for a safe environment. Minim Invasive Ther Allied Technol. 2006;15:53-64.

24. Johnston T, Moser R, Moeller K, Moriarty TM. Intraoperative MRI: safety. Neurosurg Clin N Am 2009; 20:147–153.

25. Kugel H. Safety Considerations in Interventional MRI. In: Kahn T, Busse H, Editors. Interventional Magnetic Resonance Imaging (Medical Radiology/ Diagnostic Imaging). Berlin Heidelberg: Springer-Verlag; 2012. pp. 77-88.

26. Rahmathulla G, Recinos PF, Traul DE. Surgical briefings, checklists, and the creation of an environment of safety in the neurosurgical intraoperative magnetic resonance imaging suite. Neurosurg Focus 2012; 33:E12.

27. Kanal, E, Barkovich AJ, Bell C, et al. American College of Radiology (ACR) guidance document on MR safe practices: 2013 expert panel on MR safety. J Magn Reson Imaging 2013;37:501-530.

28. Chaljub G, Kramer LA, Johnson RF III, et al. Projectile cylinder accidents resulting from the presence of ferromagnetic nitrous oxide or oxygen tanks in the MR suite. AJR Am J Roentgenol 2001;177:27–30.

29. MRI Safety 10 Years Later: What can we learn from the accident that killed Michael Colombini? In: Patient Safety and Quality Healthcare. November, December 2011. Available at: http://www.psqh.com/component/content/article/137-november-december-2011/992-mri-safety-10-years-later.html. Accessed February, 2013.

30. Joint Commission. Preventing accidents and injuries in the MRI suite. Sentinel Event Alert, 38, 2008.

31. Gilk T. Effectiveness of existing MR safety regulatory, licensure, and accreditation standards. In: Proceedings of the Magnetic Resonance Imaging (MRI) Safety Public Workshop. October 25-26, 2011, Silver Spring, MD. Available at: http://www.fda.gov/downloads/MedicalDevices/NewsEvents/WorkshopsConferences/UCM283558.pdf. Accessed February, 2013.

32. Jankovski A, Francotte F, Vaz G. Intraoperative magnetic resonance imaging at 3 T using a dual independent operating room-magnetic resonance imaging suite: development, feasibility, safety, and preliminary experience. Neurosurgery 2008;63:412-24.

33. Surgical Safety Checklist. First Edition. In: World Health Organization Patient Safety Tools and Resources. http://www.who.int/patientsafety/safesurgery/tools_resources/SSSL_Checklist_finalJun08.pdf. Accessed February, 2013.

34. Price RR. The AAPM/RSNA physics tutorial for residents: MR imaging safety considerations. Radiographics 1999;19:1641–51.

35. Shellock FG, Crues JV. MR procedures: biologic effects, safety, and patient care. Radiology 2004;232:635–52.

36. ASTM F2503. Standard practice for marking medical devices and other items for safety in the magnetic resonance environment. ASTM International, West Conshohocken, PA.

37. ASTM F2052-06e1. Standard test method for measurement of magnetically induced displacement force on medical devices in the magnetic resonance environment. ASTM International, West Conshohocken, PA.

38. ASTM F2213-06. Standard test method for measurement of magnetically induced torque on medical devices in the magnetic resonance environment. ASTM International, West Conshohocken, PA.

39. ASTM F2182-11a. Standard test method for measurement of radio frequency induced heating on and near passive implants during magnetic resonance imaging. ASTM International, West Conshohocken, PA.

40. ASTM F2119-07. Standard test method for evaluation of MR image artifacts from passive implants. ASTM International, West Conshohocken, PA.

41. ISO/TS 10974:2012. Assessment of the safety of magnetic resonance imaging for patients with an active implantable medical device. American National Standards Institute, 2012

42. Shellock FG. Metallic surgical instruments for interventional MRI procedures: Evaluation of MR safety. J Magn Reson Imaging 2001;13:152–157.

43. De Wilde JP, Grainger D, Price DL, Renaud C. Magnetic resonance imaging safety issues including an analysis of recorded incidents within the UK. Prog Nucl Magn Reson Spectrosc 2007;51:37–48.

44. Jolesz FA, Morrison PR, Koran SJ. Compatible instrumentation for intraoperative MRI: expanding resources. J Magn Reson Imaging 1998;8:8-11.

45. Schenck J. The role of magnetic susceptibility in magnetic resonance imaging: MRI magnetic compatibility of the first and second kinds. Med Phys 1996; 23:815–850.

46. DiMaio SP, Kacher DF, Ellis RE, et al. Needle artifact localization in 3-T MR images. Stud Health Technol Inform 2006;119:120-5.

47. Oppelt A, Delakis I. Safety aspects in interventional MRI. Z Med Phys 2002;2:5–15.

48. Hirose M, Kacher DF, Smith DN, Kaelin CM, Jolesz FA. Feasibility of MR imaging-guided breast lumpectomy for malignant tumors in a 0.5-T open-configuration MR imaging system. Acad Radiol 2002;9:933-41.

49. Bartels LW, Bakker CJ, Viergever MA. Improved lumen visualization in metallic vascular implants by reducing RF artifacts. Magn Reson Med 2002;47:171–180.

50. Hall WA, Truwit CL. Intraoperative MR-guided neurosurgery. J Magn Reson Imaging 2008;27:368-75.

51. U.S. Department of Health and Human Services. Food and Drug Administration, Center for Devices and Radiological Health. Guidance for the submission of premarket notifications for magnetic resonance diagnostic devices. Rockville, MD: US DHHS FDA; 1998.

52. International Electrotechnical Commission (IEC). Medical electrical equipment. Part 2. In: Particular Requirements for the Safety of Magnetic Resonance Equipment for Medical Diagnosis. International Standard 60601-2-33, Second Edition. Geneva: IEC; 2002.

53. Hardy PT, Weil KM. A review of thermal MR injuries. Radiol Technol 2010;81:606-609.

54. Knopp MV, Essig M, et al. Unusual burns of the lower extremities caused by a closed conduction loop in a patient at MR imaging. Radiology 1996;200:772–75.

55. Rezai AR, Phillips M, Baker KB, et al. Neurostimulation system used for deep brain stimulation (DBS): MR safety issues and implications of failing to follow safety recommendations. Investigative Radiology 2004;39:300-303.

56. Jackson JD. Classical Electrodynamics, Second Edition. New York: John Wiley & Sons; 2 edition; 1975. Section 2.11.

57. Yeung CJ, Karmarkar P, McVeigh ER. Minimizing RF heating of conducting wires in MRI. Magn Reson Med 2007;58:1028-34.

58. Van den Bosch MR, Moerland MA, et al. New method to monitor RF safety in MRI-guided interventions based on RF induced image artifacts. Med Phys 2010;37:814-21.

59. Reiter T, Gensler D, Ritter O, et al. Direct cooling of the catheter tip increases safety for CMR-guided electrophysiological procedures. J Cardiovasc Magn Reson 2012;14:12.

60. Hushek S. A New iMRI Suite Design. In: Proceedings of the 9th International Interventional MRI Symposium.. Boston, MA. Sept 2012. Available at: http://www.ncigt.org/publications/item/view/2234. Accessed February, 2013.

61. Martin AJ, Hall WA, Liu H, et al. Brain tumor resection: intraoperative monitoring with high-field-strength MR imaging-initial results. Radiology 2000;215:221-8.

62. Degreze P. MR Enabled Therapy. In: Proceedings of the 28th Danish Annual Congress in Biomedical Engineering; Braedstrup, Denmark; 2009.

63. Philip JH, Smith CB, Martin RF, Kacher DF. MR-compatible portable anesthesia machine with ventilator moves with patient through the magnet bore. In: Proceedings of the American Society of Anesthesiologists, 2008.

64. Hall WA, Galicich W, Bergman T, Truwit CL. 3-Tesla intraoperative MR imaging for neurosurgery. J Neurooncol 2006;77:297-303.

65. Hadani M. Development and design of low field compact intraoperative MRI for standard operating room. Acta Neurochir Suppl 2011;109:29-33.

66. Morrison PR, Silverman SG, Tuncali K, Tatli S. MRI-guided cryotherapy. J Magn Reson Imaging 2008;27:410–420.

67. Martin R. Anesthetic Concerns in the Magnetic Resonance (MR) Environment. In: Kahn T, Busse H, Editors. Interventional Magnetic Resonance Imaging (Medical Radiology/Diagnostic Imaging). Berlin Heidelberg: Springer-Verlag; 2012. pp. 89-93.

68. Henrichs B, Walsh RP. Intraoperative magnetic resonance imaging for neurosurgical procedures: anesthetic implications. AANA J 2011;79:71–77.

69. Smith JA. Hazards, safety, and anesthetic considerations for magnetic resonance imaging. Top Companion Anim Med 2010;25:98–106.

70. Tan TK, Goh J. The anaesthetist's role in the setting up of an intraoperative MR imaging facility. Singapore Med J 2009;50:4–10.

71. Shibasaki H. Human brain mapping: hemodynamic response and electrophysiology.Clin Neurophysiol 2008;119:731-43.

72. North OJ, Ristic M, Wadsworth CA, Young IR, Taylor-Robinson SD. Design and evaluation of endoscope remote actuator for MRI-guided endoscopic retrograde cholangio-pancreatography (ERCP). In: Proceedings of the International Conference on Biomedical Robotics and Biomechatronics (BioRob). Fourth IEEE RAS & EMBS; 2012. pp. 787–792.

73. Zuo S, Ymanaka N, Masamune K, et al. MRI compatible rigid-flexible outer sheath device using pneumatic locking mechanism for endoscopic ereatment. IFMBE Proceedings 2008;19:741–744.

74. Shellock, FG. Reference Manual for Magnetic Resonance Safety, Implants and Devices, 2013 Edition. Los Angeles: Biomedical Research Publishing Group; 2013.

75. Birkholz T, Schmid M, Nimsky C, Schuttler J, Schmitz B. ECG artifacts during intraoperative high-field MRI scanning. J Neurosurg Anesthesiol 2004;16:271-6.

76. Rhode KS, Sermesant M, Brogan D, et al. A system for real-time XMR guided cardiovascular intervention. IEEE Trans Med Imaging 2005;24:1428-1440.

77. Schmidt EJ, Mallozzi RP, Thiagalingam A, et al. Electroanatomic mapping and radiofrequency ablation of porcine left atria and atrioventricular nodes using magnetic resonance catheter tracking. Circ Arrhythm Electrophysiol 2009;2:695-704.

78. Vergara GR, Vijayakumar S, Kholmovski EG, et al. Real-time magnetic resonance imaging-guided radiofrequency atrial ablation and visualization of lesion formation at 3 Tesla. Heart Rhythm 2011;8:295-303.

79. Halperin HR, Kolandaivelu A. MRI-guided electrophysiology intervention. Rambam Maimonides Medical Journal 2010;1:e0015.

80. Faris OP, Shein MJ. Government viewpoint: U.S. Food & Drug Administration: pacemakers, ICDs and MRI. Pacing Clin Electrophysiol 2005;28:268-9.

81. Wu V, Benbash IM, Ratnayaha K, et al. Adaptive noise cancellation to suppress electrocardiography artifacts during real-time interventional MRI. J Mag Reson Imaging 2011;33:1184-93.

82. Haberl R. ECG Pocket, Second Edition. El Segundo, CA: Borm Bruckmeier Publishing LLC; 2006.

83. Gupta A, Weeks AR, Richie SM. Simulation of elevated T-waves of an ECG inside a static magnetic field (MRI). IEEE Trans Biomed Eng. 2008;55:1890-6.

84. Tse ZTH, Dumoulin CL, Clifford G, et al. 12 lead ECG in a 1.5 Tesla MRI: Separation of real ECG and MHD voltages with adaptive filtering for gating and non-invasive cardiac output. In: Proceedings of the Society for Cardiac Magnetic Resonance; Phoenix: Arizona; 2010.

85. Gimbel RJ, Bello D, Schmitt M, et al. Randomized trial of pacemaker and lead system for safe scanning at 1.5 Tesla. Heart Rhythm 2013;17:S1547-5271.

86. Wilkoff BL, Bello D, Taborsky M, et al. EnRhythm MRI SureScan Pacing System study investigators. Magnetic resonance imaging in patients with a pacemaker system designed for the magnetic resonance environment. Heart Rhythm 2011;8:65-73.

87. Nazarian S, Hansford R, Roguin A, et al. A prospective evaluation of a protocol for magnetic resonance imaging of patients with implanted cardiac devices. Ann Intern Med 2011;155:415-24.

88. Busse RF, Riederer SJ, Fletcher JG, et al. Interactive fast spin-echo imaging. Magn Reson Med 2000;44:339-48.

89. Makki M, Graves MJ, Lomas DJ. Interactive body magnetic resonance fluoroscopy using modified single-shot half-Fourier rapid acquisition with relaxation enhancement (RARE) with multiparameter control. J Magn Reson Imaging 2002;16:85-93.

90. Chopra SS, Rump J, Schmidt SC, et al. Imaging sequences for intraoperative MR-guided laparoscopic liver resection in 1.0-T high field open MRI. Eur Radiol 2009;19:2191-6.

91. Stattaus J, Maderwald S, Forsting M, et al. MR-guided core biopsy with MR fluoroscopy using a short, wide-bore 1.5-Tesla scanner: feasibility and initial results. J Magn Reson Imaging 2008;27:1181-7.

92. Duerk JL, Lewin JS, Wendt M, Petersilge C. Remember true FISP? A high SNR, near 1-second imaging method for T2-like contrast in interventional MRI at 0.2 T. J Magn Reson Imaging 1998;8:203-8.

93. Zhang S, Rafie S, Chen Y, et al. In vivo cardiovascular catheterization under real-time MRI guidance. J Magn Reson Imaging 2006;24:914-7.

94. Yutzy SR, Duerk JL. Pulse sequences and system interfaces for interventional and real-time MRI. J Magn Reson Imaging 2008;27:267-75.

95. Madore B, Panych LP, Mei CS, Yuan J, Chu R. Multipathway sequences for MR thermometry. Magn Reson Med 2011;66:658-68.

96. Cernicanu A, Lepetit-Coiffe M, Roland J, et al. Validation of fast MR thermometry at 1.5 T with gradient-echo echo planar imaging sequences: phantom and clinical feasibility studies. NMR Biomed 2008;21:849-58.

97. Holbrook AB, Santos JM, Kaye E, Rieke V, Pauly KB. Real-time MR thermometry for monitoring HIFU ablations of the liver. Magn Reson Med 2010;63:365-73.

98. Weidensteiner C, Kerioui N, Quesson B, et al. Stability of real-time MR temperature mapping in healthy and diseased human liver. J Magn Reson Imaging 2004;19:438-46.

99. Butts K, Pauly JM, Daniel BL, Kee S, Norbash AM. Management of biopsy needle artifacts: techniques for RF-refocused MRI. J Magn Reson Imaging 1999;9:586-95.

100. Butts K, Pauly JM, Gold GE. Reduction of blurring in view angle tilting MRI. Magn Reson Med 2005;53:418-24.

Chapter 27   Occupational Exposure During MRI

DONALD W. MCROBBIE, PH.D.

Senior Lecturer in Imaging
Imperial College London
United Kingdom and
Chief Physicist
South Australia Medical Imaging
Adelaide, Australia

INTRODUCTION

With the growth of magnetic resonance imaging (MRI), large cohorts of patients and staff members are now routinely exposed to the static, time-varying, and radiofrequency (RF) fields integral to the imaging procedure. For the millions of MRI examinations performed each year, the majority are conducted at 1.5-Tesla, but with 3-Tesla MR systems proliferating and a smaller number of 7-Tesla scanners installed in research centers around the world. Increasing technical advances have resulted in the magnitude of exposures to electromagnetic fields to steadily grow during the use of clinical MRI, which began in the early 1980s.

Many voluntary international (1-4) and national (5-8) standards or guidelines for occupational and public exposure to electromagnetic fields (EMF) are in existence and reviewed elsewhere in this textbook. It is only since the recent formulation of the Physical Agents (electromagnetic fields) Directive in Europe, that occupational exposure limits for EMF have had a potential regulatory impact (9). In turn, this has led to a renewed interest in occupational exposures in MRI. It needs to be stated here that patient safety in MRI has always been paramount within the MRI community and that publications (10,11), exposure guidelines (12-14) and operational safety standards (15-17) address its many facets, as is evident throughout this textbook.

Staff exposures mainly involve the static magnetic field and its spatial gradient, responsible for the projectile force on ferromagnetic objects. The time-varying magnetic fields from the imaging gradients and the radiofrequency (RF) excitation field are substantially confined to within the bore of the MR system, and only become significant for staff members if they remain close to the bore during the scan acquisition (18).

DEFINITIONS AND OCCUPATIONAL LIMITS

Biological effects of electromagnetic fields and their underlying physical and physiological mechanisms are described elsewhere in this textbook. In occupational exposure or hygiene it is commonplace to consider the incident and induced EMFs: the former are those generated directly from the scanner (e.g., B_0, dB/dt, B_1), the latter are those generated in tissue as a consequence of the incident exposure (e.g., induced electric fields or current densities) and which are considered to be responsible for acute effects, such as vertigo, metallic taste, peripheral nerve stimulation (PNS), and tissue heating. Accurate dosimetry for both incident and induced EMF is paramount in occupational exposure studies.

Incident Fields

In occupational hygiene, static magnetic fields are sometimes denoted by the abbreviation SMF, and time-varying magnetic fields by TVMF. The magnetic field intensity (*H*) is indicated in units of amperes per meter (A/m). However in MRI, it is more usual to consider magnetic induction or flux density, commonly called magnetic field strength B_0, measured in Tesla (T). In a medium the magnetic flux density *B* is

$$B \quad = \quad \mu_0 (1 + \chi_m) H \tag{1}$$

where μ_0, the permeability of vacuum, has a value $4\pi \times 10^{-7}$ henry/m and χ_m is the dimensionless magnetic susceptibility. Beyond the bore of the MR system, the fringe field of B_0 varies spatially and has a gradient d*B*/dt in Tesla per meter (T/m). A time-weighted average (TWA) SMF over a duration T is defined as

$$B_{TWA} = \frac{1}{T} \int_0^T B(t)\,dt \tag{2}$$

The gradient magnetic fields are defined as linear spatial variations in B_z

$$G_x = dB_z/dx; \; G_y = dB_z/dy; \; G_z = dB_z/dz; \tag{3}$$

and are specified in millitesla per meter (mT/m). The gradient slew rate (SR), or maximum switching speed is defined in T/m/sec. The rate of change of B field (dB/dt) or the step change in B (ΔB) is physiologically significant for acute sensory effects.

The RF field, B_1, is measured in microtesla (μT) but is also specified as H_1 (Equation 1) and has an electric field component E_1. Electric fields (*E*) are measured in volts per meter

(V/m). For a plane wave in the far field, the ratio of E/H has a constant value of 337-ohms and the power density is

$$P = E\,B/\mu_0 = E^2 / 337 \tag{4}$$

measured in watts per square meter (W/m^2). The specific absorption rate (SAR) is the RF power absorbed per unit body mass (W/kg). An SAR value may apply for the whole or partial body (e.g., head or extremities). For more information please refer to the relevant chapters in this textbook.

The incident fields (B, H, and their time derivatives) are vectors and may have directional components which are not utilized in the image formation process but which, nevertheless, contribute to occupational exposures. For both patient and occupational exposures, it is important to consider the magnitude of these vector fields, e.g., for B

$$|B| = \sqrt{(B_x^2 + B_y^2 + B_z^2)} \tag{5}$$

Exposure limits are often expressed as root mean square (RMS) values. The RMS value of a time-varying function (e.g., B$_1$ and the imaging gradients) is

$$B_{RMS} = \lim_{T \to \infty} \sqrt{\left(\frac{1}{T} \int_0^T [B(t)]^2\, dt \right)} \tag{6}$$

For a sinusoidal waveform the peak value is √2 times the RMS value.

Induced Fields

The generation of the induced fields in tissue is determined by Faraday's law of Induction:

$$\oint E_i\,.dl = -\frac{d}{dt}\int_S B \cdot dS \tag{7}$$

where E_i is the induced electric field around a closed path and dS is the differential area vector normal to the applied field. For a circular loop of radius, r, in a uniform medium normal to the applied field this simplifies to (19):

$$E_i = 0.5 \ r \ dB/dt \tag{8}$$

The induced electric field generates a current density J_i (A/m^2) in tissue is

$$J_i = \sigma \ E_i \tag{9}$$

where σ is the electrical conductivity of the tissue in siemens per meter (S/m). Both induced E_i and J_i vary linearly with the loop radius, and therefore increase with body size. For an elliptical body cross section perpendicular to the magnetic field, the maximum current density is (20):

$$J_{max} = \frac{a^2 b}{a^2 + b^2} \sigma \ dB/dt \tag{10}$$

where a is the semi-major axial length and b the semi-minor. The choice of axes will depend upon the orientation of the subject within the field. For a person standing close to the bore of the MR system, a would be in the head-foot direction, and b left-right, and with typical values of 0.4-m and 0.2-m, the geometric multiplier would be 0.16.

Movement through the gradient of the static field (i.e., through the fringe field) effectively acts as a time-varying magnetic field. In the simplest case of a uniform body moving with a constant velocity v (m/s)

$$E_i = 0.5 \ r \ v \ |dB/dr| \tag{11}$$

and, therefore, moving more slowly will result in lower induced fields in tissues. The elliptical geometric term (Equation 10) may also be used in place of r, with appropriate values of a and b.

Concerning the RF field, B_1, for a spatially uniform rectangular RF pulse with duty cycle D and a uniform spherical medium of density ρ (kg/m^3) (21)

$$SAR = 0.5 \ \sigma \ \pi^2 r^2 f^2 B_1{}^2 D / \rho \tag{12}$$

and, thus, SAR has a square dependence upon Larmor frequency or B_0, B_1, patient 'radius' and a linear dependence upon duty cycle or reciprocal repetition time, $1/TR$.

Occupational Exposure Standards and Limits

The numerous occupational exposure guidelines for electromagnetic fields in the frequency range 0-Hz to 300-GHz cover all aspects of work-related exposures, not just those related to MRI (1-9). Most guidelines operate under two regimes: Basic Restrictions or Exposure Limit Values are set to avoid short term acute adverse effects and are defined in terms of RMS induced electric field, E_i, in tissue. As the induced fields are not directly measurable, compliance can be demonstrated using derived Reference Levels (RL), Maximum Permissible Exposures (MPE), or Action Values specified in terms of the incident fields. Some standards include higher limits for "controlled situations." These apply in a highly organized setting with appropriately trained staff and would, therefore, be applicable in the MRI environment.

For situations where an incident field limit is not exceeded, it can be assumed that the induced field limit will not be exceeded. Compliance with a Reference Level ensures compliance with the underlying Basic Restriction or equivalent limit. However, when an incident limit is exceeded, it is necessary for the employer to demonstrate that the relevant induced field limit is not exceeded. This would normally entail modeling of the induced fields. The derivation of the incident field limits is often based upon algebraic calculations, that is, from Equations 7 to 12 using idealized body geometries with a homogeneous electrical properties.

MR system manufacturers follow the International Electrotechnical Commission (IEC) standard 60601-2-33 that includes limits for occupational exposure (1). Other chapters in this textbook review additional exposure guidelines in greater detail.

Static Magnetic Fields

Occupational limits for static fields are shown in **Table 1**. The International Commission on Non-Ionizing Radiation Protection (ICNIRP) has a 2-T limit for static magnetic field exposure but allows for peak exposures of up to 8-T in controlled situations (2). The Institute of Electrical and Electronics Engineers (IEEE) limit applies for slowly varying sinusoidal fields of less than 0.153-Hz defined as RMS (5), but as shown in **Table 1**, it is converted to a peak value for comparison. The IEC 60601-2-33 limit for workers is 4-T (1). The National Radiological Protection Board (NRPB) guidelines also have a daily time-

Table 1. Static magnetic field limits for occupational exposure. All values are peak levels.

	Whole body TWA (T)	Trunk & Head Instantaneous Ceiling (T)	Limbs (T)
IEC (1)	N/A	4	4
ICNIRP (2)	N/A	2	8
IEEE (5)	N/A	0.5	0.5
NRPB (7)	0.2	2	5

weighted average (TWA) limit of 200-mT (7).   In its original formulation, the European Union (EU) Directive had an Action Value of 200-mT, applied as a limit rather than as TWA (9).

Movement within the static field gradient is experienced as a slowly time-varying magnetic field, which will induce an electric field in tissues. For most standards, the low frequency, that is, below 1-Hz, limits can be applied. The ICNIRP is currently developing limits for movement within the static magnetic field (22).

Time-Varying Fields Up to 100-kHz

The ICNIRP and IEEE Basic Restrictions for time-varying magnetic fields up to 100-kHz are shown in **Figure 1**, along with the IEC limit for peripheral nerve stimulation. The IEEE Basic Restrictions are specific to the body part: brain, heart and other, while the ICNIRP's restrictions are for central nervous system (CNS) tissues in the head or for any tissue in a controlled situation. IEC 60601-2-33 stipulates that the MRI worker should not experience PNS and, in the absence of experimental data from a specific MR system, proposes a rheobase of 2.2-V/m or 20-T/sec. and chronaxie of 0.36-ms.

These limits pertain to single frequency sinusoidal fields. For non-sinusoidal pulses, in the region 1 to 100-kHz, one can apply the limits to each frequency component present in the waveform (23):

$$\sum_{f_{min}}^{f_{max}} \frac{B_i}{L_i} \leq 1 \tag{13}$$

where, B_i, is each individual frequency component of the field, L_i, the appropriate limit value and f_{min} and f_{max} define the frequency range. This approach may result in overly conservative limits because it assumes coherent phase between the spectral components (24). For frequency ranges where the incident field limit, B_L, has an inverse relationship to frequency, its time derivative, dB/dt, is constant and may be used to test compliance even for complex waveforms (23, 24):

$$(dB/dt)_{pk} = \sqrt{2} \; 2\pi \, f \, B_L \tag{14}$$

Applying this approach, the ICNIRP Reference Level becomes 2.6-T/sec. over the frequency range 300 to 3000-Hz. Similarly, the IEEE head and trunk MPEs below 20-Hz become 0.48-T/sec. and, for the heart, 18.4-T/sec. below 3.325-kHz as shown in **Figure 2**. This methodology is particularly useful for MRI where gradient waveforms are usually of trapezoidal form with multiple harmonics but a single peak dB/dt. **Figure 2** shows Reference Levels up to 100-kHz.

Figure 1. Induced field limits up to 100 kHz. ICNIRP and IEEE values are root mean square (RMS). The IEC limit is the 100% median PNS threshold.

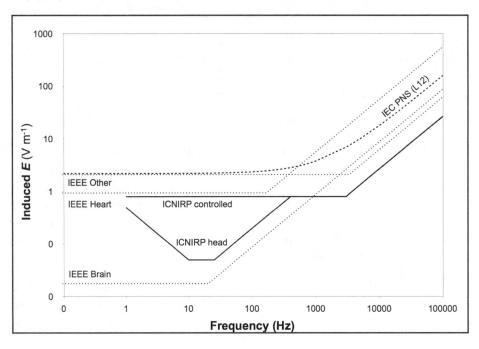

Figure 2. Incident field limits: ICNIRP reference levels and IEEE maximum permissible exposures.

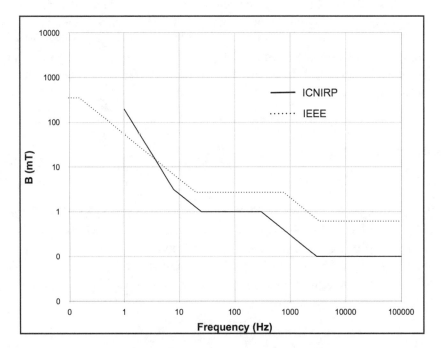

Radiofrequency Fields

Occupational limits relevant to MRI for RF exposures are shown in **Table 2**. Induced field limits are specified as SAR, with a whole body limit of 0.4-W/kg time averaged over six minutes, chosen to restrict a core body temperature rise to not more than 0.1°C. This is one tenth of the upper limit for patients. Also specified are localized (i.e., over 10-g of tissue) SAR limits of 10-W/kg for the head and trunk and 20-W/kg for the limbs. The IEEE incident field limits have a frequency and, therefore, scanner B_0 dependence. The IEC uses the same limit both for workers and patients, that is, a whole body SAR of up to 4-W/kg (1).

Table 2. RF limits for occupational exposure as applicable to MRI. All time-averaged over 6-minutes.

	Scanner B_0	Frequency (MHz)	Basic Restriction	Reference Level, Limit or Maximum Permissible Exposure			
			SAR (W/kg)	E (V/m)	H (A/m)	B ((µT)	Power density (W/m²)
IEC (1)	Any	All	4	N/A	N/A	N/A	N/A
ICNIRP (4) NRPB (7)	Any	10 to 400	0.4	61	0.16	0.2	10
IEEE (6)	1-T	42.57	0.4	61.4	0.163	N/A	55.2
	1.5-T	63.9	N/A	61.4	0.163	N/A	25.5
	3-T	127.7	N/A	61.4	0.128	N/A	10
	7-T	298.0	N/A	61.4	0.0547	N/A	10

(N/A, not applicable)

STUDIES OF INCIDENT FIELDS

Studies of occupational exposures have utilized a number of approaches. The most direct is to issue magnetic dosimeters to staff members and to record their exposures to static and time-varying magnetic fields during the working day (25-29). The second approach is to record the movements of staff members during real activities and correlate these with field maps, either from the manufacturers' data sheets, theoretical calculations, or environmental electromagnetic field (EMF) measurements (30, 31). The third approach is to simulate staff member activities while measuring the magnetic field exposure. This has the advantage of being predictive, such that worst-case movements can be investigated and peak exposures may be estimated (32-36). In a more generalized approach to occupational exposure in MRI, one can identify specific tasks and their temporal and magnitude exposures to formulate a Job Evaluation Matrix (37). This can then be used predictively to estimate occupational exposures for different staff groups over a prolonged period of time.

Personal Dosimeter Studies

Personal magnetic dosimeters utilize a combination of three axis Hall effect probes (B) and search coils (dB/dt), sometimes in conjunction with an integrator to give B readings (26, 38). Studies conducted at Oxford (25) and Queensland (26, 27) used dosimeters worn by MRI radiographers and technologists during their routine duties. Bradley, et al. (25) investigated static magnetic field exposures in four 1.5-T closed bore MR systems, one 3-T closed bore scanner, and one open 0.6-T MR system. Staff members carried the dosimeters in the pocket closest to the scanners. Peak and 24 hour time-averaged B fields were reported. In the Queensland study (26), peak B, peak dB/dt and TWA B over the shift were measured for three clinical 1.5-T scanners, and research systems at 2-T and 4-T. **Figure 3** shows typical readings of instantaneous B and dB/dt over a whole shift on a 1.5-T clinical system.

Table 3 summarizes the results from these two studies. The average maximum instantaneous exposure from both studies combined was 42% ± 24% of B_0. The TWA B was 5.2 ± 2.8-mT over all 165 shifts. Both IEEE limit (500-mT) and the ICNIRP 1-Hz Reference Level (280-mT peak) were exceeded. For the Queensland survey, the study mean of peak dB/dt exposure was 2.1 ± 1.3-T/sec. Assuming a maximum motion-equivalent frequency of 1-Hz, then the applicable IEEE and ICNIRP limits are routinely exceeded, including the draft ICNIRP movement-related limit of 1.8-T/sec. (22).

De Vocht, et al. (28) monitored occupational exposure for MR system engineering staff performing various tasks, including shimming, body coil adjustment, magnet ramping and

Figure 3. Staff dosimeter readings over one work shift from a 1.5T clinical system. Top: Instantaneous B; Bottom: Instantaneous dB/dt. Reproduced with permission from reference 26.

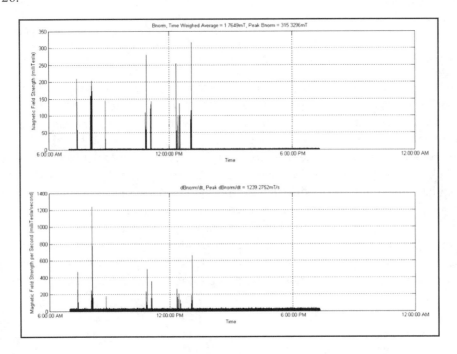

Table 3. Personal dosimetry measurements from MRI radiographers/technologists. Adapted with permission from reference 18.

B_0 (T)	No. of Scanners	No. of Shifts	Average Peak B (mT)	TWA B (mT)	Maximum B (mT)	Mean Peak dB/dt (T/sec.)	Maximum dB/dt (T/sec)	Ref.
0.6	1	19	380	5.7 ± 3.0	380	N/A	N/A	(25)
1.5	4	103	467 ± 103	5.1 ± 2.8	518	N/A	N/A	(25)
1.5	3	23	601 ± 240	5.1 ± 3.1	1281	2.2 ± 1.5	5.98	(26, 27)
2.0	1	2	561 ± 33	6.9 ± 1.2	584	1.5 ± 0.4	1.75	(26, 27)
3.0	1	12	822	4.8 ± 2.4	822	N/A	N/A	(25)
4.0	1	5	513 ± 67	6.4 ± 2.9	616	1.7 ± 0.4	2.04	(26, 27)

(N/A, not applicable)

system tests. In general, magnet shimming produced the highest exposures with TWA B values of 17-, 25- and 86-mT for 1-, 1.5- and 3-T scanners, respectively, showing a strong correlation with the strength of the static magnetic field. Peak exposures occurred in the range of 54- to 1094-mT with a mean of 549-mT ± 303-mT. The dB/dt values were up to 3.97-T/sec. and were associated with movement within the static field gradient, exceeding the draft ICNIRP limit. The peak dB/dt did not correlate well with B_0.

Other personal dosimetry studies are ongoing, with currently two under way: in the United Kingdom (F. de Vocht, Personal Communication, 2013) and in the Netherlands (29). The Dutch study involves 12 different occupations over 15 various institutions including academic, clinical and veterinary MRI facilities. At the time of writing, full results are not available, although preliminary results for peak B and dB/dt per job type are shown in **Figure 4**. While further analysis, including correction for temporal drift, needs to be made, the early results confirm that service engineers experience higher exposure levels than clinical staff members. The highest peak B and dB/dt recorded were 5-T and 5.1-T/sec. but the means were in the range of 500 to 1000-mT and less than 2-T/sec. TWA values from this study are eagerly awaited.

Environmental EMF Studies

Static Magnetic Field

Static field surveys (30, 32) show that 200-mT (the Action Value for 0-Hz in the original 2004 EU Directive and also the current ICNIRP RMS reference level for 1-Hz is exceeded at about 0.5-m from the bore opening for most 1.5-T and 3-T MR systems. The 500-mT contour (IEEE MPE for <0.153-Hz) lies in the region 0.2 to 0.3-m from the bore entrance. **Figure 5** shows measured field plots in one-quadrant outside the bore for a 1-T open, 1.5-T, 3-T and 7-T (unshielded) closed bore MR systems.

Figure 4. Preliminary results for staff dosimetry study in the Netherlands (29) for different staff groups. The boxes indicate first and third quartiles, the horizontal line is the median, the diamond symbols denotes the mean, circles are outliers. Reproduced with permission from reference 29.

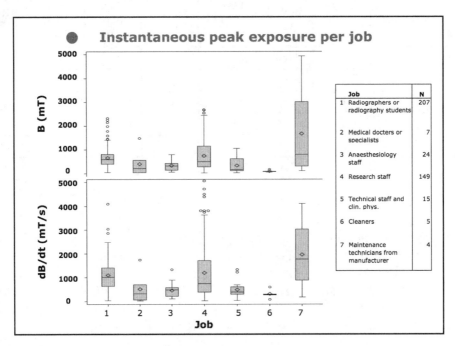

Figure 5. Single quadrant static field plots for 1-T open, 1.5-, 3- and 7-T MR systems. The dotted arrow indicates the isocenter and the solid arrow indicates the center of the bore opening. Reproduced with permission from reference 30.

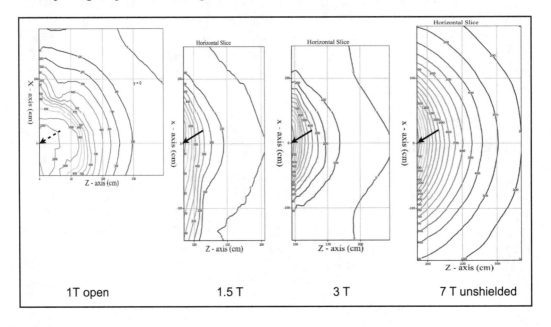

Time-Varying Magnetic Fields

Early measurements involving a single search coil established that significant gradient fringe fields exist beyond the bore of the scanner (39). These results have been extended using 3-axis calibrated meters (30, 32, 33, 35, 36). **Table 4** shows peak B, dB/dt and percentage of the ICNIRP reference levels measured outside the bore of the magnet for the worst-case sequences from the available data. In 2012, the report by McRobbie (18) presents results from all the sequences investigated. While the EU Directive's 2004 Action Values were readily exceeded for many pulse sequences, the new ICNIRP RL was rarely exceeded outside the bore of the scanner (18), rendering a staff exclusion zone unnecessary.

In general, the faster pulse sequences (e.g., EPI, b-TFE, b-FFE, TruFi) had higher peak dB/dt, although some MR systems are programmed to utilize the highest possible slew rate,

Table 4. B and dB/dt fringe field values and % limit exposures from the imaging gradients for worst-case sequences. Negative distance indicates distance into the bore of the MR system. <<RL indicates measurement very much less than the Reference Level.

B_0 (T)	MR System	|B|rms (µT)	Peak dB/dt (T/sec.)	% ICNIRP RL	Distance from Bore Entrance (m)	Sequence	Fundamental Frequency	Reference
0.6	Fonar	N/A	0.22	8.5	0.30	FSE	Unknown	25
1.0	Philips Panorama	N/A	0.32	12	0.0	B-TFE	260-Hz	30
1.0	Philips Panorama	N/A	0.1	3.8	0.0	EPI	Unknown	35
1.5	GE Signa Twin	N/A	1.14	44	0.0	EPI	Unknown	25
1.5	Unspecified A	1500	N/A	141	0.0	B-FFE	300-Hz	32
1.5	Unspecified B	700	N/A	85	0.0	B-FFE	360-Hz	32
1.5	Philips Intera	650	N/A	110	0.0	FFE	500-Hz	33
1.5	Siemens Avanto	N/A	1.99	77	0.15	TruFISP	670-Hz	30
1.5	Siemens Espree	100	0.77	29	0.3	TruFi	Unknown	36
3.0	Philips Achieva	N/A	1.69	65	0.11	EPI	1-kHz	30
3.0	Philips Achieva	N/A	1.6	62	0.0	EPI	Unknown	35
7.0	Philips Intera	662	1.78	<<RL	-0.85	Perfusion	770-Hz	30

(N/A, not applicable)

making the peak dB/dt more independent of the sequence type. Greater exposures may occur for open scanners (40). For the other MR systems, the length of the bore is important. For example, the very long bore of the 7-T scanner ensures that the fringe field of the gradients is negligible outside this MR system's bore. The exposure values scale with various factors including pixel size, field-of-view (30), slice thickness and orientation, bandwidth, echo time and acoustic noise reduction (36). **Figure 6** shows the instantaneous |dB/dt|(vector sum for all gradients) for various pulse sequences from one MR system measured at the entrance to the bore.

The fundamental frequency of the sequences ranged from as low as 80-Hz (turbo spin echo) to 1-kHz (echo planar imaging, EPI). Most of the fast pulse sequences relevant to interventional MRI (b-TFE, b-FFE, TruFi) had fundamental frequencies in the range of 300- to 500-Hz, appropriate to the application of the ICNIRP dB/dt limit of 2.6-T/sec. **Figure 6** shows the frequency components for an EPI sequence.

Radiofrequency Field

Studies of the fringe field associated with the RF field for a turbo spin echo (TSE) pulse sequence used for magnetic resonance cholangiopancreatography (MRCP) examinations and a bespoke test sequence on a range on scanners showed that Reference Levels can be exceeded close to the bore of the MR system (30), within 0.45-m for an open scanner and 0.2-m for a short-bore, closed scanner (33).

Figure 6. Instantaneous dB/dt from the imaging gradients (vector sum of all gradients) measured outside the bore 95-cm from the isocenter. Top three tracings: Turbo spin echo, balanced Turbo-Field Echo, Diffusion imaging. Lowest trace: Spectral content of the DW-EPI sequence. Reproduced with permission from reference 30.

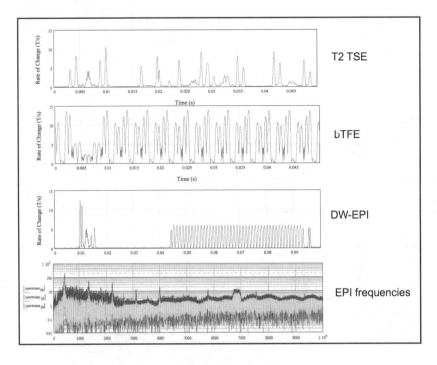

Time-Motion Studies

In a study commissioned by the European Commission, under the auspices of the European Society of Radiology and specifically designed to investigate the impact of the EU Directive on MRI, Capstick, et al. (30) observed staff members during typical clinical procedures in an open 1-T scanner and closed bore 1.5-, 3- and 7-T scanners (**Figure 7**). Staff movements were recorded by a two camera video system and their position, velocity and exposure times were determined for each procedure. The staff groups investigated included radiographers, anesthetists, interventional radiologists, cleaners (i.e., custodial workers), researchers and parent/care givers. By combining these observations with three-dimensional volumetric environmental EMF measurements, the staff exposures were estimated in terms of maximum and mean B, maximum static field gradient ($|dB/dr|$), maximum dB/dt and fundamental frequency from the imaging gradients, and TWA B_1, H_1 and E_1 (time-averaged over 6-min.).

Figure 8 and **Table 5** summarize these results and those from the other studies (25, 26, 27) for B both from the static magnetic field and the gradients shown with respect to the ICNIRP incident field limits. Static magnetic field limits were exceeded for all the activities at 7-T and a majority of the others. The ICNIRP Reference Levels for exposure from the imaging gradients were exceeded for breast biopsy clip insertion (by 7% with a sequence fundamental frequency of 260-Hz) and monitoring patients under general anesthesia (by 16% for a fundamental frequency of 670-Hz). None of the exposures exceeded the relevant IEEE or Bundesministeriums für Arbeit und Soziales (BMAS) (8) incident field limits. Most movement-related exposures exceeded the various low frequency limits. Imaging gradient dB/dt exceeded the ICNIRP Reference Level (RL) (300 to 3000-Hz) for the clip insertion by 1.9 times. In no instance was a RF field Reference Level exceeded, although for the breast interventional procedure this was largely due to the time averaging (i.e., the procedure only lasted 42-sec.). A similar study has been carried out for MR system engineers where the speed of movement for particular actions correlated with the occurrence of sensory effects (41).

Other studies have investigated exposures and induced fields from specific movements by volunteer subjects chosen to mimic actual movements performed by staff members carrying out their duties close to the MR system (32, 34, 35). The observed dB/dt values in the range of 1- to 3-T/sec. are in good agreement with the dosimetric studies. Using a unique dosimeter Glover, et al. (34) directly measured induced electric fields E_i in the range of 0.042- to 0.17-V/m for movements, compared with 2.4- to 3.8-mV/m from the gradients for a person standing next to the opening of the bore of the MR system and a gradient slew rate of 10-T/m/sec.

STUDIES OF INDUCED FIELDS IN TISSUES

As the Basic Restrictions are given in terms of induced fields or SAR, numerical simulations may be required to demonstrate compliance. Both quasi-static finite difference or finite integration numerical techniques of the field interactions for anatomically realistic models have been employed (42-49).

Figure 7. Various activities from the EU study (30). Top left: Biopsy clip insertion on a 1-T open MR system. Top Right: Pediatric general anesthesia monitoring on a 1.5-T system. Bottom Left: Tactile fMRI on a 3-T system. Bottom Right: Manual contrast administration on a 7-T MR system. Reproduced with permission from reference 30.

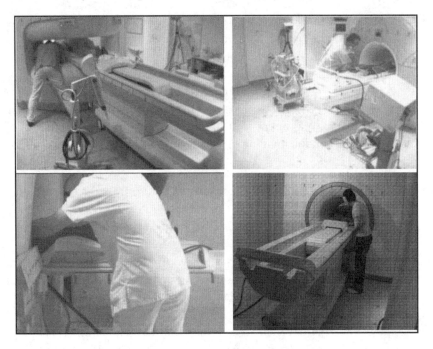

Figure 8. Static field and gradient field exposures from various studies (25, 26, 28, 30) plotted against the ICNIRP reference level.

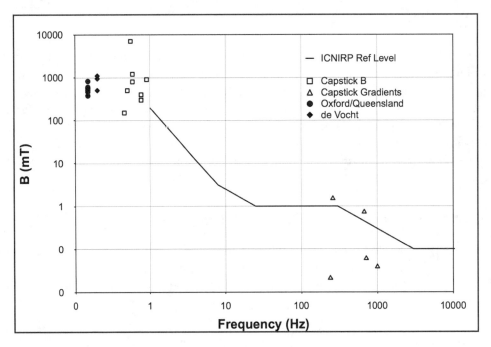

Table 5. Peak B, dB/dt and average B1 for various activities and staff groups observed in the EU study. The ICNIRP reference level for dB/dt from movement is from a draft document. Reproduced with permission from reference 30.

			Peak B (mT)	Peak dB/dt movement	Peak dB/dt gradients	TWA-B_1 (6-min. RMS)	Complies with ICNIRP Reference Levels?
			(mT)	(T/sec.)	(T/sec.)	(μT)	
ICNIRP Reference Level			280	1.8	2.6	0.2	
B_0	Activity	Occupation					
1-T	Breast biopsy	Radiologist	150	0	0	0	Yes
	Breast clip insertion	Radiologist	800	1.94	5	0.08	No
	General anesthesia child	Care giver	50	0	<<RL	<<RL	Yes
	Emergency	Radiographer	50	0.21	0	0	Yes
1.5-T	General anesthesia child	Anesthetist	500	0.13	1.89	0	No
	Manual contrast	Radiographer	200	0.13	0	0	Yes
	Emergency	Radiographer	200	0.19	0	0	Yes
	Cleaning	Cleaner	1500	0.36	0	0	No
3-T	Tactile fMRI	Radiographer	400	0.5	0.32	<<RL	No
	Cardiac stress	Cardiologist	150	0.6	0.05	<<RL	Yes
	General anesthesia	Anesthetist	300	0.72	0.39	<<RL	No
	Emergency	Radiographer	100	0.5	0	0	Yes
	Cleaning	Radiographer	3000	0.9	0	0	No
7-T	Manual contrast	Radiologist	1200	0.73	<<RL	<<RL	No
	EEG	Researcher	7000	3.7	0	0	No
	Emergency	Radiographer	900	2.5	0	0	No

Motion in the Static Magnetic Field

Studies of linear motion of workers around MR system magnets (1.5- to 7-T) have confirmed that induced field limits may be exceeded for motion at 1-m/sec. within 0.5- to 1-m of the scanner (44, 45). The induced electric field and current density scaled with B_0 (**Figure 9**). The worst-case situations associated with these occurred for motion parallel to the z-axis towards the magnet. The ICNIRP 1-Hz Basic Restrictions was exceeded in the spine and brain for 4-T and 7-T, and the IEEE basic restriction for brain was exceeded in every case. A further study of bending towards high field strength scanners revealed similar E_i in CSF with 0.16 to 0.56-V/m in the brain but much less in the spine (46).

In the study of Capstick, et al. (30) emergency evacuation which had the greatest velocities (mean 1.5 ± 0.5-m/sec.) gave a maximum J_{rms} in the range of 9.1 for 1-T to 24.6-mA/m^2 for 7-T with the maximum induced current in neural tissue approximately 60% less. RMS current densities from movement during other activities (e.g., tactile fMRI, general anesthesia monitoring, cardiac stress test, manual contrast injection) were in the range of 5.7- to 32.9-mA/m^2. Cleaning the bore of the MR system gave values up to 16.7-mA/m^2. All of these are lower than the NRPB Basic Restrictions. It is hard to estimate the maximum E_i in neural tissue from movement in these instances but using a maximum conductivity of neural tissue of 0.10-S/m, most of these activities exceed the IEEE Basic Restriction of 0.0177-V/m RMS. The only activity investigated that may exceed the ICNIRP Basic Re-

Figure 9. Induced E_i fields from movement towards 1.5-, 4- and 7-T MR systems at 1-m/sec. Reproduced with permission from reference 45.

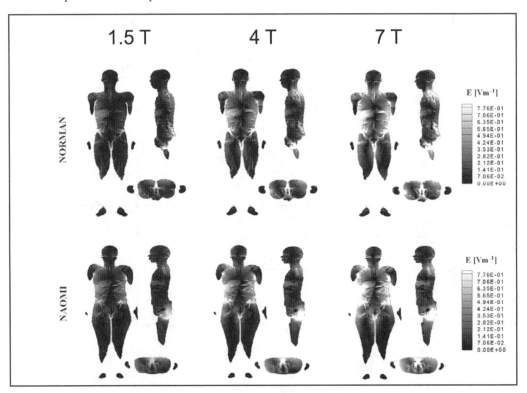

striction of 0.5-V/m RMS (0.8-V/m controlled situation) was the interventional breast biopsy clip insertion in the open 1-T MR system which gave maximum J_{rms} of 84-mA/m^2 (estimated 0.85-V/m) averaged over 1-cm^2 in neural tissue.

Induced Fields from the Gradient Magnetic Fields

Crozier, et al. (47) considered a 1-kHz trapezoidal gradient similar to that used in an EPI sequence normalized to 1-mT/m with a 0.1-ms rise time. Care is required when scaling up to higher levels because the full gradient strength assumed in this study of 40-mT/m is not typical for most clinical scans and would result in an unrealistically high slew rate. However, assuming this as a worst-case, peak E_i greater than 2.2-V/m ($J_{max} = 815$-mA/m^2) in the spinal cord was calculated on axis close to the end of the coil for combined G_x, G_y and G_z. For a more realistic gradient amplitude of 20-mT/m the ICNIRP head central nervous tissues Basic Restriction was only exceeded within 0.01-m of the end of the coil. However, other tissues also exceeded tissue limits: skin up to 0.4-m, fat 0.3-m, muscle 0.25-m and heart 0.1-m.

In a more realistically representative model, with the subject positioned 0.35-m off-axis laterally, 0.19-m from the end of the coil and exposed to a G_z of 10-mT/m at 1-kHz, Li, et al. 48), estimated E_i of 32-mV/m RMS in CNS tissue ($J_i = 20.6$-mA/m^2, 1-cm^2 average) with a maximum J_i of 59-mA/m^2 in muscle tissue and maximum E_i of 4.1-V/m in skin.

The European study (30, 49) calculated induced current densities of 60-mA/m^2 RMS for any tissue and 10-mA/m^2 RMS for neural tissue for real clinical tasks such as performing tactile fMRI and general anesthesia monitoring near closed bore 1.5- and 3-T scanners. The maximum E_i of 1.05-V/m RMS from the x-gradient occurred in the skin of the head (**Figure 10**).

The exposure to the interventional radiologist within the bore of a 1-T open scanner (**Figure 11**) produced up to 220-mA/m^2 RMS averaged over 1-cm^2 in any tissue, with 140-mA/m^2 RMS in neural tissue. The peak E_i was 0.74-V/m RMS in the skin of the head. As tissue conductivities vary considerably the maximum J_i does not necessarily coincide with the maximum E_i, nevertheless, these simulations suggest compliance with both the IEEE and ICNIRP Basic Restrictions.

Radiofrequency Exposure and SAR

The European study investigated two instances when a member of staff may exceed an RF reference level (30, 49). From their numerical simulations, a bystander standing close to the bore entrance would receive a 0.9-mW/kg whole body SAR and a 14-mW/kg peak in 10-g SAR (**Figure 12**). The second situation was an interventional radiologist within the bore of an open system, receiving 0.053-W/kg whole body SAR and 0.44-W/kg in 10-g of tissue. These are well below any occupational SAR limit.

DISCUSSION

We have seen above, that outside the bore of the MR system, exposure from the imaging gradients and RF is generally well below most incident and induced field limits. Careful

Figure 10. Induced current densities and electric fields from the gradients in a person standing adjacent to bore opening of a closed MR system from 40-mT/m x-gradient at 1-kHz. The maximum single voxel J_i is 69-mAm^2 (41-mA m^2 averaged over 1-cm^2). J_i greyscale bars are normalized to the maximum value. Reproduced with permission from reference 30.

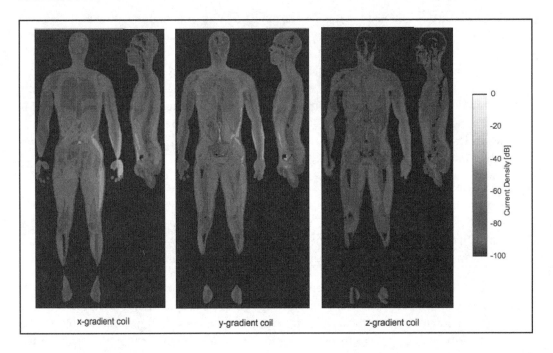

Figure 11. Induced fields in an interventional radiologist within the bore of a 1-T open MR system, z-gradient, 26-mT/m. The maximum single voxel J_i is 1.2-A/m^2 (510-mA/m^2 averaged over 1-cm^2) and occurs in the CNS. Reproduced with permission from reference 30.

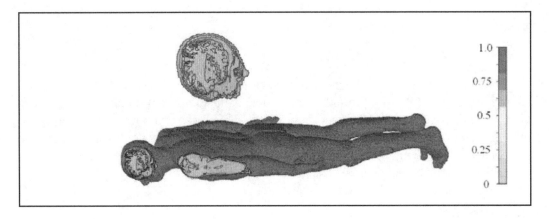

Figure 12. SAR distribution for a person standing adjacent to the opening of the bore of an MR system. The SAR 10-g is normalized to the peak value. The maximum is in the arm and has a value 10-g SAR = 0.87-mW/kg for a B_1 in the isocenter of 1-μT. The whole body SAR is 0.057-mW/kg for a B_1 in the isocenter of 1-μT. Reproduced with permission from reference 30.

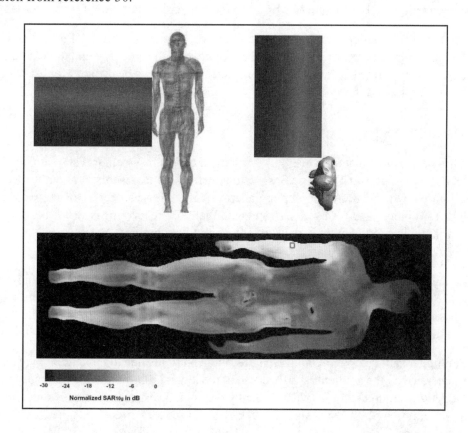

consideration needs to be given to movement around high field strength magnets for MR systems. Most activities that occur during clinical MRI will only result in significant occupational exposure in association with the static field. Special cases of particular importance include pregnant staff members, and those who must remain close to the bore of the MR system during scanning (e.g., anesthesiologists, intervention radiologists, nurses and researchers).

The current advice is for pregnant staff to avoid being in the MR system room during scan acquisition, principally on account of the risk to fetal hearing from acoustic noise (16, 17). Specific dosimetric studies for pregnant staff have not been carried out, although incident field exposures are expected to be similar to those for other staff members. Kanal, et al. (50) conducted a limited epidemiological study of pregnant MRI healthcare that demonstrated no adverse effect on pregnancy outcome.

It is estimated that approximately 3% of clinical MRI examinations require a staff member to remain within the room during scanning (51). For MRI-guided interventional radiology, the results from the previous section as one specific example, suggest that the ICNIRP

Basic Restrictions may be complied with. However, demonstration of this relies upon the accuracy of the EMF modeling, which currently has not been verified.

It is likely that the EMF exposures received by research (29, 52) and engineering (28, 41) staff members may exceed those of the clinical staff. Accordingly, further investigation of the occupational RF exposure of MR system engineering staff would be welcome.

The greatest issues concerning occupational exposure are the range of guideline limits in existence and the threat from over-zealous application of these by regulators (53-55). In particular, limits defined in terms of induced fields will always be difficult for establishing compliance or, indeed, for enforcement.

CONCLUSIONS

It has been shown that time-averaged static field exposures to clinical staff are relatively low, in the region of 5-mT, with peak static magnetic field exposures of about 40% of B_0. These figures are probably higher for engineering staff and researchers. Dosimetric surveys of dB/dt for clinical and research staff indicate that they receive peak dB/dt of around 2-T/sec. arising from movement in the static magnetic field gradient.

The current Reference Levels that exist for the imaging gradients are unlikely to be exceeded in most circumstances. The increase in the ICNIRP limits within the frequency range of the MRI gradients means that, in contradiction to the conclusions of earlier studies, RF exposure is now more likely to become an issue than the gradients for staff who remain close to the bore of the MR system during scanning (18).

For higher static magnetic field strengths, induced fields due to movement may exceed those generated by the gradients and, because of the lower limits in the low frequency range, routine activity around scanners will frequently result in the exceeding of one or more limits. For high field strength MR systems, the occurrence of sensory effects (e.g., nausea, vertigo, metallic taste, etc.) is evidence that limits are being exceeded. These induced field exposures can be minimized through staff training and appropriate control measures.

Definitive proof that EMF exposures associated with MRI to staff members are biologically safe remains elusive, although there is no evidence to the contrary. Whatever the outcome of regulatory activity in the EU or elsewhere, occupational exposure in MRI will continue to have a high profile in the medical, scientific, and engineering communities.

REFERENCES

1. International Electrotechnical Commission. Medical Electrical Equipment – Part 2-33: Particular Requirements for the Safety of Magnetic Resonance Equipment for Medical Diagnosis. IEC 60601-2-33, Third Edition. Geneva: 2009.

2. International Commission on Non-Ionizing Radiation Protection. Guidelines on limits to exposure from static magnetic field. Health Physics 2009;96:504-514.

3. International Commission on Non-Ionizing Radiation Protection. Guidelines for limiting exposure to time-varying electric, magnetic, and electromagnetic fields (up to 100 kHz). Health Physics 2010;99:818-836 and Erratum Health Physics 2011;100:112.

4. International Commission on Non-Ionizing Radiation Protection. ICNIRP statement on the "Guidelines for limiting exposure to time-varying electric, magnetic, and electromagnetic fields (up to 300 GHz)". Health Physics 2009;93:257-258.

5. Institute of Electrical and Electronics Engineers (IEEE). IEEE Standard for Safety Levels with Respect to Human Exposure to Radio Frequency Electromagnetic Fields. 0-3 kHz, C95.6-2002. New York, USA: The Institute of Electrical and Electronics Engineers, 2002.

6. Institute of Electrical and Electronics Engineers. IEEE Standard for Safety Levels with Respect to Human Exposure to Radio Frequency Electromagnetic Fields, 3 kHz to 300 GHz -Description, C95.1-199. New York, USA: Institute of Electrical and Electronics Engineers, 2005.

7. National Radiological Protection Board. Advice on Limiting Exposure to Electromagnetic Fields (0-300 GHz). Documents of the NRPB 2004;15,2.

8. Borner F, Bruggemeyer H, Eggert S, et al. Electromagnetic fields at workplaces: A new scientific approach to occupational health and safety. Bundesministeriums für Arbeit und Soziales (BMAS). http://www.bmas.de/portal/44700/fb400__elektromagnetische__felder.html Accessed January, 2013.

9. European Commission Directive 2004/40/EC of the European Parliament and of the Council of 29 April 2004 on the minimum health and safety requirements regarding the exposure of workers to the risks arising from physical agents (electromagnetic fields). Official Journal of the European Union L 159, 2004.

10. Shellock FG, Editor. Magnetic Resonance Procedures: Health Effects and Safety. Boca Raton, USA: CRC Press, 2001.

11. Partain CL, Editor. Journal of MRI special edition: MRI safety. J Magn Reson Imaging 2007;26:1175-1344.

12. Food and Drugs Administration. Criteria for significant risk investigations of magnetic resonance diagnostic devices. Rockville, MD: Center for Devices and Radiological Health, US Food and Drug Administration, 2003.

13. Health Protection Agency. Protection of patients and volunteers undergoing MRI procedures, Documents of the Health Protection Agency RCE-7, Chilton, United Kingdom: Health Protection Agency, 2008.

14. International Commission on Non-Ionizing Radiation Protection. Medical magnetic resonance (MR) procedures: protection of patients. Health Phys 2004;87:197-216.

15. International Commission on Non-Ionizing Radiation Protection. Amendment to the ICNIRP "Statement on medical magnetic resonance procedures: protection of patients." Health Physics 2009;97:259-261.

16. Medicines and Healthcare Products Regulatory Agency. Safety guidelines for magnetic resonance imaging equipment in clinical use. MHRA DB2007. London, United Kingdom: Medicines and Healthcare Products Regulatory Agency, 2007.

17. Kanal E, Borgstede JP, Barkovich AJ, et al. American College of Radiology white paper on MR safety. Amer J Roentgen 2001;178:1335–1347.

18. McRobbie DW. Occupational exposure in MRI. Br J Radiol 2012;85:293–312.

19. Budinger TF. Thresholds for physiological effects due to RF and magnetic fields used in NMR imaging. IEEE Trans Nucl Sci 1979;NS-26:2821-2825.

20. McRobbie D, Foster MA. Pulsed magnetic field exposure during pregnancy and implications for NMR foetal imaging: a study with mice. Magn Reson Imaging 1985;3:231-234.

21. Shaefer DJ, Shellock FG. Health Effects and Safety of Radiofrequency Power Deposition Associated with Magnetic Resonance Procedures. In: Shellock FG, Editor. Magnetic Resonance Procedures: Health Effects and Safety. Boca Raton, USA: CRC Press, 2001; pp. 75-96.

22. International Commission on Non-Ionizing Radiation Protection. Draft guidelines for limiting exposure to electric fields induced by movement of the human body in a static magnetic fields and by time-varying magnetic fields below 1-Hz. http://www.icnirp.de/OpenMovement/ICNIRPMovementConsultation Draft2012.pdf Accessed January, 2013.

23. International Commission on Non-Ionizing Radiation Protection. Guidance on determining compliance of exposure to pulsed and complex non-sinusoidal waveforms below 100 kHz with ICNIRP guidelines. Health Physics 2003; 84:383-387.

24. Jokela K. Assessment of complex EMF exposure situations including inhomogeneous field distribution. Health Physics 2007;92:531-540.

25. Bradley JK, Nyekiova M, Price DL, D'jon Lopez L, Crawley T. Occupational exposure to static and time-varying gradient magnetic fields in MR units. J Magn Reson Imaging 2007;26:1204-1209.

26. Fuentes MA, Trakic A, Wilson SJ, Crozier S. Analysis and measurements of magnetic field exposures for healthcare workers in selected MR environments. IEEE Trans Biomed Eng 2008;55:1355-64.

27. Chadwick P. Assessment of electromagnetic fields around magnetic resonance imaging (MRI) equipment. United Kingdom Health and Safety Executive 2007; RR570. Available from: http://www.hse.gov.uk/research/rpdf/rr570.pdf Accessed January, 2013.

28. de Vocht F, Muller F, Engels H, Kromhout H. Personal exposure to static and time-varying magnetic fields during MRI system test procedures. J Magn Reson Imaging 2009;30:1223-8.

29. Schaap K. Quantitative assessment of exposure to stray static magnetic fields from MRI devices in clinical and research environments. Proc. British Occupational Hygiene Society X2012 conference Edinburgh, 4 July 2012. http://www.bohs.org/X2012presentations/# Accessed January, 2013.

30. Capstick M, McRobbie D, Hand J, et al. An investigation into occupational exposure to electro-magnetic fields for personnel working with and around medical magnetic resonance imaging equipment. Report on Project VT/2007/017 of the European Commission Employment, Social Affairs and Equal Opportunities DG; 2008. www.myesr.org/html/img/pool/VT2007017FinalReportv04.pdf Accessed January, 2013.

31. Hartwig V, Vanello N, Giovannetti G, et al. A novel tool for estimation of magnetic resonance occupational exposure to spatially varying magnetic fields. MAGMA 2011;24:323-30.

32. Riches SF, Charles-Edwards GD, Shafford JC, et al. Measurements of occupational exposure to switched gradient and spatially-varying magnetic fields in areas adjacent to 1.5T clinical MRI systems. J Magn Reson Imaging 2007;26:1346-1352.

33. Riches SF, Collins DJ, Scuffham JW, Leach MO. EU Directive 2004/40: field measurements of a 1.5 T clinical MR scanner. Br J Radiol 2007;80:483-487.

34. Glover PM, Bowtell R. Measurement of electric fields induced in a human subject due to natural movements in static magnetic fields or exposure to alternating gradient fields. Phys Med Biol 2008;53:361-373.

35. Kannala S, Toivo T, Alanko T, Jokela K. Occupational exposure measurements of static and pulsed gradient magnetic fields in the vicinity of MRI scanners. Phys Med Biol 2009;54: 2243-2257.

36. Wilen J, Hauksson J, Hansson Mild K. Modification of pulse sequences reduces occupational exposure from MRI switched gradient fields: preliminary results. Bioelectromagnetics 2010;31:85–7.

37. Christopher-de Vries Y, Bongers S , Engels H, Pauline Slottje P, Hans Kromhout H. A generic model for estimating exposure to MRI-related static magnetic fields and its use in reconstructing historical occupational exposure. Proc. British Occupational Hygiene Society X2012 conference Edinburgh, 4 July 2012. http://www.bohs.org/X2012presentations/# Accessed January, 2013.

38. Cavagnetto F, Prati P, Ariola V, et al. A personal dosimeter prototype for static magnetic fields. Health Physics 1993;65:172-177.

39. McRobbie DW, Cross T. Occupational exposure to time varying magnetic gradient fields (dB/dt) in MRI and European limits. In: Proceedings of the International Society for Magnetic Resonance in Medicine (ISMRM) Workshop on MRI Safety: Update, Practical Information and Future Implications. McLean Virginia. Berkeley, USA: International Society for Magnetic Resonance in Medicine, 2005.

40. Bassen H, Shaefer DJ, Zaremba L, et al. IEEE committee on man and radiation (COMAR) technical information statement. Exposure of medical personnel to electromagnetic fields from open magnetic resonance imaging systems. Health Physics 2005;89:684-689.

41. de Vocht F, van Drooge H, Engels H, Kromhout H. Exposure, health complaints and cognitive performance among employees of an MRI scanners manufacturing department. J Magn Reson Imaging 2006;23:197-204.

42. Hand JW. Modelling the interaction of electromagnetic fields (10 MHz-10 GHz) with the human body: methods and applications. Phys Med Biol 2008;53:R243-286.

43. Liu F, Crozier S. A distributed equivalent magnetic current based FDTD method for the calculation of E-fields induced by gradient coils. J Magn Reson Imaging 2004;169:323-327.

44. Liu F, Zhao H, Crozier S. Calculation of electric fields induced by body and head motion in high-field MRI. J Magn Reson Imaging 2003;161:99-107.

45. Crozier S, Trakic A, Wang H, Liu F. Numerical study of currents in workers induced by body-motion around high-ultrahigh field MRI magnets. J Magn Reson Imaging 2007;26:1261-1277.

46. Wang H, Trakic A, Lui F, Crozier S. Numerical field evaluation of healthcare workers when bending towards high-field MRI magnets. Magn Reson Med 2008;59:410-422.

47. Crozier S, Wang H, Trakic A, Lui F. Exposure of workers to pulsed gradients in MRI. J Magn Reson Imaging 2007;26:1236-1254.

48. Li Y, Hand JW, Wills T, Hajnal JV. Numerically simulated induced electric field and current density within a human model located close to a z-gradient coil. J Magn Reson Imaging 2007;26:1286-1295.

49. Li Y, Hand J, Christ A, et al. Modelling occupational exposure to RF and gradient fields associated with an interventional procedure in an open 1 T MR system. In: Proceedings of the International Society for Magnetic Resonance in Medicine, 17th Annual Meeting, Honolulu, HI. Berkeley, USA: International Society for Magnetic Resonance in Medicine (ISMRM), 2009; pp. 3042.

50. Kanal E, Gillen J, Evans, JA, et al. Survey of reproductive health among female MR workers. Radiology 1993;187:395-399.

51. Moore EA, Scurr ED. British Association of MR Radiographers (BAMRR) safety survey 2005: Potential impact of European Union (EU) Physical Agents Directive (PAD) on electromagnetic fields (EMF). J Magn Reson Imaging 2007;26:1303-1307.

52. Perrin N, Morris CJ. A survey of the potential impact of the European Union Physical Agents Directive (EU PAD) on electromagnetic fields (EMF) on MRI research practice in the United Kingdom. J Magn Reson Imaging 2008;28:482-492.

53. Keevil SF, Gedroyc W, Gowland P, et al. Electromagnetic field exposure limitation and the future of MRI. Commentary. Br J Radiol 2005;78:973-975.

54. Young I, McRobbie D, Keevil S, Taylor A. Unintended consequences of an unwarrantedly cautious approach to safety. Br J Hosp Med 2006;67:174-175.

55. Hill DLG, McLeish K, Keevil SF. Impact of electromagnetic field exposure limits in Europe: Is the future of interventional MRI safe? Acad Radiol 2005;12:1135-42.

Chapter 28   MRI Standards and Guidance Documents from the United States, Food and Drug Administration

WOLFGANG KAINZ, PH.D.

Research Biomedical Engineer
Division of Physics
Office of Science and Engineering Laboratories
Center for Devices and Radiological Health
Food and Drug Administration
Silver Spring, MD

INTRODUCTION

In 1976, the United States (U.S.), Food and Drug Administration (FDA) was given the authority to regulate medical devices through the Medical Device Amendments to the U.S. Food, Drug and Cosmetic Act. The FDA's regulation of medical devices roughly coincided with the first experimental uses of nuclear magnetic resonance (MR) systems in 1979. Presently, the FDA develops guidance documents to communicate its current thinking on a particular matter and participates in the development of standards by national and international standards development organizations (SDOs) to promote methods important to the evaluation of medical devices. Following the publication of standards, the FDA's Center for Devices and Radiological Health (CDRH) has a process to publically recognize all or parts of standards that it believes are helpful to assess medical devices. The CDRH updates their list of recognized standards periodically, adding newly recognized standards for medical devices and radiation-emitting electronic products, while replacing certain recognized standards with newly recognized revisions.

In some instances, it is believed that conformance with recognized consensus standards can provide scientific evidence to support a reasonable assurance of safety and/or effectiveness. However, conformance with recognized consensus standards may not always be a sufficient basis for regulatory decisions. Conformance with recognized consensus standards is strictly voluntary for a medical device manufacturer. Therefore, a manufacturer may choose to conform to applicable recognized standards or may choose to address relevant issues in another manner. Relevant and up-to-date information related to standards used in medical device submissions can be found at CDRH's Standard website (1).

This chapter provides an overview of the FDA's statutory authority over magnetic resonance imaging (MRI) devices in the United States, the regulatory interpretations of that authority, and the limitations of FDA's authority. However, it does not establish any new FDA policies or make changes, actual or implied, to existing policies. This chapter also describes the procedures that have recently been developed to facilitate the device review process. This is followed by a discussion of the present international standard for MRI equipment (also referred to as the "MR system") safety, standards for safety of medical devices in the MRI environment, and current FDA guidance documents related to MRI. Finally, there is a discussion of possible future developments in the field of MRI safety.

Importantly, the content of this chapter does not establish any new U.S. Food and Drug Administration (FDA) policies or make changes to existing policies. Furthermore, the content in this chapter is valid only at the time of publication and subject to change. The reader is referred to the pertinent FDA and standards development organizations (SDOs) websites to obtain comprehensive and up-to-date information regarding FDA policies, submissions of medical devices, and standards updates.

FDA AUTHORITY AND REGULATORY MECHANISMS

The Medical Device Amendments of 1976 to the Food, Drug and Cosmetic Act provide the statutory authority for FDA regulation of medical devices, including those involving MRI equipment. The Medical Device Amendments established three classes of devices, which are differentiated by the degree of risk and the amount of regulatory control needed to ensure their safety and effectiveness. The three classifications are, as follows: (1) Class I devices involve minimum risk and require only general controls; (2) Class II devices are those for which general controls are insufficient to assure safety and effectiveness, but for which existing methods are available to provide such assurances. In addition to general controls, Class II devices are also subject to special controls. Class II devices require premarket clearance prior to marketing. These premarket notifications are referred to as 510(k) applications and must demonstrate that the Class II device is substantially equivalent to a legally marketed Class I or II device. (3) Class III devices are those for which insufficient information exists to assure safety and effectiveness solely through general or special controls. Class III devices are usually those that support or sustain human life, are of substantial importance in preventing impairment of human health, or which present a potential, unreasonable risk of illness or injury. Manufacturers of Class III devices must submit a Premarket Approval application (PMA) demonstrating that the device is safe and effective. A Humanitarian Device Exemption (HDE) may be submitted for devices that are intended for use in diseases that affect less than 4,000 individuals per year in the United States. A clinical study is generally required as part of a PMA. If a study involves a significant risk to patients, the manufacturer must submit an Investigational Device Exemption (IDE) to the FDA prior to beginning clinical studies.

Effective July 28, 1988, MRI was reclassified by the FDA from a Class III to a Class II device. In August 1998, the *Guidance for Content and Review of a Magnetic Resonance*

Diagnostic Device 510(k) Application was issued (2). Since that time, MRI has undergone considerable technological advances and changes.

The FDA's premarket approval authority applies to medical device distributors, usually the medical device manufacturer, a point commonly misunderstood. For example, the FDA can ask manufacturers to provide information regarding the spatial distribution of the static magnetic field associated with the MR system and to advise MRI healthcare workers to establish a controlled access zone at the 5-gauss line in the instruction manuals provided with the MR system. However, the FDA does not inspect MRI facilities and cannot require end-users to establish a controlled access zone. Authority for such activities resides with state governmental agencies or other similar entities. Another common misconception is that the FDA premarket approval, or marketing clearance, of a device ensures insurance reimbursement. The FDA's authority does not extend to reimbursement decisions, which are made by the private or public insurance providers.

Several years ago, new mechanisms were introduced at CDRH to facilitate the introduction of medical devices into the marketplace. These mechanisms include alternatives to traditional premarket notifications: the Special, and the Abbreviated 510(k), and the Third Party Review (3). The Special 510(k) is used for device modifications and utilizes the design controls. A special 510(k) may be submitted for a modification to the particular manufacturer's device that has been cleared under the 510(k) process. If a new 510(k) is needed for the modification and if the modification does not affect the intended use of the device or alter the fundamental scientific technology of the device, then summary information that results from the design control process can serve as the basis for clearing the application. Under the Special 510(k) review, 510(k) holders who intend to modify their own legally marketed device shall conduct a risk analysis and the necessary verification and validation activities to demonstrate that the design outputs of the modified device meet the design input requirements. Device manufacturers may choose to submit an Abbreviated 510(k) when: (1) Guidance documents exist, and (2) A special control has been established, or (3) The FDA has recognized a relevant consensus standard. An Abbreviated 510(k) submission must include the required elements identified in 21 CFR 807.87 [Traditional 510(k)]. However, in an Abbreviated 510(k) submission, companies elect to provide summary reports on the use of guidance documents and/or special controls or declarations of conformity to FDA recognized standards in order to expedite the review of a submission. An abbreviated 510(k) is also appropriate for an MR system because there are several applicable standards, such as IEC 60601-2-33 and the standards developed by the National Electrical Manufacturers Association (NEMA).

FDA GUIDANCE DOCUMENTS FOR MRI

Over the last decade, the FDA/CDRH has developed and implemented five guidance documents related to MRI: four related to Magnetic Resonance Diagnostic Devices (MRDDs) and one related to passive implants in the MRI environment.

Magnetic Resonance Diagnostic Device (MRDD) Guidance Documents

Effective July 28, 1988, MRDDs were reclassified by FDA from Class III to Class II and were described under 21 CFR 892.1000.

(1) Guidance for the *Submission of Premarket Notifications for MR Diagnostic Devices* issued 14 Nov. 1998 (originally published August 2, 1988)(2). The purpose of this guidance was to provide a description of the information, which should be included in a premarket notification, or 510(k) for a MRDD submitted to CDRH.

(2) The *Criteria for Significant Risk Investigations of MR Diagnostic Devices* was issued July 14, 2003 and supersedes the original guidance document from September 29, 1997 (2). This guidance describes the device operation for MRDDs that the FDA considers significant risk for the purposes of determining whether a clinical study requires FDA approval of an IDE. The FDA believes that an MRDD used under specific conditions and exposure limits of the operating conditions is a significant risk and, therefore, those studies involving such a device do not qualify for the abbreviated IDE. A sponsor should consider the following operating conditions when assessing whether a study may be considered significant risk: (1) main static magnetic field; (2) specific absorption rate (SAR), (3) gradient, time-varying fields, rate of change (dB/dt); and (4) sound level (i.e., acoustic noise). For each for the four conditions, the guidance document defines specific conditions and exposure limits for when the clinical study is considered a significant risk and so requires IDE approval.

There are two other CDRH guidance documents that also contain information possibly pertaining to MRDDs:

(3) The *Guidance for Industry, FDA Reviewers and Compliance on Off-The-Shelf Software Use in Medical Devices* issued September 9, 1999 and

(4) The *Guidance for the Content of Premarket Submissions for Software Contained in Medical Devices* issued May 11, 2005 (2).

Guidance for Passive Implants in the MRI Environment

The CDRH published one guidance document related to the safety of passive implants. The guidance for *Establishing Safety and Compatibility of Passive Implants in the MR Environment* was issued August 21, 2008 (2). This guidance addresses testing and labeling of passive implants for MRI issues (i.e., MR safe or MR conditional labeling) in the MRI environment. In preparing a premarket approval application (PMA), Investigational Device Exemption (IDE), and premarket notification (510(k) submission, this guidance document applies to passive implants (i.e., implants without the supply of electronic power). Active implants or devices that are not implants do not fall within the scope of this guidance. The main safety issues affecting the MR safe or MR conditional status of a passive implant in the MRI environment are the magnetically induced displacement force and torque, radio frequency (RF) heating, and image artifacts. The static field induces displacement forces and torque on magnetic materials. The RF fields may induce substantial heating in metallic implants. The presence of an implant may produce an image artifact that can appear as region or signal loss or as a geometric distortion of the MR image. If the image artifact is near the area of interest, the artifact could render the MR image non-diagnostic or may lead to an erroneous clinical diagnosis potentially leading to inappropriate medical action.

The guidance recommends nonclinical testing for PMA, IDE or 510(k) submissions to establish the MR safe or MR conditional status of the passive implant in the MRI environment. Testing should encompass the entire range of sizes of the device, particularly the size or implant combinations that represent a worst-case scenario. The guidance further recommends the marking terminology defined in ASTM F2503, *Standard Practice for Marking Medical Devices and Other Items for Safety in the Magnetic Resonance Environment*, for defining the safety of items in the MRI environment: MR Safe, MR Conditional, and MR Unsafe. If a passive implant is labeled as MR Safe, the submission should include a scientific rationale or adequate testing. For MR Conditional labeling of passive implants, the submission needs to include testing information. For MR Unsafe labeling of passive implants, a scientific rationale or the testing should be provided. For all passive implants, the guidance recommends the following standards to be used: ASTM F2052, ASTM F2213, ASTM F2182, and ASTM F2119. Importantly, if a medical device which is deemed MR Safe or MR Conditional in a 1.5-Tesla/64-MHz MR system, it may not be MR Safe or MR Conditional in scanner with a higher or lower static magnetic field/RF frequency. This guidance document gives also recommendations for MRI-related labeling language.

THE IEC STANDARD 60601-2-33 FOR MR SYSTEMS

The National Electrical Manufacturers Association (NEMA) has developed standards for the measurement of performance and safety parameters in MRI. Another international standard, the International Electrotechnical Commission (IEC) 60601-2-33, has been developed that addresses many of the safety issues associated with MRI examinations. In the early 1990s, work began on International Electrotechnical Commission (IEC) 60601-2-33, *Particular Requirements for the Safety of Magnetic Resonance Equipment for Medical Diagnosis*, and the first edition was finalized in 1995. The FDA participated in the development of this document, which had a significant influence on current FDA policies and guidance documents relating to MRI. This is particularly important because the FDA has the responsibility of ensuring both the safety and effectiveness of medical devices.

The latest version of IEC 60601-2-33 (Third Edition), *Particular Requirements for the Basic Safety and Essential Performance of Magnetic Resonance Equipment for Medical Diagnosis*, was published in 2010 (4). Although the title mentions "essential performance," no such requirements have been identified within the scope of the standard. The third edition mainly establishes particular basic safety to provide protection for the patient and the MRI healthcare worker. Because the IEC 60601-2-33 standard does not address performance issues, such as signal-to-noise (SNR), image uniformity, geometric distortion, and slice thickness, the FDA has specified in the *Guidance for the Submission Of Premarket Notifications for Magnetic Resonance Diagnostic Devices* from November 14, 1998, performance tests for MR imaging and spectroscopy.

NEMA STANDARDS FOR MR SYSTEMS – MS 1 TO MS 12

Standardized tests for demonstrating safety and effectiveness that have been recognized by the FDA facilitate the premarket review process for MR system manufacturers and the FDA. Without recognition by the FDA, measurement techniques submitted to the FDA need to be independently justified by each medical device manufacturer. The National Electrical Manufacturers Association (NEMA) formed the Magnetic Resonance Section and then the Magnetic Resonance Technical Committee (under the MR Section) to develop such standards. The MR Technical Committee currently has published various MRI standards that are readily available at NEMA's website (5). According to NEMA mandates, these standards must be reviewed every five years and either re-approved, updated and re-approved, or withdrawn. A standard is developed as the MR Section identifies the need. They provide standardized methods for measuring performance and safety parameters for MRDDs which can be utilized in Traditional as well as Abbreviated 510(k)s. The following information provides an overview of the currently published NEMA Standards (5):

NEMA MS 1-2008, Determination of Signal-to-Noise Ratio (SNR) in Diagnostic Magnetic Resonance Imaging

NEMA MS 1-2008 defines four test methods for measuring the signal-to-noise ratio (SNR) under a specific set of conditions, using head and body radiofrequency (RF) coils. NEMA MS 1-2008 does not address the use of surface RF coils, chemical shift imaging, or spectroscopy.

The major feature of the first method is that the SNR performance of the MR system is evaluated using a standard clinical scan sequence. However, it should be noted that, because this method involves the subtraction of two images, it can be very sensitive to MR system instabilities that may occur during the data acquisition process. If results are highly variable, the document recommends performing the alternative calculation of standard deviation, described in the first method, or using the other methods. These alternative methods have been designed to be less susceptible to MR system instabilities and can be used to determine if any variability in the SNR is due to scanner instability or genuinely poor SNR. All methods are intended to measure thermal and other broadband noise, and specifically do not address low frequency variations in an image or artifacts as defined herein.

NEMA MS 2-2008, Determination of Two-Dimensional Geometric Distortion in Diagnostic Magnetic Resonance Images

NEMA MS 2-2008 defines a method for determining the maximum percent difference between measured distances in an image and actual phantom dimensions. This standard evaluates the geometric distortion in three orthogonal planes passing through the center of the specification volume. The purpose of the defined procedure is to provide a standardized method of measuring and reporting two-dimensional geometric distortion in an MR system (i.e., the maximum percent difference between measured distances in an image and the actual corresponding phantom dimensions). Radial measurements (i.e., between points spanning the geometric center of the test object) are used to characterize the geometric distortion. Measurements should be evenly spaced with an angular separation less than 45-degrees in order to sample sufficiently the angular variation of geometric distortion.

NEMA MS 3-2008, Determination of Image Uniformity in Diagnostic Magnetic Resonance Images

NEMA MS 3-2008 defines a test method for measuring image-uniformity performance of MRDDs using head and body RF coils. NEMA MS 3-2008 does not address the use of surface RF coils, chemical shift imaging, or spectroscopy. Image-uniformity refers to the ability of an MRDD to produce an identical signal response throughout the scanned volume when the object being imaged is homogenous. Image-intensity non-uniformity in a two-dimensional MR image of a uniform test object can be caused by a number of factors (e.g., RF coil geometry and penetration), inhomogeneity of the static magnetic field (B_0 non-uniformity), non-uniformity of the transmitted RF field, inadequacies in gradient pulse calibration or eddy current corrections, and spatial positioning of the phantom. Image uniformity is defined in NEMA MS 3-2008 as the deviation of the image pixel intensities from the midrange value. The analysis of uniformity is performed over the region of interest that typically occupies clinical samples and not over the full volume of the RF coil.

NEMA MS 4-2010, Acoustic Noise Measurement Procedure for Diagnostic Magnetic Resonance Imaging (MRI) Devices

NEMA MS 4-2010 defines test conditions and parameters that approximate the worst-case acoustic noise levels that a particular magnet/gradient system combination produces when using pulsed gradient waveforms. NEMA MS 4-2010 also describes how the acoustic noise levels should be measured. In the absence of specific guidelines for sound level exposure associated with MRI equipment, this procedure references the OSHA (Occupational Safety and Health Administration) guidelines for acoustic noise exposure and the IEC standards for sound level meters.

NEMA MS 5-2010, Determination of Slice Thickness in Diagnostic Magnetic Resonance Imaging

NEMA MS 5-2010 defines two methods for determining slice thickness in diagnostic magnetic resonance imaging. The methods presented are essentially numerical in character and, consequently, will require the preparation and use of supplementary dedicated computer software to perform the computations. The methods are based on determining the slice profile, from which the slice thickness is obtained as the full width at half maximum. The slice profile is obtained either by direct measurement with a thin inclined slab of signal-producing material, or by numerical differentiation of the measured edge response function from an inclined surface of a wedge immersed in signal producing material. A correction technique is provided to compensate for errors caused by tilt of the phantom. With the inclined slab approach, better signal-to-noise ratio can be realized. However, the extremely thin slabs required for measurement of very thin slices are not practical to fabricate. Differentiation of the edge response function degrades the SNR that is obtained for the slice profile and usually requires the averaging of several measurements. Slices of any thickness, which can provide adequate signal, may be evaluated with the wedge procedure, whereas the slab method is suitable for thicker slices.

NEMA MS 6-2008, Determination of Signal-to-Noise Ratio and Image Uniformity for Single-Channel, Non-Volume Coils in Diagnostic Magnetic Resonance Imaging (MRI)

NEMA MS 6-2008 defines methods for evaluating single-channel, non-volume special purpose transmit RF coils for use with MRI. Both receive-only and transmit-receive RF coils are included. Head and body RF coils, and single-channel volume specialty RF coils, are excluded (see NEMA MS 1 and NEMA MS 3), as are RF coils requiring multiple receiver channels for operation (i.e., array RF coils, see NEMA MS 9) (5). These RF coils are used to receive signals from a limited region of interest and include linear or quadrature combined surface RF coils, flexible coils, pairs of coils such as Helmholtz coils, or RF coils that partially surround a specific tissue such as the calf or other extremity. NEMA MS 6-2008 refers to these coils as "surface coils." These RF coils achieve good signal-to-noise performance because of their increased filling factor. The purpose of the defined test procedure is to provide a standard means for measuring and reporting the signal-to-noise ratio and uniformity of signal intensity in images acquired with surface RF coils. These quantities are helpful in evaluating RF coil performance and effectiveness. Evaluations are performed on phantom images generated using standard clinical MRI sequences.

NEMA MS 7-1993 (Revision 1998, Rescinded), Measurement Procedure for Time Varying Gradient Fields (dB/dt) for Magnetic Resonance Imaging Systems

NEMA MS 7-1993 defines two independent characterization methods including test conditions and parameters that ensure that worst-case dB/dt values of time-varying gradients fields used for patient exposure regions associated with MRI are measured or calculated (5). Both methods are based on the maximum peak dB/dt that the gradient system is capable of producing, when using pulsed waveforms. If the static magnetic field lies along the z-axis, then time-varying gradient fields necessary for an MRI procedure are the dB_z/dt components produced by the x-, y-, and z-gradients.

NEMA MS 8-2008, Characterization of the Specific Absorption Rate (SAR) for Magnetic Resonance Imaging Systems

NEMA MS 8-2008 defines test conditions and parameters to measure the Specific Absorption Rate (SAR). This standard does not define a relationship between the SAR and the body temperature increase. NEMA MS 8-2008 describes two procedures for whole-body-averaged SAR measurements, the calorimetric method and the pulse-energy method. The document does not apply to gradient (low-frequency time-varying magnetic fields) safety where nerve and cardiac excitation are the primary safety issues. It is also not intended to apply to spatial peak or local average SAR, nor does it address other factors involved with patient heating. The tests are specifically developed for volume RF transmit coils that produce relatively homogeneous RF fields.

NEMA MS 9-2008, Characterization of Phased Array Coils for Diagnostic Magnetic Resonance Images (MRI)

NEMA MS 9-2008 defines a test method for evaluating phased array RF coils used with MR systems. Phased array RF coils consist of multiple receive-only coils that are used to detect signals from a limited portion of the patient's anatomy. The output of each RF coil element, or combined set of elements, is connected to the input of an independent receiver chain. Phased array RF coils may be composed of surface coils, flexible coils, pairs of coils such as Helmholtz coils, or RF coils that surround a specific anatomical region as well as combinations of these coils. Phased array RF coils achieve good signal-to-noise performance because of their increased filling factor and the use of smaller, higher signal-to-noise receive coil. The purpose of NEMA MS 9-2008 is to provide a standard means for measuring the signal-to noise ratio (SNR) and the uniformity of signal intensity in images acquired with phased array coils. These quantities are helpful in evaluating the impact of MR system changes on performance or in demonstrating effectiveness for FDA applications.

NEMA MS 10-2010, Determination of Local Specific Absorption Rate (SAR) in Diagnostic Magnetic Resonance Imaging (MRI)

NEMA MS 10-2010 defines a measurement method for local specific absorption rate (SAR). The measurement method requires construction of a radio frequency phantom for a given frequency and the use of radiofrequency transparent thermometry. The procedure is intended for local SAR measurements only and specifically does not address whole-body SAR. Local SAR is a parameter that relates to the safety of MRI scanners. The primary safety concern with transmit surface coils involves local SAR which may be highest near electrical conductors. This standard does not attempt to establish relationships between SAR and body temperature.

NEMA MS 11-2010, Determination of Gradient-Induced Electric Fields in Diagnostic Magnetic Resonance Imaging

NEMA MS 11-2010 defines measurement methods for determining the gradient-induced electric fields for each gradient axis at a radius of 20-cm off the patient axis. The measurement method requires construction of electric field dipoles, spacers, a phantom, and the use of a high impedance device for measuring voltages. The electric field measurements are done in a solution with conductivity similar to that of the human body. Numerical methods of estimating the electric field are discussed in an appendix to NEMA MS 11-2010. Gradient-induced electric fields may affect the safety and comfort of patients. Typically, stimulation requires a gradient induced electric field of more than 2-V/m. The method described in this standard makes electric field measurements inside a phantom loaded with electrically conductive material. This NEMA document defines methods for determining the gradient-induced electric fields of diagnostic magnetic resonance imaging gradient coils (head and body) under specific conditions. However, it does not address the effect of electrical inhomogeneities in the body on internal, gradient-induced, electrical fields.

NEMA MS 12-2010, Quantification and Mapping of Geometric Distortion for Special Applications

NEMA MS 12-2010 defines a method for evaluating the geometric distortion characteristics throughout a specified imaging volume. The equipment contribution to geometric distortion in MR systems is largely due to inhomogeneities of the main magnetic field and the spatially encoding gradient subsystem. In addition, the object may also induce magnetic field distortions that geometrically distort the image. Because geometric distortion is spatially variable, it is important to understand the spatial distribution of error when MR images are used quantitatively. The purpose of NEMA MS 12-2010 is to provide a standard for measuring and reporting the geometric distortion characteristics of an MR system. This information is helpful in matching MR system characteristics to clinical requirements, when geometric accuracy is crucial (e.g., for MR image-guided interventional procedures). This information is also helpful in evaluating the impact of changes in MR system performance, for quality control programs that seek to continually reaffirm system performance, or in demonstrating effectiveness for FDA submissions. The defined methods have not been designed for compatibility with existing NEMA methods. Evaluations are performed on MR images generated using standard clinical imaging protocols.

ASTM International Standards for Medical Devices and Implants

In 1997, the CDRH requested that the American Society for Testing and Materials (ASTM) (now known as the "ASTM International") develop test methods to address safety and effectiveness issues for medical devices in the MRI environment. Based on this request, the ASTM formed the task group F04.15.11 on the safety and compatibility of implant materials and medical devices in the magnetic resonance (MR) environment. This task group, F04.15.11, developed test methods for evaluating magnetically induced displacement force and torque, radio frequency (RF) heating, and image artifacts. The first ASTM MRI test method was published in 2000, F2052-00, Standard Test Method for Measurement of Magnetically Induced Displacement Force on Passive Implants in the Magnetic Resonance Environment. Presently, the ASTM International has five different documents for passive implants and devices (6), including, the following:

(1) ASTM F2052-06 defines a method for determining the displacement force or translational attraction (7). The spatial gradient of the magnetic field of the MR system produces a displacement force on magnetic objects placed in this magnetic field. This displacement force is responsible for the projectile effect that continues to cause injuries in the MRI environment. ASTM F2052 requires the test object to be suspended by a thin string and moved to the position in the magnetic field that produces the greatest displacement. The angular deflection of the device from the vertical is measured and the deflection force is calculated. If the angular deflection is less than 45°, and the magnetic force is in the horizontal direction, the deflection force is less than the device's weight and it is assumed that the risk imposed by the magnetically-induced deflection force is no greater than the risk due to the gravitational force. However, counter-forces may also need to be considered because these can be act on an implant and prevent movement or displacement of the object.

(2) ASTM F2213-06 (2011) defines a method for measuring the torque on a medical device in the MRI environment (8). The static magnetic field produces a torque on an object and forces it to align the long-axis of the object with the magnetic field. For this test procedure, the medical device with one principal axis aligned in the vertical direction is placed on a holder suspended on a torsional spring. The test fixture is then placed in the center of the MR system where the effect of torque is at a maximum. The angular deflection of the holder from its equilibrium position is recorded and the torque is calculated. The frame supporting the spring and holder is rotated through 360-degrees, and the torque, as a function of the angle of the device is determined. This measurement is repeated for the other two

principal axes of the device to determine the maximum torque. According to ASTM F2213-06 (2011), the torque is acceptable if the maximum torque induced by the MR system is less than the product of the longest dimension of the implant and its weight (8). For medical devices within the acceptance criteria, the magnetically induced torque is less than the worst-case torque on the implant due to gravity. Again, counter-forces may also need to be considered because these can act on an implant and prevent movement or displacement of the object associated with torque.

(3) ASTM F2182-11a defines a test method for measuring RF-induced heating of passive implants (9). The RF field associated with an MR system induces electrical currents in the body, which generate heat. The specific absorption rate (SAR), reported in Watts per kilogram (W/kg), is the mass normalized rate at which RF energy is coupled to biological tissue, which, if a metallic implant is present, is an important parameter to control in order to prevent excessive heating that may result in patient injury. According to ASTM F2182-11a, the implant to be tested is placed in a phantom filled with a medium that simulates the electrical and thermal properties of the human body. The implant is placed at a location with well-characterized exposure conditions. The phantom material is a gelled-saline consisting of a saline solution and a gelling agent. Temperature probes, which are typically fluoroptic thermometry probes, are placed at locations where the induced implant heating is expected to be the greatest (this may require pilot experiments to determine the proper placement of the temperature probes). The phantom is then placed in an MR system or an apparatus that reproduces just the RF field. ASTM F2182-11a recommends using an RF field producing a whole-body averaged SAR of about 2-W/kg applied for approximately 15-minutes (or other time sufficient to characterize the temperature rise and the local SAR). The test procedure is divided into two steps: (1) the temperature rise on or near the implant at several locations is measured using the temperature probes during approximately 15-minutes of RF application. The temperature rise is also measured at a reference location during Step 1. (2) The implant is removed and the same RF application is repeated while the temperature measurements are obtained at the same probe locations as in Step 1 (i.e., at the positions applied to the implant that is undergoing evaluation). From these measurements, the local SAR is calculated for each probe, including the reference location. The local SAR at the temperature reference probe is used to verify that the same RF exposure conditions are applied during Steps 1 and 2.

(4) ASTM F2119-07 defines a protocol for determining image artifacts associated with implants and devices using standardized pulse sequences (10). Although image artifacts do not generally affect the safety of a device in the MRI environment, physicians need information about the size and location of image artifacts with respect to the location of the portion of the body that is to be imaged. The test defines pairs of spin echo and gradient echo MR images generated both with and without the implant in the field of view. The image artifacts are assessed by computing the differences between the reference and implant images.

(5) ASTM F2503-13 defines the terms, MR Safe, MR Conditional, and MR Unsafe, as follows (6, 11): MR Safe — an item that poses no known hazards in all MR environments; MR Unsafe — an item that is known to pose hazards in all MR environments; and MR Conditional — an item that has been demonstrated to pose no known hazards in a specified MRI environment with specified conditions of use. The particular conditions that define

the specified MRI environment include the static field strength, spatial gradient magnetic field, time-varying field (i.e., dB/dt), radiofrequency fields, and specific absorption rate (SAR). Additional conditions, including specific configurations or operational conditions of the implants or device, may also be defined.

In addition to these definitions, ASTM F2503-8 defines icons for the three definitions (6, 11). The icons are intended for use on implants, devices, and items that may be brought into or near the MRI environment as well as in product labeling. The icons can be in color or in black and white. The MR Safe icon consists of the letters "MR" in green in a white square with a green border, or the letters "MR" in white within a green square. The MR Conditional icon consists of the letters "MR" in black inside a yellow triangle with a black border and the MR Unsafe icon consists of the letters "MR" in black on a white field inside a red circle with a diagonal red stripe. The MR Conditional item labeling must include information for the acceptable conditions that are sufficient to characterize the behavior of the item in the MRI environment. This additional information should address magnetic field interactions (i.e., magnetically-induced displacement force and torque) and RF heating. Other possible safety issues include induced currents/voltages, electromagnetic field-related issues, thermal injury, nerve stimulation, acoustic noise, interaction among different devices, the safe functioning of the device, and the safe operation of the MR system. Any parameter that affects the safety of the item should be listed and any condition that is known to produce an unsafe condition must be described in the MR Conditional labeling for the item.

THE ISO TECHNICAL SPECIFICATION (TS) 10974 FOR ACTIVE IMPLANTABLE MEDICAL DEVICES

For many years, scanning a patient with an AIMD (Active Implantable Medical Device) was contraindicated by the MR system and the AIMD manufacturers. Because performing MRI procedures in patients with AIMDs such as cardiac pacemakers, neurostimulation systems, cochlear implants, implantable infusion pumps, and other similar devices is increasingly necessary for proper patient management, the CDRH is faced with increasingly more submissions requesting MR Conditional status for AIMDs.

The issue of AIMDs in patients referred for MRI examinations became even more noticeable because of anecdotal reports of off-label scanning and the possible perception that the risk is not as significant as believed by AIMD manufacturers, MR system manufacturers, and the regulatory bodies. Interestingly, the FDA's Manufacturer and User Facility Device Experience (MAUDE) database for adverse event reporting indicates instances of device failures and/or patient injuries associated with MRI examinations performed on patients with AIMDs, despite the current contraindications (12).

While MRI test methods have been developed and published by the ASTM International for passive implants, no similar test methods for AIMDs are available. Because of the harsh electromagnetic environment associated with MRI, the testing of AIMDs in these fields is especially challenging. The development of appropriate test methods require detailed technical knowledge of the electromagnetic fields emitted by the MR system. Unfortunately most of this information is not public. Additionally, manufacturers of MR systems have contraindicated all AIMDs from scanning in their systems.

The CDRH held meetings with representatives from both MR system and AIMD manufacturers that led in 2005 to an ISO recommendation to form a liaison with the International Electrotechnical Commission (IEC, responsible for the safety standard for MRI equipment, IEC 60601-2-33, particular requirements for the safety of magnetic resonance equipment for medical diagnosis) (3), to consider recommendations that could be used to write MRI-related safety requirements for AIMDs. In 2012, the joint ISO/IEC working group published the dual logo Technical Specification (TS) 10974 entitled, "Assessment of the safety of magnetic resonance imaging for patients with an active implantable medical device" (13). This document contains novel concepts and test methods particularly developed for AIMDs in association with the use of MR systems.

THE FUTURE OF MRI SAFETY STANDARDS

The Fixed Parameter Option – FPO:B

In the current version of IEC 60601-2-33, patient safety is defined by human physiologic limits related to heating (i.e., in associated with RF power deposition, SAR), peripheral nerve stimulation, acoustic noise, venting cryogens, and magnetic forces and torques. However, safety for a patient with an AIMD may need additional controls that limit peak B_{1+}, peak dB/dt, $B_{1+,rms}$, and dB/dt_{rms} (B_{1+} is defined as the primary RF field; peak dB/dt is defined as the time varying gradient field, $B_{1+,rms}$, and dB/dt_{rms} are defined as the root-mean-square of B_{1+} and dB/dt). Therefore, the need for special MR system modes of operation, to improve testing, labeling, and scanning of AIMDs has been debated for several years. The basic concept of these new modes has been broadly supported by both AIMD and MR system manufacturers. However, until recently, the practical details have prevented rapid progress toward an effective and reasonable set of definitions and limit values for MRI parameters. A special working group of the Joint Working Group (JWG) between ISO TC150/SC6 and IEC SC/62B (the standards committee that developed TS 10974, *Assessment of the Safety of Magnetic Resonance Imaging for Patients with an Active Implantable Medical Device*) led the discussions to the following tasks: (1) Establish a new MR system mode of operation with clearly defined exposure limits of the radiated field parameters that are directly relevant to safety related interactions with AIMDs in the MRI environment, and (2) To establish values for the exposure limits that are as safe as possible for most AIMDs without unnecessary and substantially compromising the diagnostic ability of MRI examinations performed in the Normal Operating Mode of operation for the MR system. These discussions resulted in the proposal of a special MR system operation mode to limit outputs from the scanner for patients with MR Conditional AIMDs. This operation mode was given the name, "Fixed Parameter Option: Basic" or FPO:B. FPO:B is currently only being proposed for the IEC MR system safety standard 60601-2-33, subject to IEC approval, recognition by regulatory bodies, and, thus, is not yet available in the clinical setting.

FPO:B defines a set of gradient (time-varying fields) and RF field output limits, within the Normal Operating Mode and the First Level Controlled Mode of operation of the MR system, that: (1) provide exposure limits which MR systems adhere to, (2) provide 1.5-Tesla/64-MHz MRI capabilities similar to present Normal Operating Mode limits, and (3) in conjunction with IEC TS 10974, facilitates the testing to label AIMDs as MR Conditional within the FPO:B limits.

The working group analyzed the current technology for AIMD devices with regard to 1.5-Tesla/64-MHz MR systems and established practical limits for the key electromagnetic field exposure levels. AIMD characteristics and the performance of MR scanners were considered in relation to patient safety and acceptable clinical MRI needs and requirements. The new FPO:B limits are proposed to be included under the existing modes of MR system operation. Although the primary reason for the use of FPO:B is to support AIMD safety, FPO:B could also be useful for other implants and there may be additional reasons for physicians to limit patient exposure. While FPO:B is not exactly an "implant mode," FPO:B will improve and simplify scanning patients with AIMDs. However, that will only be achieved once AIMD manufacturers provide devices tested according to ISO TS 10974 or equivalent methods, labeled for the proposed FPO:B exposure values, and MR systems make FPO:B available to MRI healthcare professionals.

FPO:B is intended only for use with appropriately tested and labeled AIMDs. Thus, the use of FPO:B with AIMDs without specific FPO:B labeling could present unacceptable risks and there may be additional AIMD safety issues and labeling restrictions related to total scan time, static magnetic field spatial gradients, and other considerations to make certain AIMD safe in the FPO:B mode. Initial details pertaining to FPO:B have been presented recently at an MRI safety workshop sponsored by the International Society for Magnetic Resonance Imaging (14).

RF Power Absorption and Controlling the SAR

MRI is deemed safe for patients if the potential hazards, such as magnetic field interactions, peripheral nerve stimulation, and local and whole-body tissue heating by radiofrequency (RF) fields are carefully managed. Tissue heating is controlled for transmit RF coils according to IEC 60601-2-33 by limiting the whole-body-averaged SAR, the head-averaged SAR, and the partial-body SAR. Induced eddy currents are the primary RF absorption mechanism of the B_1 magnetic field exposures or interactions with the human body. Therefore large-scale anatomical properties may significantly influence the energy absorption.

The induced eddy currents depend mainly on the cross-sectional area of the body and the field strength normal to the cross-section and are, therefore, largely independent of birdcage RF coil design and the X-Y position of the patient within the birdcage. In general, the B_1 field, being rather homogenous in the field of view, is larger near the metallic structure and decreases along the Z-axis. The formation of RF loops formed by the extremities may dramatically increase local SAR, which is currently neither controlled nor limited by MR systems and, thus, should be avoided. The secondary RF absorption mechanism is the capacitive coupling of stray E-fields, predominantly close to the matching capacitors. The stray E-fields expose the tissues in close proximity to the rungs and end-rings of the RF coil, and strongly depend on the actual RF coil design (e.g., the number and location of the capacities in the rungs, distance of the shield, etc.). The size of the body has no direct influence on the stray E-field absorption pattern.

The actual deposited energy is a superposition of the B_1-induced eddy current absorption and the localized stray E-field exposure. The effects of the stray E-fields are typically limited to the arms for typical (centered) postures and, therefore, have a minor influence on trunk exposure and the whole-body averaged SAR. However, to accurately estimate safe local

SAR levels, which are the presumed to be the primary reason for burns in patients undergoing MRI procedures, anatomically correct human models for the entire patient population are needed. Therefore, the local deposition of RF energy must be carefully managed and limited to prevent local tissue damage, particularly in the consideration of modern, multi-channel transmit RF coils.

While the whole-body- averaged SAR is typically monitored and controlled by the MR system, the local SAR levels cannot be directly monitored or limited (i.e., it can only be accurately determined by full-wave simulations). Various studies have investigated local SAR hotspots in realistic human anatomical models. However, the influences of anatomical variations of these models have been incompletely quantified. Because the RF field-induced eddy currents increase with the radial dimension of the patient, the RF absorption increases with the large-scale anatomical property.

Recent computational studies performed in collaboration with the FDA have shown that for a fixed B_1 incident field, the whole-body averaged SAR can be up to 2.5 times higher in obese adult models compared to small children, while the local SAR increases by a factor of up to 7 (15, 16). The prediction of these increases using the large-scale anatomical properties (i.e., their correlation) is only partially reliable. A fixed B_1 field generally yields a strong correlation between anatomy and the local SAR, but it cannot accurately predict the whole-body-averaged SAR.

The Future of IEC Standard 60601-2-33

Before working on the Fourth Edition of 60601-2-33 the Committee (IEC 62/62B/MT40) plans to release two Amendments to the Third Edition. The first Amendment is expected for release sometime in 2013 with formal updates to the latest general and collateral standards. The planned major changes for the Second Amendment is the introduction of the Fixed Parameter Option (FPO:B) and the increase of the static magnetic field limit in the First Level Controlled Operating Mode from 4-Tesla to 8-Tesla (although, it should be noted that currently there is no 8-Tesla MR system in operation, however, more than fifty 7-Tesla scanners exist). The Committee believes that the increase of the static magnetic field limit to 8-Tesla is supported by several new studies providing evidence of safety and efficacy of ultra-high-field systems and that since 2003, the FDA no longer classifies field strengths up to and including 8-Tesla as a "significant risk" for most populations (17). Also ICNIRP introduced a controlled operating mode for static magnetic field strengths up to 8-Tesla and permits exposure up to 8-Tesla for healthcare workers in a "controlled environment" (18).

Plans for the Fourth Edition of 60601-2-33 include a major revision of RF power control. The motivation behind this revision is that new multi-channel RF transmit coil technology needs new safety concepts insofar as there is a growing need to focus on local exposure (i.e., local SAR and temperature hot spots) rather than the whole-body-averaged SAR. Importantly, computer simulations have shown inconsistencies in the relation between whole-body-averaged SAR and local SAR, but there is no empirical data to substantiate this. One possible idea is to introduce a new thermal dose safety concept to control the local temperature as a function of time and tissue based on the CEM 43 (Cumulative Equivalent Minutes) model (19). This new thermal dose safety concept considers not only the SAR, but also the exposed tissue characteristics, the thermoregulatory behavior and local temperature distribution, and, more importantly, the exposure duration.

CONCLUSIONS

In the past twenty-five years, MRI technology has developed into a major radiological modality to the point where it has become the gold standard for the diagnosis of a number of disorders and conditions. During this period, there have been major changes in safety standards and guidelines. In general, recommended exposure limits have risen significantly as a result of the increased knowledge regarding the biological effects of the static, RF, and time-varying magnetic fields employed in MRI. One of the most important lessons learned is that it is important to include flexibility and alternatives in safety standards and guidelines so that the benefits of technical advances in MRI are available to patients as soon as possible without compromising their safety.

Disclaimer

The mention of commercial products, their sources or their use in connection with material reported, herein, is not to be construed as either an actual or implied endorsement of such products by the U.S., Food and Drug Administration.

REFERENCES

1. Standards (Medical Devices). In: CDRH standards program/standards management staff. Available via http://www.fda.gov/MedicalDevices/DeviceRegulationandGuidance/Standards/default.htm. Accessed March, 2013.

2. Guidance documents (Medical devices and radiation-emitting products). Available via http://www.fda.gov/MedicalDevices/DeviceRegulationandGuidance/GuidanceDocuments/. Accessed March 2013.

3. 510(k) Submission methods. Available via http://www.fda.gov/MedicalDevices/DeviceRegulationandGuidance/HowtoMarketYourDevice/PremarketSubmissions/PremarketNotification510k/default.htm. Accessed March, 2013.

4. International Electrotechnical Committee (IEC). 60601-2-33 Edition 3.0, Medical electrical equipment - Part 2-33: Particular requirements for the basic safety and essential performance of magnetic resonance equipment for medical diagnostic.

5. National Electrical Manufacturers Association (NEMA). Available via http://www.nema.org/. Accessed March, 2013.

6. Shellock FG, Woods TO, Crues JV 3rd. MR labeling information for implants and devices: explanation of terminology. Radiology 2009;253:26-30.

7. American Society for Testing and Materials (ASTM) International. ASTM F2052-06 Standard test method for measurement of magnetically induced displacement force on medical devices in the magnetic resonance environment. 2006.

8. American Society for Testing and Materials (ASTM) International. ASTM F2213-06 (2011) Standard test method for measurement of magnetically induced torque on medical devices in the magnetic resonance environment. 2011.

9.   American Society for Testing and Materials (ASTM) International. F2182-11a, Standard test method for measurement of radio frequency induced heating on or near passive implants during magnetic resonance imaging. 2011.

10. American Society for Testing and Materials (ASTM) International. ASTM F2119-07 Standard test method for evaluation of MR image artifacts from passive implants. 2007.

11. American Society for Testing and Materials (ASTM) International. ASTM F2503-13 Standard practice for marking medical devices and other items for safety in the magnetic resonance environment. 2013.

12. Center for Devices and Radiological Health. MAUDE - Manufacturer and user facility device experience database. Available via http://www.accessdata.fda.gov/scripts/cdrh/cfdocs/cfmaude/search.cfm. Accessed March, 2013.

13. ISO TS 10974/Ed.1, Requirements for the safety and compatibility of magnetic resonance imaging for patients with an active implantable medical device. 2012.

14. Steckner M, Venook R, Frese G, Olsen J, et al. Proposed fixed parameter option: limiting MRI scanner outputs for patients with MR conditional active implantable medical devices. Proceedings of the International Society for Magnetic Resonance Imaging, Scientific Workshop - MR Safety in Practice: Now and In the Future. Sweden 2012:5-7.

15. Murbach M, Neufeld E, Capstick M, et al. Thermal damage tissue models analyzed for different whole-body SAR and scan duration for standard MR body coils. Magn Reson Med 2013 Feb 14.

16. Murbach M, Neufeld E, Kainz W, Pruessmann KP, Kuster N. Whole-body and local RF absorption in human models as a function of anatomy and position within 1.5T MR body coil. Magn Reson Med 2013 [Epub ahead of print].

17. Guidance for industry and FDA staff: criteria for significant risk investigations of magnetic resonance diagnostic devices. Available via http://www.fda.gov/downloads/MedicalDevices/DeviceRegulationandGuidance/GuidanceDocuments/UCM072688.pdf. Accessed March 2013.

18. International Commission on Non-Ionizing Radiation Protection (ICNIRP). Guidelines for limiting exposure to time-varying electric, magnetic, and electromagnetic fields (up to 300 GHz). Health Phys 1998;74:494–522.

19. Sapareto SA, Dewey WC. Thermal dose determination in cancer therapy. Int J Radiat Oncol Biol Phys 1984;10:787–800.

Chapter 29   MRI Standards and Safety Guidelines in Europe

STEPHEN F. KEEVIL, PH.D.

Consultant Physicist
Head of Magnetic Resonance Physics
Department of Medical Physics
Guy's and St Thomas' NHS Foundation Trust
London, England
and
Professor of Medical Physics
Department of Biomedical Engineering
King's College London
London, England
United Kingdom

INTRODUCTION

Since 2003, the magnetic resonance imaging (MRI) community in Europe has engaged in a campaign about a portion of European Union (EU) health and safety legislation, the Physical Agents (Electromagnetic Fields, EMF) Directive (1), which poses a substantial threat to the use of MRI in clinical practice and research (2, 3, 4). This contentious debate has served to highlight the question of how MRI safety issues are currently addressed by regulations and official guidance in Europe. While the EMF Directive is concerned purely with worker safety, it is also important to consider patient safety in any discussion of this kind.

In this chapter, the existing body of EU safety legislation, international standards and guidelines that impact the use of MRI in Europe are discussed. In addition, the legislation and guidance that exist in individual European countries and how current developments with the EMF Directive might lead to greater harmonization in the future is presented. Although Europe and the European Union (EU) are neither synonymous nor coterminous, this chapter will be concerned mainly with the situation in the EU. Notably, in some policy areas, including occupational health and safety, EU legislation also applies in the wider European Economic Area (EEA) (encompassing Iceland, Liechtenstein and Norway), often also in Switzerland, and in some instances even more widely [e.g., the Medical Devices Directive (see below) applies in Turkey]. Since there will be considerable discussion of EU legislation in this chapter, background information is needed for readers outside the EU (and for many within it).

NATIONAL AND SUPRANATIONAL LEGISLATION IN THE EUROPEAN UNION

Currently, the EU is a partnership of 27 sovereign countries, each with its own independent government, legislature, and body of law. However, under the treaties establishing the EU, these "member states" have conferred certain powers on the EU collectively, including the power to make laws that are binding on all of them, in order to advance the objectives of the treaties. The mechanism by which EU law is made varies between different policy areas but, in general, it involves the European Commission, the European Parliament, and the Council of the EU. The Commission is composed of permanent officials and provides the EU's "civil service". It is headed by the College of Commissioners, a group of politicians forming the "cabinet" of the EU. There is one Commissioner from each member state, each having different policy responsibilities. Only the Commission has the power to propose new legislation, which is then passed to the Parliament and Council for amendment and approval. The European Parliament is composed of members (MEPs) directly elected by citizens of EU member states for terms of five years. Like most national legislatures, it contains a variety of political groupings and carries out much of its work through a system of committees focusing on different policy areas. The Council is made up of government ministers from each member state, with the minister attending changing depending on the area of policy under discussion. In practice, much of its work is carried out in committees and working parties made up of civil servants and diplomats.

Most EU legislation (for our purposes) takes the form of *directives* and *regulations*, which become law in member states in different ways. Once the Parliament and Council have adopted a directive, all member state governments are required to implement its provisions in their domestic law (a process known as "transposition") by a fixed date. If a member state fails to meet the transposition deadline, the Commission may take "infraction proceedings" against that country in the Court of Justice of the EU. A regulation, by contrast, is legally binding in all member states as soon as it comes into force, without the need for transposition. EU law takes priority over individual national law, although, importantly in our context, member states are able to introduce more stringent laws in some policy areas, including worker protection.

Several EU directives have implications for MRI safety. The most significant of these are discussed below, but others that may need to be taken into account in the context of MRI include the Physical Agents (Noise) Directive (2003/10/EC) and the Pressure Equipment Directive (97/23/EC), as well as more general legislation dealing with issues such as electrical and mechanical safety, manual handling, use of display screens, and others. Most of these issues will not be discussed further in this chapter, where the focus is primarily on the management of hazards arising from electromagnetic fields (EMF) with an emphasis on MRI.

THE PURPOSE OF STANDARDS AND GUIDELINES: DIRECT AND INDIRECT HAZARDS ASSOCIATED WITH MRI

The hazards of MRI are discussed in detail elsewhere in this textbook. Briefly, MRI safety discussions often focus on direct and indirect hazards of EMF. *Direct hazards* are those arising directly from exposure of the human body to EMF (the static magnetic field, time-varying magnetic fields and radiofrequency radiation), primarily peripheral nerve stimulation (PNS) and radiofrequency (RF) heating. There are also transient sensory effects such as magnetic field-induced vertigo and (rarely in MRI) magnetophosphenes. There is debate in Europe as to whether or not these phenomena should be regarded as adverse health effects. Most in the MRI community would take the view that they should not, but some commentators argue that the World Health Organisation (WHO) definition of health as "complete physical, mental and social well-being..." (5) encompasses transient disturbances of this kind. Direct hazards are often prevented by setting exposure limits in order to avoid or to minimize the effect in question. These limits may be specific to MRI, or may apply to all sources of EMF exposure.

Indirect hazards arise when electromagnetic fields interact with an object or device in such a way that it then poses a hazard to patients or workers. Examples are ferromagnetic projectiles attracted by the strong static magnetic field and effects on biomedical implants. By far, these are the more serious type of hazards in MRI and are best prevented through adoption of rules for safe working, worker training etc. This may be an entirely local matter, but in some countries there are national guidelines on MRI safety to provide more effective and uniform protection. Both types of hazard may also be minimized through proper equipment and facility design.

THE EU HEALTH AND SAFETY FRAMEWORK DIRECTIVE: RULES AND RESPONSIBILITIES

Most European countries do not have specific laws addressing MRI safety, or indeed EMF safety, in general. However, generic legislation to protect worker health and safety exists in each EU member state, based on the health and safety framework directive (89/391/EEC) (6). Under this legislation, employers (which in this context would encompass hospitals, private clinics and universities) have a duty to ensure the safety and health of workers in every aspect related to the work. For example, they must conduct risk assessments of each work process, adopt appropriate protective measures, and provide workers with adequate training. There are also requirements placed on workers to take care of their own health and safety, and that of other persons, and to make correct use of work equipment. However, this is explicitly dependent on the training and instructions received so, again, the primary responsibility rests with the employer. These provisions apply to MRI just as much as to any other occupational setting. In the United Kingdom (UK), the Health and Safety Executive (HSE), the government agency responsible for occupational health and safety, has in recent years conducted inspections of MRI facilities, requiring an evaluation of risk assessment and other evidence of safe working practices.

Risk assessment is an important aspect of compliance with the framework directive. A variety of approaches exist for assessing and quantifying risk and the impact of risk miti-

Table 1. A simple risk assessment matrix. Performance of risk assessments in all workplaces, including MRI facilities, is a requirement of the EU health and safety framework directive (89/391/EEC).

		Consequences (severity of injury / financial loss / reputational damage)				
		Minimal	Minor	Moderate	Major	Catastrophic
Likelihood (within a year)	Almost certain	Moderate risk	Significant risk	High risk	Extreme risk	Extreme risk
	Likely	Low risk	Moderate risk	Significant risk	High risk	Extreme risk
	Possible	Low risk	Low risk	Moderate risk	Significant risk	High risk
	Unlikely	Low risk	Low risk	Low risk	Moderate risk	Significant risk
	Rare	Low risk	Low risk	Low risk	Low risk	Moderate risk

gation, often taking the form of a matrix in which the risk of an event is categorized (and sometimes quantified) according to its likelihood and the severity of its outcome (**Table 1**). In the case of MRI, a projectile incident, for example, might be categorized as an "extreme risk" event in the absence of appropriate safety procedures and training, but with that mitigation in place might then be downgraded to a "moderate risk".

THE MEDICAL DEVICES DIRECTIVE: SAFETY BY DESIGN

EU legislation relating to medical devices also creates health and safety responsibilities for both manufacturers and users of MRI equipment. Many classes of product require a "CE mark" before they can be placed on the market in the EU. These include products as diverse as gas appliances, refrigerators, weighing instruments, fireworks, and toys. The process of obtaining a CE mark requires the manufacturer to ensure that the product conforms to the "essential requirements" of applicable EU directives. In the case of "medical devices", a broad term that encompasses everything from bandages to MRI scanners, this means the Medical Devices Directive (MDD) (7). The very first essential requirement of the MDD is that "the device must be designed and manufactured in such a way that... they will not compromise the clinical condition or the safety of patients, or the safety and health of users or, where applicable, other persons...". Demonstrating safety is therefore an important aspect of the CE marking process and, hence, a prerequisite for marketing a medical device in Europe.

The MDD is currently undergoing revision to improve harmonization across member states. This is as a result of concerns entirely unrelated to MRI. It is expected that the replacement legislation will take the form of an EU regulation, giving less leeway for variation in member state implementation. However, there is unlikely to be a major impact on users of MRI equipment.

THE IEC/EN 60601 STANDARD SERIES

The International Electrotechnical Commission (IEC) 60601 standard series provides the usual means whereby medical device manufacturers demonstrate compliance with the MDD. The European Commission recognizes these standards as harmonized standards for the purposes of the MDD, so that satisfying their requirements gives a "presumption of conformity" with the essential requirements of the directive. These are global standards, not specific to Europe. They underpin the design and manufacture of MR systems sold throughout the world and are recognized by many national medical device regulatory agencies, including the United States (U.S.) Food and Drug Administration (FDA). However, they have a particular importance in Europe because of their close relationship to the MDD and, therefore, are discussed in some detail here. Strictly speaking, it is the version of the IEC standard adopted by the European Committee for Electrotechnical Standardization (CENELEC), known as an EN standard, that is harmonized to the MDD but this is practically identical to the IEC original.

The IEC/EN 60601 series consists of a general medical device safety standard (60601-1) (8), "collateral standards" covering specific aspects of device performance, some of which are relevant to MRI such as electromagnetic compatibility (60601-1-2) and usability (60601-1-6), and "particular standards" in the 60601-2 series dealing with specific device types. Standard 60601-2-33 is the particular standard for MRI equipment (9) and is maintained by a group of MRI experts drawn from industry, clinical users, regulators and the academic community.

IEC/EC 60601-2-33 sets out criteria for equipment safety and details of measurement procedures for manufacturers to demonstrate compliance. Importantly, it also describes the "Instructions for Use" that manufacturers must provide to purchasers of MR systems. These include mandatory safety information and create obligations for the end user in areas such as safe system operation, worker training, control of access to the scanner, and patient handling. Much of this material is intended to prevent indirect hazards.

Unusually for a standard of this type, 60601-2-33 also contains EMF exposure limit values, addressing direct hazards. These limits are summarized in **Table 2**. They apply equally to patients and to MRI workers, with the rationale that the intention to avoid adverse effects in patients ensures that workers are also protected. The standard adopts a tiered approach to EMF exposure limitation, with three operating modes defined by exposure thresholds. In the *Normal Operating Mode*, there is considered to be no risk of "physiological stress" to patients. In the *First Level Controlled Operating Mode*, the threshold for physiological effects may be approached, and medical supervision is recommended. In the *Second Level Controlled Operating Mode*, there may be significant risk and local regulatory approval is required (e.g., from a research ethics committee), which should explicitly state the permitted levels of exposure. The instructions for use passed to the end user must refer to the hazards associated with EMF and to these exposure limits. They must also give advice on worker training to mitigate transient effects, such as vertigo, that may occur at higher exposure levels, and explain that national laws may set lower exposure limits for workers in some countries, as is discussed later in this chapter.

Table 2. Exposure limits for patients and MRI workers according to the IEC standard 60601-2-33.

	Static magnetic field	Switched gradients*	Radiofrequency field**		
		Gradient output as a percentage of directly determined mean PNS threshold level	Maximum core temperature (°C)	Maximum local tissue temperature (°C)	Maximum rise in core temperature (°C)
Normal Operating Mode	≤ 3-T	≯ 80%	39	39	0.5
First Level Controlled Operating Mode	> 3-T, ≤ 4-T	≯ 100%	40	40	1
Second Level Controlled Operating Mode	> 4-T	> 100%	> 40	> 40	>1

*Default limits are also defined, in terms of induced electric field strength and gradient switching rate, as an alternative to direct determination.

**Various specific absorption rate (SAR) limits are also defined to ensure compliance with these temperature limits

There are two points worthy of particular note. First, the static magnetic field limits in the IEC standard are relatively low, so that any use of a 7-T scanner requires both local regulatory approval and medical supervision. This may change in the near future in a proposed amendment to the standard. Second, the main approach to limiting exposures to time-varying magnetic fields focuses on direct determination of the physiological threshold for peripheral nerve stimulation (PNS) (which is merely a tactile sensation at the onset level) in a group of healthy volunteers, with the *Normal Operating Mode* limit set at 80% of this threshold. This differs from most other guidelines in avoiding the unwanted physiological effect directly, rather than by means of an exposure limit expressed in terms of physical quantities that is inevitably a conservative proxy. There are also default limits on induced electric field and gradient switching rates for use when direct determination has not been employed, but these are also derived from an empirical equation describing PNS thresholds.

ICNIRP GUIDELINES ON EMF EXPOSURE

The EMF exposure limits contained in IEC/EN standard 60601-2-33 are designed specifically for use in MRI and, as far as possible, they are incorporated into MRI equipment in the form of hardware and software interlocks and other safety features. There are also international guidelines on EMF exposure of more generally applicability. The International Commission on Non-Ionizing Radiation Protection (ICNIRP) is the main organisation active in this area and its guidelines have significant influence in Europe.

The ICNIRP develops guidelines and exposure limits to address adverse health effects of exposure to all forms of non-ionizing radiation, including EMF. The ICNIRP issued guidance on static magnetic field exposure in 1994 (10), which was updated in 2009 (11). Guidance on time-varying magnetic fields in the frequency range up to 300-GHz was published in 1998 (12), and updated in 2010 for the frequency range 1-Hz to 100-kHz (13). All of these guidelines contain exposure limits for workers, and also lower limits for members of the general public, which do not concern us directly here. At the time of this writing, the ICNIRP is preparing to publish new guidance on exposure to time-varying magnetic fields with frequencies below 1-Hz (primarily to prevent sensory effects associated with movement in static magnetic fields) and revision of guidance in the radiofrequency range (100-kHz to 300-GHz) is also underway. There is also a specific statement from the ICNIRP on protection of patients in MRI, published in 2004 (14) and revised in 2009 (15).

The ICNIRP bases its exposure limits, known as "basic restrictions", on the thresholds for "established adverse effects", determined by critical review of the literature (16). The biological effects of EMF on the human body vary dramatically with frequency. In the low frequency range relevant to the switched gradients in MRI (around 1-kHz), the relevant effect is stimulation of nervous tissue. The obvious manifestation of this is PNS, but historically there has been a tendency to regard magnetophosphenes (which only occur over a narrow frequency range around 10- to 50-Hz) as a possible indication of EMF interactions with the central nervous system over a much wider frequency range (17), resulting in much lower exposure limits than are justified by the desire to avoid PNS alone. This is more of an issue with the 1998 guidelines than with those issued in 2010, where a helpful distinction has been drawn between adverse effects (PNS) and transient disturbances (magnetophosphenes). In the radiofrequency range the critical effect is tissue heating and setting a limit is simply a matter of deciding how much heating is acceptable. Basic restrictions are often expressed in terms of quantities that cannot be readily determined, such as the electric field or current density induced in the body by a time-varying magnetic field, so the ICNIRP also defines "reference levels" in terms of quantities that are easier to measure, such as static magnetic field strength. These are derived from the basic restrictions using conservative models, so that complying with the reference level ensures that the relevant basic restriction is satisfied.

With the exception of those related to the static magnetic field, the ICNIRP's basic restrictions on occupational exposure are more restrictive than the exposure limits contained in the IEC standard. This is mainly because the ICNIRP applies reduction factors to adverse effect thresholds in order to arrive at the basic restrictions. The rationale is that this reflects uncertainties in scientific knowledge about adverse effects and their thresholds, and also accounts for biological variations in effect thresholds that may exist between individuals. Also, the ICNIRP adopts a broad definition of health, based on that of the WHO (5), so that effects resulting in annoyance or discomfort, affecting a person's wellbeing but otherwise harmless, may be regarded as potential health hazards (16). To add to this, because it is often impractical to demonstrate compliance with the basic restrictions, there is a tendency to treat the more conservative reference levels as default exposure limits.

Table 3 summarizes the ICNIRP basic restrictions for workers, insofar as they are relevant to MRI. For clarity, reference levels, general public limits and the complexities of

Table 3. ICNIRP basic restrictions for occupational exposure to EMF relevant to MRI.

Static magnetic field	Movement in static magnetic field (< 1-Hz representative frequency)	Switched gradients (1-kHz representative frequency)	Radiofrequency field

1994
- Time average: 200-mT
- Head and trunk: 2-T
- Limbs: 5-T
 	
2009
- Controlled environment: 8-T
	1998
	Induced current density (RMS)
	- Head and trunk:
	  40-mA m^{-2}
	  ($\approx$ 200-mV m^{-1})
	
	New guidelines expected in 2013
		1998
		Induced current density (RMS)
		- Head and trunk:
		  10-mA m^{-2}
		  ($\approx$ 50-mV m^{-1})
		2010
		Induced electric field
		- Head and body:
		  800-mV m^{-1}
			1998
			SAR*
			- Whole body:
			  0.4-W kg^{-1}
			- Localized, head and trunk: 10-W kg^{-1}
			- Localized, limbs:
			  20-W kg^{-1}

*SAR values averaged over 6-minutes; Localized SAR values averaged over 10-g of tissue.			

frequency dependence have been omitted. Where guidelines allow, it has been assumed that MRI is a "controlled environment" in which workers have been adequately trained. In some instances higher limits apply in such circumstances. In the case of switched gradients, which have complex non-sinusoidal waveforms, the ICNIRP limits at a representative frequency of 1-kHz have been used. Values have also been included for frequencies less than 1-Hz, because movement of persons through the temporally static but spatially varying magnetic field around an MR scanner results in exposure to a time-varying magnetic field in this frequency range and, therefore, falls within the scope of the guidelines. Values from the superseded 1994 and 1998 guidelines are included, for reasons that will become clear later.

Table 4 summarizes the ICNIRP guidance on exposure limits for MRI patients. In its MRI statements, the ICNIRP takes a similar approach to that adopted in IEC 60601-2-33. Three tiers of exposure are defined: *Normal Operating Mode*, *Controlled Operating Mode* (requiring medical supervision) and *Experimental Operating Mode* (requiring ethical approval). The gradient exposure limits are based on PNS perception thresholds derived from the same equation as is used to generate the IEC default limit values. Thus, they are based on actual effect thresholds, although direct determination is not embraced. RF heating limitations are also similar to those in the IEC standard and, again, there are a number of derived SAR limits. However, crucially, these limits apply only to patients undergoing MRI. MRI workers remain subject to the ICNIRP occupational basic restrictions shown in **Table 3**.

THE EU EMF DIRECTIVE: CURRENT STATUS AND FUTURE PROSPECTS

Article 16 (1) of the framework directive (6) envisages adoption of additional individual directives to address specific health and safety hazards. The Physical Agents (EMF) Directive (2004/40/EC) (1), the eighteenth of these individual directives, was adopted by the European Parliament and Council on 29th April 2004, with a deadline of 30th April 2008 for member state transposition. It is one of a set of four physical agents directives (the others relate to noise, vibration and artificial optical radiation). Its objective is to protect workers from the "known short-term adverse effects in the human body" of exposure to EMF. It is

Table 4. ICNIRP recommended limits for patient exposures during MRI.

	Static magnetic field	Switched gradients	Radiofrequency field			
		Gradient switching rate (dB/dt) as a percentage of mean perception threshold for PNS*	Maximum core temperature rise (°C)	Maximum local tissue temperature (°C)		
				Head	Trunk	Extremities
Normal Operating Mode	≤ 4-T	⇗ 80%	0.5	38	39	40
Controlled Operating Mode	> 4-T, ≤ 8-T	⇗ 100%	1	38	39	40
Experimental Operating Mode	>8-T	> 100%	>1	>38	>39	>40

*The peripheral nerve stimulation (PNS) mean perception threshold is derived from an empirical equation.

concerned only with occupational exposure, not exposure of MRI patients or of the general public.

The directive incorporates the 1998 ICNIRP exposure limits for time-varying magnetic fields. Transposition of the directive would have the effect of making the ICNIRP basic restrictions, referred to as "exposure limit values" (ELVs) in the directive, into legally binding limits throughout the EU. The ICNIRP reference levels become "action levels" in the directive, with the same purpose of providing a more practical way of ensuring compliance with the ELVs. The ICNIRP 1994 static magnetic field limits were not included because it was known that this guidance was due for revision. However, somewhat illogically in the absence of an ELV, there is a static magnetic field action value of 200-mT, based on the ICNIRP time-averaged exposure limit (**Table 3**).

Members of the European MRI community became aware of the directive shortly before it was adopted. It was quickly realized that the ELVs are exceeded in a number of situations in MRI and that the directive would have serious consequences for both clinical and research activity. A campaign was launched, led by the European Society of Radiology (ESR), to lobby the EU institutions to change the directive. The Alliance for MRI was established, bringing together professional bodies, patient groups, research funding organisations, and individual scientists as well as politicians united in their concern about the issue. There were also campaigns in individual member states and a parliamentary inquiry in the United Kingdom (UK) (18). After considerable effort and the publication of research showing that the ELVs are indeed exceeded by MRI workers (19, 20, 21), the community's argument about the impact of the directive was accepted. Specifically, research showed that the ELV for frequencies below 1-Hz was exceeded by a factor of up to 10 for workers moving through the static magnetic field near the MR system (18), and the ELV in the gradient frequency range by a factor of 20 or more for workers standing close to the scanner during imaging (19) (note, RF exposure is rarely, if ever, a problem). Thus, providing clinical care to a patient during MRI, all forms of interventional MRI, some research activities, or even walking at a normal speed close to an MR system, would have become illegal throughout the EU following transposition of the directive.

Of course, this does not mean that workers in these situations are placing themselves at risk of direct EMF effects: IEC 60601-2-33 ensures that this is not the case. The problem is the large safety factors built into the ICNIRP basic restrictions and, hence, the ELVs, particularly in the gradient frequency range. These may have a place in industrial settings with highly variable EMF outputs, but are unnecessary and highly problematic in the context of MRI, where EMF outputs are precisely controlled and adverse effects are already addressed under the more specific IEC standard.

Late in 2007, the European Commission proposed postponement of the transposition deadline by four years to allow time for a solution to be found. In June 2011 the Commission proposed a new directive, based on the new 2009 and 2010 ICNIRP recommendations but also incorporating a "derogation" to exclude MRI workers from the exposure limits and a mechanism to develop harmonized safe working practices for MRI throughout the EU. However, this proposal has not yet been accepted, and, indeed, has encountered significant opposition, particularly in the Council. In April 2012, a further transposition delay of 18 months was announced.

The final outcome of this lengthy saga remains unknown at the time of writing. It seems certain that the MRI derogation will survive the legislative process, but various conditions are likely to be imposed. The exemption will probably only apply to CE-marked scanners, which may be problematic for 7-T and some other research MR systems. The new directive is likely to be adopted during 2013, and before the transposition deadline during 2016, EU-wide guidelines on safe working practices will be developed in collaboration with the MRI community. (Note: The new directive was adopted in June 2013 as 2013/35/EU.)

EXPOSURE LIMITS AND GUIDELINES IN INDIVIDUAL COUNTRIES

Individual European countries take a variety of approaches to EMF exposure limitations. It is difficult to find an authoritative and up-to-date source of information on this topic, although WHO maintains a partial list (22), and the situation can only be summarized briefly here.

In some countries (e.g., the Czech Republic), the ICNIRP 1994 and 1998 guidelines are legally binding, but generally (e.g., in Austria, France, Ireland, the UK and Malta), the ICNIRP guidelines are regarded purely as recommendations to be taken into account for example in risk assessments. In some jurisdictions (e.g., Bulgaria and Poland), limits have been adopted that are even more conservative than those recommended by ICNIRP. If properly enforced, the ICNIRP or these more stringent limits are clearly problematic for MRI and there will be no requirement for countries with such limits in place to relax them following passage of an amended EMF directive. When EMF exposure limits based on the ICNIRP guidelines were introduced in Germany in 2001 (23), the implications were realized in time and an exemption for MRI was included following lobbying by the imaging community. In other countries (e.g., Portugal and Finland) ICNIRP limits are mandatory only in frequency ranges that do not impact on MRI.

A few countries have adopted specific guidance on MRI safety. The UK Medicines and Healthcare Products Regulatory Agency (MHRA) guidance covers issues such as safety infrastructure, safe working practices, worker training, and control of access to MRI facilities (24). In the Netherlands, safe working guidance was issued in 2008 with the support of the relevant professional bodies and government agencies (25). The prospect of harmonized EU-wide MRI safety guidelines in the wake of the amended EMF directive has triggered initiatives such as development of standards on the role and training of MRI safety officers in Austria (26, 27).

SUMMARY AND CONCLUSIONS

Protection of patients and workers from hazards associated with EMF related to MRI requires both appropriate equipment design and use to ensure that the thresholds for direct effects are not exceeded and appropriate working practices and training to minimize the probability of indirect effects are in place. The combination of the Medical Devices Directive, supported by the IEC 60601 series standards, and the framework health and safety directive should be sufficient to ensure that these conditions are met in Europe. In practice, however, it is unclear how uniformly the obligations created by the framework directive are applied in MRI facilities and there is certainly a case for specific guidelines in this area, which ideally should be harmonized across Europe. The ICNIRP occupational exposure guidelines are a blunt instrument in our context, designed to apply across very wide frequency ranges and incorporating safety factors that are both unnecessary and problematic. A critical difference between the IEC and ICNIRP approaches is that the IEC standard recognizes that MRI equipment designed to ensure patient safety is also safe for workers at the same exposure levels, whereas the ICNIRP applies different exposure limits for patients and workers. The derogation for MRI proposed in the revised EMF directive will ensure that MRI activities can continue in Europe, while workers remain protected by the IEC standard and, hopefully, by new EU-wide guidelines on safe working and training.

REFERENCES

1. Directive 2004/40/EC of the European Parliament and of the council of 29 April 2004 on the minimum health and safety requirements regarding the exposure of workers to the risks arising from physical agents (electromagnetic fields). Official Journal of the European Union. Available at: http://eur-lex.europa.eu/LexUriServ/LexUriServ.do?uri=OJ:L:2004:159:0001:0026:EN:PDF. Accessed December 2012.

2. Keevil SF, Gedroyc W, Gowland P, et al. Electromagnetic field exposure limitation and the future of MRI. Br J Radiol 2005;78:973-975.

3. Keevil SF, Krestin GP. EMF directive still poses a risk to MRI research in Europe. Lancet 2010;376:1124-1125.

4. Keevil SF. The European union EMF directive and MRI: Is a solution in sight at last? Diagnostic Imaging Europe 2012;28:8-12.

5. Preamble to the Constitution of the World Health Organization as adopted by the International Health Conference. New York: 1946.

6. Council Directive 89/391/EEC of 12th June 1989 on the introduction of measures to encourage improvements in the safety and health of workers at work. Official Journal of the European Communities. Available at: http://eur-lex.europa.eu/LexUriServ/LexUriServ.do?uri=OJ:L:1989:183:0001:0008:EN:PDF. Accessed December 2012.

7. Council Directive 93/42/EEC of 14 June 1993 concerning medical devices. Official Journal of the European Communities.1993. Available at: http://eur-lex.europa.eu/LexUriServ/LexUriServ.do?uri=OJ:L:1993:169:0001:0043:EN:PDF. Accessed December 2012.

8. International Electrotechnical Commission (IEC). Medical electrical equipment – Part 1: general requirements for basic safety and essential performance, IEC 60601-1, 3rd Edition. Geneva: IEC, 2005.

9. International Electrotechnical Commission. Medical electrical equipment – Part 2-33: particular requirements for the safety of magnetic resonance equipment for medical diagnosis, IEC 60601-2-33, 3rd Edition. Geneva: IEC, 2010.

10. International Commission on Non-Ionizing Radiation Protection. Guidelines on limits of exposure to static magnetic fields. Health Physics 1994;66:100-106.

11. International Commission on Non-Ionizing Radiation Protection. Guidelines on limits of exposure to static magnetic fields. Health Physics 2009;96:504-514.

12. International Commission on Non-Ionizing Radiation Protection. Guidelines for limiting exposure to time-varying electric, magnetic, and electromagnetic fields (up to 300 GHz). Health Physics 1998;74:494-522.

13. International Commission on Non-Ionizing Radiation Protection. Guidelines for limiting exposure to time-varying electric and magnetic fields (1 Hz - 100 kHz). Health Physics 2010;99:818-836.

14. International Commission on Non-ionizing Radiation Protection. Statement on medical magnetic resonance (MR) procedures: protection of patients. Health Physics 2004;87:197-216.

15. International Commission on Non-Ionizing Radiation Protection. Amendment to the ICNIRP "Statement on medical magnetic resonance (MR) procedures: protection of patients". Health Physics 2009;97:259-261.

16. International Commission on Non-Ionizing Radiation Protection. General approach to protection against non-ionizing radiation. Health Physics 2002;82:540-548.

17. Attwell D. Interaction of low frequency electric fields with the nervous system: the retina as a model system. Radiat Protect Dosimetr 2003;106:341-348.

18. House of Commons Science and Technology Committee. Watching the directives: scientific advice on the EU Physical Agents (Electromagnetic Fields) Directive. London: The Stationery Office Limited; 2006. pp.140. Available at: http://www.publications.parliament.uk/pa/cm200506/cmselect/cmsctech/1030/1030.pdf. Accessed December 2012.

19. Crozier S, Trakic A, Wang H, Liu F. Numerical study of currents in workers induced by body-motion around high-ultrahigh field MRI magnets. J Magn Reson Imaging 2007;26:1261-1277.

20. Crozier S, Wang H, Trakic A, Liu F. Exposure of workers to pulsed gradients in MRI. J Magn Reson Imaging 2007;26:1236-1254.

21. Capstick M, McRobbie D, Hand J, et al. An investigation into occupational exposure to electromagnetic fields for personnel working with and around medical magnetic resonance imaging equipment. Geneva: IT'IS Foundation; 2008. pp: 287. Available at: http://www.itis.ethz.ch/assets/Downloads/Papers-Reports/Reports/VT2007017FinalReportv04.pdf. Accessed December 2012.

22. International EMF Project. EMF worldwide standards. Available at: http://www.who.int/docstore/peh-emf/EMFStandards/who-0102/Worldmap5.htm. Accessed December 2012.

23. Professional Associations (BG). Regulation for Occupational Health and Safety at Work. BGV B11 Accident prevention regulation electromagnetic fields. Berlin: Hauptverband der gewerblichen Berufsgenossenschaften; 2001:25

24. Medicines and Healthcare Products Regulatory Agency. Device bulletin DB2007(03). Safety guidelines for magnetic resonance imaging equipment in clinical use, 3rd Edition. London: MHRA, 2007. Available at: http://www.mhra.gov.uk/Publications/Safetyguidance/DeviceBulletins/CON2033018. Accessed December 2012.

25. MRI Working Group. Using MRI safely: practical rules for employees. Available at: Ministerie van Sociale Zaken en Werkgelegenheid. Available at: http://docs.minszw.nl/pdf/92/2008/92_2008_1_22102.pdf. Accessed December 2012.

26. Austrian Standards Institute. ÖNORM S 1125-1: Safety officer for magnetic resonance equipment for medical diagnosis - part 1: Responsibilities and competences. Vienna: Austrian Standards Institute, 2009. Available at: https://www.astandis.at/shopV5/Preview.action;jsessionid= 5411938848EBC85559C0D51F 240F6DDE?preview=&dokkey=305935&selectedLocale=de. Accessed December 2012.

27. Austrian Standards Institute. ÖNORM S 1125-2: Safety officer for magnetic resonance equipment for medical diagnosis - part 2: Requirements on training. Vienna: Austrian Standards Institute, 2009. Available at: https://www.astandis.at/shopV5/Preview.action;jsessionid=5164FB96391EEFCEA351D097601A8EE1? preview=&dokkey=305936&selectedLocale=de. Accessed December 2012.

Chapter 30   MRI Standards and Safety Guidelines in Canada

KAREN SMITH, M.S., (RTMR)

Life Member
Canadian Association of Medical Radiation Technologists
Regional Practice Lead, MRI
Integrated Medical Imaging
Vancouver, British Columbia, Canada
and
Instructor
MRI Program
British Columbia Institute of Technology
Burnaby, British Columbia, Canada

INTRODUCTION

This chapter focuses on the standards and safety guidelines recommended for practice in Canada, particularly those designed to ensure magnetic resonance imaging (MRI) safety for the patient, staff, and others entering the MRI environment. It is very important to implement these guidelines for both MRI safety and excellence in patient care. The major concerns and risks to the patient and staff members are those related to the powerful static magnetic field, gradient magnetic fields, and radiofrequency (RF) fields. Accordingly, these are the main factors to consider for MRI safety:

- Approval of the MR system, RF coils, and peripheral equipment as safe medical devices in Canada by Health Canada
- Health Canada Safety Code 26 and the Health Canada Safety Code 6
- Other MRI safety resources
- Acceptance testing of the MRI facility
- Accreditation of the MRI facility
- Quality Improvement Program
- General MRI safety, guidelines, and policies

- Careful screening and preparation of the patient or individual before entering the MRI environment

- Appropriate qualified medical personnel

- Quality control program

- MRI contrast agent use and safety

- Clinical standards optimized for clinical indications following the Canadian Association of Radiologists (CAR) MRI guidelines

MEDICAL DEVICES

The approval of the MR system as a medical device is the responsibility of Health Canada, through its Health Products and Food Branch (HPFB). The HPFB monitors and evaluates the safety, efficacy, and quality of diagnostic and therapeutic medical devices, so that consumers and healthcare professionals can use them with confidence. The HPFB works to balance the risks associated with any new health science innovation with the benefits that medical devices can provide to Canadians. All medical devices in Canada are subject to the *Food and Drugs Act* and its regulations.

In Canada, medical devices are categorized into four classes based on the level of risk associated with their use. Class I devices present the lowest potential risk (e.g., oral thermometers) and Class IV devices present the greatest potential risk (e.g., cardiac pacemakers). Class II, III, and IV devices receive increasingly rigorous reviews, and must be licensed before being sold in Canada. By comparison, Class I devices do not require licenses, but manufacturers must ensure that these devices are designed and manufactured to be safe, as required by the *Medical Devices Regulations*. Of note is that an MR system is classified as a medical device Class II by these regulations (1).

In order to determine if a particular MR system is approved for use in Canada, a searchable database called Medical Devices Active Licensing Listing (MDALL) is available that lists Class II, III, and IV medical devices licensed in Canada. Both active and archived licenses can be viewed at the website: http://www.mdall.ca

The *Medical Devices Regulations* for Class II, III, and IV medical devices were last amended December, 2011. The pertinent information from regulations 26 to 32 are applied to MR systems and these are provided from the Government of Canada's website, as follows (2):

Class II, III, and IV Medical Devices
Prohibition

26. Subject to section 37, no person shall import or sell a Class II, III or IV medical device unless the manufacturer of the device holds a license in respect of that device or, if the medical device has been subjected to a change described in section 34, an amended medical device license.

27. No person shall advertise a Class II, III or IV medical device for the purpose of sale unless

(a) the manufacturer of the device holds a license in respect of that device or, if the device has been subjected to a change described in section 34, an amended medical device license; or

(b) the advertisement is placed only in a catalogue that includes a clear and visible warning that the devices advertised in the catalogue may not have been licensed in accordance with Canadian law.

Medical Devices Deemed Licensed

28. If a system is licensed, all of its components or parts that are manufactured by the manufacturer of the system are deemed, for the purposes of its importation, sale or advertisement, to have been licensed.

29. If a test kit is licensed, all of its reagents or articles that are manufactured by the manufacturer of the test kit are deemed, for the purposes of its importation, sale or advertisement, to have been licensed.

30. If a medical device or a medical device group is licensed and forms part of a medical device family or a medical device group family, as the case may be, all other medical devices or medical device groups in the family are deemed to have been licensed.

31. (1) If all the medical devices that form part of a medical device group are licensed, that medical device group is deemed to have been licensed.

(2) If a medical device group is licensed, all the medical devices that form part of the medical device group are deemed, for the purposes of its importation, sale or advertisement, to have been licensed.

Application for a Medical Device License

32. (1) An application for a medical device license shall be submitted to the Minister by the manufacturer of the medical device in a format established by the Minister and shall contain the following:

  (a) the name of the device;
  (b) the class of the device;
  (c) the identifier of the device, including the identifier of any medical device that is part of a system, test kit, medical device group, medical device family or medical device group family;

  (d) the name and address of the manufacturer as it appears on the device label; and

  (e) the name and address of the establishment where the device is being manufactured, if different from the one referred to in paragraph called (d) above

(2) An application for a Class II medical device license shall contain, in addition to the information and documents set out in subsection (1), the following:

  (a) a description of the medical conditions, purposes and uses for which the device is manufactured, sold or represented;

  (b) a list of the standards complied with in the manufacture of the device to satisfy the safety and effectiveness requirements;

  (c) an attestation by a senior official of the manufacturer that the manufacturer has objective evidence to establish that the device meets the safety and effectiveness requirements;

(d) an attestation by a senior official of the manufacturer that the device label meets the applicable labeling requirements of these Regulations;

(e) in the case of a near patient *in vitro* diagnostic device, an attestation by a senior official of the manufacturer that investigational testing has been conducted on the device using human subjects representative of the intended users and under conditions similar to the conditions of use; and

(f) A copy of the quality management system certificate certifying that the quality management system under which the device is manufactured satisfies National Standard of Canada CAN/CSA-ISO 13485:03, Medical devices — Quality management systems — Requirements for regulatory purposes.

The MR system specifications and performance should meet all provincial and federal guidelines, including Health Canada guidelines. Other MRI safety resources and recommendations are also followed to ensure MRI safety.

HEALTH CANADA'S SAFETY CODE 26 AND 6

Health Canada's Safety Code 26 is the *Guidelines on Exposure to Electromagnetic Fields from Magnetic Resonance Clinical Systems* (3), which was developed in 1987 when both magnetic resonance imaging (MRI) and magnetic resonance spectroscopy (MRS) gained widespread acceptance as well as many applications in clinical settings.

Because the fields produced by MR systems (i.e., static, gradient, and RF fields) can create detrimental biological effects, questions have been raised regarding the safety of these devices. This aforementioned document briefly reviews the biological effects of the electromagnetic fields used in MR devices and provides general guidance on exposure levels to the patient and to the operator. The levels cited should not be considered as strict limits which, if exceeded, could result in a dangerous situation, but rather indicate the established levels in 1987 below which potential hazards, if any, are considered minimal. Higher exposure levels may still be safe, depending on various factors. For patient exposures exceeding the specified safe limits, the usual risk versus benefit assessment must be made. Interpretation and further details of the recommendations of this safety code may be obtained from the Non-Ionizing Radiation Section, Bureau of Radiation and Medical Devices, Environmental Health Directorate, Health Protection Branch, Ottawa, Ontario, K1A 0L2.

As with any technology, even when beneficial in medical applications, it is necessary to carefully consider the potential health hazards and to develop and implement proper safety precautions. There are several safety factors that have to be considered with respect to the clinical use of MR for human subjects. In this safety code, besides a brief review of the biological effects of electromagnetic fields used in MRI, information is also provided on guidelines regarding the use of MRI in other countries. General guidance is presented regarding what patient and operator exposure levels are considered safe, at the present time. Advice is also provided with respect to cardiac pacemakers and metallic implants. However, other safety issues not directly related to human subject exposure to electromagnetic fields are not addressed here. These include possible injury by projectiles (i.e., because of the forces from the static magnetic field acting on ferromagnetic objects), injury due to the quench of a cryogenic magnet, and electromagnetic interference by MRI-related electromagnetic fields with other medical devices (e.g., patient monitoring systems) (3). Another related document, Health Canada's *Safety Code 6, Limits of Human Exposure to Radiofrequency Electromagnetic Energy in the Frequency Range from 3 kHz to 300 GHz*, was updated in 2009 and is available on-line (4).

OTHER MRI SAFETY RESOURCES PROVIDING STANDARDS AND GUIDELINES

Canadian sites refer to other sources for current MRI safety guidelines and information, which include, the following:

- The Canadian Association of Radiologists (CAR) Standards for Magnetic Resonance Imaging, Approved April, 2011 (5).

- The Reference Manual for Magnetic Resonance Safety, Implants, and Devices annual edition by Dr. Frank G. Shellock (6). This medical textbook provides a comprehensive resource that includes guidelines and recommendations for MRI safety based on peer-reviewed literature, labeling information on devices from manufacturers, and documents developed by International Society for magnetic Resonance in Medicine (ISMRM), American College of Radiology (ACR), the Food and Drug Administration (FDA), the National Electrical Manufacturers Association (NEMA), the International Electrotechnical Commission (IEC), the Medical Devices Agency (MDA) and the International Commission on Non-Ionizing Radiation Protection (ICNIRP), and other agencies (6).

- The MRI safety website, www.mrisafety.com, which was developed by Dr. Frank G. Shellock (7). This website is updated on a regular basis.

- The latest document from the American College of Radiology (ACR), Guidance Document on MR Safe Practices: 2013 (8).

ACCEPTANCE TESTING FOR MR SYSTEMS

Acceptance testing of an MR system is intended to measure quantifiable system parameters that may then be compared to the manufacturer's specifications. According to the document, *Acceptance Testing of Magnetic Resonance Imaging Systems*, complete evaluation of the scanner's performance shall be conducted by a medical physicist after completion of installation and prior to regular patient imaging (9). The medical physicist is preferably someone on-site, but may also be contracted to perform this testing. The credentials of the medical physicist should include a doctorate (Ph.D.) in MRI physics. Furthermore, this individual should be accredited by either the Canadian College of Physicists in Medicine (CCPM) or one of the affiliated professional engineering societies in Canada, with specific training and experience in MRI. Training and experience shall include detailed knowledge of MRI physics, MR system components and performance, safety procedures, acceptance testing, and quality control testing. Acceptance testing may be performed by a team of medical physicists as long as at least one of the group members has the aforementioned credentials and can vouch for the testing quality of the team.

The acceptance testing should include a detailed description and inspection of the entire MRI facility. This should include assessment of the MRI equipment room, control room, MR system room, patient preparation area, and patient waiting area. This general assessment should be conducted for construction irregularities and incomplete features, locations and functionality of lighting, safety switches, patient and staff flow, safety features (e.g., MR safe or MR conditional fire extinguishers, emergency off switches, patient monitoring, security, etc.), Faraday shield grounding and integrity, installation neatness and completion. The fringe field associated with the MR system also needs to be detailed by the physicist (even though a similar document may have been provided by the MR system manufacturer). Fringe field lines must be measured using a tri-directional Hall effect magnetometer and reported on a site drawing.

The performance tests conducted on the MR system should be repeated as a routine part of the acceptance test. While the MR system manufacturer does these tests during the installation process, the tests also need to be repeated with the independent physicist present. There are overall manufacturer-specific system tests and tests to characterize many features of the scanner including the shim, eddy currents, stability, quadrature ghosting, system performance, signal-to-noise ratio, white pixel, coherent noise, geometric distortion, slice cross talk, slice position and thickness accuracy, low contrast object detectability, high contrast spatial resolution tests, ghosting tests, and RF linearity. A general evaluation of specialized pulse sequences (i.e., sequences that are not routinely on all MR system) is required. Testing of all pulse sequences is not possible, nor practical, and, therefore, would be part of clinical acceptance testing which is done after the scanner has been "handed over" by the manufacturer and physicist to the clinical MRI facility. Sequences that should be assessed include those used for MR spectroscopy. MR spectroscopy provides a revealing signature of the MR system's "health" because it is an extremely sensitive technique. In addition to evaluating specialized sequences, parallel imaging and acceleration (in both phase encode directions) should be verified and tested for speed, signal-to-noise, and artifacts. Lastly, patient monitoring associated with the scanner (e.g., pulse oximeter and respiratory bellows) should be verified for functionality and sensitivity. If the physicist has access to a portable waveform generator, this can be used to test functionality of the electrocardiograph system.

All RF coils need to be tested for functionality and have a signal-to-noise measurement performed as a baseline. Individual elements of multichannel RF coils also need testing to verify each element. This evaluation provides a valuable baseline measurement for future comparisons of the scanners integrity.

Hard copies of the acceptance report should include information for all tests and measured values, data evaluation graphs, and photographs showing deficiencies described in the text. Additionally, hard copies of the report should be provided to the MRI facility (one for the control room and one for the managing director of the diagnostic imaging department) and one to the MR system manufacturer vendor. The physicist should also provide a digital copy of the report, with all baseline data acquired in the tests and any vendor specific reports from the MR system. The written report should include a list of recommendations and suggested changes. It is the responsibility of the MR system manufacturer to ensure that all hardware and software as well as any technical issues defined in the deficiency list are addressed immediately and prior to clinical use of the scanner. It is the responsibility of the MRI facility to address all other aspects of the recommendations. The report should be evaluated and discussed by representative(s) of the vendor (e.g., the field engineer), the managing director of MRI in the diagnostic imaging department, the MRI technologist manager, and the lead physician of the MRI facility (5).

ACCREDITATION OF MRI FACILITIES

In Canada, the Minister of Health is the Minister of the Crown in the Canadian Cabinet who is responsible for overseeing the federal government's health department, which is Health Canada, and enforcing the Public Health Agency of Canada, the Canada Health Act, which is the law governing Medicare. Though the Canada Health Act provides national guidelines for healthcare, the provinces of Canada have exclusive jurisdiction over health under the constitution and are free to ignore these guidelines. If they ignore the guidelines, the federal government may deny funding for healthcare in that province. The federal government has no direct role in the delivery of medicine in the provinces and territories so each province or territory has its own independent public health insurance program. Under the Canada Health Act, each province and territory must provide services to members of plans in other provinces and territories (11). The administration and delivery of healthcare services, such as MRI, is the responsibility of each province or territory. This is guided by the provisions of the Canada Health Act. The Ministry of Health is a provincial government department and each is responsible for a specific province's health services. Each province has a Minister of Health responsible for health services in that province or territory. In 2004, the First Ministers directed the Health Ministers to work on the following additional healthcare reform initiatives: patient safety, health human resources, technology assessment, innovative research, and healthy Canadians.

At the provincial level, there are the Colleges of Physicians and Surgeons. As the radiologist in each province reporting on MRI examinations belongs to the College of Physicians and Surgeons, one of the goals on the provincial level is to establish programs and committees that promote high standards in diagnostic medical facilities. Diagnostic facilities are accredited to provide a diagnostic imaging service, such as MRI. In order to maintain accreditation, the diagnostic facility must fully participate in ongoing assessment activities. This is done differently in each province or territory. There is no national accreditation standard for MRI facilities, but these are done on a provincial level (12, 13). One of the benefits of accreditation of the MRI facility is that it increases compliance with quality and safety standards (10). Accreditation also promotes a quality and safety culture and facilitates the sharing of policies, procedures and best practices among healthcare organizations and facilities (14).

QUALITY IMPROVEMENT PROGRAM FOR MRI

The Canadian Association of Radiologists (CAR) recommends that a documented, systematic quality improvement program should be established under the direction of the supervising physician radiologist in order to monitor and evaluate such problems as claustrophobia, sedation, administration of contrast agents, equipment malfunctions and accidents (such as metallic objects entering the scan room) endangering patients or workers. Monitoring such activities should include the evaluation of the accuracy of radiologic interpretations as well as the appropriateness of examinations. The incidence of complications and adverse events should be recorded and periodically reviewed in order to identify opportunities to improve patient care. Data should be collected in a manner that complies with statutory and regulatory peer-reviewed procedures in order to protect the confidentiality of the peer-reviewed data.

In 2010, the Royal College of Physicians and Surgeons of Canada, the Canadian Medical Protective Association (CMPA), the Canadian Medical Association (CMA), and the College of Family Physicians of Canada (CFPC) co-sponsored the program, *Getting It Right: A Policy Forum to Advance Quality Improvement in Canada*. The discussions amongst these groups pertained to how to facilitate quality improvement in healthcare and promote a just culture of safety. Notably, healthcare executives, physicians, and other providers all have a collective responsibility to ensure that they create and maintain a supportive and fair culture in which everyone can fully learn from adverse events and help prevent their reoccurrence. The need for change and for improvements in quality and safety are increasingly being recognized (15).

GENERAL MRI SAFETY GUIDELINES, PRACTICES, AND POLICIES

The Canadian Association of Radiologists (CAR) recommends that MRI safety guidelines, practices, and policies shall be written, enforced, documented, and reviewed at least annually by the supervising radiologist and the MRI technologist manager. All technologists and other supporting staffs working in the MRI department are expected to review safety policies annually. It must be understood that these safety practices are important not only for the patients but also for others who will be accompanying the patient or entering in the MR system room. All MRI safety incidents or 'near incidents' must be reported to the lead physician of the MRI facility in a timely fashion and should be analyzed and used in future quality improvement processes.

These guidelines take into consideration potential interactions of the strong static magnetic field of the MR system with ferromagnetic objects in the environment of the scanner that might result in projectiles leading to injuries or damages. MRI safety information for any external device should never be assumed if the item is not clearly documented in writing. All necessary information must be obtained before bringing the device (e.g., wheelchairs, gurneys, IV poles, etc.) into the MR system room.

The risks to the patient could be related to the electromagnetic field used for the MRI procedure. Implants and devices must be screened thoroughly, as detailed below. It is important to note that practices should be in place to decrease the possibility of patient burns while scanning. This includes optimization of scanning protocols that do not exceed the recommended specific absorption rate (SAR) limit, the use of adequate padding, proper patient positioning, and appropriate placement of patient monitoring devices. Extra care must be taken with sedated or anesthetized patients and those who are unable to maintain communication with the MRI technologist. Recognized contraindications include, but are not limited to, the presence of certain cardiac pacemakers, ferromagnetic intracranial aneurysm clips, certain neurostimulation systems, and ferromagnetic foreign bodies in critical anatomic locations (e.g., the eye).

With regard to using MRI in a pregnant patient, according to the Canadian Association of Radiologists (CAR) Standard for Magnetic Resonance Imaging (5), "The safety of MRI scanning during pregnancy has not been established. The decision to scan during pregnancy should be made on an individual basis after consideration of medical necessity and alternate imaging methods. This particularly applies to scanning during the first trimester." Notably, this information is different from the pregnancy information recently presented by the American College of Radiology (8), which indicates, "Present data have not conclusively documented any deleterious effects of MR imaging exposure on the developing fetus. Therefore, no special consideration is recommended for the first, versus any other, trimester in pregnancy. Nevertheless, as with all interventions during pregnancy, it is prudent to screen females of reproductive age for pregnancy before permitting them access to MR imaging environments. If pregnancy is established consideration should be given to reassessing the potential risks versus benefits of the pending study in determining whether the requested MR examination could safely wait to the end of the pregnancy before being performed."

Patients require thorough screening prior to scanning (i.e., to include completion of a screening form and a verbal interview). Importantly, it is recommended that referring physicians be aware of MRI screening protocols. Screening should initially be performed at the referring physician's office, upon registration at the clinical MRI facility, and, again, by the MRI technologist who will scan the patient. Screening should also be noted and reviewed at the scheduling office of the Diagnostic Imaging Department. Even with four levels of screening, it is well known that patients will either forget to mention something or possibly not mention anything at all for fear of losing their scan slot. Therefore, patients must be educated as to the importance of the screening process.

Implants and devices found in patients must be carefully screened and investigated to determine the exact type, which may or may not be safe for the MRI examination. It is the responsibility of the radiologist to confirm the exact type of device in consultation with the referring physician. Screening patients with implants and devices may be facilitating using the latest edition of the *Reference Manual for Magnetic Resonance Safety, Implants and Devices* or researched online at the website, www.mrisafety.com (6, 7). As a last resort, MRI technologists should contact the manufacturer of the device in order to obtain the specific MRI labeling information for the product.

In Canada, we rely on these sources for assessing what is safe to go into the MRI environment, whether it is in the patient or equipment needing to be placed in the MR system room. The following is what usually happens and constitutes the procedure for verifying if implants and devices are MR safe, MR unsafe, or MR conditional. First, information on the implant from the patient, medical records, or surgical reports is reviewed. The next step is to refer to the *"Reference Manual for Magnetic Resonance Safety, Implants and Devices"* or www.MRIsafety.com (6, 7). Additionally, notices are considered that are obtained from the Health Protection and Food Branch of Health Canada to see if the implant or device is contraindicated. If the relative safety for the implant is not found on these resources, then the MRI technologist contacts the manufacturer. If still unable to determine the safety for the implant or device, consultation occurs with the radiologist and the end result may be that the patient is not scanned unless the benefit outweighs the risk.

Other MRI safety concerns associated with the MRI procedure are thermal issues and MRI-related acoustic noise. For these issues, prevention whenever possible is the key. It is important to communicate with patients throughout the examinations to make sure they are not having any unusual experiences. For example, if the patient feels any heating, this should be addressed immediately by checking to make sure there is no excessive heating. It is best to have patients change into hospital gowns to prevent burns that may be caused from metallic threads in the clothing and to ensure that all metallic objects are removed prior to the MRI examination. To prevent issues related to acoustic noise, it is important to provide the patient with properly fitting earplugs or other hearing protection device.

QUALIFIED MEDICAL PERSONNEL

In order to have a high quality MRI facility, a team of appropriately trained medical personnel is essential. This team should consist of radiologists, a physicist, and MRI technologists. Physicians involved in the performance, supervision and interpretation of MRI procedures should be Diagnostic Radiologists and must have documented experience, Fellowship training, or a Certification in Diagnostic Radiology from the Royal College of Physicians and Surgeons of Canada and/or the Collège des médecins du Québec, or an equivalent. Also acceptable for this matter are fellowship-trained physicians, as well as those with foreign specialist qualifications if the physician so qualified holds an appointment in Radiology from a Canadian University or appropriate licensing authority.

As new imaging modalities and interventional techniques are developed, additional clinical training, under supervision and with proper documentation, should be obtained before radiologists independently interpret or perform such examinations or procedures, independently. Such additional training must meet with pertinent provincial and/or regional regulations. Continuing professional development must meet with the requirements of the Maintenance of Certification Program of the Royal College of Physicians and Surgeons of Canada. A properly trained, MRI physicist should perform initial acceptance testing of the MR system immediately following installation, and prior to any clinical scanning, as previously indicated.

The technologist must be certified by the Canadian Association of Medical Radiation Technologists (CAMRT) in the discipline of magnetic resonance (RTMR) and, in some provinces, be registered with the provincial regulatory body and authorized to work in the discipline of MRI (16). The technologist is primarily responsible for performing the MRI procedures and maintaining the overall safety of patients, staff and equipment within the MRI environment. This includes careful screening and preparation of patients, ensuring patient comfort, adjustment of protocols (if required) to produce high quality, diagnostic scans, technical and quality evaluation of images, and relevant quality assurance. MRI technologists are also responsible for the MR room safety and ensuring that no maintenance staff member enters the area without direct supervision. All personnel must be screened and educated about MRI by the MRI technologist. MRI technologists, if adequately trained, may also perform intravenous gadolinium-based contrast injections requested by the responsible physician. Continued education of MRI technologists is encouraged by the CAMRT and should meet pertinent provincial regulations.

Last and certainly not least is the MR system service engineer. The service engineer should be responsible for system installation, calibration, and preventive maintenance (PM) at regularly scheduled intervals. The schedule is to be dictated by the specific MR system manufacturer and clearly described prior to purchase of the scanner. The service engineer's qualification must be ensured by the corporation responsible for service and the manufacturer of the MR system used at the site. It is highly recommended the site use a field engineer who is employed by the manufacturer of the MR system. The field engineer should be in routine communication with the site MRI technologist manager and physicist. Preventive maintenance shall be scheduled, performed, and documented by a qualified service engineer on a regular basis.

QUALITY CONTROL PROGRAM

The objective of an MRI quality control (QC) program is to provide a series of tests and measurements that may be performed on a regular basis to determine if the MR system is performing in a reproducible, predictable, and reliable manner. Protocols for routine system performance testing continue to evolve. Quality control testing should be conducted under the supervision of the medical physicist (if present on-site), with review at least every six months by the supervising radiologist. A preventive maintenance program is recommended as a means to minimize unscheduled down time and/or poor scanner performance.

Following acceptance testing, each MRI site is required to maintain its level of scan quality through the performance and assessment of weekly quality assurance/quality control (QA/QC) testing, where appropriate. Acquisition of the test data can be done by an MRI technologist who has been trained by the MRI physicist in the QA/QC acquisition procedure. Testing is optimally done on a routine schedule, first thing in the morning, prior to clinical scanning. It is highly recommended the site follow the American College of Radiology (ACR) guidelines for this procedure. This requires an ACR phantom and MRI physicist or other properly trained individual. In absence of ACR accreditation, other weekly QA/QC procedures can be followed as recommended by the specific MR system manufacturer. Similar to acceptance testing, an MRI physicist, certified either through the Canadian College of Physicists in Medicine or one of the Canadian Professional Engineering societies, and having specific training and experience in MRI is required to analyze and maintain a record of the QA/QC data.

A quality control program with written procedures and logs should be maintained at the MRI facility. The ongoing quality control program assesses relative changes in system performance as determined by an MRI technologist and medical physicist (if present on-site). It is highly recommended that a qualified MRI physicist (see above for qualifications) be consulted at least once per year to assess QA/QC results and provide recommendations, as needed. The Canadian Association of Radiologists recommends that the following quality control tests shall be performed and documented, as follows:

- measurement of center frequency
- measurement of system signal-to-noise ratio on a standard head or body RF coil
- table positioning
- geometric accuracy
- high and low contrast resolution
- artifact analysis

The Canadian Association of Radiologists also recommends that the following quality control tests must be reviewed by the medical physicist annually and after any major upgrade or major change in equipment:

- review of daily quality control testing records
- measurement of image uniformity
- measurement of spatial linearity
- measurement of high contrast resolution
- measurement of slice thickness, locations and separations
- assessment of image quality and image artifacts
- eddy current compensation
- system shim

All quality control testing shall be carried out in accordance with specific procedures and methods. Preventive maintenance shall be scheduled, performed, and documented by a qualified service engineer on a regular basis. Service performed to correct system deficiencies must also be documented and service records must be maintained by the MRI facility (5).

MRI CONTRAST AGENT USE AND SAFETY

There are many potential indications for the use of MRI contrast agents in patients. In general, contrast agents are used for both intra- and extra-vascular compartments to achieve, the following: (1) detection of lesions, (2) characterization of lesions and to assess perfusion, and (3) evaluation of vascular lumen patency and/or to improve visualization of endothelial or intramural abnormalities. In general, it is desirable to acquire T1-weighted images [either spin echo (SE), turbo spin echo (TSE), or gradient echo (GRE)] using the same technique both before and after the administration of gadolinium-based contrast agents. Tissue specific contrast, combined contrast and delayed imaging techniques are strategies that could improve the yield of contrast-enhanced studies.

Gadolinium-based contrast agents should not be administered to patients with known or suspected hypersensitivity to the product or with severe hepatic or renal insufficiency (17). Nephrogenic systemic fibrosis (NSF) is a fibrosing disease, primarily involving the skin and subcutaneous tissues but also known to involve other internal organs. This is associated with gadolinium-based contrast agent use in patients with severe renal insufficiency. For further safety recommendation, please refer to the Canadian Association of Radiologists (CAR) National Advisory on Gadolinium Administration and Nephrogenic Systemic Fibrosis (17).

The same concerns regarding allergic reactions and nephrogenic systemic fibrosis (NSF) exist in children as they do in adults, and pediatric cases of NSF have been reported by Penfield, et al. (18). Importantly, it should be noted that serum creatinine as a marker of renal function may be unreliable in infants. There are hypothetical concerns regarding the safety of gadolinium-based contrast agents in neonates and infants less than one year of age, due to their immature renal function. Therefore, the risks and benefits of contrast enhancement must be weighed carefully in this population, and consideration should be given to nephrology consultation before making the decision to proceed with enhancement (17).

CLINICAL STANDARDS FOR MRI

The Canadian Association of Radiologists committee has attempted to enumerate the currently accepted techniques for MRI, based on clinical experience, as summarized in the peer-reviewed literature (5). Because the clinical application of MRI is still under development, it is not intended that the enumerated techniques (and indications in the reference document) be all-inclusive. It is very important that each site offering MRI has documented procedures for the indications and technical factors for each anatomic site. These procedures will need to be reviewed frequently. The final judgment regarding appropriateness of a given examination for a particular patient is the responsibility of the radiologist. The indications for scanning could include any part of the human body, depending on the MRI software and hardware available and the efficacy and availability of competing imaging methods. To accomplish its clinical purposes, MRI must be performed with adequate attention to technical abilities of the MR system.

Spatial resolution, slice thickness, signal-to-noise, and acquisition time are all inter-related sequence parameters that have a major influence on the quality of the images and, thus, the ability to detect disease or abnormalities. In the performance of any MRI examination, major decisions have to be made regarding the appropriate RF coil, the imaging plane(s), the field of view (FOV), the slice thickness and slice gap, the imaging matrix, the number of excitations, bandwidth selection, and the pulse sequence parameters which maximize signal as well as contrast-to-noise, and the requirement for cardiac gating and respiratory compensation.

The purpose of these guidelines is not to prescribe the details of individual techniques, but rather to address the spectrum of recognized MRI applications and to outline the minimum requirements necessary to undertake these, and to which the radiologist, in conjunction with ancillary staff, should aspire.

Gadolinium-based contrast agents and sedation shall be administered in accordance with institutional policy, and provincial and federal law by a physician who has been trained in cardiopulmonary resuscitation (CPR) and the potential for contrast agent-induced adverse events. As mentioned, MRI technologists, if adequately trained, could also perform intravenous gadolinium injections supervised by the responsible physician. An appropriately equipped emergency cart and designated trained staff must be immediately available to treat serious adverse reactions. MR conditional ventilators and appropriate patient monitoring should be available at those MRI facilities undertaking general anesthesia and sedation examinations.

Sedation is an issue of particular concern in pediatric imaging, where sedation is often required to achieve immobility during relatively prolonged imaging sessions. It is essential that the members of the team providing sedation are trained in pediatric cardiac life support and that drugs and support equipment necessary for resuscitation of children of all ages and sizes are readily available. Gadolinium-based contrast agents should be used judiciously in neonates and infants less than one year of age, due to theoretical concerns based on their immature renal function (5, 6).

Developing clinical standards, maintaining and reviewing them is important for striving for the best image quality, diagnosis, and management of the patient and for prevention of MRI safety issues. Imaging techniques may vary from site to site but similarities will be seen with the clinical indication and clinical applications. The radiologist ultimately determines the appropriateness of a given examination for a particular patient and what is safe and best for the management of the patient (19).

SUMMARY AND CONCLUSIONS

In the past thirty years, there has been a major growth in MRI technology. MRI has become a common diagnostic procedure and, in many cases, is considered to be the most appropriate and best test for specific clinical indications. In Canada, we have seen both radiologists and physicists specialize in the speciality of MRI. We have experienced the development of a new modality for MRI technologists through the Canadian Association of Medical Radiation Technologist and the Canadian Medical Association. The MRI technologist is primarily responsible for performing the MRI procedures and for maintaining the overall safety of patients, staff, and equipment within the MRI environment. There have been major changes and developments in safety standards and guidelines regarding the effects of the static, time-varying magnetic, and RF fields. MRI technology continues to evolve. Therefore, we will be presented with additional challenges within the realm of MRI safety. In Canada, we have benefited from the great contributions from researchers and clinicians in the United States and elsewhere around the World.

As MRI technology advances, so will what is implanted in patients referred for MRI examinations. Let's hope that when these devices are developed, some thought is given that most patients will need to have MRI examinations at some point in their lives. Importantly, there is evidence that this has occurred since specially designed, electronically-activated implants (including cardiac pacemakers and neuromodulation systems) now exist with approved labeling that permit MRI procedures to be conducted in patients with these devices.

The challenge lies ahead to develop consistent practices in order to prevent MRI-related incidents and to continuously attempt to decrease the "near-misses" and adverse events. Remember, the reason for this sophisticated and complicated technology with all its MRI safety concerns is to provide a high quality diagnostic examination for the optimal management of the patient.

DISCLAIMER

The content of this chapter reflects the opinions of the author and not of her places of employment. The information contained in this chapter is publicly available on the Health Canada, Government of Canada Justice Laws, Canadian Association of Radiologists, and Canadian Association of Medical Radiation Technologists websites. Importantly, this information is valid only at the time of publication and is subject to change. Therefore, reader is referred to the pertinent Health Canada, Government of Canada, Canadian Association of Radiologists and Canadian Association of Medical Radiation Technologists websites to obtain comprehensive and up-to-date information regarding

Health Canada policies, submissions of medical devices in Canada, and other information related to Canadian standards.

REFERENCES

1. Health Canada, Health Products and Food Branch. Issued 2006. Available at: http://www.hc-sc.gc.ca/ahc-asc/branch-dirgen/hpfb-dgpsa/3kit-fiche/factsheet_fiches-info_14-eng.php

2. Government of Canada Justice Laws Website. Updated 2011. Available at: http://laws-lois.justice.gc.ca/eng/regulations/SOR-98-282/page-5.html#docCont

3. Guidelines on Exposure to Electromagnetic Fields from Magnetic Resonance Clinical Systems - Safety Code 26, Health Canada 1987. Available at: http://www.hc-sc.gc.ca/ewh-semt/pubs/radiation/87ehd-dhm127/index-eng.php#a51

4. Limits of Human Exposure to Radiofrequency Electromagnetic Energy in the Frequency Range from 3 kHz to 300 GHz, Safety Code 6, Health Canada, Consumer and Clinical Radiation Protection Bureau, Environmental and Radiation Health Sciences Directorate, Healthy Environments and Consumer Safety Branch, 2009. Available at: http://www.radiationsafety.ca/wp-content/uploads/2012/06/Safety-Code-6.pdf

5. Canadian Association of Radiologists (CAR) Standard for Magnetic Resonance Imaging, 2011. Available at: http://www.car.ca/uploads/standards%20guidelines/20110428_en_standard_magnetic_resonance.pdf

6. Shellock FG. Reference Manual for Magnetic Resonance Safety, Implants, and Devices: 2013 Edition. Biomedical Research Publishing Group, Los Angeles, CA, 2013.

7. www.MRIsafety.com. Accessed, May 2013.

8. Kanal E, Barkovich AJ, Bell C, Borgstede JP, et al. ACR guidance document on MR safe practices: 2013. J Magn Reson Imaging 2013:37:501-30.

9. Acceptance Testing of Magnetic Resonance Imaging Systems. Report of American Association of Physicists in Medicine (AAPM) Nuclear Magnetic Resonance, Task Group No. 6. Medical Physics 1992:19:217-219.

10. International Accreditation (IAC) Standards and Guidelines for MRI Accreditation, Updated 2013. Available at: www.intersocietal.org/mri/standards/IACMRIStandards2013.pdf

11. Government of Canada, Health Canada. Canada's Health Care System (Medicare) - Health Canada. Available at: www.hc-sc.gc.ca/hcs-sss/medi-assur/index-eng.php

12. College of Physicians and Surgeons British Columbia Bylaws Health Professions Act RSBC 1996, c.183, 2009; Revised, 2013)

13. College of Physicians and Surgeons of Manitoba. Manitoba Diagnostic Imaging Standards. 2013. Available at: cpsm.mb.ca/cjj39alckF30a/wp-content/uploads/DI-Standards-April-2013.pdf

14. Greenfield D, Pawsey M, Braithwaite J. What motivates professional to engage in the accreditation of healthcare organizations? International Journal for Quality in Health Care 2011;23:8-14

15. Canadian Patient Institute, 2011. Canadian Disclosure Guidelines: Being Open with Patients and Families. Available at: http://www.patientsafetyinstitute.ca/english/toolsresources/disclosure/pages/default.aspx

16. Canadian Association of Medical Radiation Technologists, Magnetic Resonance Competency Profiles. Available at: http://www.camrt.ca/certification/canadian/competencyprofiles/

17. Canadian Association of Radiologists (CAR) National Advisory on Gadolinium Administration and Nephrogenic Systemic Fibrosis, 2008. Available at: http://www.car.ca/uploads/standards%20guidelines/advisory_nsf_en.pdf

18. Penfield JG. Nephrogenic systemic fibrosis and the use of gadolinium-based contrast agents. Pediatric Nephrology 2008;23:2121-2129.

19. Governance Steering Group. Effective Governance for Quality and Patient Safety: A toolkit for healthcare board members and senior leaders. Version 2. Edmonton, AB: Canadian Patient Safety Institute; 2011. p. 2. Available at: www.patientsafetyinstitute.ca/English/toolsResources/GovernancePatientSafety/Pages/MessagefromtheCo-Chairs.aspx

Chapter 31   MRI Safety Standards and Guidelines in Australia

GREGORY BROWN, A. DIP. RAD. TECH. (DIAG.), A. DIP. ADMIN. (HEALTH), FSMRT

Centre for Advanced Imaging
The University of Queensland
St. Lucia, Queensland
Australia
and
Department of Radiology
Royal Adelaide Hospital
Adelaide, South Australia
Australia

INTRODUCTION

The practice of safety with regard to the use of magnetic resonance imaging (MRI) technology must deliver a practical level of protection for patients and staff by avoiding harm, and balancing all risks against the benefits of the examination. While the technology and the potential hazards of the MRI environment are essentially common to the practice of MRI globally, there are jurisdictional and regional differences, which can impact local differences in practice. These stem from variations in regulatory structures, professional standards and education (i.e., for radiologists and radiographers), levels of participation in international professional and scientific communities, the implants and devices found in the respective market place, legal structures, and local public expectations regarding medical risk and redress. This chapter describes and reviews the relevant documented material underpinning the patterns of clinical MRI safety practices in Australia.

MRI IN AUSTRALIA

Australia is an island nation covering an area of land similar to that of continental United States (U.S.) but with a population of approximately 23 million people. The population is predominately urban and focused heavily on the east coast. There are also population clusters in the middle of the southern coast (2 million), at the southern and northern extent of the west coast (4 million), as well as a small population center on the northern coast and on a large island state (Tasmania), south of the east coast. Capital cities and regional centers are well serviced by MRI facilities that operate within a modern western healthcare system. The Organization for Economic Co-operation and Development (OECD) reported that, in 2011, Australia had 5.7 MR systems per million people (127 scanners) (1), but the Australian Government figures in 2012 shows 345 fully and partially funded scanners (15.7 per million people) (2). By comparison the OECD country average is 12.5 MR systems per million people, and the U.S. is equipped with 31 scanners per million. The apparent discrepancy is probably because the 2011 figure only included Medicare funded scanners. There was a significant change in governmental policy during 2012, expanding the number of Medicare funded scanners. There are also an uncertain number of additional MR systems providing clinical MRI services without being eligible for Medicare payments. Several universities and research institutes operate human MR systems operating at 1.5-Tesla to 4-Tesla, but the majority of MRI examinations are performed for clinical indications in hospitals or stand-alone radiology practices at 1.5-Tesla. The bulk of the installed scanners are less than 10 years old, operating with high performance gradient systems, comprehensive phased-array radiofrequency (RF) coils, and advanced applications software. About 20% of MR systems operate at 3-Tesla. There are a small number of lower field strength and vertical-field scanners, as well as a few intra-operative MR systems in major Australian hospitals. In 2013, several hospitals will install clinical MRI-Positron Emission Tomography (PET) systems, and two research centers will install 7-Tesla, whole-body MR systems.

MRI Funding

Australia operates a "fee for service" healthcare model supported by a universal health insurance system called Medicare. Medicare is the major source of all medical service funding, including that used for MRI examinations. Under the associated Commonwealth Medical Benefits Schedule (MBS) scheme, a fixed fee is paid for a defined range of MRI procedures, carried out by specifically licensed sites, for specified clinical indications. Virtually all of the 345 Medicare funded sites also perform variable numbers of MRI examinations for indications that are not eligible for Medicare payments. Some of those examinations are billed to the patient while others are performed at no charge depending on local contractual and commercial factors. Currently the MBS fees for MRI examinations are between $179 and $690 Australian dollars (3), with small additional rebates paid for the use of MR spectroscopy, contrast media, sedation, and general anesthesia support during MRI. Many MRI facilities charge the patient more than the MBS fee, and require so-called "gap" payments out of pocket, and at other sites the terms of their Medicare contracts prohibits gap billing. MRI scans for some motor vehicle and workers compensation funded claims fall outside of the Medicare MBS arrangements, but there are similar administrative and legal limitations on examination fees charged for these examinations and they generally approximate the MBS fees.

MRI Facility Ownership

Clinical MRI facillities are almost exclusively operated within radiology departments and practices. The Royal Australian and New Zealand College of Radiologists (RANZCR) has established simple accreditation of Radiologists performing MRI and a Quality Assurance Accreditation program. Each of these elements will be explored in detail later in this chapter. Independent cardiologist owned MR systems are rare in Australia, although many sites offer time for cardiology-directed examinations on systems owned by radiology practices. Thus, cardiologists may be the responsible healthcare group for site and patient safety at certain times.

MRI Staffing and Radiographer Training

In Australia, clinical MRI procedures and most human subject research scanning is performed by radiographers (known as MRI technologists in other parts of the world) who are nationally registered as Medical Radiation Practitioners. Bachelor level radiography courses are now mandatory and the curriculum is approved by a peak professional body, the Australian Institute of Radiography (AIR). The courses for the degree include topics such as basic MRI principles, MRI safety, and clinical applications. However, graduates are not expected to be independently competent in MRI until they complete further clinical training and supervised imaging. Therefore, to gain MRI competency, radiographers undertake site-based "on the job" training or pursue post-graduate education. Unlike graduate level radiography courses, site and post-graduate training curricula are not standardized. Adequate skills and competency can be decided administratively by the MRI practice, or through a two level professional accreditation program administered by the AIR. AIR Level 1 MRI accreditation is gained by passing an exam, and evidenced completion of 300 MRI examinations in a twelve-month period. AIR Level 2 MRI accreditation, intended for MRI supervisors, is granted on presentation of a portfolio of professional development activities. Details of the program are available at the AIR website (4).

The MRI safety module of the Level 1 accreditation curriculum requires knowledge of MRI bioeffects, and the potential hazards associated with the static, time-varying, and RF electromagnetic fields. MRI safety questions, in combination with general patient care topics, accounts for 15% of the examination marks (5). This is not to say that knowledge of MRI safety topics are examined in depth by the Level 1 accreditation process. Issues of motion through static magnetic fields, the spatial gradient of the static field and interactions between devices and the scanner are not included. The MRI Study Guide (available to AIR members only) contains a number of unfortunate and significant errors in its MRI safety section that can confuse candidates. AIR Level 2 MRI accreditation is gained through a log of MRI-related educational, and experiential activities.

Despite the lack of a clear curriculum from the traditional professional body, Australian MRI radiographers tend to take the lead role in understanding MRI technology, pulse sequences, and imaging principles as well as the comprehensive issues of MRI safety. There is a very high level of membership of the International Society for Magnetic Resonance in Medicine's (ISMRM), Section for Magnetic Resonance Technologists (SMRT) amongst Australian MRI radiographers.

The International and Australia & New Zealand (ANZ) chapter of the SMRT provides a continuing stream of quality MRI safety education through annual national and international meetings, and via on-line educational materials. Very few Australian clinical MRI facilities employ Medical Physicists due, in part, to a chronic shortage of suitably trained professionals. A recent Australian government report suggests this situation will worsen progressively over the predicatable future unless new programs of training reforms, and recruitment through immigration are initiated (6).

MRI SAFETY PRACTICES IN AUSTRALIA

Australia has few absolute requirements regarding MRI safety practices. The legal and clinical responsibilities to keep public, staff, patients and other individuals free from harm are supported by equipment and device standards, professional and regulatory body guidelines, and publications from government departments and authorities. This section will explain and review the key documents applicable in MRI safety.

Australian Standards for MRI Equipment and Patient Exposure

The Australia/Standards New Zealand (AS/NZS) document, AS/NZS 3200.2.3.2005 (Medical electrical equipment: Particular requirements for safety - Magnetic resonance equipment for medical diagnosis) (7) is essentially equivalent to the International Electrotechnical Commission (IEC) document IEC60601-2-33:2002. Because of this, Australian MR systems are programmed to observe the European limits for the static magnetic field strength, radio frequency (RF), specific absorption rate (SAR), and time-varying, magnetic field limits (TVMF) related to patient exposures.

Key MRI Safety Points From AS/NZS 3200.2.33:2005

The IEC model of three-tiered operating modes is used in Australia. In the *Normal Operating Mode*, none of the scanner outputs may cause physiological stress to patients. In the *First Level Controlled Mode*, one or more of the scanner outputs are at values that may cause physiological stress to patients. Before employing the *First Level Controlled Operating Mode*, a medical decision must be made to confirm that the patient can handle the increased exposures. Medical supervision is required to control any physiological stress caused by the MR system. The standards require scanners operate in a way that needs a deliberate action by the MR system operator before enabling the *First Level Controlled Mode*. A *Second Level Controlled Operating Mode* also exists, where one or more of the scanner outputs reach levels that may cause significant risk for patients. Operation in this mode requires explicit local ethical approvals, and most clinical MR systems cannot be easily switched to *Second Level Controlled Operating Mode*. The standards specify thresholds for the static magnetic field strength, RF power deposition, and time varying magnetic fields at each operating mode (**Table 1**).

MR System manufacturers bear the primary onus of implementing many requirements of the IEC and AS/NZS standards in these regards (8). The AS/NZS 3200.2.33:2005 has not been revised since 2005 and is now out of step with the parent standard (third edition, 2013). Most notably, the Australian standards classify all MRI above 2-Tesla as the *First Level Controlled Operating Mode* (i.e., requiring a medical decision and supervision). The current European standard IEC60601-2-33:2013 3.1 (9) sets 3-Tesla as the upper limit of the *Normal Operating Mode*.

Table 1. Key Australian exposure limits for MRI.

Parameter	Normal Operating Mode	First Level Controlled Operating Mode	Second Level Controlled Operating Mode
RF Power	Averaged over 6-min.	Averaged over 6-min.	Averaged over 6-min.
Whole Body SAR	2-W/kg	4-W/kg	Above 4-W/kg
Head SAR	3.2-W/kg	3.2-W/kg	> 3.2-W/kg
Local SAR Head	10-W/kg	10-W/kg	>10-W/kg
Local SAR Trunk	10-W/kg	10-W/kg	>10-W/kg
Local SAR Extremities	20-W/kg	20-W/kg	>20-W/kg
Static Magnetic Field Strength	≤ 2-Tesla	>2-Tesla, ≤ 4-Tesla	>4-Tesla

(SAR, specific absorption rate; W/kg, Watts per kilogram)

The AS/NZS and IEC standards can be purchased on-line or accessed through some academic libraries. The MRI Safety Guidelines of The Royal Australian and New Zealand College of Radiologists, discussed later in this chapter, include description of the operating modes, and the threshold values defined by AS/NZS 3200.2.33:2005. Despite the technically dry language, AS/NZS 3200.2.33:2005 contains substantial appendices and discussions addressing the rationale of the selected patient exposure limits. It also provides insights into occupational exposure issues, specific requirements for the documentation provided with scanners, patient screening, acoustic noise levels, and several test methodologies. The AS/NZS 3200.2.33:2005, or the IEC counterpart, are important reading material for advanced MRI practitioners.

Therapeutic Goods Administration

Compliance with an Australian standard is not compulsory unless enforced by law or regulation. Compliance with AS/NZS 3200.2.33:2005 is required indirectly by the regulations and processes of the Therapeutic Goods Administration (TGA). The TGA is empowered by Federal law (The Therapeutic Goods Administration Act 1989) to control the import, export, manufacture, and supply of all therapeutic goods in Australia including medical devices, medicines and biological products.

All MR systems, must obtain registration on the TGA's Australian Registry of Therapeutic Goods (ARTG) before they can be imported, or sold in Australia. Certified conformance with the IEC60601-2-33:2013 or AS/NZS 3200.2.33.2005 can be accepted as sufficient evidence to place an MRI scanner on the ARTG.

The ARTG system also approves all implanted medical devices used in Australia. The registration process assesses information provided by a device sponsor against a set of defined "essential principles". The essential principles require that use of the sponsored device does not compromise health and safety, that it has been designed and constructed to comply with safety principles, that the device remains safe throughout its useful life, and that the benefits of the device outweigh any undesirable effects. There are also additional essential principles regarding design and construction that include specific information to be supplied by the manufacturer. These requirements define the content of Australian Information for Use (IFU) documents for implants and medical devices, requiring them to include "Any warnings, restrictions on use, or precautions that should be taken, in relation to the device." The TGA regulations are similar to those of the European Union (EU), and the TGA will accept conformity assessments issued by specific EU Notified Bodies or other evidence of compliance with Australian or international standards, as evidence of compliance with many of the essential principles (11). The ARTG requirements to provide warnings, restrictions on use, and precautions, includes exposure to MR systems, but the TGA does not prescribe a format for information regarding MRI and device interactions in the way that the U.S. Food and Drug Administration (FDA) has done since 2005. As a result, the nature and quality of information concerning interactions between devices and MR systems is variable but, increasingly, device Instructions for Use include FDA-style statements of MRI conditions for safe scanning, and the use of American Society for Testing and Materials (ASTM) International symbols for MR Safe, MR Conditional and MR Unsafe. The Royal Australian and New Zealand College of Radiologists made a submission to a recent TGA enquiry on operational transparency, asking that it require MRI information in the Instructions for Use in line with international best practice, and making several other suggestions that would aid daily decision- making regarding MRI safety matters (12).

Professional Standards

The Royal Australian and New Zealand College of Radiologists (RANZCR) Standards of Practice for Diagnostic and Interventional Practice (Version 9.2) details the professional standards expected by the RANZCR Medical Imaging Accreditation Program. The current version was published in 2012 and is freely available on-line (13). Members of the RANZCR are expected to respect the Standards of Practice, and non-observance can lead to professional consequences. In addition, Medicare funding is conditional, in part, on observance of these professional standards through the RANZCR Quality Assurance Program. For these reasons, the Standards of Practice arguably define the Australian minimum acceptable position on MRI safety.

Section 12 of the document includes several specific standards and indicators regarding MRI safety (14), which state that the general public is excluded from areas where the field is 0.5-mTesla or higher. The designated liaison MRI radiologist is responsible for establishing and enforcing MRI safety practice. Patient screening must be performed in accordance with the RANZCR MRI Safety Guidelines and the 1991 Australian guidelines for safety in MRI facilities (15), and must consider potentially dangerous interactions with the static magnetic field of the scanner by objects in proximity, and objects within patients and personnel. An MRI-accredited radiologist must be available for consultation on safety questions within 10-minutes of patient screening, directly or by telephone. The MRI facility must maintain records of any unauthorized entry of objects into the MR system room and handle this as an adverse event within a quality improvement program. Appropriate [described as "MR compatible", a term abandoned in 2005 (16)] patient monitoring systems are to be available for use in the MRI examination room in conjunction with sedation, and MRI "appropriate" anesthesia equipment must be located in the room when anesthesia support is provided. All staff with access to the MR system room must have undergone MRI safety training. Safety policies must be reviewed annually.

Beyond these points, the RANZCR Standards of Practice refer to the RANZCR Guidelines on MRI safety for most matters. The standards of practice display a superficial and dated approach to MRI safety issues. There is no serious consideration of interactions beyond that of the static magnetic field, and the standards of practice make no reference to the primary Australian standard (AS/NZS 3200.2.33:2005) regarding safety for MRI equipment and patient exposure limits. The RANZCR Standards of Practice are next due for revision in 2015.

RANZCR MRI Safety Guidelines, 2007

The RANZCR MRI Safety Guidelines support the RANZCR Standards of Practice by offering a broad range of guidance material regarding MRI safety (17). Beyond the obligations created by the Standards of Practice that were detailed above there are no enforced consequences for non-adherence with the guidelines. It is an advisory document only.

The RANZCR guideline has many similarities with the American College of Radiology (ACR) White Papers and Guidance documents on MRI safe practice (18-20). It is divided into formal sections that address practical issues faced in MRI safety, such as site design and access, pre-MRI screening, MRI staff training, implants and foreign bodies, and basic patient management issues specific to the MRI environment. Readers should note that Section I, dealing with contrast media was superseded by a 2009 guideline on gadolinium-based contrast agents (21). Each section consists of notes, discussion and some guidance of a basic kind, but because some topics are dealt with over several different sections, the document is difficult to follow as a rapid reference source. The opportunity for this document to present a coherent approach to MRI safety practices, or describe a clear paradigm for safety decision-making, is lost within a patchwork of varying text styles, unreferenced statements, and confusing typographical errors. Readers may need to understand international best practices in MRI safety, such as the 2013 version of the ACR guidance document, before being ready to critically consider the contents of the Australian counterpart. The most important sections of the document are reviewed below.

Section A: MR Equipment – General

This section describes the central components of the IEC standard, IEC 60601-2-33:2002, and given the price of a copy of that document or the Australian Standards equivalent, the RANZCR guidelines are the most accessible description of the exposure limits applied in Australia. The three operating mode model (*Normal, First Level Controlled*, and *Second Level Controlled*), SAR, static magnetic field and time varying magnetic field limits for MRI examinations are addressed in the opening section and again in Appendix 1. Curiously, the document makes no mention of the equivalent Australian and New Zealand Standard AS/NZS 3200.2.33:2005, or any of the revisions to the IEC document since 2002.

Section C: Site Design

The guideline adopts the four zone model described by the ACR guidelines (18-20) for controlling access to the MRI environment, in contrast to the two zone model described in the Australia document. It also recommends that MRI facilities provide for the safe storage of cryogens and create a safe resuscitation or patient management area outside the MR system room.

Section E: Screening of Patients and Others

The RANZCR Guideline differs in several ways from the ACR approach and is generally less stringent, apart from screening the patient at four time instances up to the performance of the MRI examination (17). The referring physician is asked to confirm, on the request, that the patient has no major contraindication to MRI. The MRI practice is advised to carry out three additional screening steps using a locally designed screening form, and to record information including the patient's weight, possible pregnancy, breastfeeding, seizures, medications, allergies, asthma, diabetes, and a checklist of items of potential concern (e.g., implants and devices). At least two of the screenings should be performed on site by MRI personnel specifically trained in access control measures, and there must be a review of the safety checklist with the patient by a senior MRI staff member (radiographer or radiologist) trained in screening, MRI principles, safety, and the applicable exposure limits. These screening steps should take place at the time of scheduling, on arrival at the MRI facility, and immediately before accessing the MR system (17). The RANZCR Standards of Practice additionally require the opportunity for the patient to discuss any points of concern, at least by telephone, with an MRI-accredited Radiologist.

The guidelines suggest that, in high risk situations where the medical history and screening information may be incomplete or inaccurate, speaking with family members, performing a physical examination, reviewing skull and chest radiographs, or obtaining other appropriate radiographs or computed tomography (CT) are appropriate to detect or exclude implants (17).

Other individuals entering the MR system room (i.e., the area described in the ACR documents as Zone IV) must be fully screened at least once. People entering the area immediately outside the MR system room (i.e., Zone III) must be screened for cardiac pacemakers at a minimum, and then supervised by a Senior MRI staff member. Alternately, these individuals must be trained in the rules of the controlled areas and local emergency procedures to obviate the need for constant expert supervision, but they must still be prevented from entering the MR system room until they have been fully screened (17).

Section F: Management of Implants and Foreign Bodies

This section should present clear guidance on day-to-day MRI safety decision-making, but the RANCR guidelines contain an incomplete discussion without effective advice. For example, section F.1 only focuses on documenting the *presence* of implants and foreign bodies. It suggests, but does not require, reference to implant documentation to identify devices. Furthermore, the RANZCR guidelines suggest that where documentation cannot be obtained, then old, or limited imaging should be used to detect implants and foreign bodies even though the text acknowledges that such imaging will not positively identify an implant.

The RANZCR guidelines do not effectively advocate positive identification of implants. They do not adequately describe the use of available information from MRI safety reference sources or product information when determining the MR Safe or MR Conditional status of an implant. They do not discuss active decision-making. By contrast, the ACR document has plainly stated that implants must be positively identified, and the potential device-MRI interactions should be determined from "best effort assessments" of pre-implant records, product information, and peer-reviewed literature on MRI safety testing (18-20).

When we consider how much the RANZCR guidelines emulate the format and content of the ACR documents in most other regards, this departure is very difficult to understand. Section F.2 of the RANZCR 2007 document purports to address documentation of a device's "compatibility status", however, it only contains a simple recount of the ASTM International definitions for MR Safe, MR Conditional and MR Unsafe, and an outline of standard sources of device-specific, MRI safety information.

Besides not advocating diligent assessment of the suitability of implants for patients undergoing MRI examinations, the RANZCR guidelines also fail to offer advice on how to make the decision to scan or exclude particular patients or how to modify an examination to keep scanner outputs within known safe limits for scanning. This omission is another significant problem undermining the utility of the guidelines as a reference for reasonable professional practice. The need for safety-based decisions can be implied from the RANZCR Standards of Practice requirements for a radiology practice, "to conduct all examinations in a manner ensuring safety of patients and personnel" (14). The RANZCR MRI Safety Guidelines could, therefore, express the responsibility of the MRI radiologist or the designated "MRI liaison radiologist" to make, or approve, safety decisions. If the RANZCR document accepts that, after careful screening, a safety decision must be made, it would also be valuable to include guidance about how reasonable decisions might be made, and by whom. Delegation of decision-making, within limits of training, expertise, and a written practice policy document is allowed in the ACR guidance document and is the proposed model by European medical physicists, but the RANZCR MRI Safety Guidelines are relatively silent on the matter. The RANZCR Standards of Practice does provide for delegation of appropriate duties to MRI radiographers (14). This delegation could be adapted to expressly include implementation of standardized decisions regarding safe scanning of patients with specific implants and foreign bodies according to an in-house set of policies approved by the MRI Director (i.e., the Liaison MRI Radiologist), thus, reducing inconsistent or on the spot decision-making, and removing repetitious research of implant scanning information that presently occupies a lot of time at many MRI sites.

Section J: Noise Protection

The AS/NZS 3200.2.33 2005, and equivalent IEC standards, require that MR systems shall not produce an un-weighted peak sound pressure limit above 140-dB in any accessible area. These documents further specify that hearing protection is to be used to limit the sound levels for the patient to 99-dB(A). This level is still extreme when considered in light of the Australian standards on occupational noise exposure set to avoid hearing damage (14), as on simple analysis, the occupational limit [85-dB(A) averaged over 8 hours] would be exceeded by only 15-minutes of exposure at 99-dB(A). The RANZCR MRI Safety Guidelines advocates the provision of hearing protection for all MRI examinations above 1.5-Tesla and illustrates that in the most extreme setting [140-dB(A)], a combination of earplugs and earmuffs may be necessary to achieve the required 40 to 50-dB reduction in acoustic noise levels.

The RANZCR guidelines do stress that MRI staff members must be trained in the correct placement and use of hearing protection devices and that noise exposure to pregnant patients should be minimized to protect the fetus. The RANZCR advises that hearing protection be *considered* in the light of acoustic noise levels below 0.5-Tesla, and *encouraged* when scanning at, or above 1.5-Tesla, but the nexus between acoustic noise levels and static magnetic field strength may not be reliable. Hearing protection for patients and others in the MR system room must be used in all situations where there is potential for injury. These may occur at any static magnetic field strength, depending mainly on the pulse sequences used and the specific area containing the MR system.

Section K: Thermal Risks and Injury

Section K presents the commonly accepted advice regarding surface coil and other cable routing, avoidance of conductive loops, and providing insulating padding between the skin surfaces and padding between the patient and the bore of the MR system. Direct quotation from the IEC and Australian documents emphasize how SAR limits assume a specific environment within the scanner (temperature, <24°C and relative humidity, <60%), and explain that MR systems may not automatically compensate for room conditions above those limits. There is also an important discussion of the groups of patient who may be at risk of thermal stress and for whom it may not be appropriate to use the *First Level Controlled Operating Mode* with regard to RF power. Both these points are significant considerations for clinical MRI safety, which are not often brought into daily discussion.

The current RANZCR guidelines were published in 2007 and are freely available on line (13). This document is due for revision (Ferris NJ, Personal Communication, 2013), but there is no information regarding when the revision may be commenced. Despite several shortcomings, the RANZCR MRI safety guidelines should be required reading for all Australian MRI radiologists and radiographers, and their contents actively considered and debated by Australian MRI professionals.

RANZCR 2010 MR Conditional Pacemaker Update

Appendix 2b of the 2007 RANZCR guidelines presents out dated material regarding scanning patients with cardiac pacemakers. The general contraindication on scanning pacemakers is stated, along with "emerging" approaches drawn from a 2001 course held at the scientific meeting of the Radiological Society of North America (RSNA). The appendix describes the option of carefully controlled and restricted scanning of patients with conventional (i.e., non-MR conditional) cardiac pacemakers with appropriate support and consent.

In 2010, the RANZCR MRI Reference Group issued an MRI safety update addressing the arrival of one brand of MR conditional pacemaker in the Australian market (22). It directs readers to the appropriate website for the details of its conditional use and information relevant to the use of MRI. Since 2010, two more companies market MR conditional pacemakers in the Australian market. Each device has different conditions that must be followed to ensure safe scanning, but the information regarding these newer MR conditional pacemakers has not prompted further advice or safety updates from the RANZCR.

AUSTRALIAN GOVERNMENT SCIENTIFIC AUTHORITIES

Patient, Public, and Occupational Exposure Limits

Exposure limits for static magnetic, time-varying magnetic fields, and RF heating have been defined in Australian standards for the patient undergoing an MRI procedure, where the patient receives some benefit from undergoing the examination. Exposure limits for the general public or occupational exposures are often set lower than a patient limit to reflect the lack of benefit from that exposure.

In the early period of MRI use in Australia, prior to adoption of the IEC standards, the main Australian scientific body, the National Health and Medical Research Council (NHMRC) commissioned production of the "Safety guidelines for magnetic resonance diagnostic facilities (1991)". Such publications were in line with its objective to "advise the Australian community on the achievement and maintenance of the highest practicable standards of individual and public health" (15). The NHMRC guidelines were published in a radiation health series, and placed the responsibility for MRI safety in the hands of the Australian Radiation Protection and Nuclear Safety Agency (ARPANSA). ARPANSA is the body responsible for monitoring ionizing radiation from medical exposure, solar radiation exposure, environmental non-ionizing radiation (such as microwaves and low frequency electromagnetic fields), the uranium mining industry, and Australian nuclear reactors. This delegation mirrors similar decisions in the United Kingdom and Europe.

The 1991 document drew its material largely from original publications and international scientific bodies of the period. It recognized a paucity of information regarding repeated exposure to the electromagnetic fields used by MR systems, and established some conservative recommendations. After a period of public comment, it was published and then seemed to be largely ignored or to go unnoticed by clinical MRI users.

Section 6 contained most of the recommended limits and actions to support patient safety during MRI, including the need to establish that the responsible physician expected the potential clinical advantage would outweigh any perceived risk, or that volunteer subjects underwent informed consent. MRI facilities were to ensure MR system operators were appropriately trained in the principles of MRI, indications and contraindications for use, and safety precautions. Furthermore, it was recommended that sites conduct a survey of magnetic and RF fields prior to imaging patients. Exposure to the static field was limited to 2-Tesla for the head and trunk, and 5-Tesla for limbs. Occupational exposure to static magnetic fields was limited to a daily time weighted average of 200-mTesla (2000-gauss) and the public was to be excluded from stray fields above 10-mTesla (100-gauss). Individuals with cardiac pacemakers were to be restricted from areas at or below 0.5-mTesla (5-gauss), while all other individuals with implants were to excluded from fields greater than 1-mTesla (10-gauss), and those with ferromagnetic implants were excluded above 50-mTesla (500-gauss).

The confusion over static magnetic field limits was not present in the time-varying magnetic fields (TVMF) limit which was set at 20-Tesla/second. Specific absorption rate (SAR) limitations (i.e., for RF power deposition) were initially set higher than the subsequent IEC standards, at 4-W/kg head, 8-W/kg for the trunk. Limits were reduced 50% for infants or patients with cardiovascular conditions. The "general considerations" section supported strict access control for people and objects, warning signs, and the need for local testing of any equipment to be used in the MR system room. The rationale for these recommendations is explained in an appendix, and there is a bibliography of the relevant literature of the time. The limits established by the NHMRC guideline in 1991, were superseded in 1996 by Australia's creation of the AS/NZS 32000.2.33.23 standard and, in principle, ARPANSA was released from direct responsibility for setting MRI exposure limits.

ARPANSA has returned obliquely to matters that impact MRI exposures with its work to establish an Australian radiation protection standard establishing maximum exposure levels for electric and magnetic fields 0-Hz (static) to 3-Hz. This work was initially intended to address public concerns regarding the safety of proximity to electrical power lines and was to replace a 1989 statement on 50/60-Hz field exposures (23). The working group responsible for drafting the radiation protection standard was dominated by representatives of the power generation and distribution industry. A draft was released for public comment in late 2006 (24). The document was focused on power line field exposure, but also set out to establish mandatory restrictions for general public and occupational exposure over the full range of activities that produce extremely low frequency (ELF) fields. In another chapter in this textbook which pertains to MRI safety in Europe, Dr. Stephen Keevil illustrates how efforts to address safety concerns public concerns over exposure to extremely low frequency (ELF) time-varying electrical and magnetic fields (EMF) from sources such as power transmission lines, and specific industrial exposures, can impact the practice of MRI. Scientific consideration of an extensive literature review in the draft focused on certain information on peripheral nerve stimulation (PNS) that may develop in association with MRI, but by suggesting a public exposure levels 5 times lower than the PNS threshold, it contained a very conservative occupational restriction level.

The 2006 consultation document did not recognize any potential impact on the practice of MRI (even though it included an occupational limit of 2-Tesla at a time when 3-Tesla MR systems were being installed) and the committee responsible for the proposed exposure limits failed to make any connection with the European Union (EU) debate raging at that time (and which still continues in 2013). MRI professional organizations including the ISMRM, SMRT and RANZCR (25) were mobilized and approximately one third of all submissions made to the ARPANSA working group came from MRI professionals and MRI equipment suppliers concerned that the proposed exposure limits would interfere with important diagnostic technology and practice. By February 2008, ARPANSA was taking note of the concerns regarding MRI (26) and apparently considered increasing the static magnetic field limits and adopting an the International Commission on Non-Ionizing Radiation Protection (ICNIRP) approach of exempting certain professional activities (27). The release of a final radiation protection standard was expected by the middle of 2010.

ARPANSA has since stepped away from producing a radiation protection standard in the ELF range. This organization undertook an internal review of public comments and moved to release the so-called, "Guidelines on managing exposure to electric and magnetic fields 0- to 3-kHz" in 2013. These guidelines will not carry the level of compulsion associated with a radiation protection standard. ARPANSA expects its guidelines will be closely aligned with the ICNIRP 2010 guidelines in the 1- to 100-kHz range (28) and the ICNIRP 2009 guidelines on limits of exposure to static magnetic fields. (ARPANSA Secretariat, Personal Correspondence, 2013). The later restricts static magnetic field exposures to 2-Tesla except in "work applications where exposure above 2-Tesla is deemed necessary" and "appropriate work practices are implemented to control movement-induced effects" (29). In this regard, ICNIRP 2009 is at odds with the 2013 IEC standard on magnetic resonance equipment (ISE60601-2-33:2013 3.1) and it is likely that ICNIRP will review its guidelines during 2013, although it is less clear if ARPANSA will wait for or incorporate any ICNIRP revisions. ARPANSA has also announced an intention to produce a safety guide on MRI, once the final ELF document has been released (30).

Reporting MRI Safety Incidents

MRI safety incidents can be recorded on at least two Australian databases but currently, their utility is limited because there is no facility for public interrogation of the records.

Incident Reporting and Investigation Scheme (IRIS)

The TGA operates the medical devices Incident Reporting and Investigation Scheme (IRIS). Reports of adverse events associated with MRI can be made on-line. The reports receive a thorough risk assessment procedure and are reviewed by a panel of scientific, engineering, and clinical experts who may recommend further investigation. The event reports and findings recorded in the IRIS database can be used by the TGA to initiate a range of responses such as recalls, user education, or compliance testing. The system is well described on its website (31). The IRIS does not facilitate public or researcher access to reports. However, IRIS is the primary place to report MRI-related safety incidents because it is managed by the government agency responsible for medical device registration and safety.

Database of Adverse Events Notifications (DAEN)

The TGA manages the Database of Adverse Events Notifications (DAEN) to collate adverse events surrounding the use of medications, drawn from reports to the Australian Adverse Drug Reaction Reporting Scheme (ADRRS) (32). Adverse events related to MRI contrast agents or medications given during MRI should be reported using this system. The DAEN system is relatively transparent, and provides for public searches by product name. Two hundred eighty five DAEN notifications have been made for gadolinium-based contrast agents since 1986.

Radiology Event Registry (RaER)

The RANZCR in conjunction with the Australian Patient Safety Foundation and funding from the Australian federal government, operate the Radiology Event Registry (RaER) where radiologists, radiographers, and those involved in medical imaging are invited to report incidents (www.raer.org). The scheme has been operating since 2006 and is considered by the RANZCR as part of their quality assurance efforts. Reports can be made anonymously. Trainee radiologists are instructed in the use of the system, and required to demonstrate experience with it as a component of their training. Most of the 760 reports lodged during six years of operation have been made by radiologists in the public sector. The uptake in the private sector and by other professionals appears minimal. Reports entered into RaER are analyzed by a team of radiologists focused on quality improvement but that activity is not transparent. The only comprehensive report made by the RaER was presented in 2009. That report did not show any reports of MRI safety incidents, despite the RANZCR requirements for MRI sites to maintain records of all MRI-related safety policy breaches. The RaER continues to operate and it should be the appropriate secondary site to use in case of an actual or near miss MRI safety incident.

Electromagnetic Radiation Health (EMR) Health Complaint Register

ARPANSA provides an on line mechanism for making submissions to its Electromagnetic Radiation Health (EMR) Complaint Register (33). The register was opened in 2003 to provide a vehicle for Australians to register any health issues they believe they may have suffered from exposure to electromagnetic radiation (EMR) from 0 to 300-GHz. The register was initiated by an Australian Senate enquiry into EMR exposure held in late 2000. This enquiry considered that collection of data from the public may provide insight on the issue and indicate future research needs. The register is poorly subscribed with only 49 complaints lodged in nine years. Only one complaint mentions MRI exposure.

Patients or staff members who believe they may have suffered a health issue from exposure to EMR associated with MRI can lodge complaints with the EMR Health Complaint Register.

AUSTRALIAN MRI SAFETY ACTIVITIES AND EDUCATION

Research Regarding Australian MRI Safety Practice

There have only been two published attempts to research the practice of MRI safety in Australia. Ferris, et al. (34) published a survey of Australian MRI safety practices following the release of first RANZCR MRI Safety Guidelines in 2004. A series of questions was sent to supervising MRI radiologists at all known MRI facilities in Australia that sought to examine general and difficult aspects of MRI safe practices in the field through anonymous or attributed responses. Ninety-two of 115 sites (80%) responded after diligent follow up. The study reported selected results including the observation that the new RANZCR and ACR guidelines were considered equally influential (38% each) and ten sites reported using external consultation to review their MRI safety procedures (34).

Seven sites reported inadvertent scanning of eight cardiac pacemaker patients. One of these events resulted in a death in 2000. Eight MRI facilities were willing to accept requests to scan patients with non-MR conditional pacemakers but did not specify their precautions. Four sites had intentionally imaged cardiac pacemaker patients with undisclosed precautions. There was a general refusal to scan patients with retained pacemaker leads (77 sites) and twenty MRI facilities refused to scan patients with any type of intracranial aneurysm clip. Of the seventy-one MRI facilities that would scan patients with intracranial aneurysm clips, virtually all (70/71) relied on documented evidence of the clip's identity. Additionally, ten sites insisted that the aneurysm clip was in its original packaging before insertion, and four MRI facilities reported that they did their own testing on clips prior to implantation. With regard to patients with metallic implants, the manufacturer's product information and third-party sources were used equally to justify the decision to perform and MRI examination (34).

The variations in MRI safety practices prompted discussions between the radiology and neurosurgical professional bodies, as well as with the TGA, but there were no concrete results from these interactions. The study method did not probe the site's understanding, or use of, post-2005 FDA-style statements of conditions for safe MRI examinations in patients with implants. Eighty-six percent of the sites reported procedural delays while MRI safety issues were resolved and these situations occurred frequently and on a constant basis. The investigators concluded that dealing with MRI safety questions continues to be difficult and increased vigilance including requiring the referring physician to supply critical MRI safety information at the time of the examination request is required to prevent the inadvertent scanning of cardiac pacemaker patients (34). Ferris, et al. (34) also indicated there may be a role for an MRI safety advisor providing an external audit of site policies and procedures.

In 2007, Burwell and Davidson (35) offered another insight into MRI safety policy and procedures in Australia. Their qualitative questionnaire that was sent to all known Australian MRI sites investigated who established site safety policies, who was considered the local final authority, requested details pertaining to pre-scan screening, and determined how often policies were reviewed. This study also asked about safety breaches, although many participants chose not to respond to that section, perhaps reflecting a culture of non-disclosure (35). A total of 110 surveys were sent out and 46 were returned. Considering the growth of MRI in Australia and the similarity in the number of sites identified by these two studies, it is quite likely that data for the Burwell and Davidson (35) report was collected in 2005, about the time of the survey by Ferris, et al. (34).

The Burwell and Davidson (35) survey observed that experienced MRI radiographers and radiologists created site safety policies independently or collaboratively. In contrast to the Ferris, et al. (34) investigation, this survey indicated that the ACR white paper on MRI safety and the various works by Dr. Frank G. Shellock were most commonly referred to when creating a site policy. Screening, which the RANZCR documents required at four points before examination, were typically performed only twice or three times, and only 62% of the sites reported using written processes to follow up questions raised by the patient screening questionnaire.

In general, safety policies were reviewed "as required", rather than on a regular schedule and 80% of the respondents claimed to maintain the required log of safety violations and near misses, but few were prepared to respond to a question that asked if there had been an incident during which a patient was harmed. The undisclosed number who did respond reported that ten contrast reactions occurred, eight MRI-related burns, two problems related to "incompatible" implants, and one projectile injury. This report concluded, without clear justification, that a large number of sites did not meet the simple RANZCR safety standards of the time (35).

MRI Safety Education for Radiologists

Given that the primary responsibility for creating MRI safety policies and procedures, along with individual clinical decision-making rests with the credentialed MRI radiologists (14), it is useful to examine the evidence on their training in this area. Australian radiologists who completed their training after January 2005 were automatically certified as MRI radiologists for as long as they maintained MRI-specific continuing professional development (CPD) credits. Importantly, they carry the primary responsibility for MRI safety at their respective facilities. According to the radio-diagnosis curriculum for Australian Radiologists (36), MRI safety is addressed in the Applied Imaging Technology (AIT) syllabus. Hazards and bioeffects of the electromagnetic field-related contraindications for MRI, and Environmental issues are listed as category 1 ("must know") topics. Yet the evidence is that the understanding of MRI safety is not closely tested. An MRI safety question has only appeared in two of the sixteen AIT exam papers since 2004, and there has never been a clinical level question regarding MRI-related interactions with implants, missile effects, MRI-related burns, or MRI exposure limits. Similarly, the programs of RANZCR Annual Scientific meetings from 2007 to 2012 have only included two speakers on MRI safety issues, one international expert providing a 25-minute overview of implant and MRI interactions in 2009 and a local expert providing a review of nephrogenic systemic fibrosis (NSF) literature in 2007. These points combined make it difficult to determine where Australian radiologists are gaining their MRI safety knowledge.

SUMMARY AND CONCLUSIONS

Australia has an MRI safety system, standards, and regulatory approach that are aligned more closely with European models than those of the United States. However, the Australian professional guidelines are based more closely on the clearly expressed professional standards from the American College of Radiology, despite the significant omissions previously discussed. Anecdotally, Australian MRI sites are trying to make use of the codified statements of conditions for safe scanning of implanted devices that have been generated in response to the 2005 U.S. Food and Drug Administrations (FDA) requirements. The limited research on the practice of MRI safety in Australia confirms that the ACR guidance documents on MRI safe practices, and the resources provided on-line, and in print by U.S.-based authoritative authors, appear to be more influential on MRI practitioners than the local professional guidelines.

Despite the lack of a workable professional guideline document, a well-subscribed or transparent method of reporting and monitoring MRI safety incidents, or a model of medical device approval that considers MRI issues explicitly, MRI safety in Australia appears to be conducted with regard to the world's best practice. This may result from radiologists accessing information at international conferences, in print and on-line. The large cohorts of MRI radiographers who maintain international awareness and connections regarding MRI safety through regular attendance at international MRI conferences, and participation in educational forums and meetings of the Section for Magnetic Resonance Technologists (SMRT) may also play a strong role in the process.

In any case, there is an immediate need for revision of the RANZCR MRI Safety Guidelines in order to realign them with the international best practices expressed in the 2013 version of the ACR guidance document (20). The RANZCR MRI Safety Guidelines and the standards of practice are currently compromised by a lack of currency, recognition of the Australian regulatory scene and the omission of the directed responsibility to make a reasoned decision regarding safe scanning practices and how to proceed after diligent detection and identification of implants in patients. The RANZCR could consider the use of MRI facility policies that would produce consistent decisions on commonly encountered implanted devices in the Australian market place. MRI practitioners should also urgently consider the question of delegating common MRI safety decisions to appropriately experienced and educated MRI personnel such as advanced MRI radiographers, Medical Physicists, or other appropriately designated MRI safety officers. This last initiative will require much clearer statements of reasoned decision-making than are currently under discussion and it should identify specific training needs for radiologists, radiographers, and physicists. It should also clarify the position of non-clinicians (primarily MRI radiographers) who are currently relied upon to provide meaningful advice on particular MRI safety situations to radiologists. Furthermore, it should deliver an appropriate level of recognition and professional as well as organizational protection against the potentially serious criticisms of practicing beyond their role, while bringing a more considered and transparent approach to MRI safety.

REFERENCES

1. Organization for Economic Co-operation and Development. Stats Extract, Health Care Resources, 2012. Available at: http://stats.oecd.org/Index.aspx?DataSetCode=HEALTH_REAC. Accessed May 2013.

2. Department of Health and Ageing. Diagnostic Imaging. Magnetic resonance imaging (MRI) Canberra Australia: Department of Health and Ageing. Available at: www.health.gov.au/internet/main/publishing.nsf/Content/pathol-di-mri-index2 Accessed March 2013.

3. Department of Health and Ageing. Medicare Benefits Schedule Book Category 5 Canberra Australia: Commonwealth of Australia; 2013. pp. 185.

4. Australian Institute of Radiography. MRI Accreditation. Melbourne: Australian Institute of Radiography. Available at: www.air.asn.au/mri.php Accessed May 2013.

5. Medical Imaging Advisory Panel 1. MRI study and resource guide level 1 and level 2, 2010. Available at: www.air.asn.au/cms_files/05_Accreditation/MRI_Accreditaion_and_StudyGuide.pdf Accessed March 2013.

6. Health Workforce Australia. Medical Physicist Workforce Study Adelaide, 2012. Available at: www.hwa.gov.au/sites/uploads/20120912_FINAL_Medical%20Physicists%20Report_M1_0.pdf Accessed May 10 2013.

7. Australian/New Zealand Standard. Medical electrical equipment Part 2.33: Particular requirements for safety- Magnetic resonance equipment for medical diagnosis. AS/NZS 3200-2-33:2005 Standards Australia / Standards New Zealand; 2005.

8. Bottomley PA. Turning up the heat on MRI. Journal of the American College of Radiology 2008;5:853-5.

9. International Electrotechnical Commission. IEC 60601-2-33, Edition 3.1 2013-04. 2013.

10. Therapeutic Goods Administration. Information Document 23. Devices Forms, essential principles checklist. 2011. Available at: www.tga.gov.au/pdf/forms/devices-forms-essential-principles-checklist.pdf Accessed April 2013.

11. Therapeutic Goods Administration. Australian regulatory guidelines for medical devices (ARGMD) 2011. Available at: http://www.tga.gov.au/pdf/devices-argmd-01.pdf Accesses May 2013.

12. Ferris NJ. RANZCR Submission to TGA review panel information on MRI safety testing of medical implants [submission]. 2011. Available at: www.tga.gov.au/pdf/submissions/review-tga-transparency-1101-submission-ranzcr.pdf Accessed March 2013.

13. The Royal Australian and New Zealand College of Radiologists. Professional Guidelines. Available at: www.ranzcr.edu.au/resources/professional-documents/guidelines Accessed March 2013.

14. The Royal Australian and New Zealand College of Radiologists. Standards of Practice for Diagnostic and Interventional radiology. Version 9.2. Sydney Australia: The Royal Australian and New Zealand College of Radiologists; 2012. Available at: www.ranzcr.edu.au/component/docman/doc_download/510-ranzcr-standards-of-practice-for-diagnostic-and-interventional-radiology Accessed March 2013.

15. National Health and Medical Research Council. Safety Guidelines for Magnetic Resonance Imaging Facilities. Radiation Health Series. Canberra Australia: Australian Radiation Protection and Nuclear Safety Agency - Radiation Health Section. 1991. Available at: http://www.arpansa.gov.au/pubs/rhs/rhs34.pdf Accessed March 2013.

16. Shellock FG, Woods TO, Crues JV, 3rd. MR labeling information for implants and devices: explanation of terminology. Radiology 2009;253:26-30.

17. The Royal Australian and New Zealand College of Radiologists. RANZCR MRI Safety Guidelines 2007. Available at: http://www.ranzcr.edu.au/component/docman/doc_download/512-mri-safety-guidelines Accessed February 2013.

18. Kanal E, Borgstede JP, Barkovich AJ, et al. American College of Radiology white paper on MR safety. Am J Roentgenol 2002;178:1335-47.

19. Kanal E, Borgstede JP, Barkovich AJ, et al. American College of Radiology white paper on MR safety: 2004 update and revisions. Am J Roentgenol 2004;182:1111-4.

20. Kanal E, Barkovich AJ, Bell C, et al. ACR guidance document on MR safe practices: 2013. ACR guidance document on MR safe practices: 2013. J Magn Reson Imaging 2013;37:501-530.

21. The Royal Australian and New Zealand College of Radiologists. RANZCR Guidelines on the use of gadolinium containing MRI contrast agents. The Royal Australian and New Zealand College of Radiologists, 2009. Available at www.ranzcr.edu.au/component/docman/doc_download/553-revised-college-guidelines-for-gadolinium-containing-mri-contrast-agents- Accessed March 2013.

22. MRI Reference Group. News Update: introduction of MRI conditional pacemaker to Australasia 2010. Available at: www.ranzcr.edu.au/quality-a-safety/radiology/practice-quality-activities/mri-accreditation Accessed March 2013.

23. National Health and Medical Research Council. Interim guidelines on limits ofexposure to 50/60 Hz electric and magnetic fields (1989). Australian Radiation Laboratory; 1989. Available at: www.ranzcr.edu.au/quality-a-safety/radiology/practice-quality-activities/mri-accreditation Accessed March 2013.

24. Australian Radiation Protection and Nuclear Safety Agency (ARPANSA), Radiation Protections Standard. Exposure limits for electic & magnetic fields - 0 Hz to 3 kHz public consultation draft. Australian Radiation Protection and Nuclear Safety Agency 2006. Available at: www.arpansa.gov.au/pubs/comment/dr_elf_ris.pdf Accessed March 2013.

25. Ferris NJ. RANZCR submission to ARPANSA re draft ELF exposure. 2007.

26. Martin L. Limits & precautionary measures for reducing exposure to electric & magnetic fields - 0khz to 3 khz. Magnetic Resonance Imaging Issues 2008. Available at: www.arpansa.gov.au/pubs/events/lm_mri.pdf Accessed April 21 2013.

27. ARPANSA. Website. Forum on Development of ELF Standard. Yallambie Victoria: Australian Government, 2008. Available at: http://www.arpansa.gov.au/news/events/elf.cfm

28. International Commission on Non-Ionizing Radiation Protection. Guidelines for Limiting Exposure to Time-Varying Electric and Magnetic Fields (1 Hz TO 100 kHz). Health Physics 2010;99:818-36.

29. International Commission on Non-Ionizing Radiation Protection. ICNIRP guidelines on limits of exposure to static magnetic fields. Health Physics 2009;96:504-14.

30. ARPANSA. Publications list. 2012. Available at: www.arpansa.gov.au/pubs/rps/pub_list.doc Accessed May 2013.

31. Therapeutic Goods Administration. Medical Device Incident Reporting and Investigation Scheme (IRIS): Australian Government Department of Health and Ageing; 2013. Available at: http://www.tga.gov.au/safety/problem-device-iris.htm Accessed May 2013.

32. Therapeutic Goods Administration. Database of Adverse Events Notification (DAEN) Canberra 2012. Available at: www.tga.gov.au/safety/daen.htm Accessed April 2013.

33. Australian Radiation Protection and Nuclear Safety Agency. Electromagnetic Radiation Health Complaint Register Available at: www.arpansa.gov.au/radiationprotection/emr/index.cfm Accessed May 2013.

34. Ferris NJ, Kavnoudias H, Thiel C, Stuckey S. The 2005 Australian MRI safety survey. Amer J Roentgenol 2007;188:1388-94.

35. Burwell J, Davidson R. An evaluation of safety policies and procedures in Australian magnetic resonance imaging departments. The Radiographer 2007;54:4-7.

36. The Royal Australian and New Zealand College of Radiologists. Radiodiagnosis Training Program Curriculum. Sydney: The Royal Australian and New Zealand College of Radiologists. 2009. Available at: www.ranzcr.edu.au/component/docman/doc_download/154-radiodiagnosis-curriculum-document-full Accessed April 2013.

Index

A

A-weighted, 91-92, 112
Abandoned leads, 390, 409, 411, 416
Acoustic noise, 21-22, 28, 64, 84, 88-92, 94-108, 110-112, 114-130, 198-199, 205-206, 208-209, 219-220, 554-555, 659-660, 686-687
Active acoustic shielding, 119
Active implant, 485-486, 488-489, 498, 511
Active noise control, 106, 123, 128
Active shielding, 17-18, 172-173
Active vibration control, 109, 125, 128
Acute reactions, 242-250, 252, 254
Adverse reactions, 199, 242-244, 252-254, 289, 535, 690
Alliance for MRI, 674
American College of Radiology, ACR, 356
AMIGO Suite, 594-597, 599-600, 603, 605, 609, 616, 618
Amorphous magneto-resistive, 310
Anaphylactic, 244, 250-251, 253-254, 289, 603
Anaphylactoid, 248, 250, 254
Anaphylaxis, 244, 251-252, 254-255
Anesthesia delivery, 611, 614
Aneurysm clips, 43, 47, 56, 60, 152, 291, 371, 374-375, 386, 430, 518, 603, 685, 708
Annuloplasty ring, 378
Anti-phase noise, 106-107, 119
Anxiety, 88, 124, 195-196, 198-200, 202, 204-206, 208, 210-216, 450, 534, 552
Apnea, 330-331, 338-339, 353-354, 362-363, 365
ASTM International, 134, 194, 373, 464, 475, 483, 513, 576-577, 591, 604
Asynchronous pacing, 390, 392-393, 395-396, 403, 405, 410-411
Athermal effects, 156
Auditory perception, 122
Australian Radiation Protection and Nuclear Safety Agency, 704, 711-712

B

Barbiturates, 362
Basic restrictions, 628-629, 637, 640-641, 644, 671-674
Biopsy needles, 468, 617
Birdcage coils, 143
Blood pressure, 160-162, 164, 168, 246-250, 252, 333, 338, 344, 357-358, 362, 391, 396, 532, 569, 607
Body piercing jewelry, 375-376
Body temperature, 52, 62, 148-149, 158, 162-163, 169, 341-342, 344, 350, 555-557, 569, 614, 631, 655-656
Breastfeeding, 289-290, 701
Bronchospasm, 244, 247, 249, 251
Bullets, 295, 380-381, 387, 588
Burn, 290, 349, 430, 568-569, 577, 600

C

Canadian Association of Radiologists, 679, 682, 684-685, 688-692
Capnometer, 339
Cardiac excitation, 85, 655
Cardiac pacemaker, 395, 397-400, 415, 418-419
Cardiac stimulation, 73-74, 78, 80, 84
Cataractogenic, 165
Catheters, 246, 334, 338, 357-358, 371, 382, 384, 430, 452, 468, 615, 617
CE Mark, 441, 444, 668
Center for Devices and Radiological Health, 56, 86, 152, 421, 457, 461, 621, 645, 648, 664
Checklist, 395-396, 551, 553, 556-557, 585, 600-602, 620, 701, 711
Children's hospital, 282, 540-544, 546, 548-552
Chloral hydrate, 362, 366
Circularly polarized waves, 137
Class I devices, 649, 679
Class II devices, 649
Class III devices, 649

N

O

P

Q

Transmetallated gadolinium, 224
Transmission line theory, 491, 493
Transmit RF coil, 22, 132, 140, 147-148, 157, 219,
    335, 371, 390, 409-411, 414, 426, 432, 437,
    453, 462-464, 474, 483, 509, 534, 577-578, 608

U

Urticaria, 244, 247, 249, 251-252

V

Vagal reaction, 248, 250
Vagus nerve stimulation, 434, 449-450, 459, 486,
    488, 511, 513
Vascular access port, 384
Vascular clips, 379
Ventilator, 345-346, 348, 350, 616, 621
Verbal interview, 214, 291, 293-294, 297, 603, 686
Verbal screening procedures, 294
Vertigo, 37, 52, 55, 71, 196, 234, 608, 625, 644, 667
Visitor screening, 536

W

World Health Organization, 53, 62, 600, 620, 676
www.MRIsafety.com, 384-385, 391, 398, 426-427,
    434, 531-532, 603, 614

X

X-axis, 176

Y

Y-axis, 43, 75, 176

Z

Z-axis, 6-8, 43-47, 65, 114, 145, 176
Z-magnetization, 8
Zipper artifact, 606
Zone of quiet, 107
Zones, 181-182, 190-191, 515, 517, 531-532